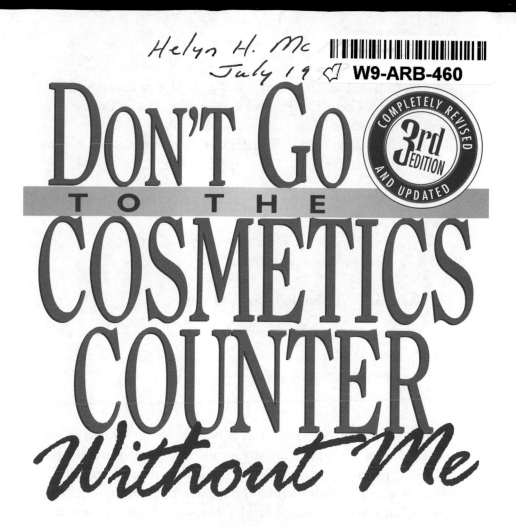

DON'T GO TO THE

COMPLETELY REVISED
3rd EDITION
AND UPDATED

TO THE

COSMETICS COUNTER

Without Me

~

An Eye-Opening Guide To Brand-Name Cosmetics

by

Paula Begoun

Editors: Miriam Bulmer, Sherri Schultz, and Laura Kraemer
Art Direction, Cover Design, and Typography: Studio Pacific
Printing: Publishers Press, Salt Lake City, Utah
Research Assistants: Kristin Folsom, Elizabeth Janda, Laura Kraemer,
and Rachel Permann

Copyright 1991, 1992, 1993, 1994, 1995, 1996 Paula Begoun
Publisher: Beginning Press
          5418 South Brandon
          Seattle, Washington 98118

First Printing for this edition: August 1996

ISBN   1-877988-18-9
       1 2 3 4 5 6 7 8 9 10

This book is distributed to the United States book trade by:

          Publishers Group West
          4065 Hollis Street
          Emeryville, California 94608
          (800) 788-3123

and to the Canadian book trade by:

          Raincoast Books Limited
          8680 Cambie Street
          Vancouver, B.C., CANADA V6P 6M9
          (604) 323-7100

Table of Contents

Chapter One—Taming the Beauty Beast

Chapter Two—Skin Care Update

TABLE OF CONTENTS

Chapter Eight—The Best Products

Chapter Nine—Beauty That Respects Nature

Publisher's Note

The intent of this book is to present the author's ideas and perceptions about the marketing, selling, and use of cosmetics. The author's sole purpose is to present consumer information and advice regarding the purchase of makeup and skin care products. The information and recommendations presented strictly reflect the author's opinions, perceptions, and knowledge about the subject and products mentioned. Some women may find success with a particular product that is not recommended or even mentioned herein, or they may be partial to a $250 skin care routine. It is everyone's inalienable right to judge products by their own criteria and standards and to disagree with the author.

More important, because everyone's skin can, and probably will, react to an external stimulus at some time, any product could cause a negative reaction on your skin at one time or another. If you develop a skin sensitivity to a cosmetic, stop using it immediately and consult your physician. If you need medical advice about your skin, it is best to consult a dermatologist.

CHAPTER

O • N • E

TAMING THE BEAUTY BEAST

Why You Need This Book

If you've read my book *Blue Eyeshadow Should Be Illegal* (now in its third edition) or a previous edition of *Don't Go To The Cosmetics Counter Without Me*, or if you subscribe to my newsletter, *Cosmetics Counter Update*, read my syndicated newspaper column, or have seen me on television, you know that I have strong feelings about the quality of information and products the cosmetics industry provides for women. My research has proven that, from almost every corner of the $45 billion cosmetics industry, in one form or another, women receive an immense amount of misleading, deceptive, or just plain false information. Whether it comes from cosmetics advertising, cosmetics salespeople, cosmetics companies' brochures, or so-called editorial pieces in fashion magazines, women are continually given distorted, inaccurate, and specious explanations about skin care and makeup products. Is there a woman anywhere who hasn't purchased a cosmetic that didn't do what it said it would? Haven't most of us felt upset when we bought an all-day lipstick that didn't last all day, a wrinkle cream that didn't change a wrinkle, or an oil-control product that didn't control oil?

My goal has always been to tell you everything the cosmetics companies won't tell you and everything the fashion magazines leave out or can't tell you because of the control cosmetics and fashion companies assert via their advertising dollars. There's a lot to tell. Some of it you may find shocking, funny, enlightening, and, depending how much money you've wasted, disheartening. What I can assure you is that I will always be as straightforward and thorough as possible. I do the best I can to present both sides of the picture, so you can make more informed decisions in an industry where the consumer is so vulnerable and easily taken advantage of. In the long run, this book will help you save money, take better care of your skin, and look more beautiful—all at the same time.

This edition of *Don't Go To The Cosmetics Counter Without Me* presents product-by-product reviews of cosmetics from more than 100 of the most popular lines, which is 40 more lines (and 10,000 more products) than I covered in the first edition of the book. I have to admit that maintaining my reputation as the "Ralph Nader of Rouge" is not always thrilling: I find the cosmetics counters as frustrating, intimidating, and annoying as you do. I don't relish the prospect of spending $40 on a foundation that isn't any better than a $10 foundation, nor do I savor dealing with the salespeople. I know that most of the "information" they give me will be nothing more than sales pitches, hype, anecdotes, and scientific "cosmebabble," and if they recognize me, they might even ask me to leave! It's not my favorite way to spend a hundred afternoons, but it's the only way to gather information for this book.

If you've ever felt uncertain or too short of time or energy to figure out for yourself which foundations are too pink or too orange, which eyeshadows are too shiny or too difficult to use, which powders go on too chalky, which cleansers are too greasy, which toners are too harsh, or what makes one moisturizer different from another, look no further. As you read the reviews in this book, you will start to better understand how the cosmetics industry really works. I've included a summary chapter of best finds and best buys, but don't jump to that one first. It is important to read the individual product reviews so you understand *exactly* what you are buying. I might recommend 20 good mascaras, but each one might be good for a different reason.

In the reviews, each product is described in terms of its reliability, value, texture, application, and effect. Within every category of product—foundations, mascaras, blushes, eyeshadows, concealers, pressed powders, lipsticks, and pencils—I established specific criteria, and I evaluated products using those standards. For example, a foundation meant for someone with oily skin, according to my criterion, should be matte, contain minimal to no oil, blend easily, leave a smooth, even finish, and have no ingredients known to cause breakouts. All foundations must match skin exactly: they cannot be any shade of orange, peach, rose, pink, or ash, because people are not orange, peach, rose, pink, or ash. I made the same determinations for mascaras, blushes, eyeshadows, concealers, pressed powders, lipsticks, and pencils. I relied on my ten years as a professional makeup artist to help establish the quality of a product.

Skin care products were evaluated almost entirely by analyzing the ingredient list and comparing it to the claims made about the product. If a toner asserts that it is designed for sensitive skin, it shouldn't contain ingredients that irritate the skin. If a moisturizer claims it can hydrate the skin, it should contain ingredients that can do just that. I have also made a point of challenging the inflated claims made about such ingredients as yeast, herbal extracts, botanicals, seaweed extracts, placenta extracts, alpha hydroxy acids, vitamins, DNA, RNA, hyaluronic acid, liposomes and other much-hyped ingredients. I also explain why some of these and other seemingly impressive-sounding ingredients might indeed benefit the skin.

The First Time

A number of you have asked how I happened into this unusual line of work. It's not as if you can answer an ad for this kind of job. Clearly, the cosmetics industry and fashion magazines aren't interested in hiring someone to do what I do (for the same reasons the insurance industry doesn't want to employ Ralph Nader), but somewhere along the line it became clear to me that someone needed to be doing this job.

It all started in 1977, when I took my first job at a department-store makeup counter to supplement my income as a free-lance makeup artist. As a young makeup artist in Washington, D.C., I had built up a list of celebrity clients and was doing quite well, both financially and professionally. I found the artistry of creating beautiful makeup styles for women intriguing, and the world of fashion and glamour was thoroughly exciting. At the age of 24 I was thrilled with my career. My clients wanted only me, and they were some of the most powerful and formidable women in Washington. The constant ego reinforcement was great. But, as with any business, it had its ups and downs, and shoring up my income once in a while became necessary. A store at a mall in Silver Spring, Maryland, had an opening for a cosmetics salesperson. They hired me on the spot because, I was told, I looked the part, wearing nice makeup and dressing well. It was also made crystal clear that, while my previous experience was a plus, it was completely unnecessary for employment as a cosmetics salesperson.

Even though I was enthusiastic and loved the dynamic and glamorous world of makeup and skin care, I already knew something was awry with a substantial number of cosmetics and their advertising, particularly in the skin care area. Having struggled for years with oily skin and acne, I knew from experience that astringents didn't close pores, that products claiming not to cause breakouts made me break out, and that most products that promised to clear up acne only made my skin more red and irritated. I didn't yet know all the technical details of why this was so, but it was blatantly obvious that plenty of mascaras that claimed to be flakeproof weren't, toners that boasted they could close pores didn't, and creams that were supposed to eliminate scarring and lighten "age spots" didn't. The claims made about the products rarely matched their performance. It seemed unmistakable that much of the cosmetics industry was grossly misrepresenting its products, but at the time there was no way to confirm my suspicions.

On my first day on the job, I was assigned to work behind the Calvin Klein (in those days, Klein had a makeup line) and Elizabeth Arden counters. With no previous training or information about these lines, I was told to sell the products. I did the best I could. Unfortunately, my notion of how to help customers was completely different from that of the other salespeople and the line manager. My first mistake was telling several customers not to bother using an astringent because alcohol-based products could cause something called a "rebound effect." By irritating the skin, these products could actually stimulate oil production and make oily skin worse. I then recommended 3% hydrogen peroxide, available for 50 cents at the drugstore. By the end of the second day, the woman working next to me was mortified. She called in the line representative, who made it clear I should keep my personal opinions to myself and just sell the products. I said I would do my best. This was only my second day. Things had to get better, I thought.

The fourth day on the job, thinking I was doing what I was supposed to do, I assisted a customer who wanted help putting together a makeup look. I went about this seemingly ordinary task by assembling a selection of products from several different lines. I noticed that the saleswomen behind the other counters didn't appear happy as I took products from their stock, but I thought maybe it was because I was making the sale instead of them. That was only the half of it. Although the women I helped that day bought almost everything I suggested, the other saleswomen complained to the head of the department, who subsequently ordered me to stay behind the counters I was assigned to. I protested that the two lines I was assigned to didn't always have the best makeup colors or skin care products for every woman I talked to. Without hesitation, she said, "That's just the way it is, so you'd better get used to it." That was the fourth day. It couldn't get any worse, I thought, sighing. But it did.

At the end of my second week, I finally met the woman who was responsible for training. At last, I was going to learn how to sell the products assigned to me, and what to say about each product's benefits. I truly wanted to find out everything I could, but apparently my approach was unacceptable. When the trainer explained that I was supposed to sell Elizabeth Arden Eight Hour Cream as a product designed to help heal the skin, I asked her what the product contained that made it able to do that. She said what it contained wasn't important. I disagreed, saying that it would help me sell the cream better if I knew what made it heal skin; surely the customer would want to know. She said, "All the customer wants to know is what you tell her; the customers never ask questions, because they trust the products."

"How can that be," I insisted, "when all the cosmetics lines say the same thing? Why should they trust us any more than someone else?"

"Because they do," she said. Finally, she threw the product down and said, "Just say it! There's nothing else to discuss." To my dismay—but not surprise—that turned out to be my last day. It was a relief to return to the world of free-lance makeup.

Shortly after that incident, I read *The Great American Skin Game* by Toni Stabille. It changed my life. This landmark book conveyed in clear, concise terms the processes and techniques the cosmetics industry used to sell hope to gullible and uninformed consumers. In fact, Ms. Stabille was largely responsible for proposing many Food and Drug Administration (FDA) regulations involving cosmetics, including advertising guidelines, safety regulations, and mandatory ingredient lists. Her work confirmed what I had already reasoned to be true, and significantly changed the way I approached cosmetics.

Although it sounds a bit melodramatic, I couldn't continue selling something I knew to be a waste of money or bad for the skin. Consumers (including myself) deserved better. I wasn't anti-makeup—just the opposite—but I was (and am) anti-hype and anti–misleading information. As one newspaper reporter recently commented, "She's not Mother Teresa, but it does seem to be just Ms. Begoun against these huge cosmetics companies." Thus I took my first steps on a long career path—longer than I ever imagined—that went from owning my own cosmetics stores to working as a TV news reporter to owning my own publishing company. With every step, my goal has been to do what it takes to find out and expose the truth behind the ads and the literally unbelievable claims thrown about by the cosmetics world. After all, one good sales pitch about an "exclusive patented secret" or a revolutionary new formula, and your pocketbook could easily be $50 to $250 lighter for a one-ounce jar of standard cosmetics ingredients or ingredients that can't live up to their claims.

Me Versus Them

Now that I have sold quite a few "beauty" books and write a syndicated newspaper column, the cosmetics companies have begun to take notice of me. (I think they would prefer to have never heard of me.) Of course, they direct their outrage at me only when I criticize their products; apparently I'm very accurate when I praise their products. Whenever I get an aggrieved letter from a cosmetics company, my response is always the same: I list my reasons for what I've written and offer to share all my research, sources, and documentation. In return, I ask them to send me documentation of their research and evidence. If I receive sufficient information establishing my error or the existence of contrary information that warrants publicizing, I am more than willing to retract, change, or add to my statement. In light of this, you will find the section containing some of the letters I've received from the cosmetics industry quite fascinating.

For the most part, I have found it a challenge to get an interview, assistance, information, a press kit, ingredient lists, or even prices from any of the public relations people at the major cosmetics companies. I've asked many times to be treated like any other beauty editor. (You should see the products and information beauty editors from newspapers and fashion magazines are lavished with. Their desks are covered with perfume, foundations, mascaras, moisturizers, and lipsticks from every company imaginable.)

In all fairness, I must say that over the years the situation has changed for the better. An increasing number of cosmetics companies have been incredibly cooperative. They acknowledge that we don't always agree, but are earnestly concerned about providing me with their research, data, and even, on occasion, products, and I would like to extend my deepest appreciation to them. Although I don't like all of the products from these companies, I do like many of them, and you should be aware of their willingness to be helpful on the behalf of the consumer. Almay, Neoteric (Alpha Hydrox), Aveda, Avon, BeautiControl, Beauty Without Cruelty, Bobbi Brown, Borghese, Chanel, Chesebrough-Pond's, Clinique, Color Me Beautiful, Freeman, Galderma, Hydron, L'Oreal, M.A.C., Maybelline, M.D. Formulations, Murad, NeoStrata, Neutrogena, Noevir, Nu Skin, Oil of Olay, Physicians Formula, Pond's, Revlon, and Ultima II: Thank you for being willing to take the risk that your products would receive an honest evaluation.

Before I go much further, I must mention that I don't have the last word when it comes to makeup and skin care. The last word is yours. This book is not about my being right, it is about disseminating independent ideas and opinions so that the cosmetics industry is not your only source of information. My fantasy is that you will take this book with you to cosmetics counters, drugstores, and in-home sales demonstrations, and have it nearby when you are watching an infomercial on TV. Then, when the salesperson carries on about how superb this or that product is, you can say, "Excuse me, I would like to see what Paula has to say about this product." You may not agree with me, but you will have more input than just advertising and marketing slogans.

The Crazy Things Cosmetics Salespeople Say

I know many cosmetics salespeople wish I would shrivel up and go away like the Wicked Witch of the West in *The Wizard of Oz*. I understand their animosity. My job is to try to make the consumer's life easier and stop the cosmetics industry from misleading the public, which has to get in the way of anyone selling a wrinkle cream or an overpriced lipstick. Although my efforts are directed more at cosmetics executives and their advertising departments, they affect the people selling makeup and skin care products as well. I sincerely apologize to these people for putting them in an awkward position, but it is essential that consumers get information from someone who is willing to present both sides of the picture.

The consumer also needs to talk to people who are truly knowledgeable about the products, and insufficient education is a recurring complaint of the cosmetics salespeople I've interviewed. They receive minimal makeup-application lessons, and the skin care information they are given is almost entirely sales jargon, leaving little room for questions or skepticism. If salespeople have any doubts or concerns about what they are selling, they cannot tell management—they could get fired just for asking. This lack of training leaves the uninformed consumer at the mercy of the cosmetics salesperson—or, turning it around, the uninformed cosmetics salesperson is at the mercy of the informed consumer. There isn't much a cosmetics salesperson can do about this until the cosmetics companies change their direction. As long as the cosmetics companies believe they can continue fooling the consumer, they have no incentive to provide their staff with more expertise than the little they currently receive.

In March 1996, I did a spot on NBC's *Today* show in which the show sent a hidden camera to cosmetics counters with reporter Janice Lieberman, who asked different salespeople what kinds of products they had for stopping wrinkles. It was my job to look at the videotape and discuss whether the outlandish information they offered was true or false. (Also appearing on the show was a dermatologist, who agreed with my evaluations.) Without question, the best sales pitch (or the worst, depending on your point of view), amid a deluge of crazy, false claims, was from the Clarins counter.

The saleswomen at several different Clarins counters all explained at length that Clarins Serum Multi-Tenseur Raffermissant Skin Firming Concentrate was superior to other products because it contained pineapple concentrate. Every one of them stated that there were studies showing that pineapple workers lost their fingerprints after handling pineapples for long periods. According to their story, the lack of fingerprints was a result of repeatedly coming in contact with pineapple extract. That's why Skin Firming Concentrate could get rid of wrinkles because it contained the same ingredient that erased fingerprints from the hands of pineapple workers. Well, this claim is utterly false! First of all, pineapple is the last ingredient in the list on the product label; it is less than 1 percent of the product, which isn't enough to peel a handful of cells from your face. Furthermore, fingerprints are not wrinkles and are not related to them in any regard. I was curious to hear what the official word from Clarins would be. I found it hard to believe that several of their salespeople would make up the same story on their own.

I called Clarins immediately and asked to see the study of pineapple workers. Clarins said the company had no such studies; the story about the pineapple workers who lost their fingerprints was purely anecdotal, used by Clarins to help its sales force learn how the product could work. In exasperation, I said, "You knowingly trained your salespeople with a false story that you never intended them to use?"

Interestingly, despite the absurd selling tactics, Clarins Skin Firming Concentrate *is* a decent moisturizer; however, it is hardly worth even half of its overblown price tag.

Clarins had the misfortune to get on the air, but it's not the only company misleading consumers. Just about every time I hit the cosmetics counters, watch an infomercial, or listen to in-home salespeople describe their line, I hear them say the most preposterous things. Cosmetics salespeople will tell you that only *their* moisturizer can make your skin produce better cells; that *their* firming cream contains the right kind of elastin and collagen to reinforce the structure of your skin; that the specially formulated amino acids in *their* toner can merge into the deepest layers of your skin, where it will fuse to your own DNA, building new layers of stronger cells that will make your face look younger in only two weeks. I've even heard cosmetics salespeople describe a freshener as a "liberating liquid that can purify the toxins from your skin and improve circulation, helping the skin to regenerate younger skin, because old skin is caused by poor circulation to the face." Or how about this one: "Our products are all natural, because synthetic ingredients can't merge into the natural layers of skin." Of course, neither statement is the least bit true.

And the claims don't stop there. I've heard facial masks—standard clay masks with some herbs or oils thrown in—described as nothing less than the answer to women's prayers to remove blackheads and drastically reduce oil production. One of the spiels I heard recently claimed that the mask in question pulls the water and garbage (garbage?) right out of your skin and automatically reduces puffiness and blemishes; that the botanicals and essential oils in it reduce the stress and tension that build up in the face and cause wrinkles (sounds like Valium for the face); and (this is the best one) that it combats pollution by feeding the skin nutrients and vitamins that the environment has depleted, and once your skin is fed properly it can generate new, youthful skin that can't be harmed by pollution again—as long as you use the mask once a week, that is.

I recently overheard a woman questioning a cosmetics-line representative about the effects of a specific eye gel. I know you'll appreciate her reply: "We can't even tell you everything it can do for your skin, because then it would be a drug and it would cost the company too much money to keep it on the market." The epitome of cosmetics insanity is this type of sales pitch. What they're really saying is that the cosmetics company saves millions of dollars risking your skin because it won't do what is required by the FDA to prove its claims. Aspirin is $4 a bottle, and extensive research has been done to prove its efficacy and safety. The multibillion-dollar cosmetics industry could do the same if it really had something to prove.

Perhaps you've heard a moisturizer described as follows: "This night cream penetrates down to the birth area of the skin, where cells are produced, and feeds it oxygen so the cells have the ability to make healthy new cells. Oxygen is essential to making new cells, and because of pollution there's so little oxygen left in the air that it destroys the skin, and you can't have good skin without oxygen." It's amazing any of us can breathe! But it is even more unbelievable that a skin cream or lotion could provide any significant amount oxygen for the skin. How much air can be stored in side a two-ounce skin care product that isn't released once you open it or used up the second it touches the skin? Even if there were some amount of oxygen in these products it isn't enought to help even a handful of skin cells.

The most popular ruses at the cosmetics counter these days are distortions about alpha hydroxy acid (AHA) products and products containing vitamins A, C, and E. It isn't surprising that AHA products are getting so much ballyhoo. AHAs can temporarily smooth the skin, but in no way can they alter, restructure, or permanently improve the skin; they are just very good moisturizing ingredients that in higher concentrations also exfoliate. Nevertheless, cosmetics salespeople will tell you that AHA can "rearrange the fibers of the skin to make them firmer and more elastic" or that it "works in harmony with the skin's own natural balance, returning it to a younger state."

The hype concerning vitamins in skin care products is nearly as bad: "There are conclusive studies that show free-radical damage is tearing down our skin, causing wrinkles, and the only way to stop the damage is to use products that contain vitamins." There are no conclusive studies on this subject anywhere. Just ask if you can see them; I have, and, more often than not, they don't exist. There are some theories and fascinating research, but no conclusive evidence. But more about that later.

Then there's the assertion that one line's ingredients are better than the next one's, regardless of what they are—AHAs, protein, sea salts, collagen, herbs, or oils. Many companies act as if no other cosmetics manufacturer has access to the same distributors of these trendy little gems, or as if only one distributor is selling the good stuff and the rest are selling inferior ingredients. Perhaps the most absurd notion is that only one or two cosmetic chemists know any of these secrets and they are employed for the rest of natural life to that one company. That just isn't the way things happen, especially not in the world of cosmetics.

As wonderful as these and millions of other sales pitches sound, they all lead you to believe what isn't true: that a cosmetic can change the inherent nature of your skin. It cannot. Or that a cosmetic can feed the skin from the outside in. It cannot. Or that a cosmetic can in any way permanently alter the wrinkles on your face. It cannot.

Why do the salespeople get away with it? Because the FDA is unable to monitor the thousands of people selling cosmetics, and is barely able to monitor the ads and product labels. Why does the cosmetics industry get away with it? Because, according to the FDA, cosmetics companies do not have to prove their claims. They can say just about anything they want, and they do not have to demonstrate that any part of their claim is true.

In order to comply with the FDA's ruling with regards to cosmetics advertising, the claims made for any given product can only *suggest* that your skin will be better; it can't say that it actually will be. A company cannot claim that a cosmetic will change the skin's structure (if it could, it would be a drug and therefore subject to radically different federal regulations). So if a cosmetics company can lead you to believe that its products can change your skin, without actually stating such a claim, it is not breaking the FDA rules. In other words, misleading consumers is perfectly legal. And because the number of products is vastly greater than the number of FDA inspectors, bending the rules too far is part of the game. The Federal Trade Commission (FTC) *is* concerned with claim support, but it doesn't take much for cosmetic chemists to create research and studies that prove just about anything they want it to, or to for copy writer to use language that demonstrates the truthfulness of a claim. (See "Declarations of Independence"). Phrases like "light-reflecting color" are always true because all color reflects light. Another one I like is "increases your skin's capacity to hold moisture by 240%." Just sit in a bathtub and your skin will absorb more moisture than that. I could go on, but you get the picture.

You may wonder which products made the excessive claims mentioned above. I didn't include the names of those products for two reasons. First, I didn't want you to think for one second that any of that sales gibberish is true, causing you to run out and buy it for yourself. Second, *many* cosmetics salespeople, regardless of the product line, say crazy things that are either blatantly false or so misleading as to be essentially false. Why pick on one line when all are guilty of the same offense?

Patented Secrets?

Are there really any secret formulas at the cosmetics counters? After all, if you're spending $45 to $65 or more for a moisturizer or foundation with impressive claims, you want to believe that you're purchasing an exclusive product that justifies the exorbitant price. The salespeople make much ado about patented or patent-pending formulas to which only their line has access. And when you look at the product label, there it is in black and white: "patented" or "patent-pending" formula. It must be special.

You think to yourself, "Finally, something I can bank on," because you know that patent law is very strict, and the cosmetics industry couldn't lie about this, particularly when it comes to patent infringement laws. Right? Well, yes and no. I had a long talk with William Nugent, an attorney who specializes in U.S. patent law, and he had some revealing insights.

A U.S. patent is a contract between an inventor (in this instance, a cosmetics company) and the government. Once a patent is accepted, the inventor has exclusive use of the new invention (or, when it involves a cosmetic, a new formula) for 17 years. In exchange for the government's protection of that restricted use, the inventor discloses to the government all the information concerning the product. After the 17 years are up, the product or formula is available to the world.

In order for an inventor or company to get a patent, the product must be truly new and different from what is already available. The Patent and Trademark Office staff does an extensive examination to ascertain whether the formula or new ingredient is genuinely unique. In essence, that makes patents pretty reliable when it comes to the concept of originality. It would appear, then, that when it comes to patented cosmetics formulas, you might be getting a product that is verifiably special.

But the important question, and one that the patent office makes no attempt to answer, is what, if anything, can the new formula do for the skin? A cosmetics patent is no guarantee that the product can do anything new or unique for the skin. According to Mr. Nugent, there are millions of cosmetics patents, but they have no meaning when it comes to effectiveness. Often the patent is granted for formulation procedures or for combining two standard ingredients in a new way—say, in alcohol instead of wax, or heated instead of at room temperature. The variations are endless (which is why there are millions of patents).

Even when a patented product or formula actually does do something positive for the skin, which is the case for glycolic acid (alpha hydroxy acid), liposomes, and ceramides, it's often easy for another company to come up with a similar formula. L'Oreal and

Lancome were the first to patent liposomes, but several other companies created different versions of the same formula. Glycolic acid is patented, and any company that uses glycolic acid must pay the patent holders a licensing fee for usage. That is why you find so many different combinations of AHAs in cosmetics—everything from lactic acid to citrus acid, and other versions or derivatives of glycolic acid. That way the companies can sell a pretty effective AHA product without having to pay a licensing fee. And the list goes on.

So the next time a cosmetics salesperson carries on about an exclusive patented formula, remember that a patent doesn't tell you anything about how well the product works, and it definitely doesn't tell you whether there is a similar product on the market that does a better job.

Beauty Note: "Patent pending" means just what it says: a patent has been filed but has not yet been approved (and may not ever be approved). Companies like to say "patent pending" because they want you to think their products are unique.

Declarations of Independence

When fashion magazines and the media in general don't question the biases and methods of medical or scientific sources, they perpetuate and even enhance the illusion that something significant is taking place in the cosmetics industry. Repeatedly, uninvestigated stories fuel consumer demand for misrepresented products that can't live up to their claims. Package an ordinary product with unsubstantiated, highly questionable studies by impressive sources that aren't even remotely independent, and consumers will shell out their hard-earned money in the blink of an eye. (Remember the fuss about thigh creams a year or two ago?)

When are sources not independent? When they have financial ties to products for which they provide information. Cynthia Crossen, a *Wall Street Journal* editor and author of *Tainted Truth: The Manipulation of Fact in America,* says, "If you say you're independent, that gives more credibility than if you say, 'I was paid by a big cosmetics company.' But it takes a lot of effort to prove a source isn't all it is cracked up to be."

One cosmetics authority often quoted in fashion magazines as being independent is Gary Grove, vice president for research and development at the Skin Study Center in Broomall, Pennsylvania. Although Grove insists his work is independent, his clients, who include L'Oreal, Elizabeth Arden, Avon, Christian Dior, and Estee Lauder, pay him a speaking fee and reimburse his travel expenses so he can talk to trade groups about the "positive results" of his tests. When asked if any of his test results could be examined, Grove says they are not available to the public.

In 1986, Grove was quoted in the *New York Times* as saying, "There's more truth in [cosmetics] ads than there has been in the past. No longer can the cosmetics companies really make false claims." That was one year before the FDA cracked down on several major cosmetics companies for making exaggerated anti-aging claims. One of those companies, Avon, came under FDA fire for making unproven anti-aging claims about their product BioAdvance—claims that were, according to Grove, based on his research.

"Independent means without a conflict of interest. You can't be independent if you're beholden enough to only report positive results. . . . It all must be reported—positive and negative," says Dr. Lawrence Solomon, head of dermatology at the University of Illinois in Chicago.

"What if some products deserve criticism?" asks Michael Jacobson from the Center for Science in the Public Interest. Grove defends his refusal to reveal negative information by stating that his research for the cosmetics industry is "proprietary. . . . Seldom is that information made public. That's just the way American business is." But that's not the way science is, at least according to the standards of the independent dermatologists and researchers who talked with me. "Openness is one of the basic doctrines of science, and concealment is a sign that something is wrong," Crossen says.

Grove isn't the only cosmetics scientist referred to as independent in the media. Dr. Peter Pugliese's firm, Milmark Research, has been described in fashion magazines as an independent source of scientific research on cosmetics. Pugliese insists he is independent because he works on a contract basis with many cosmetics firms. But he too will not expose his data to public scrutiny, because, he says, the cosmetics companies he works for won't allow it, and "the public couldn't even begin to know how to read the data." But there are many other professionals who could, and that is how real scientific research is done.

Keeping Up with Aging

One of the best ways to curb our appetite for wrinkle creams is to understand that the skin's aging process is more complicated than we can ever imagine. Researchers generally agree that the visible signs of aging on the surface of the skin—deep wrinkles, lines, and discolorations—are only one aspect of a multilevel composite of events. Surprisingly, furrowed, leathery skin and brown "liver" spots are directly caused by sun exposure and are not genetically predetermined. What does seem to be genetically predetermined is a vast range of occurrences in the skin that can cause it to look older.

Looking at the issue objectively can help us to better understand what is happening to our skin, and therefore gain insight into why wrinkle products make the claims they do, and why it is most unlikely that they can actually live up to their claims. For example, while we might know that collagen and elastin are the support structures of the skin and that they break down and flatten as a result of exposure to the sun, we should realize that they also become less pliant and more hardened with age, so the skin becomes less elastic. Even if a product could build more collagen or elastin, if it isn't pliant and flexible, what good is it? Some products claim to build only collagen or only elastin. That is much like building a house with only cross beams and no support beams. One without the other is useless, because the house won't stay erect. But, for the sake of argument, let's say these products *can* build more collagen or elastin. Regardless, just rebuilding elastin or collagen or any other single part of the skin isn't enough to halt or reverse the intricate, convoluted aging process and its effect on our faces.

A notable difference between older skin and younger skin is that younger skin has more fat cells in the dermis than older skin. That is one reason older skin looks more transparent and thinner than younger skin. Furthermore, for some unknown reason, the skin keeps growing and expanding as we age, despite the fact that the fat tissue in the lower layers of skin is decreasing. That is why the skin begins to sag. Too much skin is being produced, but there isn't enough bone (remember, bone also deteriorates with age) and fat to shore it up. Simultaneously, facial muscles lose their shape and firmness, giving the face a drooping appearance. All the exercise in the world can't stop that from happening; just ask any bodybuilder.

Certain components of the skin also become depleted with age. The water-retaining and texture-enhancing elements such as ceramides, hyaluronic acids, and polysaccharides are exhausted. Older skin is also more subject to allergic reactions and skin sensitivities than younger skin, which suggests that older skin is less capable of defending itself against irritants because of a weakening autoimmune system.

On a deeper molecular level, the DNA codes of the skin get lost or rearranged. This change in the DNA (the fundamental cornerstone of why the entire body ages) prevents our skin cells from reproducing as they did when we were younger. Cells become abnormally shaped, which further changes the skin's texture and prevents the cells from holding on to water. This inability to retain water is why older skin tends to be drier than younger skin. Companies that stick DNA and RNA in their products want you to believe they can help rectify this deterioration. They can't, and even if they could do something, do you really want to mess around with your genetic coding?

Cosmetics companies target many of these factors of aging by adding cosmetic ingredients that claim to counteract the effect of these specific depletions. Ceramide, hyaluronic acid, and other components of skin are popular in wrinkle creams. The problem is you can't put ceramide or hyaluronic acid back into the skin from the outside in (or even from the inside out); their molecular structure is too large to penetrate the skin. Moreover, even when these ingredients are chemically altered so they can penetrate skin, they can't merge with and augment what you have; instead, they simply pass through and are eliminated, just like any other cosmetics ingredient absorbed by the skin.

Like collagen and elastin, ceramide and hyaluronic acid are good water-binding agents and therefore useful in moisturizers. Unfortunately, the cosmetics industry loves to use phrases such as "Replaces what skin has lost," leading you to believe that these ingredients can affect skin structure. Even DNA, on occasion, shows up in skin care products. But stop and think. Your genetic structure cannot be affected or replaced by a cosmetic, nor would you want it to be. If you could tamper with DNA, you could wreak havoc on the entire human system. Besides, if it did have an effect on your DNA, it would be classified as a drug, not a cosmetic, and you would absolutely want that to be the case.

Facial exercises are another popular way to prevent muscles from sagging, but there comes a time when all the exercise in the world isn't going to stop the muscles from breaking down. It seems to be genetically encoded; even weightlifters lose their tone with time. Besides, we already use our facial muscles more than any other muscles in our body, and extra activity isn't going to make them bulge out to support the skin.

Growing old cannot be reversed by the right skin care routine, by jerking your face into funny shapes, or by stimulating muscles with machines. As far as anti-aging products are concerned, you are never going to get what you think you've paid for, unless it's a sunscreen, because sunscreens can truly prevent a great deal of what is causing our skin to wrinkle, and thats sun damage.

The Agony and the Ecstasy

I spend a lot of time at department-store cosmetics counters, watching infomercials, perusing makeup displays at drugstores, and shopping in-home cosmetics lines. My average yearly expenditure on cosmetics research exceeds $60,000. That probably doesn't shock you. But what may shock you is that I find the experience just as daunting today as I did when I started. I am consistently dismayed by the degrading and scandalous way cosmetics are sold to women every day by the more than 600 cosmetics lines available in the United States and Canada.

The typical information given out by the cosmetics companies is heavily seasoned with pubescent models selling wrinkle creams; smooth-skinned teens selling acne preparations; salespeople dressed in smocks to make them look like clinicians; and sales rhetoric, on labels and in ads and brochures, that is indecipherable and, for the most part, unbelievable, at least if you have enough information to realize what is really being said. Every line has its share of astounding and wondrous products that promise perfect skin. How do we sort out the claims? Unfortunately, we often end up believing that the expensive lines are telling the truth, or at least their products are more likely to work. In our minds, "expensive" somehow translates into "honest." But confusion and exaggeration are the standard regardless of how much money we spend.

In spite of my genuine resentment of the cosmetics industry's exaggerated claims and promises, including products that simply don't work or are just not very good, I am often rather impressed by the many improvements that have taken place in most of the lines reviewed for this book. (Of course, my ego would like to believe that I sparked some of these changes.) What is wonderful in the world of cosmetics? The good news is that you'll find a growing number of matte eyeshadows, a wide variety of water-soluble cleansers that don't irritate the skin or burn the eyes, an ample assortment of toners that really are irritant-free, an outstanding number of sunscreens that can block a great deal of ultraviolet radiation (thus preventing wrinkles and sun damage), great mascaras that don't smear or clump, an improved selection of foundation colors (particularly for women of color), a large array of silky, matte blush colors, lightweight moisturizers that are capable of keeping the skin moist and soft without feeling slick or greasy, and lipsticks that stay for most of the morning (which isn't all day, but it's still pretty good).

What you still have to watch out for is the array of wrinkle creams and oil-control products that sound as if they have just the answer for your skin. I could list thousands of examples, but the emphasis is always the same: a woman's skin is being attacked and is in desperate need of help, requiring penetrating moisture, nourishment, rebalancing, and cell regeneration.

What is never mentioned, although the information is there in black and white, is that moisturizing ingredients are surprisingly similar and acne-product ingredients are surprisingly similar. Even when there are differences, and of course there are differences between products, more often than not they are minor compared with the similarities. Furthermore, what you are supposed to believe about these products is almost embarrassing; there seem to be more miracle ingredients in the world of cosmetics than in any other industry. Isn't it amazing, with the thousands of wrinkle creams promising wrinkle- and blemish-free skin, that anyone still has wrinkles? And even though some things can make a difference (such as alpha hydroxy acids, antioxidants, liposomes, benzoyl peroxide, vitamins, and minerals), they never live up to the sensational claims made for them. Most miraculous skin care wonders only last a few seasons, until a new product is introduced, with new, improved claims. Why would any of them be needed, unless the last remarkable answer to your skin care woes didn't work?

The agony and the ecstasy of all this is that many skin care and makeup products work, and work beautifully, but just because a product works or is good for the skin doesn't mean it will get rid of one wrinkle or stop breakouts or that another line doesn't have something almost identical for much less money. A product may temporarily make your skin look smoother, and may even clear up a blemish or two, but that doesn't warrant a $25 to $200 price tag, especially when the same thing may be available around the corner for under $10.

Wrinkle creams, moisturizers, and products that eliminate breakouts are the most expensive and the most emotional cosmetics purchases most women make. If the cosmetics industry can persuade you that something in the environment (such as pollution) or something inside of you (such as stress) causes wrinkles, acne, or any other skin problem, they can further convince you that they have creams, lotions, and gels to combat it. It doesn't matter whether or not they work, and it doesn't even matter whether or not pollution or stress can affect your skin; convincing you that they can, even in the smallest, almost imperceptible, way, is all it takes to get your money. Propagating myths about skin care is one of the things the cosmetics industry does best. There is no evidence that pollution or stress causes wrinkles, or that any products can stop oil production. Yet the number of cosmetics being sold to combat these skin maladies is remarkable.

Cosmetics Seduction

Whenever you shop for makeup, the choices are dazzling, provocative, and extensive, and the sales methods fetching and slick. You notice the display for a new foundation or eye cream at the department-store, or you hear enthusiastic exclamations from a celebrity endorsing an infomercial line of skin care products, or a friend selling a new line of cosmetics rattles off a litany of scientific-sounding information that sounds too good to be true. Enticing names and colors suggest the very essence of beauty. Tantalizing claims sound too good to pass up. The thoughts flicker: "If I buy that, I will look really great; if I use that, my skin may really look younger." Elegance, glamour, and sensuality, all in one small bottle. How can you not at least try it? What difference does price make when all that matters is looking and feeling beautiful? Your hand is in your wallet before you know it.

That is when the déjà vu should begin. You should be saying to yourself, "Didn't this happen a few months or a year ago? Did the last wrinkle cream I bought really make a difference? Why should this one work? Didn't the last lipstick I bought, which said it wouldn't bleed but did, convince me to be more skeptical?" Even if you like the products you are using, the next eye-catching ad can make you doubt them. Perhaps there is something better out there that you're missing. Another $50, $75, $100, or $200 later, you have a collection of new products at home, and the cycle continues.

I understand the pull generated by creative cosmetics advertising. But chasing after every new anti-wrinkle product or anti-acne product that comes on the market would cost thousands upon thousands of dollars a year. At the Lancome counter, the salespeople tout the miraculous results of their new Primordial Lotion, giving it the same kind of hype they gave their Bienfait Total a few months before. In fact, you can hear similar claims no matter where you stop to get advice, whether from Chanel, Prescriptives, Arden, Orlane, Christian Dior, L'Oreal, Nivea, Almay, Amway, Murad, or Cellex-C. All cosmetics companies promote their skin "miracles."

They also use vague language that can't be proved or disproved, so they don't have to worry about claim substantiation. How does skin "act young"? That can be defined in a hundred different ways. Additionally, even if the company can substantiate the claim, what they substantiate may not be what you were hoping for. This cycle gets you nowhere, and that's why you need me.

There are several major obstacles to overcome when tackling the cosmetics-buying process: (1) the vast number of choices; (2) the vast number of products that are a waste of time and money; (3) the vast number of products that really work and help you look wonderful; (4) salespeople who are trained to sell products, and not how to honestly evaluate your skin care needs or apply makeup colors; and (5) the difficulty of knowing what really works and what doesn't, as well as what looks good on you and what doesn't.

The purpose of this book is to help you narrow down the choices. Yes, it's hard to know what looks the best and what skin care products really do work, but the more information you have, the easier it gets and the less money you will waste. In all honesty, shopping the cosmetics counters may never be truly easy, but it can be a fun, challenging adventure that you can approach with confidence and more knowledge then most any salesperson you will ever meet.

What Should Be Illegal, Besides Blue Eyeshadow?

Even though I am impressed by many improvements on the cosmetics front, there are still many disappointments. Some of the more ineffective, unnecessary, and unflattering products you may encounter are shiny eyeshadows (they make the skin look wrinkly); wrinkle creams; rejuvenating creams; astringents; toners that contain irritating ingredients; special eyelid foundations (they are almost always unnecessary); bright green, lavender, or pink eyeshadows (check out any fashion magazine and see how many women are wearing these colors); eye-lift creams; firming lotions; eyeshadow sets (you always use just one or two colors and the others go to waste); sponge-tip eyeshadow applicators (something professional makeup artists never use); compact-size brushes (too small for almost any cheek); models under the age of 30 posing for wrinkle-cream ads; models with perfect skin posing for skin care ads; tanned models posing for sunscreen ads; ingredient names no one understands; "all-day" lipstick claims; mascaras that clump and flake; water-soluble mascaras that don't rinse off completely; overly aggressive cosmetics salespeople; poorly lit makeup counters; miracle ingredients; "dermatologist-tested" claims; "hypoallergenic" claims (these aren't regulated terms so a cosmetics company can, and do, include any ingredients they want regardless of their potential for irritation or skin sensitivity); "noncomedogenic" and "nonacnegenic" claims (these terms are also not regulated and many cosmetics labeled as such absolutely contain ingredients that can cause breakouts or blackheads); "all natural" claims; pink- and orange-colored foundations (there are no pink or orange people); and tanning powders, bronzers, and tinted moisturizers.

Beauty Note: In the past I have complained emphatically that eye creams are a waste of money, and for the most part that is still true. Most face creams and lotions are completely suitable for use around the eyes. In fact, many moisturizers contain virtually identical ingredients, regardless of the area they are "supposed" to be used on. There are some notable exceptions to that rule, though. When the eye area is drier than the skin on the rest of the face, a more emollient moisturizer may indeed be necessary. If that is the case, it is completely acceptable to use an emollient eye cream over that area. Some women may prefer a gel or a lighter-weight moisturizer for the eye area; in that case as well, an eye gel or lotion is perfect. My major concern about eye creams is that most women believe they can somehow firm skin, get rid of bags, or eliminate wrinkles around the eye. That is simply not the case.

For Women of Color

Many cosmetics lines are trying to make up for their past inequities by adding makeup products appropriate for women of color. Previously, the foundations offered in this area were too orange and greasy, the eyeshadows were strictly shiny, and the skin care products were fairly drying. It seems unbelievable that it's taken so long for the major cosmetics companies to finally acknowledge and try to meet the needs of such a large group of women. Maybelline, Revlon, Prescriptives, M.A.C., and Lancome are the leaders in this area, and they are to be commended. Not only are their color products appropriate, but they offer a large number of choices. Although some lines designed specifically for women of color, such as Flori Roberts and Fashion Fair, offer limited options, some new lines now available, including Black Opal, Posner, and Iman, have incredible color selections and high-quality products.

An area where these specialty lines often fail is when it comes to skin care. Although, Black Opal or Flori Roberts would lead the consumer to believe that their products are specially formulated for African American skin, there is nothing in the formulation supporting that claim. In fact, often products for African American women are formulated to be either greasy with heavy moisturizers and wipe off cleansers, or drying with alcohol-based toners. Both of these product types pose problems for darker skin tones. Alcohol can dry out the skin and increase ashiness, and greasy products can cause breakouts.

A handful of cosmetics lines coming on the scene claim they are designed for Asian women. The brochures say Asian skin is supposedly so different from Caucasian, Latin, and African-American skin that it requires a separate product line. Nothing could be further from the truth, and the products in these lines are just like those in all the other lines on the market. Creating a special marketing niche where none exists might be good business, but it isn't necessarily good for the consumer. As it turns out, according to marketing surveys most Asian women do not want a line directed specifically at them; they would rather buy mainstream cosmetics, just as they have always done.

Cosmetics Counter Reality

1. **All the makeup and skin care products in the world can't cover up an unhealthy lifestyle of no exercise, smoking, and/or a high-fat diet.** This first point is essential.

2. **There is no such thing as the perfect cosmetic or cosmetics line.** There are a lot of good products available, but no miracle products. That search can cost you a lot of money and won't help your skin one iota.

3. **Spending more money does not mean you will look more beautiful.** Buying expensive cosmetics may make you feel as if you're doing something good for yourself, but don't be fooled. Expensive, shiny eyeshadows or irritating toners with alcohol won't make anyone look good.

4. **Do not get sucked into the elite craze of spa treatments for the skin.** Spas have no more information about skin care than other companies. The suggestion that you'll be getting the same products the rich and famous use is a come-on you'll be better off resisting.

5. **It is a waste of money to buy more than two or three shades of any color.** No one needs eight shades of pink lipstick or coral blush.

6. **There is nothing wrong with shopping for makeup.** But keep in mind how much energy you spend trying to look glamorous instead of getting out and being beautiful by living life.

7. **You must be willing to change some of your beliefs about the world of skin care and makeup.** If you are willing to buy stuff that is overpriced, doesn't work, or isn't fashionable, the cosmetics industry will keep selling it, because there is no reason for them to change.

8. **Every cosmetics line has good and bad products.** Of course, the products that work are often still overpriced.

9. **Give up line loyalty.** It is great when you find a product that you like. That doesn't mean that every other product in that line will please you or be good for you.

10. **Do not buy impulsively or quickly.** Take notes, wear a color for a while, take a sample of a skin care item, and then make a decision. In fact, buying a product you've just tried on and haven't worn for at least an hour or two is almost always a mistake. You have nothing to lose if you take your time.

11. **Cosmetics advertising may be alluring and interesting, but it is advertising, not a documentary.** Just because the ads are sensual and the models beautiful doesn't mean the products featured in the ads will make you more sensual or beautiful. Accept seductive ads for what they are—seductive ads, not a reliable source of facts.

12. **Don't assume you can remain unaffected by cosmetics advertising.** Advertising sells products, and sells them very well, because the cosmetics companies wouldn't keep throwing money at something that produced no financial return. The next time you think you are not affected by cosmetics advertising, think again.

13. **Truly superior mascaras, foundations, lipsticks, blushes, and eyeshadows can be found in inexpensive lines.** Formulations might vary and some products are better than others, but on the whole, a product's quality is not reflected in its price. I find just as many great products at the drugstore as I do at the department store.

Marketing creates the mystique of makeup. If spending $50 on foundation makes you look $50 better, then I guess it's worth it. But if spending $50 makes you look the same as if you had bought the $5 product, then you should reconsider your decision-making process.

14. **Return products that you have allergic reactions to or that don't live up to their claims.** Returning products and explaining our preferences and complaints is a great way to educate manufacturers. We can tell them what we think, but companies of any kind listen better when it affects their bottom line. If the FDA isn't going to make cosmetics companies live up to their claims, then we can by returning products that don't do what they say they can do. (See the appendix for a list of phone numbers for many of the major cosmetics companies.)

15. **Celebrities and models are not skin care or makeup experts.** This one speaks for itself.

SKIN CARE UPDATE

Helps Skin Look Younger?

Many times ad copy goes on at length about what a product can do, with a disclaimer at the very end or tucked in somewhere inconspicuous to prevent the company from running afoul of the FDA. Take Clinique's Moisture On-Call, for example. Moisture On-Call, according to the brochure, is supposed to help skin cells "remember" how to produce their own moisture barrier. Clinique calls this memory booster "mnemonic."

Can you make skin cells remember to produce better moisture barriers over time? Yes. You can do it with the daily use of any moisturizer, which is the only claim Clinique is really making; if you read further in the pamphlet that accompanies the product, it clearly states, "As for the more long-term benefits, it will take your skin about four weeks of constant reminding. . . Then daily prompting will help keep skin's memory refreshed." How inane. The daily use of any moisturizer will keep the skin "refreshed" and moist.

Examining the claims of packaged youth or flawless skin is the one of the most fascinating parts of dissecting the cosmetics business. There is a stark difference between the things said at the counters and the things said on TV and in magazine ads. Unlike the claims made by cosmetics salespeople, which vary wildly from person to person and, as a result, are hard to pin down and refute, the claims of cosmetics advertising and promotional literature are bold, direct, and accompanied by full-color illustrations. The one- and two-page ads or 30-minute television infomercials make definite claims for an individual product or product line. Most of these ads are beautiful and beguiling, with all the trappings of authenticity and veracity. But more often than not, the claims couldn't be further from the truth, or at best they're misleading. What isn't smothered in scientific jargon is shrouded in confusing rhetoric. Anyone who has heard phrases such as "a two-week treatment synchronized to your skin's natural rhythm" or "cellular balancing complex" knows that it all sounds good, but what does it mean? Are your cells imbalanced? Exactly which cells are we talking about? Does skin have a rhythm? And if it does, how can the product play everybody's tune?

See how many of the most typically used, catchy, albeit meaningless, phrases you recognize: "appears to" (doesn't say it will, just that it can seem to); "leaves the skin looking smoother" ("looks smooth" doesn't mean it *is* smooth); "changes the appearance of" (doesn't say it changes the skin structure, only the way it looks, which any moisturizer can do); "lessens the signs of" ("signs" refers to dryness, and almost any moisturizer can do this too); "reduces the chances of" ("chances" can mean that in 1 of 100 cases it actually will reduce, but that's still a "chance"); "reduces the temporary signs of aging" ("temporary" means dryness), "anti-aging" (as opposed to pro-aging? This term has no meaning at all); "affects the visible signs of aging" ("visible" means superficial, as in dry skin, not anything deeper); "reverses the visual damage of aging" ("visual" also means what you can see on the surface and refers only to dry skin); "accelerates cell renewal" (if something helps peel the skin, it can affect cell turnover, but so can a washcloth); and "independent studies show" (these studies are rarely truly independent; they are almost always paid for by the cosmetics company and the results are never published, which makes them scientifically untenable).

The number of products that make claims like these is staggering. Just remember that nothing specific, long-lasting, or permanent can be guaranteed, because nothing specific, long-lasting, or permanent can be proved.

The Greening of Cosmetics

As never before, the value of a product today lies not only in how natural it appears to be but in how sincerely natural it is. Everything from volcanic minerals to mangoes, Dead Sea salts to oatmeal, sea kelp to vitamins, DNA to plant oils, when added to an ordinary effective moisturizer, can make it seem sensational. It's still ordinary, but perception is everything in cosmetics.

Now, if every cosmetics company adding food to their products, how do you make your company's products stand out? How much more natural can you get? The Body Shop has taken the search for (and marketing of) "green" ingredients to the seemingly ultimate degree, obtaining oils through native peoples of foreign countries, including the Maasai of Africa and the Kayapo Indians of the Amazon rain forest. Has this search produced better products? There is no evidence that the oils and herbs they've used provide any benefit for the skin or for the earth. In fact, the use of nonrenewable resources such as sandalwood is a problem, and the rain forest may end up being overcultivated for the purpose of harvesting these plants and trees. It isn't happening yet, but it could if consumers demand more and more exotic-sounding natural ingredients. Exotic ingredients serve nothing more than the emotional needs of the consumers, who want to believe that "natural" products will keep their skin young.

What you really need to know is whether a natural ingredient (particularly anything labeled "botanical" or an essential oil) interacts better with the skin than a synthetic ingredient does. Even substances found in human skin that have been manufactured synthetically for cosmetics cannot become a permanent part of your skin, nor do they necessarily provide any better protection. All the collagen, hyaluronic acid, protein, vegetable oils, plant extracts, or amino acids in the world cannot perform wonders for your skin. They can keep water in the skin, add texture to a product, and perform a number of other functions, but they are not automatically better for the skin simply because they originated from the earth, a plant, a person, or an animal.

According to the June 1992 issue of *Household and Personal Products Industry* magazine, "The concentration of plant extracts used in cosmetics is rarely enough to make a difference in a product. . . . [Cosmetics companies] use a little [amount of botanicals] and then rely on consumer perceptions." Although cosmetics companies vow they are using botanicals due to their effect and not as a sales tool, the jump-on-the-bandwagon evidence is hard to ignore.

My favorite quote is from the March 1992 issue of *Drug and Cosmetics Industry* magazine, which stated, "Aromatherapy . . . is a newly emerging science that isn't yet understood. But why lose time by waiting until scientists can prove that essential oils work." That is basic cosmetics industry logic: convince the public, whether there is any supporting evidence or not. As long as the consumer believes you, what else counts? It doesn't matter whether it works.

Another significant comment comes from Robert L. Goldemberg, a longtime columnist for *Drug and Cosmetics Industry* as well as a cosmetics chemist. In the November 1995 issue of the magazine, he wrote, "The actual level of the 'naturals' is usually rather low for various reasons which include cost, discoloration, poor odor, and difficulty of preservation. As a result, some less-than-ethical marketers are tempted merely to buy herbal extract mixtures containing five or six [plant] ingredients, and use only 0.1% to 0.5% of this mixture in their cosmetic. . . . While legally correct, nevertheless such window dressing is unfortunate. Its prime purpose is not to remedy a poor skin condition but rather, a means of selling product to gullible women who believe that 'natural' is safer and more efficacious than synthetic. Thus we must read product labels that contain grape root, Irish moss, and licorice. Since licorice sticks were found in King Tut's tomb, licorice must be good, right? No, of course not."

Think twice before purchasing tiny amounts of creams and lotions in attractive containers for a large amount of money. Traces of plant extracts suspended in standard cosmetics ingredients are not worth $30 to $100 for one ounce when they make up less than 1 percent of the product. When was the last time you bought an assortment of herbs for several thousand dollars a pound? Presently there are hundreds of plant extracts in varying combinations being used in skin care products. The cosmetic industry, without any substantiation or proof is able to convince women that any concoction of plants they come up with is a curative for every skin woe imaginable.

Many cosmetics companies use the concept of all-natural and pure ingredients as one of the primary inducements to buy their products. Over the years this has been an exceedingly effective sales gimmick, and combined with scientific jargon it is too much for many consumers to ignore. "Pure and natural" fused with anything that sounds like modern technology can make products jump off the shelf into a woman's purse.

I'm not saying that pure and natural ingredients aren't good, but they aren't essential or necessarily the best options for good skin care. Additionally, many cosmetics ingredients that sound completely unnatural are naturally derived. You might not realize it from their names, but ingredients such as cetyl alcohol, stearic acid, stearyl alcohol, acetic acid, sodium cocoyl isethionate, oleoresin, cocamidopropyl, and caprylic glycerides are all derived from natural sources. On the other hand, although you're probably familiar with ingredients such as chamomile, lavender oil, and vegetable oil, which sound quite natural, the label doesn't tell you what kind of processing that plant went through to get into the cosmetic. Even something that starts out as natural doesn't resemble anything natural once it gets into a cosmetic. First, synthetic chemical ingredients are used to obtain a plant extract or oil. Extracts that have been processed through formaldehyde or acid lose some of their allure. Over and above the chemical extraction process, there is the chemical process of combining ingredients. When plants have been mixed together with preservatives and other synthetic chemicals, their natural status is irrevocably altered. Further, saying an ingredient is natural or derived from natural sources doesn't tell you anything about its value or irritation potential. "Natural" is just too vague a term; it gives you no consequential information. A number of natural ingredients can even be bad for the skin.

Many ingredients, such as mineral oil, get a bad rap because they are derived from coal tar, which sounds unnatural but is actually as natural as any plant. Mineral oil is actually one of the better, least irritating, least problem-causing ingredients for the skin.

Remember, the question isn't whether something sounds good or appears to be good for your skin, but whether it is genuinely good.

It is interesting to note that the terms "natural" and "pure" are not regulated by the FDA. Cosmetics manufacturers use the terms as they see fit. "Natural" can mean that the ingredient in question is part natural and part synthetic, that the product itself has some natural ingredients and some synthetic ones, or that all the ingredients are natural but have been synthetically extracted. To hold the blind belief that "natural" means good and "chemical" (synthetic) means bad is to ignore a wide range of substances that can be combined to make great skin care and makeup products. In fact, there is little evidence that natural ingredients significantly improve a product. A bunch of herbal extracts and essential oils without standard cosmetics ingredients wouldn't be much of a product, and they would also probably be smelly and moldy. You can do without the extracts and oils, but you can't make a cosmetic without the usual ingredients that sound, and usually are, anything but natural, such as preservatives and thickening agents. Natural ingredients are almost always synthetically treated so they can be blended into a cosmetic. Besides, synthetic isn't necessarily bad. Table salt consists of sodium and chloride, which separately would eat through the surface of a car.

If you are to make wise decisions at the cosmetics counter, it is essential that you stop falling for the erroneous belief that plant extracts, botanicals, essential oils, or any other pure- or natural-sounding ingredients are automatically good for the skin. They aren't, and they aren't all that natural to begin with. Do not let the cosmetics industry entice you with meaningless language.

Friend or Foe?

In my battle against the flagrantly ambiguous information surrounding natural ingredients and the frequently inconclusive studies heralded as indisputable truth, I feel I have inadvertently ignored some worthwhile natural ingredients. Conversely, I have also neglected to point out the specific natural ingredients that can cause problems for some skin types. Given the abundance of these ingredients and the fact that they aren't going away, it is crucial to point out both the beneficial and the harmful natural-sounding ingredients. I'm not suggesting you should run right out to find any of these ingredients in products, or automatically avoid them either. But when you do see the ones that may be helpful in a moisturizer or toner, you can think of them as friendly naturals that could be an asset for your skin; when you see the ones that may be irritants, you may want to consider staying away if you have sensitive skin.

I have read summaries of several different studies demonstrating that green tea, kola extract, bisabol (from trees), licorice root, and glycyrrhetinic acid (derived from licorice) are very good anti-irritants. Kojic acid may lighten the skin (especially when used in combination with an alpha hydroxy acid) as well as or better than hydroquinone, a skin-lightening agent that doesn't work all that well and has irritating side effects. Kojic acid purports to cause less irritation, but there hasn't yet been enough research to make a definitive statement about this new ingredient.

Antioxidants, which I will discuss at greater length in a later section in this chapter, may help the skin by slowing free-radical damage. Antioxidants derived from natural sources include vitamin A (retinyl palmitate), vitamin B (riboflavin), vitamin C (ascorbic acid), vitamin D (calciferol), vitamin E (tocopherol, tocopherol acetate, tocopherol succinate), vitamin K, selenium, superoxide dismutase (from protein), bioflavonoids, glutathione, cysteine, lecithin, and zinc.

There are a whole host of natural water-binding agents that provide very good protection for the skin: collagen, elastin, mucopolysaccharides, hyaluronic acid, NaPCA (sodium PCA), amino acids, protein, glycosphingolipids, glycoproteins, plant oils (some of which, unfortunately, can be potential skin irritants), phospholipids, lecithin, and shea butter.

All of the following natural extracts or oils can cause skin irritation and/or sun sensitivity: allspice, almond, angelica, arnica, balm mint, balsam, bergamot, chamomile, cinnamon, citrus, clove, clover blossom, cocoa butter, coriander, corn oil, cornstarch, cottonseed, fennel, fir needle, geranium, grapefruit, horsetail, jojoba, lavender, lemon, lemongrass, lime, marjoram, melissa, oak bark, papaya, peppermint, rose, sage, tea tree, thyme, wintergreen, and ylang ylang. The label might say "pure and natural," but you could be buying a purely natural irritating product. If you tend to have allergies, many plant extracts can be especially irritating.

Understanding the Ingredients

Fortunately, the cosmetics companies have provided all of us with the very tool we need to implement an objective evaluation—the ingredient list. Every skin care item (and makeup item, for that matter) lists the exact contents, in descending order of amount, on the box or container. The ingredient list can be your best friend, because it can't mislead you. All of the information in that one small spot (often covered up by the price tag, unfortunately) has to be accurate, by law.

Below is a list of some typical cosmetics ingredients. I briefly describe what each ingredient is and what it can or cannot do for the skin. This information is truly the nuts and bolts of the cosmetics industry. Understanding the ingredient list may not change the way you buy skin care products, but I hope it will make you more aware of what you're buying. My major sources for this list were *A Consumer's Dictionary of Cosmetics Ingredients* by Ruth Winter (Crown Trade Paperbacks); the *International Cosmetic Ingredient Handbook* and the *International Cosmetic Ingredient Dictionary* (Cosmetic, Toiletry, and Fragrance Association); and several past issues of *Drug and Cosmetics Industry* magazine and *Cosmetics & Toiletries* magazine. Keep in mind that this list is not complete; there are potentially thousands of cosmetics ingredients.

Acetone: Used in some astringents and toners for its ability to remove oil from the surface of the skin. Extremely drying; can cause severe irritation.

Acetylated lanolin: *See* Lanolin.

Alcohol, SD alcohol 10-40: Alcohol is found in many types of skin care products. It can irritate and dry out the skin. **Cetyl** and **Stearyl** alcohols are <u>not</u> the kind of alcohols you need to worry about. These are simply emollient thickening agents.

Algae extract: Derived from seaweed. It is considered a good protective and emollient agent for the skin. All the miraculous claims about it healing the skin or getting rid of wrinkles are unsubstantiated.

Allantoin: Considered a good soothing agent.

Allspice: Whether as an oil or an extract, can be a skin irritant.

Almond: Whether as an oil or an extract, can be a skin irritant.

Aloe vera: Well known, legitimately, for its ability to soothe the skin.

Alpha hydroxy acids (AHAs): *See the section on alpha hydroxy acids later in this chapter.*

Amino acids: Constitute the protein in human skin. Twenty-two of these extremely complex substances are used in cosmetics. Proteins provide a smooth covering on the skin and are considered beneficial in helping the skin absorb water. They provide no other benefit, such as building or supplementing the protein in your own skin. *See* Protein.

Ammonium glycerhizinate: A very good anti-inflammatory agent. Helps soothe skin and reduce irritation.

Ammonium lauryl sulfate: *See* Sodium laureth sulfate.

Amniotic fluid: Derived from the liquid surrounding an animal embryo. Some cosmetics companies claim this fluid can rejuvenate the skin. There are no independent studies that support this claim.

Angelica: Whether as an oil or an extract, can be a skin irritant.

Animal extracts: Animal extracts include the following: spleen, matrix, neural lipid, epidermal lipid, thymus, and animal tissue. These are dead fat or skin tissues from the thymus, testes, ovaries, udder, placenta, or other parts of a cow, pig, or sheep. The cosmetics industry would like you to believe that they have some rejuvenating effect on the skin. There is no evidence that these extracts can do anything for the skin, especially make it look younger. There is some evidence that these ingredients may be water-binding agents, however, which is good for the skin but hardly unique or unusual.

Animal thymus extract: *See* Animal extracts.

Animal tissue extract: *See* Animal extracts.

Arnica: Whether as an oil or an extract, can be a skin irritant. However, some studies indicate that arnica in small concentrations can be a healing agent.

Ascorbic acid: Considered a good antioxidant.

Avocado oil: A plant oil that is a good emollient and water-binding agent.

Balm mint: Whether as an oil or an extract, can be a skin irritant.

Balsam: Whether as an oil or an extract, can be a skin irritant.

Bentonite: A clay that can help to absorb oil but can also be a skin irritant.

Benzalkonium chloride: Used as a disinfectant in cosmetics, but can be a potent skin sensitizer if it is found near the beginning of an ingredient list.

Benzoyl peroxide: A disinfectant. There has been some controversial evidence that benzoyl peroxide may have a negative impact on the skin. That research is not widely supported, and other research has disputed it. In my opinion, benzoyl peroxide is an effective option for someone with acne.

Bergamot: Whether as an oil or an extract, can be a skin irritant.

Beta hydroxy acids: *See* Salicylic acid.

Bioflavonoids: Considered a good and effective antioxidant.

Bisabol: Considered a good and effective anti-irritant.

Butylene glycol: *See* Glycerin.

Camphor: Found in many products intended to treat acne and chapped lips, but can cause contact dermatitis and be a potent skin irritant.

Caprylic/capric/lauric triglycerides: An oily substance derived from coconut oil; helps keep water in the skin.

Carrot oil: A plant oil that is a good emollient and water-binding agent.

Castor oil: A plant oil that is a good emollient and water-binding agent.

Ceramide: A component of skin. When used in cosmetics, can be a good water-binding ingredient.

Chamomile: Whether as an oil or an extract, can be a skin irritant if there is a lot of present in a product.

Cholesterol: Found in most living tissue, both plant and animal. An antioxidant, it is also considered a good emollient.

Cinnamon: Whether as an oil or an extract, can be a skin irritant.

Citrus: Whether as an oil or an extract, can be a skin irritant.

Clove: Whether as an oil or an extract, can be a skin irritant.

Clover blossom: Whether as an oil or an extract, can be a skin irritant.

Cocoa butter: A thickening agent and emollient. Considered very effective for dry skin but may cause skin irritation.

Coconut oil: A plant oil that is a good emollient and water-binding agent.

Collagen: A component of skin, and a well-known ingredient that helps keep water in the skin. The belief that somehow collagen and elastin rubbed on the skin will help rebuild the collagen and elastin in your own skin is, I hope, a thing of the past. The collagen and elastin found in cosmetics, because of their structure, cannot even penetrate the skin.

Coriander: Whether as an oil or an extract, can be a skin irritant.

Corn oil: Can be a skin irritant.

Cornstarch: Used as a thickening agent in cosmetics; can be a skin irritant.

Cottonseed oil: Can be a skin irritant.

Cyclomethicone: One of the many silicone oils used in cosmetics because of the incredibly soft, silky feel they leave on the skin and because of their versatility. They also are good water-binding agents. Cyclomethicone evaporates quickly, so it leaves little residue on the skin.

Dimethicone: *See* Cyclomethicone.

Dmdm hydantoin: A common preservative in cosmetics that is also considered one of the more potentially irritating for the skin.

Elastin: A component of skin; when used in cosmetics, can be a good water-binding ingredient. *See also* Collagen.

Epidermal lipid extract: *See* Animal extracts.

Eucalyptus oil: Found in many products meant to treat acne and chapped lips, but can cause contact dermatitis and be a potent skin irritant.

Fatty acids: Stearic acid, the most popular fatty acid used in cosmetics, is a substance found in skin tissue. Used in a cosmetic, it helps keep water in the skin.

Fennel: Whether as an oil or an extract, can be a skin irritant.

Fennel oil: A plant oil that can be a good emollient but may also be a skin sensitizer.

Fir needle: Whether as an oil or an extract, can be a skin irritant.

Geranium: Whether as an oil or an extract, can be a skin irritant.

Glutathione: Considered a good antioxidant.

Glycerhizinate: Considered a good anti-irritant.

Glycerin: A fairly standard skin care ingredient that helps attract water to the skin (an ingredient that can do this is called a humectant) and also helps deliver other ingredients into the skin. In large amounts, can be a skin sensitizer. Butylene, hexylene, and propylene glycol have similar properties.

Glycolic acid: *See the section on alpha hydroxy acids later in this chapter.*

Glycoprotein: *See* Protein.

Glycosamnioglycans: A basic element found in skin tissue. When used in creams and lotions, helps water penetrate the skin. There is no evidence that glycosamnioglycans can aid the skin in any way besides keeping the surface soft and helping bind water to the skin.

Glycosphingolipids: A component of skin. When used in cosmetics, can be a good water-binding ingredient.

Grapefruit: Whether as an oil or an extract, can be a skin irritant.

Green tea: Considered a good and effective anti-irritant for the skin.

Hexylene glycol: *See* Glycerin.

Horsetail: Whether as an oil or an extract, can be a skin irritant.

Hyaluronic acid: A component of skin; when used in cosmetics, can be a good water-binding ingredient.

Hydrolyzed animal protein: A component of skin; when used in cosmetics, can be a good water-binding ingredient. *See* Protein.

Hydroquinone: A skin-lightening agent considered most effective when combined with alpha hydroxy acids. Can be a skin sensitizer; many consider its skin-lightening effects to be minimal.

Imidazolidinyl urea: A common preservative that is also considered to have more potential for irritating for the skin, then other preservatives.

Isopropyl lanolate: A thickening agent and emollient. Studies show that it can cause breakouts or acne; however, it should not cause any problems if it is found at the end of an ingredient list.

Isopropyl myristate: A thickening agent and emollient. Studies show that it can cause breakouts or acne; however, it should not cause any problems if it is found at the end of an ingredient list.

Jojoba oil: A plant oil that is a good emollient and water-binding agent but can be a skin irritant or sensitizer.

Kaolin: A clay that can help absorb oil but can also be a skin irritant.

Kojic acid: Some studies indicate this is a skin-lightening agent. Considered most effective when used combined with alpha hydroxy acids.

Kola extract: Considered a good and effective anti-irritant.

Lactic acid: *See the section on alpha hydroxy acids later in this chapter.*

Lanolin: A superior emollient and lubricant for dry skin. There is evidence that it can be a skin sensitizer or can aggravate breakouts. Other than that, it is very effective at keeping the skin moist and supple. You will see several forms of lanolin on skin care ingredient lists: lanolin oil, hydroxylated lanolin, lanolin alcohols, lanolin oil, and acetylated lanolin. All of these work as well as or better than pure lanolin to keep moisture in the skin.

Lanolin alcohol: *See* Lanolin.

Lanolin oil: *See* Lanolin.

Lavender: Whether as an oil or an extract, can be a skin irritant and a photosensitizer.

Lecithin: Found in most living tissue, both plant and animal. An antioxidant, it is also considered a good emollient.

Lemon: Whether as an oil or an extract, can be a skin irritant.

Lemongrass: Whether as an oil or an extract, can be a skin irritant.

Licorice root: Considered a good and effective anti-irritant.

Lime: Whether as an oil or an extract, can be a skin irritant.

Linoleic acid: A component of skin and plants known as a fatty acid. Considered excellent for keeping water in the skin.

Liposomes: Not a specific ingredient you would see on an ingredient list; rather, it is a unique delivery system that allows the penetration and slow release of water and lipids (oils and fats that act as water-binding agents) into the layers of skin.

Macadamia oil: A plant oil that is a good emollient and water-binding agent.

Magnesium laureth sulfate: *See* Sodium laureth sulfate.

Marine extracts: Seaweed, algae and other marine plants are used in cosmetics with claims of wrinkle prevention. None are substantiated and they are definitely not a unique or preferred source for antioxidants or water-binding agents.

Marjoram: Whether as an oil or an extract, can be a skin irritant.

Melissa: Whether as an oil or an extract, can be a skin irritant.

Menthol: Although found in many products meant to treat acne and chapped lips, can cause contact dermatitis and be a potent skin irritant.

Methylparaben: *See* Propylparaben.

Methylacrylate: Forms a film or coating over the skin, similar to ingredients found in hairsprays that hold hair in place. It can temporarily make skin look smooth and hold it in place. Can be a potent skin irritant.

Mineral oil: This widely used cosmetics ingredient has had a bad reputation in the past. In spite of the occasional bad press, mineral oil is considered one of the most nonirritating cosmetics ingredients available and is superior at keeping water in the skin.

Minerals: Minerals such as salt (sodium chloride), iodine, magnesium, chloride, and potassium are potential skin irritants when found in the first part of a cosmetic's ingredient list. However, minerals such as zinc, selenium, and choline are considered good antioxidants.

Mucopolysaccharides: A component of skin; when used in cosmetics, can be a good water-binding ingredient.

NaPCA: A component of skin; when used in cosmetics, can be a good water-binding ingredient.

Neural lipid extract: *See* Animal extracts.

Oak bark: Whether as an oil or an extract, can be a skin irritant.

Oil: In general, oils of all kinds, whether plant, animal, or mineral, help keep water in the skin. A wide variety of oils are used in skin care products, including plant oil, egg oil, lanolin oil, castor oil, mineral oil, and silicone oil. If you have dry skin, buy a moisturizer that contains one or more oils as the primary ingredients.

Palm oil: A plant oil that is a good emollient and water-binding agent.

Panthenol: Well known, legitimately, for its ability to soothe the skin.

Papaya: Used in skin care products as an exfoliant; can be a skin irritant.

Peppermint: Although found in many natural products, can cause contact dermatitis and be a potent skin sensitizer.

Petrolatum: One of the more effective moisturizing ingredients around. Study after study indicates it performs as well as or better than any other skin care ingredient for keeping water in the skin, and it does not clog pores. Mineral oil is derived from petrolatum. *See also* Mineral oil.

Phospholipids: Found in human and plant tissue. In cosmetics, helps bind water to the skin and keep it there, and is considered a good emollient.

Placenta extract: *See* Animal extracts.

Plant extracts: An endless array of plant ingredients that range from algae to chamomile. By far the most overly hyped of all cosmetics ingredients. Some do benefit the skin, but no more or less than many other ingredients. More often than not, these ingredients offer little benefit other boosting the appeal (and price) of a product. Many plant extracts can be skin sensitizers, particularly for people with plant allergies.

Plant oils: For the most part, these have a positive effect on the skin, helping to keep water in and lubricating and smoothing the surface. However, many plant oils can be skin irritants.

Polyacrylamide: *See* Methylacrylate.

Polyethylene glycol (PEG): At least one member of this vast group of skin care ingredients is present in practically every cleanser, toner, lotion, cream, and specialty product you will ever buy. These ingredients help attract moisture to the skin, help the product spread evenly, keep the other ingredients mixed together, and are good water-binding agents.

Propylene glycol: *See* Glycerin.

Propylparaben: A standard preservative. All parabens are considered to be the least irritating of the preservatives used in cosmetics.

Protein: A component of skin. When used in cosmetics, can be a good water-binding ingredient, but won't add to the protein content of your skin.

PVP: *See* Methylacrylate.

Quaternium-15: A common preservative that is also considered to be potentially irritating for the skin.

Retinol: A derivative of vitamin A. Vitamin A is also the source of the prescription drug Retin-A. This association with Retin-A misleads many consumers into believing that products containing retinol can provide benefits similar to those of Retin-A. At this time, there is no conclusive evidence to support this idea, although studies are being conducted. For the most part, vitamin A, retinyl palmitate, and retinol are simple but good antioxidants and help prevent free-radical damage. They may also have some benefits in terms of allowing moisture to penetrate the skin, but that's about it.

Retinyl palmitate: *See* Retinol.

Rice bran oil: A plant oil that is a good emollient and water-binding agent.

Sage: Whether as an oil or an extract, can be a skin irritant.

Salicylic acid: A beta hydroxy acid (BHA) that is an effective exfoliant, but it doesn't have a drop-off rate (meaning it doesn't stop exfoliating the skin), as AHAs do. Salicylic acid just keeps exfoliating, which can be too irritating for skin on a regular basis. Also, salicylic acid doesn't have the additional benefit of water-binding properties the way AHAs do.

Sandalwood oil: A plant oil that can be a skin sensitizer.

Seaweed: *See* Marine extracts.

SD alcohol: *See* Alcohol.

Selenium: Considered a very effective antioxidant.

Serum protein: Derived from the blood of cows or pigs and used as a moisturizing ingredient. It may be a water-binding agent, but it isn't some miracle for the skin, despite its exotic sound.

Shea butter: A thickening agent and emollient. Considered nonirritating and very effective for dry skin.

Sodium C14-16 olefin sulfate: *See* Sodium lauryl sulfate.

Sodium laureth sulfate: Along with a dozen or so similar-sounding ingredients, sodium laureth sulfate is considered a very gentle detergent cleansing agent. It is found most often in shampoos and water-soluble skin cleansers. It can be gentle, but it can also be somewhat drying.

Sodium lauroyl sarcosinate: *See* Sodium laureth sulfate.

Sodium lauryl sulfate: A cleansing agent found mostly in shampoos and skin cleansers. It is considered quite drying and potentially irritating when used as the primary ingredient in a skin cleanser.

Sodium PCA: *See* NaPCA.

Soybean oil: A plant oil that is a good emollient and water-binding agent.

Spleen extract: *See* Animal extracts.

Squalane: A plant oil that is a good emollient and water-binding agent.

Squalene: *See* Squalane.

Sunflower seed oil: A plant oil that is a good emollient and water-binding agent.

Superoxide dismutase: Considered a very effective antioxidant.

Sweet almond oil: A plant oil that is a good emollient and water-binding agent, but can be a skin sensitizer.

TEA-lauryl sulfate: *See* Sodium lauryl sulfate.

Tea tree: Also known as melaluca; almost identical to menthol. *See* Menthol.

Thyme: Whether as an oil or an extract, can be a skin irritant.

Tissue matrix extract: *See* Animal extracts.

Tocopherol: The chemical name for vitamin E. Used in cosmetics as an antioxidant, which means it helps keep the air off the face, which helps prevent dehydration and possible free-radical damage. Vitamins do not feed the skin in any way from the outside in. The amount used is rarely enough to provide much benefit.

Triclosan: A disinfectant.

Triethanolamine: Typically used as a pH adjuster in cosmetics as well as, in combination with other ingredients, a detergent cleansing agent. Because triethanolamine is such a strong alkaline ingredient, it is also considered to quite irritating.

Triglycerides: Found in human and plant tissue. In cosmetics, helps bind water to the skin and keep it there.

2-bromo-2-nitropane-1,3-diol: A less than common preservative that is considered potentially irritating.

Vitamin A: *See* Retinol.

Vitamin C: *See* Ascorbic acid.

Vitamin E: *See* Tocopherol.

Water: Dry skin and mature skin contain an increased number of dried-out skin cells. Water rehydrates these cells. Water is water—whether it is fancy water from the Swiss Alps, natural spring water, demineralized water, or water extracted from plants or flowers—and it must be present in your skin cells, or in your skin care product, if you want to see positive effects on your face.

Wheat germ oil: A plant oil that is a good emollient and water-binding agent.

Wintergreen: Whether as an oil or an extract, can be a skin irritant.

Witch hazel: A compound that is about 15% to 20% alcohol. Considered a mild skin irritant. Many products that claim to be alcohol-free contain witch hazel.

Ylang ylang: Whether as an oil or an extract, can be a skin irritant.

Zinc: Considered an effective antioxidant.

Is It Really Oil-Free?

Cyclomethicone and dimethicone are showing up in everything from foundations and moisturizers to shampoos and conditioners. These two popular cosmetics components aren't anything new, but they are gaining incredible popularity. What are they? They are silicone oils with unique properties that make them very desirable in cosmetics, and they are fast replacing their kissing cousin, the unjustly maligned mineral oil. Although there is nothing wrong with mineral oil in cosmetics, especially for those with dry skin, some people perceive it as a problem. What's a cosmetics manufacturer to do when mineral oil does such a terrific job of keeping moisture in the skin, with little chance of causing skin sensitivity, not to mention being inexpensive to use? Dimethicone and cyclomethicone to the rescue.

Unlike mineral oil, which is derived from petrolatum, dimethicone and cyclomethicone are derived from sand or rock. Mineral oil has a greasy after-feel, while dimethicone and cyclomethicone both have a texture reminiscent of silk. While mineral oil and petrolatum have a tendency to spread somewhat unevenly over the skin, dimethicone and cyclomethicone leave a thin, even layer wherever you place them. After all that praise, are there any drawbacks to silicone oils? For most skin types they shouldn't pose a problem, and they can have exceptionally desirable effects For the most part, silicone oils evaporate and leave little to no after-feel, but women with oily skin might have problems with the feel of silicone oil on their skin. This doesn't mean someone with oily skin should absolutely avoid products containing silicone oils. What it does mean is that you should be aware of what you are buying. A so-called oil-free product might still contain oil—a silicone oil—and have an oily or slippery feeling, no matter how slight. Dimethicone has properties that make it better for dry skin than oily skin; cyclomethicone and phenyl trimethicone among others, because they evaporate and leave almost no perceptible finish behind, can be better for someone with normal to combination/oily skin.

Above and beyond the claim of being oil-free, label after label promises that the product inside is "noncomedogenic" or "nonacnegenic." Most of us have bought products with this assurance, only to find that they did cause breakouts. A product may truly be oil-free, even free of silicone oil, but there are many, many other ingredients that can aggravate acne. Standard to most cosmetics are wax-like thickening agents that are notorious for clogging pores. The terms "noncomedogenic" and "nonacnegenic" have slowly but surely begun to replace "hypoallergenic" on cosmetics labels. By now, most consumers who tend to break out or have oily skin have had flare-ups with products claiming to be noncomedogenic or nonacnegenic. Those are meaningless marketing words, just like "oil-free."

Empty Hype for Oily Skin

Most of us have sought relief from the emotional pain and humiliation that often accompany acne, whether it be one blemish or many, by going to drugstores or cosmetics counters where acne products and skin care regimes line the shelves. Myriad products promise clear skin, and several pledge to zap zits, dry up blemishes, and drink up oil. The commercials and ads sound fairly convincing, but a closer look reveals that these products can't zap zits or dry up oil, much less stop either from occurring, and the irritation they cause can create more problems than they clear up.

These products claim they are designed for skin that breaks out, offering choices for women with oily, dry, or sensitive skin. But when you read the ingredient list, where the real information is, you find an array of ingredients that can make acne worse and cause problems for sensitive skin. Ingredients that show up repeatedly include alcohol; salicylic acid (a peeling agent); benzoyl peroxide (a disinfectant); sulfur (a mild antiseptic); boric acid (a toxic antiseptic); and camphor, menthol, eucalyptus, and clove oil. All of these are potential skin irritants. Some of these ingredients do make sense. Sulfur and benzoyl peroxide can help to disinfect skin that breaks out, and salicylic acid can peel the skin, which can keep pores from getting clogged. My concern is that almost all of these ingredients are too strong for the face and end up overly irritating the skin, making things even worse than before. There are gentler ways to do the same things. For example, alpha hydroxy acid products can do the same thing as salicylic acid with much less irritation.

But what are alcohol, boric acid, and menthol, camphor, eucalyptus, and clove oil doing in acne products? From everything I've read, they have no positive effect on acne whatsoever. They only irritate and dry the skin, which serves no purpose for any skin type, and they can make oily skin oilier through something called a "rebound effect": irritation stimulates oil production, which makes oily skin worse.

Alcohol is a very irritating and drying ingredient. It is not even a good disinfectant, because the concentration used in skin care products isn't strong enough. Alcohol is something people of every skin type should avoid. Bottom line: If an acne product is working for you, stay with it. If your skin is red and irritated and still oily, and you still have blemishes (as do most people who use these products), reconsider what you are doing.

It is harder to heal oily, acned skin than we would like to believe, but there are steps you can take to calm down acne as well as steps you shouldn't take. But you can't completely eliminate the problem with products from the cosmetics counters or the drugstore—those of us who have acne and have tried everything have come to understand this.

I am reluctant to list ingredients to avoid if you have oily skin. Some of you are using products right now that contain several of these ingredients, and you may feel that your skin is doing just fine. So much for tests, and so much for my opinion. As I said, this is a complicated, tricky area. But if your skin is not doing well or you are experiencing skin irritation and you're wondering what to do about it, you may want to start by eliminating products that contain the questionable ingredients mentioned above.

Sensitive Skin

First of all, let me state plainly that, to one extent or another, we all have sensitive skin. Do not skip this section because you think you have a tough exterior. At some time almost all of us will experience a skin reaction to something. You can prevent some reactions, however, if you are aware of what can cause them.

The best part of the cosmetics world is that many products just feel good on the skin. Silky-smooth creams and lotions glide on, leaving a dewy, moist gloss that can make skin look and feel beautiful and provide a blissful emotional lift as well. The same thing happens with makeup. As you artfully, or even not so artfully, apply an appealing shade of eyeshadow to your lids in a velvety soft tone that sets off the depths of your eyes perfectly, you may feel a surge of self-esteem as you admire the way you look. That's what skin care and makeup should be all about.

Unfortunately, for those of you with even slightly sensitive skin, finding products that enhance but don't irritate is a challenge. I would love to list ingredients that I could guarantee won't cause your skin to react, but there is no single ingredient or combination of ingredients that can live up to that sweeping claim. Because of the almost limitless combinations, in all sorts of mixtures and formulations, it is virtually impossible to know what, when, or how a cosmetic will react on your skin. Your only recourse, and this is not the best news, is to keep experimenting until you find what works for you. If you do get a reaction, stop using the product immediately, consult your physician if the reaction is serious or prolonged, return the products that are suspect, and keep track of the ingredients included in products to which you seem to be allergic. Also, just because you've used a cosmetic for a long time doesn't mean you won't develop an allergic reaction to it.

Although some ingredients tend to be more sensitizing than others, remember that the amount of a specific problem ingredient can determine how a product will affect your skin. The less there is of an ingredient—the farther down in the ingredient list it is—the less likely you are to have a reaction to it. Just because the ingredient is suspect or may have a potential for causing skin sensitivities doesn't mean it will always cause problems. Listen to your skin and be cautious.

It is also important to understand that some potentially irritating ingredients, such as the many preservatives present in cosmetics, are critical to the products' stability, but are not good for skin and are known to cause allergic reactions. But chemists have literally no other option when it comes to preventing microbes from taking up residence in their products. Fragrances are another known source of skin irritations, and while they are frequently used to mask the unpleasant odor of many cosmetics ingredients, more often they are added to increase sales. Apparently many cosmetics consumers want their lotions and creams to exude an obvious bouquet. This isn't the fault of the cosmetics companies, although it does reflect a need for consumer education. If you want perfume, use perfume, but choose skin care products that are fragrance-free.

It is impossible to predict with any accuracy why, where, when, and how a single ingredient or combination of ingredients in a particular product will affect your skin. When you consider the hundreds of chemicals a woman places on her face in such varied products as cleansers, toners, moisturizers, foundations, blushes, lipsticks, eyeshadows, and mascaras, it is surprising to realize how safe and nonirritating cosmetics usually are.

I'm sure that many of you already are aware of this, but it can never be said too often: if you have an allergic reaction of any kind to a cosmetic product, stop using it immediately and consult your physician if the problem persists. Do not hesitate to return the product to the place where you purchased it and get your money back. It is not your fault that the product caused problems. Also, returning the product gives the cosmetics company essential information about how their formulas are working.

Alpha Hydroxy Acids

Surely by now everyone has heard about alpha hydroxy acids (AHAs), the most amazing ingredients of all time. They aren't the most amazing because they can perform miracles on the skin. Rather, what makes them so remarkable is the number of products they have spawned over the past four years. More than any other cosmetic ingredient, alpha hydroxy acids have created an industry unto themselves. Over the past four years, ever since Avon launched Anew, one of the first AHA products, in the latter part of 1992, products containing these exfoliating agents have appeared by the hundreds. What can this small group of acids do? You would think nothing short of a supernatural phenomenon. In reality, AHAs are hardly a phenomenon, but they are an effective exfoliant for many different skin types.

Most of the companies producing these products, and independent sources—including dermatologists, plastic surgeons, and cosmetic chemists—claim that regular AHA use can make skin smoother, diminish wrinkles, and unclog pores. Quite a lot for a group of ingredients derived from such sources as sugarcane and milk or synthesized from a mixture of formaldehyde and monoxide, but more about that later. The bottom line is, do AHAs work? The good news is that many of the AHA products on the market, from drugstore brands to infomercial products to department-store lines, do, to some extent, live up to those basic claims. But once the cosmetics companies fire up their marketing smoke screens, the whole topic gets exaggerated and quite confusing. It's not easy to undo the pretense, but it can be done.

There are five types of AHAs on the market: glycolic, lactic, malic, citric, and tartaric acids. There is also a group of hydroxy acids called beta hydroxy acids (BHAs). When BHAs are used instead of—or in tandem with—AHAs, the BHA is almost always salicylic acid. The most commonly used AHAs are glycolic and lactic acids, because of their special ability to penetrate the skin. All of these are derived from very inexpensive natural sources such as sugarcane, sour milk, citrus fruits, apples, grapes, and wintergreen leaves. AHAs and BHAs have been used in cosmetics for quite some time. What these acids can do is "unglue" (or burn off) the outer layer of dead skin cells and help increase cell turnover (exfoliation). Removing this dead layer can impro___ and color, unclog pores, and allow moisturizers to be better absorbed by ____ ___ ___ difference is that AHAs (and, to a much lesser extent, BHAs) have more in common with Retin-A and Renova (the cream form of Retin-A—tretinoin acid derived from vitamin A) than with cosmetic scrubs, yet they are not a drug, so no prescription is necessary.

AHAs and BHAs work much the way Retin-A does (Retin-A and Renova are discussed later in this chapter), in a chemical rather than a physical process, ungluing the substance that holds skin cells together. That means AHAs and BHAs can possibly produce better results than cosmetic scrubs (which work only on the surface), and they are more readily available than Retin-A or Renova.

Even though AHAs and BHAs work similarly and are most effective at the same concentrations and pH, AHAs also have water-binding properties, so they can be less irritating than BHAs. Additionally, AHAs have a drop-off rate: their ability to exfoliate decreases (which is also true for Retin-A). BHAs, on the other hand, continue to exfoliate at a constant rate. (According to Dr. Walter Smith, an independent and respected authority on cosmetics, writing in the May 1995 issue of *Cosmetics & Toiletries*, salicylic acid keeps the stratum corneum—top layer of skin—in a state of high turnover; AHAs' effect decreases once the stratum corneum has been exfoliated to a certain level.) Constant exfoliation can have a negative impact on the skin by maintaining a permanent level of irritation. And repeated irritation may actually *cause* wrinkles.

To sum it up: Salicylic acid is an effective exfoliant, but it doesn't have a drop-off rate (meaning it doesn't stop exfoliating the skin), as AHAs do. Salicylic acid just keeps exfoliating, which can be too irritating for skin on a regular basis. Also, salicylic acid doesn't have the additional benefit of water-binding properties the way AHAs do. For these reasons, I strongly recommend using products that contain AHAs instead of BHAs.

Many experts, including Dr. Albert Kligman, the inventor of Retin-A, suggest that it is best to use any chemical exfoliant on a consistent basis for about six months to a year and then reduce usage by 50 percent, meaning every other day instead of every day, or once a day but for alternate months, or three months of daily usage and then three months of no usage, and so on.

Meanwhile, cosmetics companies are jumping on the AHA bandwagon with both feet. Some of these products can be purchased from drugstores and cosmetics counters; others are available through aestheticians, physicians, infomercials, and in-home sales. What make this crowded field so troublesome is that so many cosmetics companies supply grossly misleading or completely inane information about their products.

Particularly annoying is the fact that many companies announce proudly that their products contain AHAs or BHAs, but say nothing about (or even refuse to tell consumers) how much AHA or BHA is in the product, even though this basic information is the key to knowing what you are buying and has everything to do with a product's effectiveness and potential for irritation. Chanel's consumer relations department first told me their Day Lifting Refining Complex ($45) contains glycolic acid, but it isn't in the ingredient list; when asked, they said the name of the ingredient and the percentage used are confidential. Of course, the ingredients aren't confidential; they have to be disclosed on the ingredient list. According to that, my best guess is that Chanel's product contains about 3% lactic acid and about 1% or less salicylic acid.

Elizabeth Arden's Ceramide Time Complex Moisture Cream contains HCA (hydroxycaprylic acid), a synthetic form of AHA that does not penetrate the skin the way glycolic or lactic acid can. HCA is good for moisturizing, but not much else. (Arden's Alpha-Ceramide, however, is an excellent, albeit expensive, AHA product.) Sodium lactate, another form of AHAs, is used in many products. The salespeople will tell you it is the same as lactic acid, but it isn't the same at all; it can be a good moisturizing ingredient, but it won't exfoliate the skin. Other AHA sound-alikes include sugarcane extract, mixed fruit acids, and fruit extracts. You may think you've purchased a more natural or better AHA product, but that isn't the case. Without knowing exactly what type of AHAs you are buying, there is no way to know exactly what you are putting on your skin or how effective it really is.

Revlon introduced its Revlon Results with Alpha ReCap at the height of the AHA craze. Surprise: despite its name, Alpha ReCap didn't contain one smidgen of AHA. It did contain a very good water-binding agent, but if you wanted the exfoliation effects of AHAs, you were out of luck. Estee Lauder's Fruition was one of the first department-store lines to launch an AHA product. It was an overnight success, but not because of its AHA content: Fruition contains less than 2% AHA. At that percentage it is little more than a good water-binding agent. That isn't bad; it just isn't what makes AHAs and BHAs such fascinating ingredients.

I could go on listing the comparative contents of the myriad AHA and BHA products, but that is what the product review section of this book is for. What is more to the point for this section is whether there is a difference between all these products and the nature of these differences. The crucial information is the percentage, type, and pH of the AHAs or BHAs used. Dr. Walter Smith, in his summary report on AHA and BHA products and their effectiveness in a paper published in the *Cosmetics and Toiletries Ingredient Resource Series*, suggests that AHAs and BHAs work similarly at percentages of 5% and above and at pH levels of 3 to 5.5. Their effectiveness drops considerably as a product's pH level goes up and the concentration goes down. Once again, he points out that BHAs (salicylic acid) continually exfoliate without a drop-off rate and therefore continually irritate. That is not a problem at a lower pH and reduced concentration, but then effectiveness in exfoliation and skin smoothing is also reduced.

As a general rule, it is best if the AHA ingredient is either second, third, or fourth on the ingredient list. That makes it likely that you are getting a 5% or higher concentration of AHAs at a good pH. Glycolic and lactic acid are the two AHAs with the most research behind them. Tartaric, citric, and malic acids may perform the same way, but there hasn't yet been enough research to make any conclusive statements.

Most important, none of these AHA or BHA product on earth, regardless of concentration, pH, or type, that can prevent aging or change a wrinkle. These products can smooth the skin, improve texture, and unclog pores, but when you stop using them, the skin goes back to the way it was before you started. Some research indicates that AHAs, and possibly BHAs, can increase collagen and elastin, much as Retin-A and Renova can. But the amount of collagen and elastin produced, if any, is not permanent or significant, because it too reverts to previous levels once you stop using these products.

Should You Use AHAs?

A plethora of evidence suggests that AHA products (depending on the percentage, type, and pH level) can work quite well for two categories of skin problems: sun-damaged skin and skin that breaks out. How can AHAs help such disparate skin conditions as dry skin and acne, generally thought to be at opposite ends of the skin continuum? Good question.

Dry skin suffers from "hyper" skin-cell production, which causes cells to stack up on the skin's surface, creating a flaky, dull appearance. Oily, acne-prone skin is aggravated by thick dead skin cells that block the pores and trap the oil inside, causing the pores to become clogged. With increased exfoliation, both dry skin and skin that breaks out can be improved by removing dead skin cells that block absorption of moisturizers (dry skin) or block pores (oily skin).

Depending on your skin type, AHAs can be wonderful. Most experts recommend applying the AHA lotion, cream (for dry skin), or liquid solution (for oily skin) to your face or any other area 15 minutes after cleansing, and then waiting 15 minutes more before applying any other product such as your foundation, sunscreen, or additional moisturizers. Why the 15-minute wait between product application? Because AHAs are acids, and if the other products you are using, such as soap or moisturizers, are slightly alkaline, they can negate the effectiveness of the AHA product. Waiting 15 minutes allows your face to return to its own acid balance, which does not adversely affect the AHAs or BHAs. You can experiment with the waiting period, however, to see what works for you. It is most likely that the other skin care products you use, except for soap, have a pH of 7 or less, which probably will not interfere with AHAs or BHAs.

Depending on your skin type, you can apply an AHA product once or twice a day. Apply the AHA product first, or just after your toner has dried, then apply any other product, such as additional moisturizer, eye cream, sunscreen, and/or foundation. It is not essential to wear a moisturizer over an AHA product. That totally depends on your type of skin and how it reacts to AHAs. If you find the AHA product is slightly drying, you will probably want to wear a moisturizer, but the AHA product may be all you need. (Of course, the cosmetics salespeople will tell you to use the AHA products along with their complete program, including two or three other moisturizers and Lord knows what else.)

Be prepared for the hard sell when it comes to AHA products. Many cosmetics companies treat them like the fountain of youth. Some companies deal in specialty AHA products that contain higher percentages (from 8% to 15%). If your skin can handle these higher percentages, these products may be beneficial. However, higher percentages may also guarantee higher irritation, and there is little research indicating what kind of risk or harm that might pose over time.

Many AHA products designed for oily skin contain alcohol; I do not recommend these because of the risk of increased irritation and sensitization they pose. Oily skin types need to look for AHA products that are irritant-free (meaning no alcohol) and do not come in a moisturizing base. More of these are becoming available, but the pickings are still relatively slim if you're looking for a good, reasonably priced AHA product that won't adversely affect oily skin types. In short, listen to your skin; it will tell you what to do and what other products you need.

As a general rule, you should not use other cosmetic scrubs or a washcloth at the same time you are using an AHA or BHA product. Also, be aware that many cosmetics companies put AHAs and BHAs in everything they make. Remember, the skin can handle only so much irritation; one effective exfoliant is all that is necessary for anyone's skin. Be sure to review the list of cautions in the section on Retin-A and Renova, all of which apply to AHAs as well.

Frequently Asked Questions about AHAs

What does the FDA say about the AHA products?

The majority of AHA products, even the professional-strength versions (except for the prescription-only Lac-Hydrin-5 and Hydrin-12), are currently classified as cosmetics, and that's exactly where the manufacturers would like to keep them. Safety reviews and legal standards are almost nonexistent for cosmetics manufacturers. Safety testing for drugs is vastly more stringent. According to Dr. John Bailey, the FDA's director of colors and cosmetics, his department has an active interest in AHA products. His main concerns are: (1) What are the effects on people with sensitive skin? (2) What are the long-term side effects? (3) What levels of concentration are safe and effective? These are good questions, but it will take some time before we have all the answers.

Are there any side effects? Should I take any precautions?

Most people have a tingling or slight stinging sensation when they use glycolic acid products with concentrations of 5% or greater. Some people have had minor to severe problems with dryness and flaking when using glycolic acid products. This is to be expected, given the nature of the AHA ingredient. Most of the products tell you not to use them on your eyelids. Listen to your skin: if it gets dry and flaky, consider using a moisturizer; if it gets red and irritated, use the AHA product less frequently; if it gets very dry and irritated, consider stopping altogether. Severe irritation is not the goal or the desired result. And, as you probably already know, wearing a sunscreen of at least SPF 15 during the day for protection from sun damage is best no matter what else you use on your face.

What about the data indicating that some products that claim an 8% concentration of AHAs really contain just an 8% concentration of a 70% solution of AHAs?

The issue of concentration is one of the trickiest parts of the AHA equation, because there are no unified regulations. In their undiluted form, AHAs are crystallized and therefore hard for a cosmetics formulator to use. Most cosmetic chemists use a 70% solution of AHAs, which means 70% pure AHAs to 30% water (and other trace ingredients). Most companies that quote a percentage are referring to concentration from a 70% solution, not a 100% one. Thus, most, if not all, 8% AHA products actually contain a 5.6% concentration (8% of 70% is 5.6%). Is that misleading? Should we be looking for an 8% concentration from a 100% solution? Probably not (and in any case, the cosmetics companies don't have to tell us what kind of raw material they are using, which means there is no way to know for sure). A 70% solution of AHAs is fairly standard in the cosmetics industry.

Which type of AHA product is best: lotion, gel, cream, or liquid?

That depends on what you want it to do and the ingredients in the specific product. Gels and liquids that contain alcohol can irritate the skin and cause more problems. (Alcohol can allowing deeper penetration of the AHAs, which could be good for a stronger initial impact, but also increases the possibility of many more unwanted side effects.) They should be avoided at all costs for all skin types. Gels and liquids that contain no other irritants besides the AHAs are best for someone with normal to oily skin. Creams and lotions slow down absorption of the AHAs, but they also cushion the skin and protect it from possible irritation. Creams and lotions can be best for someone with dry skin; however, applying a separate liquid AHA product and then a moisturizer allows some flexibility. For example, you could alternate the AHA product with your moisturizer—using each one every other night, say.

What about the long-term effects of these products and the notion of skin fatigue?

There isn't much information about the long term use of AHAs or BHAs. We've been told that within a few months AHAs stop working the way they did when they were first used. Is that good or bad? AHAs exfoliate the top layer of skin that has thickened because of sun damage or simply because some people produce more top layers of skin than others. Once that top layer has been exfoliated, AHAs no longer have the same effect (again, this is not true for BHAs). If AHAs continued to have the same effect, there is a potential for skin fatigue. Skin fatigue is where the exfoliated skin grows back immediately, becoming thick again, even if you continued using the product, almost like building a callous. But that doesn't seem to happen with AHAs. It appears they have no other affect on any other skin layer. If you stop using AHAs, the skin reverts to its original state, but slowly, over a period of time. Using AHAs regularly for a while and then alternating applications appears to be the key to keeping things smooth and exfoliated.

Skin Peels

Aestheticians, dermatologists, and plastic surgeons from coast to coast are pouncing on the latest trend in "anti-aging" skin care: salon-administered deep-peeling glycolic acid treatments for the face. Cosmetic peels generally consist of a series of exfoliating masks in concentrations of 15% all the way up to 70% glycolic acid. A typical salon series usually uses a 15% to 30% concentration of glycolic acid and may require the client to visit the salon once a week for six consecutive weeks; the mask procedure itself takes from one to two hours. Dermatologists and plastic surgeons often perform higher-concentration peels using between 30% and 70% glycolic acid, in one-time visits that can be repeated as you and the doctor see fit. The skin initially reddens, as with a sunburn, then darkens, and finally peels away, revealing what manufacturers claim is a "new skin." The boast is that deep acid peeling "attacks only the top few layers of skin" and works cumulatively to "improve texture and reduce wrinkles and blotchiness." Prices for the salon treatment can range from $180 to $400 for six applications; a physician's series of six treatments can range from $600 to $900.

For the most part, women who have had peels are thrilled with the results. Their faces look smoother and feel softer almost instantaneously—after the redness and flaking subside. Have any wrinkles been erased? No, not a one. The exfoliation smooths the skin, and the irritation plumps out wrinkles. But after a few months (or sometimes after only one month), the skin is back to the way it was.

For the most part, the FDA is not at all happy with the safety aspect of salon glycolic acid peels. The agency has fielded reports of skin burns, scarring, and hospitalization due to salon and mail-order skin peelers, and has issued a warning to consumers about these hazards. "We are warning consumers about the use of skin peelers because they can cause serious injuries, particularly when used without the supervision of a physician," FDA commissioner Dr. David A. Kessler has said. Glycolic acid peels are a concern of cosmetics watchdogs these days.

Do you need these expensive glycolic acid peels? Not really, although the praises sung by women who have had them make that statement hard to believe. Glycolic acid peels definitely have positive results for most women. However, the concern is not immediate benefits but long-term results. Women who have these peels done monthly (as opposed to once or twice a year) face a distinct possibility that the repeated intense irritation can damage skin and produce wrinkles. Moreover, many experts say that regular, twice-daily use of AHA products (particularly those containing glycolic acid) with concentrations of 8% to 15% produce the same results without the risk of severe irritation.

By the way, glycolic acid peels are not to be confused with medically performed face peels that use use such chemicals as phenol or trichloracetic acid and put you out of the public eye for at least four to seven days and sometimes up to a month. With the glycolic acid peels, some people have no problem at all, while others might experience varying amounts of flaking and peeling.

What about the AHA and BHA products doctors and plastic surgeons are selling these days? Skin care products sold by doctors are not any more medically based or reliable than any other cosmetics line available through drugstores, cosmetics counters, or infomercials. The problem is that most consumers feel that the products sold by their dermatologist or plastic surgeon are nothing short of a prescription mandate.

As I have said before, I consider it a major problem that so many plastic surgeons and dermatologists are getting into the cosmetics business. For example, a dermatologist should say to you, "I recommend that you use a gentle, nonalkaline, water-soluble cleanser twice a day. I sell one here that is very good, but there are others on the market. It is your choice. These are not prescription items, these are cosmetics, and they are regulated in that manner." But what seems to be happening more and more often is that doctors are selling their products by playing on their patients' belief that they are somehow better than typical cosmetics products or that they are medically necessary. That is simply not the case. I'm not saying these products are bad, but they definitely aren't any better than other skin care products found at drugstores or department stores, and they're usually much more expensive.

Retin-A and Renova

Most of you probably recall the hoopla that erupted regarding Johnson & Johnson's little-known acne drug Retin-A (tretinoin acid in a gel or a matte cream base) when, back in 1987, a study released to the media seemed to show that acne was not the only thing this prescription drug could tackle. Rather dramatic before-and-after pictures seemed to indicate scientists had finally found the fountain of youth. All forms of the media had a field day with this one. Every news channel, talk show, newspaper, and fashion magazine featured pictures from the study and interviews with Dr. John Voorhees, the doctor who performed the study, and Dr. Albert Kligman, the inventor of Retin-A.

If this kind of media blitz had been in the form of advertising, it would have been illegal, because prescription drugs can't be advertised without a vast range of restrictions and constraints. Drugs of any kind are tightly controlled by the FDA, with strict guidelines as to what the manufacturer can and cannot say about the product. (At that time, Retin-A was approved for use as an acne medication only. If an individual doctor wanted to let a patient use it for wrinkles, that was fine, but it was not sanctioned by the FDA, and the company could make no claims to the contrary.) A free publicity event was another story altogether.

All that media coverage helped sales of Retin-A soar into the millions, which didn't hurt Johnson & Johnson's stock price either. What was the bottom line after the dust settled and all the prescriptions were filled? It turned out that the study that generated all the publicity was paid for by Johnson & Johnson, the study was too small to be significant, and many women who used Retin-A were not necessarily enthralled with the results, at least not when it came to a change in their wrinkles.

Now it is almost ten years later, and in that time Johnson & Johnson has labored long and hard to produce studies that would convince the FDA that Retin-A should be approved for use as a wrinkle cream. Convince them they did: the FDA has approved a version of Retin-A called Renova (which is simply Retin-A, tretinoin acid, in an emollient base) for use as a wrinkle cream. That makes Renova the first medicine ever approved by the FDA for the treatment of sun-damaged skin, meaning wrinkles.

Should you run right out for your new prescription? Well, the press release I received from the FDA wasn't all that thrilling. Only a small percentage of users, about 16 percent in one study and less than that in another, were pleased with their results. More than two-thirds thought the results were either mediocre or nonexistent. Regardless, while using either Retin-A or Renova can have a positive effect by changing how skin cells are formed and shed and by making skin feel smoother, both products are useless when it comes to preventing wrinkles if women do not wear a sunscreen as well. Not a wrinkle cream in the world, even the one approved by the FDA, can have lasting results if you don't use a sunscreen.

Incidentally, Renova isn't cheap; it costs about $60 for a 40-gram tube (a two-month supply), and that doesn't include the cost of a visit to your doctor. The big question is, Are AHA and BHA products a replacement for Retin-A or Renova? It depends on who you talk to. Some "experts" recommend using AHA products *and* Retin-A or Renova, while others say AHA products can be used totally alone instead of Retin-A or Renova. They do work in a similar fashion (both are acids that unglue dead skin cells and encourage new cell growth), and both can help sun-damaged skin as well as skin that breaks out, by exfoliating the skin. Some say the major difference is simply that one is a relatively expensive prescription drug and the other is a cosmetic available over the counter. But others say that Retin-A and Renova do effect a change in the structure of the skin. There is evidence that Retin-A and Renova can help the skin to produce collagen. Many dermatologists and plastic surgeons are prescribing Retin-A or Renova for use in the evenings and AHAs or BHAs during the day. Of course, it is hard to say to what degree that recommendation may be inspired by financial gain, because many of the doctors making this recommendation sell skin care products that contain AHAs and BHAs.

What is true with Retin-A, Renova, AHAs, and BHAs is that once you stop using them, your skin will revert to the way it was before. No permanent change is produced or generated from using any of these products. The smooth exterior lasts only as long as you use them. This is one of the major reasons that researchers don't believe AHAs, BHAs, Retin-A, or Renova change the deeper layer of the skin. If they did create more collagen and elastin in the skin, the effects wouldn't be quite so temporary.

If you do choose to get a prescription for Retin-A or Renova (or if you cross the border into Mexico to get it over the counter), it is important to be careful when using them and/or AHA and BHA products. Review and remember the following list of cautions.

1.   It is dangerous to tan after you start using Retin-A, Renova, or an AHA or BHA product that contains a 5% or greater concentration. As the skin peels and becomes somewhat thinner, it becomes more sensitive to sunlight and is therefore more subject to serious sunburn. Also, tanning will negate any positive effects you hope to gain from using these exfoliators. If you are using any of these products, it is essential to wear a sunscreen whenever you venture outside and to keep your sun exposure to a minimum.

2.   Retin-A, Renova, and AHA and BHA products can irritate the skin. If you use any other irritant on the skin at the same time, you will exacerbate the initial negative side effects of the product. You must eliminate all of the following from your skin care routine during your first months of using these products (it's probably best for your skin to *always* avoid these, by the way): washcloths; hot water; cold water; all astringents, toners, fresheners, clarifying lotions, refining lotions, and the like that contain irritants; scrubs; clay facial masks; bar soaps; skin care products that contain fragrances or strong preservatives; saunas; and steam rooms (used on a regular basis, saunas and steam rooms can cause spider veins on the face).

3.   If you want Retin-A, Renova, or AHA or BHA products to work, you must use them regularly. To sustain the results, you must continue using them for the rest of your life. The changes that take place on the skin are not permanent. Once you stop using the product, the skin slowly reverts to its original condition. Using something forever is a tremendous commitment. But according to the majority of women I've interviewed and who have written to me, the difference is positive enough to warrant a long-term relationship.

4.   If you want to use Retin-A or Renova with an AHA or BHA product, most doctors recommend using AHAs during the day, under a sunscreen, and Retin-A or Renova at night, under a moisturizer if you need one.

Mad Dogs and Englishmen Go Out in the Midday Sun

The cosmetics playing field is getting more and more crowded with sunscreens of all kinds, so let's go over the basics, review new research, and look at which products are good or bad for your skin type. Perhaps the most confounding aspect is that because the competition for consumers' dollars has grown more intense, sunscreens now claim to do more than just protect the skin from UV radiation. Today's sunscreens contain everything from antioxidants to alpha hydroxy acids to plants and vegetables. And what about nonchemical sunscreens versus inorganic sunscreens (that is, titanium dioxide–based sunblocks versus synthetic-ingredient sunscreen agents). How do you choose? That's a very good question.

First of all, it *is* possible, at least theoretically, for a sunscreen to contain AHAs. In the second edition of this book, I indicated that it was not possible; I had misunderstood some conflicting information but was corrected in my correspondence with Chanel (printed in the March 1996 issue of my newsletter, *Cosmetics Counter Update*). (I had assumed that sunscreens weren't compatible with AHAs because of the difference in the two components' effective pH levels.) In any case, only a limited number of products on the market today contain both AHAs or BHAs and sunscreen, and I have yet to see one with a high enough concentration of AHAs or BHAs to be an effective exfoliant. Few, if any, higher-percentage AHA or BHA products (over 5%) incorporate sunscreen, especially not at SPF 15. Additionally, according to cosmetic chemists at Neoteric, Chesebrough-Pond's, M.D. Formulations, GlyDerm, and elsewhere, sunscreens and AHAs or BHAs are not happy together in the same product. Sunscreens' solubility at lower pHs makes these two important skin care ingredients a difficult combination.

Sunscreen ingredients can be irritating no matter what the product's label says. The way these ingredients work can cause a reaction on the skin. Experiment to find the one that works best for your skin type. For instance, although nonchemical sunscreens use titanium dioxide, which is considered completely nonirritating, as the active ingredient, this substance can clog pores and aggravate breakouts and acne.

How long do sunscreens last? Should you throw them away after a year or two if you haven't used them up? The FDA considers sunscreens to be over-the-counter (OTC) drugs, meaning they are subject to much more stringent guidelines and regulations than cosmetics. According to the FDA's OTC regulations, sunscreens should be stamped with an expiration date. From the time a sunscreen is packaged it has about a two-year period of efficacy. Unfortunately, the cosmetics industry is sort of loosey-goosey with this one, and not all products have expiration dates on their labels. That's a risk for the consumer, because there is no telling how long that product has been sitting around the warehouse or on the shelf. Look for, and ask for, sunscreens with expiration dates whenever possible, and avoid sunscreens that don't have them.

Broad-spectrum protection is considered paramount these days. Most sunscreens are rated according to how long they allow you to stay in the sun without burning, and they also help prevent tanning, which wards off leathery-looking, sun-damaged skin. However, many studies over the past ten years show that skin cancer has not declined despite the increased use of sunscreens. We now know that sunscreen ingredients protect mostly against UVB rays, which burn the skin, and only minimally against UVA rays, which are responsible for cells mutating and can cause cancer. Ironically, because they keep burning to a minimum, sunscreens have given people the ability to stay in the sun longer. But that means people are exposed for longer periods to the kind of cancer-causing rays that it's hard to protect against. One of the best broad-spectrum sunscreens, admittedly a controversial one, is **Shade UVAGuard with Parsol 1789** *($7.89 for 4 ounces)*. Parsol 1789 is one of the few sunscreen agents that protect almost equally against UVA and UVB rays. There is some evidence that Parsol 1789 can be a skin irritant, but, according to recent findings, no more so than many other sunscreen agents. This issue is still under deep scrutiny by the FDA, and exactly how to determine and evaluate what is broad-spectrum sun protection is still somewhat up in the air. To be certain, it is probably best, at least for long-term sun exposure, to use a product like Shade UVAGuard or a physical sunblock such as those with titanium dioxide (these are often called "nonchemical," but titanium dioxide is definitely a chemical). There are many of the latter on the market, including **Neutrogena Chemical-Free Sunblocker, SPF 17** *($9.73 for 4 ounces)*, **Physicians Formula Sun Shield Chemical Free Sunscreen Cream SPF 15 Sensitive Skin Formula** *($7.19 for 2 ounces)*, and **Physicians Formula Sun Shield Sensitive Skin Formula SPF 25 Chemical Free Sunscreen** *($8.50 for 4 ounces)*. For daily use you will probably be just fine with most of the sunscreens on the market.

As many of you already know, wearing a foundation with a high SPF is an excellent idea, particularly for women with oily skin who don't want to wear any more layers of skin care products than they absolutely have to. The one negative thing about using a foundation that contains sunscreen is that you might forget that you also need to use a sunscreen on your hands, neck, throat, chest, and any other area of your body that is exposed to the sun on a daily basis. Those brown "age spots" are really sun-damage spots. Like wrinkles, they can't be prevented or stopped without daily use of sunscreen, and that means reapplying your sunscreen every time you wash your hands. My favorite foundations with sunscreen are **Clinique Sensitive Skin Foundation with SPF 15** *($18.50)*, **Clinique Almost Makeup with Nonchemical SPF 15** *($18.50)*, **Estee Lauder Enlighten Skin-Enhancing Makeup with SPF 10** *($27.50)*, **Lancome Maqui Libre SPF 15** *($30)*, **Maybelline Natural Defense Makeup with SPF 15 Nonchemical Sunscreen** *($5.26)*, **Physicians Formula Sun Shield with Nonchemical SPF 15** *($4.28)*,

Physicians Formula Le Velvet Powder Finish SPF 15 *($4.28)*, a cream-to-powder makeup, and **Prescriptives 100% Oil-Free Liquid Foundation SPF 15** *($28.50)*.

By the way, my favorite sunscreens for oily skin are still **Lancome Body Protective Spray with SPF 15** *($21 for 4.2 ounces)*, **Origins Silent Treatment Nonchemical SPF 15** *($15 for 1.7 ounces)*, **Almay Oil Control Lotion, Step 3, with SPF 15** *($7.27 for 4 ounces)*, **and Clinique Zero-Alcohol Sun Block with SPF 25** *($15 for 4 ounces)*.

Of course, there is little difference between expensive and inexpensive sunscreens (except the price tag). However, if using an expensive sunscreen means you are not slathering it on before spending long periods of time in the sun, you might not be getting enough protection. It isn't a problem to use it less generously when running errands or going to and from the office, but it must be liberally applied when you will be spending the day outside. And speaking of slathering, *it is essential to apply sunscreen at least 20 minutes before you go outside.*

By the way, I've modified my original position on whether SPF 8 to SPF 12 is OK for minimal daily sun exposure. If you are only going from your car to the office and then to the store, and then driving in your car pool, you will probably be just fine in terms of sun protection. Nevertheless, I still strongly recommend using SPF 15 on a daily basis, because you never know how much sun you're really going to get on any given day.

Sun Basics

1.   **SPF 15 is the best bottom-line protection for most skin types.** Lesser numbers are fine for minimal exposrue, but because you never know how much sun you will be getting, I still feel strongly, as does the Skin Cancer Foundation and the American Academy of Dermatology that anything less the SPF 15 is cheating yourself and your skin.

2.   **When it comes to sunscreens, price is meaningless.** Expensive and inexpensive SPF 15 products all work the same.

3.   **There is no such thing as a healthy tan.** Tanning causes wrinkles and may lead to skin cancer.

4.   **Burning is bad for the skin, but so is tanning.** Avoiding a sunburn but still getting a tan does not prevent wrinkles.

5.   **Most sunscreens protect against UVB rays, which cause the skin to burn, and are less effective against UVA rays, which cause cancer.** Long exposure to sun is a risk to the health of your skin.

6.   Most sun damage (especially for Caucasians) occurs within the first 10 to 20 minutes of exposure. That means your skin is vulnerable when you walk to your car or from your car to wherever you are going. **Apply sunscreen at least 20 minutes before you go outside,** and don't forget your hands, neck, legs, and chest if they are exposed to the sun.

7.   Sunscreens that contain titanium dioxide (often erroneously labeled as nonchemical) are a great way to protect skin from the sun. Because titanium dioxide works as a block (instead of absorbing the sun's rays, as other sunscreen ingredients do), it protects the skin nicely from sun damage. Unfortunately, titanium dioxide can cause breakouts in acne-prone individuals and often leaves a whitish layer on the skin.

8.   **If you have oily skin and need a sunscreen, experiment until you find one that doesn't make your skin more oily or cause it to break out.**

9.   **Almost all SPF products can be used all over, from head to toe.** Some cosmetics companies complicate matters by making separate sunscreen products for the eyes, face, and body—sometimes all with the same SPF number. That is totally unnecessary and a waste of money.

10. **All self-tanning creams contain the same ingredient: dihydroxyacetone (DHA).** Regardless of the price tag, they all work the same way.

11. **Avoid self-tanning creams with sunscreen.** You should wear sunscreen every day, and if you are spending concentrated time outdoors either playing, exercising, or swimming, you need to reapply it frequently. If you apply self-tanning cream too often, it can make your skin look blotchy and streaky and will discolor your fingernails.

12. **Tanning beds (beaches-in-a-box) are just as lethal as the sun, if not more so.** Concentrated UVA rays can damage skin in less time than direct exposure to the sun can. The very skin types that want to be tan year-round are usually the ones that can least afford the damage.

13. **Ultraviolet radiation is present all year long.** Wearing sunscreen every day, as you would wear a moisturizer, is the only way to adequately stop the sun from damaging your skin. It doesn't help to think, "I'm not in the sun that much, I don't have to worry." Damage begins in the first 10 to 30 minutes of exposure.

14. **Regardless of the price or promises, all SPF-rated products are created equal as long as the SPF numbers are the same.** There is positively no difference between

an expensive sunscreen with an SPF of 15 and an inexpensive sunscreen with an SPF of 15.

15.   **There is no reason to use a sunscreen with an SPF greater than 20, because there just isn't enough daylight to warrant a larger number.** Remember, a larger number doesn't mean greater protection, it only means *longer* protection. If there aren't that many hours of sunlight in a day, the protection is wasted. The higher number also means the product contains a greater amount of sunscreen chemicals, with a stronger likelihood of an allergic reaction or at least a more sticky-feeling product.

Self-Tanners

Remember the long-running Clairol hair dye ads that asked, "Does she or doesn't she?" Somebody ought to revive that catchy campaign and use it for the very successful new self-tanning products now on the market.

Gone are the horrible old days of ManTan, the early self-tanner that left you looking as if you'd eaten too many carrots. The technology is much improved these days—good news for all of us who haven't quite been able to give up wanting a tan. Once you get the hang of using a self-tanner, people will be wondering if your lovely, natural-looking tan is real or fake. Well, maybe not.

The new self-tanners provide a way to look tan without suffering any of the discomforts and negative effects of prolonged exposure to the sun. And self-tans are temporary; they disappear gradually and imperceptibly in a few days, and you're back to your own natural color—with no permanent changes to your skin.

The difference between an artificial tan and a real tan is simply explained. A real tan is dangerous; it is a sign that your skin has actually been "burned" and has reacted by producing melanin—brown pigments that are created as a molecular response to the penetration of harmful rays into the middle and lower layers of your epidermis. The skin produces melanin and sends it to its outermost layer as a "brown" protective cover to protect the inner layers from additional burning.

An artificial tan is quite different. Self-tanners contain a tanning agent called dihydroxyacetone. DHA is considered safe by dermatologists and the FDA; indeed, it is not even categorized as a color additive and therefore is not required to undergo testing for toxicity. A very few people have reported skin rashes from DHA, but in general DHA products are nonirritating to almost all skin types. DHA does have a distinctive sweet odor, which you may not like. Some companies scent their DHA products to try to disguise the smell, but in any case the odor dissipates quickly and shouldn't bother you after a few minutes.

DHA is a colorless powder that comes mixed into a cream, a lotion, a gel, or a spray—usually at about 2% to 5% of the total formulation. Only a little DHA is needed to produce a tan, which is why it is generally among the last ingredients on a product label.

When the self-tanner is smoothed onto the skin, the DHA interacts chemically with the protein amino acids in the outer layer of the skin to form a new chemical compound, a sort of "dye," that is orangy brown. This is your artificial, temporary tan. Think of it as similar to a temporary color rinse for your hair. The keratin protein in your hair (like the protein molecules in your skin) "grabs" the color, and for a time your hair is that new color. But as you continue washing your hair, the temporary color washes out and your hair returns to its normal shade.

DHA interacts only on the epidermis, the scaly outer layer of your skin. DHA does not penetrate into the lower layers of the epidermis and does not cause or affect the creation of melanin. And because your body is constantly sloughing off that outer layer, which is actually "dead" skin anyway, a DHA-created tan is very temporary. Your natural sloughing gets rid of it as you bathe and walk around "shedding" skin naturally.

The color of the tan you achieve depends on the proportion of DHA to "carrying" solution in the self-tanner, your complexion color, and your application skill.

All self-tanners suggest that you exfoliate your skin before use; this serves to smooth out dry, rough patches and facilitates an even application of the cream. The stuff is tricky to use. Go easy on ankles and elbows; their thickened texture absorbs more DHA, which can cause staining and streaking. Protect fair eyebrows with a coating of petroleum jelly—otherwise they may turn orange.

The best time to use a self-tanner is right after bathing, when your skin is still slightly damp—the cream will go on more easily and evenly. Shave first, exfoliate everywhere—a dry loofah works well—and use a nail brush to really scrub under fingernails and cuticles when you're finished applying the product. Apply it in very thin coats—like nail polish. A dime-sized dollop will cover your whole face. You get more even and controllable color by using less of the product at a time. You will see color in two or three hours. Apply more self-tanner the next day, and your artificial tan will be a gradual, "natural" acquisition.

Most product packages warn that the product takes 30 minutes to dry, and that you should avoid any contact with clothes during this wait. Actually, if you apply the self-tanner in an appropriately thin coat, it shouldn't take more than about 15 minutes to be absorbed. If your skin still feels sticky after half an hour, you're using too much. Next time, apply it more sparingly.

Remember to wash your hands carefully after each application; self-tanners will stain your cuticles and nails very easily. Also be aware that fabrics "tan" just as people do, because fabrics, including synthetics, contain amino acids that combine with the DHA to produce color. The tan on your clothing or bedsheets will *probably* wash out, but why take a chance? Just flap around naked for 15 minutes, and you should be fine.

That said, I give up when it comes to self-tanners. Maybe practice makes perfect, but I've had blotchy brown ankles, orange-striped legs, and dirty-looking knees, elbows, and hands too many times. Even when I have been ever so careful to exfoliate and apply self-tanner evenly and sparingly, the result is still poor. It may look good at first, but after a couple of showers or after shaving, rather than looking sun-kissed I look as if I'm suffering from a rare skin disease.

Is all this hassle really worth it? I think not. Spending so much time, energy, and money on looking tan suggests that being tan is a necessary part of being attractive, which is absolutely not true. Sure, self-tanning is a safe alternative to sunbathing, but why promote this attitude?

Using a self-tanner with an SPF, such as Physicians Formula Sunless Tanning Cream SPF 20 or Revlon's Self-Tanner for Face SPF 6, confuses two issues. Self-tans offer no protection during sun exposure; they are not "chemically" a real tan. Nor will you tan faster while you have on a self-tanner. Indeed, you may not see a burn building, and you could burn badly. It's much safer to use self-tanners indoors, out of the sun, and more convenient to apply a sunless tan product at night, when you have time to let it dry. Then use a sunscreen during the day to protect your skin. You can't kill two birds with this one stone.

How to Complement a Self-Tan

If by some good fortune you end up with a good artificial tan, consider supplementing it with a slightly "tanner" foundation, a bronzing blush, or a tinted moisturizer.

Best option: Choose a foundation color that matches your newly acquired tan or is a hint darker. Risky option: Bronzers often contain so much mica and iron oxides (shine) that you end up looking like a Las Vegas chorine. Bronzing blushes can look too shiny, too orange (orange is a poor blush color for practically everyone., or too brown, making your face the wrong color or too pale, even with a tan. Possible option: Tinted moisturizers are OK, but the selection is generally too small to accommodate a wide range of skin colors. They go on sheerer than foundation, so they aren't a bad idea, but if you use a tinted moisturizer as your foundation and moisturizer all in one, get one that is SPF 15.

Tan Accelerators

Tan accelerators purport to help speed up the skin's natural production of melanin, the compound formed naturally during the skin's exposure to sun. Whether or not they are safe is unclear.

The FDA has sent warning letters to several companies about the claims being made for tan accelerators. These companies are seeking to comply with the FDA's complaints by rewording the package promises.

Bottom line: Don't use tan accelerators. They are designed to help your skin tan in the sun, and that is the wrong thing to be doing. Spend your money on a sunscreen, and get a life without a tan. It's healthier and safer that way.

Free-Radical Damage and Antioxidants

Many women nowadays are fairly certain that free-radical damage is bad for the skin, and they are right. It is bad for the skin. It is also well known that oxygen and UV rays (not pollution and smog, as you may have heard from cosmetics salespeople) are the main catalysts of free-radical damage. Theoretically, free-radical damage can cause deterioration of the skin's support structures, decreasing elasticity and resilience. What may, and I emphasize the word *may*, have a part in slowing down free-radical damage is the presence of antioxidants in both the diet and skin care products. Antioxidants are ingredients such as vitamins A, C, and E; superoxide dismutase; bioflavonoids; beta carotene, glutathione; selenium; and zinc. Although, technically there are thousands (yes, thousands) of viable antioxidant compounds in the plant world. Despite the proliferation of skin care products containing antioxidants, according to many researchers, including Dr. Jeffrey Blumberg, Chief of Antioxidants Research at Tufts University, "there is no conclusive scientific evidence that antioxidants really prevent wrinkles, nor is there any information about how much antioxidant(s) or exactly which one(s) has to be present in a product to have an effect," if any noticeable effect is even possible. Agreeing with Dr. Blumberg are such skin care experts as Retin-A inventor Dr. Albert Kligman, from the University of Pennsylvania, and Dr. Jim Bollinger, from Galderma Laboratories, who both have stated emphatically that "everything we know about antioxidants is theoretical, and there is no proof they can do anything to stop wrinkling."

Despite this lack of hard evidence, fashion magazines have heralded the elimination of free-radical damage as the fountain of youth for the '90s. The excitement around antioxidants is understandable. According to many skin experts (both legitimate experts and those endorsing specific products), all aspects of aging, including wrinkling, are caused by free-radical damage. Vitamin companies and cosmetics companies alike use the term antioxidants and want you to believe their products can eliminate it. The evidence is fairly convincing that free-radical damage is an insidious "natural" process that causes the body to break down. What isn't known is whether you can really stop free-radical damage inside and outside of a human being from taking place.

Explaining free-radical damage is like trying to explain how television works. No matter how many times I'm told how transmission and reception happen, all I know is that I can watch television whenever I turn on the set, and nothing else makes sense. Nevertheless, here's a simplified explanation of free-radical damage.

Free-radical damage has to do with oxygen and ultraviolet radiation. Oxygen molecules are generally stable, but when they become unstable, due primarily to the presence of ultraviolet radiation and other unspecified molecules, the unstable oxygen molecules grab other molecules as a way to become stabilized. What happens then is that those other molecules also become unstable and grab more molecules to become stabilized. This chain reaction can go on indefinitely and there seems to be primarily one way to stop it, but I'll get to that in a minute.

A good, but extremely simplified, example of how free-radical damage takes place involves paint. When paint is shut off from air (oxygen) in a sealed container, it remains liquid. When it is exposed to air, however, it hardens. What takes place is that an unstable oxygen molecule gets into the exposed paint and interacts with specific parts of the paint's molecules, changing their form. The paint molecules become unstable, creating free radicals, which in turn grab all the other molecules, resulting in solid paint. Actually, referring to this process as damaging can be misleading. Free-radical damage is a major life function, in plants as well as for the human body. Immune systems, metabolism, cells communicating with each other, and collagen production are all affected both positively and negatively by the presence of free-radical damage.

So what does that have to do with aging? When the free-radical reaction continues unrestrained, it can cause systems to break down. Instead of building collagen or other components of skin, free-radical damage destroys it, and it has a similarly bad effect on all other aspects of human physiology. How can you control free-radical damage so you get only the good results and none of the bad? The answer to that question will make someone a very wealthy individual, but in the meantime it just means women are wasting their money in hopes that there really is an antioxidant fountain of youth.

What is thought to stop free-radical damage from going too far is the presence of free-radical scavengers. As silly as that sounds, they really do exist, and they stop, or, a better term, "eat" free radicals. These scavengers are better known as antioxidants.

Antioxidants keep air (specifically, unstable oxygen molecules) from interacting with other molecules and causing them to degenerate. The only problem with this theory is that free-radical damage is constant and extensive. How could you ever use enough antioxidants to stop it, and how much oxygen or sunlight can you really keep away from all skin cells, or even some skin cells? In relation to the skin, free-radical damage from sun exposure is a life long process that starts from birth and continues into old age. Targeting the problem for the short term is pointless, this is ongoing, and the world of skin care makes it sound like antioxidants are a quick fix and not in any way shape or form is that possible.

Major investigation is indeed being done in this fascinating area of human aging that most unquestionably influences wrinkling. Even though a lot of respected researchers are working on this kind of research, to suggest that the research is anything but in its infancy, is sheer fantasy. For now, in relation to your present skin care routine, check the back of your moisturizer and see if it contains any free-radical scavengers such as the ones I mentioned above and make sure they are in closer to the top of the ingredient list and not the end. Almost every company makes moisturizers that contain antioxidants, so they aren't hard to find. You won't see any difference in your skin, but if free-radical damage, and thus the destruction of the skin's structure, can be slowed, the antioxidants should help. It's a long shot, but many scientists think if there is a fountain of youth, this could be it. As Dr. Blumberg pointed out most eloquently, "just because it is in nature doesn't mean it's good for the skin," and "cosmetics companies are not known for doing the work it takes to prove anything, more or less a products reliability or efficacy." For now, it's all theoretical, no one can give you any definitive amounts or specific ingredients to look for despite the cosmetics industry's attempt to do so.

Hydrogen Peroxide

Now if this isn't crazy, I don't know what it is. Many cosmetics products contain antioxidants, ingredients that keep oxygen off the face, yet these same products also contain hydrogen peroxide (H_2O_3), which releases an extra oxygen molecule when it comes into contact with skin. It seems natural to wonder, If the antioxidants work, won't they "scavenge" up the free-radical oxygen from the hydrogen peroxide? The answer is that, even if it were possible, the amount of oxygen trapped inside cosmetics isn't enough to blow out a candle.

Why the concern about supplying oxygen to the skin? Oxygen depletion is one of the things that happens to all older skin, regardless of whether the skin is affected by sun damage or any other health issue. Yet, to point to oxygen as the way to prevent skin from aging is so much nonsense it is almost laughable. How the skin ages is very complicated and extremely interdependent. There isn't any one cause that can be addressed with a cosmetic to erase or minimize the inevitable. Skin ages in more than 50 known ways, so adding some oxygen solves, at best, only one-fiftieth of the problem—not enough to make a difference, even if it could make a difference. Besides, if extra oxygen were the answer, we would all simply live in oxygen tents, and no one would wrinkle. But it isn't just oxygen depletion, free-radical damage, collagen depletion, reduced cell turnover, abnormal cell formation, decreased fat content, or on and on, that affects the way skin ages—it is all of these things combined. What we know for sure is that the sun is the biggest culprit in causing the wrinkles associated with aging, and that using a good sunscreen can really make a difference in how our skin looks as we age.

You may be interested to know that my recommendation of 3% hydrogen peroxide as a disinfectant for acne does not increase free-radical damage or increase the oxygen content of the skin. The release of the oxygen molecule is not penetrating or lasting; it has no more impact on the skin than does the air around us. Whatever slight—I repeat, *slight*—negative impact the 3% hydrogen peroxide might have on the skin is outweighed by the positive effects of its ability to disinfect and reduce blemishes. (Be forewarned, however, that hydrogen peroxide lightens hair, so avoid contact with your eyebrows and hairline.)

Enzymes

Whether in the form of a papaya or in a substance such as papain (a proteinase in unripe papaya that's used in medicine), enzymes have been around for quite some time and are nothing more than exfoliants—not as good as AHAs, but exfoliants nonetheless. The new enzymes being put in skin care potions are supposed to stimulate your skin's own biological processes that have slowed down because of age or sun damage.

Enzymes are proteins that function as biological catalysts. They accelerate chemical reactions in a cell that would proceed minimally or not at all if they weren't there. Most enzymes, and a lot of different enzymes affect skin cells, are rather finicky about how they interact. Sometimes it takes several enzymes to produce a chemical reaction. Some enzymes depend on the presence of smaller enzymes called coenzymes in order to function. What that all boils down to is that it is pretty complicated to stimulate enzyme activity in the skin. One little enzyme in a skin care product won't turn on your skin's ability to create, say, collagen or elastin. It's a nice idea, but the theory is much more impressive than the effect, if any, on the skin.

Propylene Glycol

While most cosmetics consumers are very interested in which plants or vitamins are mixed into their creams and lotions, cosmetic chemists are very interested in an entirely different category of ingredients that have no status in the natural or pure realm. One of the more difficult aspects of product formulation is finding ingredients that have more than one function, yet aren't finicky (meaning they don't require extra preservatives, they mix well with other ingredients, they don't change their form over time, and a host of other considerations that never make it into advertising copy). This is why propylene glycol, a superior lightweight ingredient that has some water-binding capacity and can also help other ingredients penetrate the skin, has been an extremely popular cosmetics ingredient. Probably well over 50 percent of the products in your makeup and skin care arsenal right now contain propylene glycol.

In the past I have been reluctant to recommend products that contain propylene glycol because research indicated it had a high probability of causing skin irritation or sensitivity. Many cosmetics companies concurred, and substituted butylene or hexylene glycol, which are kin to propylene glycol but supposedly less irritating. Unfortunately, they are not as effective as propylene glycol. Now it seems that propylene glycol has been misjudged. According to new findings by the Cosmetic Ingredient Review panel (a division of the Cosmetic, Toilietry, and Fragrance Association in association with the FDA), and a past article in *Cosmetic Dermatology*, propylene glycol is now "recognized as safe" and listed in Category I (as determined by the FDA), a reliable category for any cosmetics ingredient. I'm convinced, and my reviews have been adjusted accordingly.

DOING WHAT'S BEST FOR YOUR SKIN

What Works and What Doesn't?

By now your skepticism about cosmetics and the cosmetics industry should be firmly in place. However, you must be wondering, if the cosmetics industry's promises and claims aren't real—then what is real? What is and isn't possible when it comes to your skin? If you can ask these questions and accept the following premises, you are much less likely to waste money on overpriced or ineffective skin care products or be swayed the next time you hear a sales pitch for a miraculous-sounding skin care product.

1. **You can clean your skin, but you can't "deep-clean" it.** You can't get inside a pore and clean it out like a dentist with a drill. Expensive water-soluble cleansers will not make your face any cleaner, nor are they necessarily any gentler, than the less expensive water-soluble cleansers. In fact, the handful of standard cleansing agents are the same across the cosmetics spectrum. What is essential is to find a gentle water-soluble cleanser that doesn't dry out the skin or leave it feeling greasy and that can remove eye makeup without irritating the eyes. Many cleansers that claim to be water-soluble are really too greasy to rinse off completely and can cause clogged pores.

2. **Spending more money does not affect the status of your skin.** The amount of money you spend on skin care has nothing to do with how your skin looks. What you use does, however. An expensive soap by Erno Lazlo is no better for your skin than an inexpensive bar soap such as Dove or Cetaphil Bar; on the other hand an irritant-free toner by Neutrogena can be just as good as, or may even better than,

an irritant-free toner by Orlane or La Prairie, and any irritant-free toner is infinitely better than any toner that contains alcohol or other irritants, regardless of the price. Spending less doesn't hurt your skin, and spending more doesn't necessarily help it.

3. **Getting a tan is foolish.** If you are exposed to the sun, even for as little as 10 to 20 minutes a day, which includes walking to your car or talking to a neighbor outside, that cumulative exposure over the years will wrinkle your skin, and no skin care products except a sunscreen with a high SPF can change that. If that minimal exposure can wrinkle the skin, imagine how much worse is the impact of sunbathing. In short, there is no such thing as careful, safe, or wrinkle-proof tanning.

4. **A great number of skin care problems are caused by the skin care products used to prevent them.** Overly emollient moisturizers can clog pores; temporary face-lift products can cause wrinkles because of the irritation they generate on the skin; and products designed to control oily skin can make skin oilier. Allergic reactions are often caused by products that are too irritating, too drying, or too thick and creamy, or that contain plant extracts and oils.

5. **Dry skin doesn't wrinkle any more or less than oily skin.** Oily skin may look less wrinkled, which means it can have a smoother appearance, but wrinkles are caused by sun exposure, genetic inheritance, or illness, not dry skin. All the moisturizers in the world won't change a wrinkle, although moisturizers can temporarily, day to day, make dry skin look smoother.

6. **Your skin may become inflamed, dry, and blemished if you use too many scrubs, products that contain potentially irritating ingredients, or several AHA or BHA products, either at the same time or in combination with one another.** For example, the following combinations can hurt the skin: a granular cleanser used with a loofah, a washcloth used with an abrasive scrub, an AHA product used with a granular scrub, or an astringent that contains alcohol used with an AHA product. If you use too many irritating products at the same time, you are likely to develop skin irritations, breakouts, dryness, and, possibly, wrinkles.

7. **Exfoliating the skin does not regenerate skin or build collagen.** It is good to exfoliate the skin, and it is very important for many skin types, but exfoliation doesn't create new skin or get rid of wrinkles. It can smooth the skin and help it absorb moisturizers better, but the effects are temporary, and it doesn't alter the actual structure of the skin.

8. **For the most part, the fewer products you use on your skin, the better.** The more you use, the greater your chances of allergic reactions, cosmetic acne, and/or irritation.

9. **Do not automatically buy skin care products based on your age.** Many products on the market are supposedly designed for women who are 30, 40, or over 50. Before you buy into these arbitrary divisions, ask yourself why the over-50 group always gets lumped together. Isn't it unlikely that women between the ages of 20 and 49 have skin that requires three categories, but women over the age of 50 need only one? There are a lot of years between 50 and 90. According to this logic, someone who is 40 shouldn't be using the same products as someone who is 50, but someone who is 80 should be using the same products as someone who is 50. Categorizing products by decades is nothing more than a marketing device that sells products; it does not benefit the skin. Skin has different needs based on how dry, sun-damaged, oily, sensitive, thin, blemished, or normal it is, and that has little to do with age. Plenty of young women have severely dry skin, and plenty of older women have oily skin. Turning 40 does not mean a woman should assume that her skin is drying up and begin using overly emollient moisturizers or skin creams.

10. **Do not automatically buy skin care products based on your skin type.** I know that sounds strange, but there are several reasons for this. It's not that skin type isn't important, but more often than not, your skin type is not what you think it is. Possibly your skin type has been created by the products you are already using. Soap can severely dry the skin; a wrinkle cream can clog pores and cause blemishes; an alcohol-based toner can irritate the skin, causing combination skin. The only way to know what your skin type really is, is to start from square one with the basics: a water-soluble cleanser, an irritant-free toner (or a disinfectant if you break out), an exfoliator (such as an AHA product), a sunscreen for the daytime (which can be included in your moisturizer or foundation), and a moisturizer at night. If your skin is truly dry or you really are prone to breakouts, you can do the extra things, such as using a more emollient moisturizer at night, or a more emollient foundation or a moisturizer with sunscreen during the day. For breakouts you can try a stronger AHA product and/or use 3% hydrogen peroxide twice a day over blemishes.

Another problem is that products designed for a specific skin type may not really be good for that skin type. Most skin care products made for people with oily skin contain harsh ingredients that can make the skin oilier or cause breakouts. The same is true of products designed for people with dry skin; the products can be so greasy they actually make the skin look dull and can also cause breakouts.

A final consideration is that skin type can fluctuate. Skin care routines based on a specific skin type don't take into consideration the fact that your skin changes according to the season, your emotions, the climate (humidity, dryness, cold, and heat all affect your skin), and your menstrual cycle. Pay attention to what your skin tells you it needs at any given time. This month you might need a moisturizer morning and night, next month only at night. The same is true for oily skin and breakouts. Don't hold fast to the idea that your skin fits into only one group—it changes, and so should your skin care routine. That doesn't mean you need new products, it just means you may need to use less of one item or more of another.

11. **Teenagers are not the only ones who have acne.** One of the biggest fallacies around is that women over the age of 20 should not have blemishes. What a joke! Women in their 30s, 40s, and 50s can have acne just like teenagers. Not everyone who has acne as a teenager will grow out of it, and even if you had clear skin as a teenager, that's no guarantee that you won't get acne later in life.

12. **Oily skin types rarely require a moisturizer.** Specialty products such as oil-free moisturizers aren't always good for someone with oily skin. Most women with oily skin have enough of their own oil, so they don't need to worry about dry skin (unless the products they are using dry out their skin). Oil-free moisturizers can be good for someone with normal to slightly dry skin, but they are often a waste for someone with truly oily skin or someone who tends to break out. When should you consider using a moisturizer (hopefully a nongreasy one)? Whenever your skin feels dry, particularly around the eye area. If the dryness is caused by other skin care products, stop using those first before you decide to use a moisturizer.

Skin Care Basics—What You Really Need

Here are the skin care basics: a water-soluble cleanser (never use an eye makeup remover or wipe-off cleanser; pulling at the eye stretches the skin and makes it sag); an exfoliating product (a scrub such as baking soda or an AHA product); a disinfectant if you have blemishes (such as 3% hydrogen peroxide or benzoyl peroxide) or an irritant-free toner if you don't; and a moisturizer or a nongreasy product, for use during the day, that contains a sunscreen with an SPF of 15 (or a foundation that contains an SPF of 15 if you don't want to use a moisturizer or nongreasy lotion).

If you have dry skin, you may want to use a different moisturizer at night, but it isn't essential. The only real reason to use different daytime and nighttime moisturizers is if your daytime moisturizer contains a sunscreen or if you want to use an AHA product at night only (you can wear an AHA product during the day, but you still need a sunscreen in a foundation or another moisturizer). It isn't necessary to have a sunscreen in your nighttime moisturizers, for obvious reasons. If you have very dry skin, you may prefer to use a more emollient moisturizer at night than the one you use during the day, but again that is strictly personal preference. Same for the eye area: if the skin around your eyes is different than the rest of your face, you need a different moisturizing product for that area. Otherwise, most face products can be used around the eye area, regardless of what the cosmetics companies claim.

Among the vast number of cleansers, toners, exfoliators, AHA products, moisturizers, and sunscreens on the market are many good products. Yet we agonize over which company has developed the best ones, or which product contains the latest secret ingredients for procuring a perfect complexion. Perfect skin—that carrot of hope dangled in the form of beautiful, overpriced containers and jars—is not possible. Spending a lot of money in the hope to achieve a more perfect skin is perhaps one the biggest deceptions at the cosmetics counters. Even if you can afford the cost, it is still a waste, because being mislead never feels or looks good.

If I can convince you that there is no reason to spend money on wrinkle creams, you will save vast sums of money over the long haul. Of all of our cosmetics concerns, worrying about wrinkles lasts the longest because it takes quite a while to grow older, and our skin is always there for the ride. But if you stop spending money on expensive wrinkle creams—many women waste an average of $200 to $300 a year on them—over a 30-year period, you will have saved $6,000 to $9,000. With interest, that can really add up, and eventually pay for a face-lift that really gets rid of wrinkles.

A Good, Realistic Skin Care Routine

Most skin care regimes are unrealistic at best. They are either too complicated or too contrived. I want you to let go of the fantasy and the hype and discover what is honest and reliable. Getting real isn't about getting back to basics, which is a comment I hear from a lot of cosmetics-weary women. They think soap and water is all they need, but soap and water dry the skin and offer no protection from the sun. Getting real also doesn't mean mixing honey and avocado together in your kitchen; because who has time for all that, it isn't convenient, food isn't great for the face, and what about sun protection? Getting real means doing what it takes to be good to your skin without wasting money, even if you have money to waste, and buying only products that live up to their claims.

The following is a realistic, viable skin care routine that's free from gimmicks and selling techniques.

Step 1

Even at night, when you're removing makeup, always wash your face with a water-soluble cleanser that rinses off completely and doesn't irritate the eyes. Your eye makeup should come off with the same water-soluble cleanser that cleans your face. Do not use an extra product to wipe across the eye, pulling the skin and eyelashes unnecessarily. (Wiping off makeup is never good for the skin; it pulls at the skin, and rubbing with a tissue or washcloth, no matter how gentle you try to be, can irritate skin.)

Use only tepid to slightly warm water. Hot water burns the skin, and cold water shocks it. Repeated use of hot water, saunas, or Jacuzzis can cause broken capillaries to surface on the nose and cheeks.

Step 2

Exfoliating the skin helps unclog pores and removes dead skin cells, benefiting both dry and oily skin. There are two ways to exfoliate: with a physical exfoliant such as a scrub, and with a chemical exfoliant such as AHAs or BHAs.

Scrubs: If your skin is oily and tends to break out, after you've rinsed off your water-soluble cleanser but while your face is still wet, pour a scant handful of baking soda into the palm of your hand. Add a small amount of water to create a paste, gently massage your entire face with this paste, then rinse generously with tepid water. (You can also mix 1 or 2 teaspoons of baking soda with a 1 or 2 tablespoons of a good water-soluble cleanser such as Cetaphil. This alternative is good for any skin type.) Be extra careful not to get carried away: overscrubbing can cause more problems than it solves. The operative word for all skin care is "gentle."

If you have combination skin, massage only those areas that tend to break out, and avoid the areas that are dry. If you have normal skin, use the baking soda scrub only two to three times a week. If you have dry skin, use the baking soda mixed with Cetaphil only about once or twice a week, and rinse very well. If you have extremely dry skin, follow the advice for dry skin, but use more Cetaphil and just a pinch of baking soda in your mixture, and be very, very gentle when massaging your face.

Chemical exfoliates: An effective alternative to scrubs is products that contain at least a 5% or greater concentration of AHAs or BHAs. (AHA and BHA products with an emollient base can double as a moisturizer.) The AHA or BHA product is applied after the face is washed and dried (see Step 4).

Once your face is clean, gently squeeze any blackheads or blemishes you want to remove. One way to get rid of blackheads is to squeeze them; they don't usually leave on their own, and they can be stubborn even if you are using a good AHA product or Retin-A. Blemishes, on the other hand, can heal on their own, but relieving the pressure and removing the contents can help them heal faster. If you are shocked by this suggestion, that's OK; you don't have to do this, but it does help. This is what most facialists do best for your skin; however, it is cheaper to do it yourself. Many people worry about making matters worse. The only way to prevent that from happening is to NEVER, absolutely NEVER, oversqueeze. If the blemish or blackhead does not respond easily, stop and leave it alone. Squeezing does not cause problems on the face; in fact, it is one of the best ways to clean out the skin. The problems occur when you massacre the skin by squeezing until you create scabs and sores.

Step 3

When your face is completely rinsed and dried and you've finished any squeezing you need to do, take a cotton ball soaked in 3% hydrogen peroxide and swab it over those areas that break out to disinfect them (but avoid the hairline and eyebrows because the 3% hydrogen peroxide over time can lighten the hair). You can use the 3% hydrogen peroxide in place of an astringent or toner once or twice a day. Avoid the hairline and eyebrows when using 3% hydrogen peroxide, or you will inadvertently lighten them.

If you have normal to dry skin that does not break out, rinse your face completely and, if you wish, go over it with a skin freshener or toner that does not contain alcohol or any other irritants. Many irritant-free toners provide a pleasant sensation, but the more expensive ones are not worth their exorbitant price tags (especially when you consider that the basic ingredients are usually the same).

If you have extremely oily skin or skin that breaks out frequently, try a facial mask of plain Phillips' Milk of Magnesia. Milk of Magnesia is a mixture of magnesium and water. Magnesium is a good disinfectant, and it can absorb oil. The clay masks for oily skin have no disinfecting properties, and their ingredients cannot absorb oil as well as magnesium can. Your skin type and reaction to the mask will determine how often you can use it. Those with severely oily skin can use it every day; those with slightly oily skin should need to use it only once a week.

Step 4

After your face is clean and the toner or 3% hydrogen peroxide has dried, this is the time to apply Retin-A, Renova, or an AHA or BHA product if you have chosen to use any of these.

Step 5

During the day it is essential to wear a sunscreen with an SPF of 15 (SPF 8 can be acceptable if you know for certain you will experience only minimal sun exposure). If you have normal to dry skin, wear a sunscreen that comes in a moisturizing base. If you have normal to oily skin, you do not need a moisturizer, but you still must wear a sunscreen with an SPF of 15. Either your foundation or a nongreasy sunscreen product are the best options for an oily skin type.

Step 6

Unless you have dry skin or want to improve the appearance of your wrinkles, it is not necessary to wear a moisturizer at night. If you choose to do so, apply a layer over a thin mist of water and allow it to be absorbed into your skin rather than rubbing it in. Heavy, creamy moisturizers are best only for extremely dry skin. Try the less expensive moisturizers before you venture into the higher-priced brands. You can use a thicker, more emollient-type moisturizer for the drier areas of your face.

If you want to use an AHA product that comes in a moisturizing base at night, apply it after the toner. If you use a liquid or gel type AHA product apply it after the toner but before the moisturizer.

CLEARING THE AIR ON ACNE

Over-the-Counter Acne Products

Horror of horrors! Another blemish. Why me? I'd give anything for clear skin. But instead I've got blackheads galore, and you could drill for oil on my face. I thought I had outgrown this stuff; doesn't it ever end? My skin was doing so well—where did these blemishes come from?

Does any of this sound familiar? It happens to a lot of us at one time or another; to many of us it happens all the time (as it did to me before I took Accutane; see that section in this chapter), and it doesn't go away at age 20 or 30. It can even start for a lot of us at 40 or 50. Whenever breakouts besiege the face, we usually begin a counterattack almost immediately. More often than not, we arm ourselves with heavy artillery from the drugstore shelves or cosmetics counters where the acne products reside.

In our search for relief from the emotional and physical discomfort that often accompanies acne, we first turn to one of the myriad products that promise to "zap zits" and give us clear skin. The commercials and ads sound fairly convincing, but a closer look reveals that these products can neither zap zits nor effectively prevent them from occurring, and the irritation they cause can create more problems than they clear up. Which is no surprise, really: if these products really worked, why would any of us still break out?

The companies use clever marketing language to sell products to people who want to reduce blemishes and fight oily skin. Neutrogena advertises its Clean Pore Advantage as fighting acne because it "cleans all 218,000 pores on your face." Technically, any cleanser can make that claim, because whenever you clean your face you're cleaning every single pore, but this sounds so meticulous and thorough. You also get the impression that if you miss a pore, your skin will break out. The truth is, blemishes and blackheads have nothing to do with "unclean" skin. In fact, overcleaning can make acne worse. In the same ad Neutrogena claims its Antiseptic Cleanser is good because it's alcohol-free, and alcohol can strip the skin dry. Well, Clean Pore Advantage contains alcohol; does that mean they think their own product is bad? And the Antiseptic Cleanser, even though it doesn't contain alcohol, does have irritating ingredients such as camphor, eucalyptus oil, and peppermint oil. It is still fairly drying and can irritate the skin and burn the eyes.

This scenario is repeated in acne product after acne product to one degree or another. What is perhaps most shocking, is that regardless of the acne product, regardless of the price tag, whether it is sold at the drugstore, department store, inhome sales, or infomercial they virtually all contain the same ingredients. Pick up just about any acne product and read the ingredient list, where the only factual information is, and you'll find an array of ingredients that can may make oily skin worse, irritate and dry the skin (which doesn't change oil production, but adds another skin problem), or cause problems for sensitive skin. Several primary ingredients show up repeatedly, regardless of how inexpensive or expensive the product is: salicylic acid (a peeling agent); benzoyl peroxide (a disinfectant); sulfur (a mild antiseptic); boric acid (a toxic antiseptic); camphor, menthol, eucalyptus, and clove oil (all irritants with no actual benefit for skin); and alcohol (a strong skin irritant that is rarely present in concentrations effective for disinfecting). While I believe there are compelling reasons to avoid almost every single one of these ingredients, some of them do make sense. Sulfur and benzoyl peroxide can help to disinfect skin that breaks out, and salicylic acid can peel the skin, which may keep pores from getting clogged.

My concern is that almost all of these ingredients are too strong for the face and can over-irritate the skin, making things worse than before. There are gentler ways to do the same things. For example, alpha hydroxy acid products can do the same thing as salicylic acid, and with much less irritation; sulfur is an OK disinfectant, but the possibility of irritation causes more problems for the skin than it helps, making 3% hydrogen peroxide a better choice. And what are menthol, camphor, eucalyptus, clove oil, and boric acid used for in acne products? I have yet to find a satisfactory answer to that one. According to everything I've read, these ingredients do nothing whatsoever to combat acne. The only thing I've consistently seen them do is temporarily make the skin feel drier and tingly, which makes a person with problem skin think that the product is doing something beneficial.

Bottom line: If an acne product is working for you, stay with it. If your skin is red and irritated, still oily, and still has blemishes, reconsider what you are doing. And don't assume, because one or two acne products didn't work, that another one might. As you read the product reviews below, notice how similar they all are. Bouncing from one product to another won't help when they all contain basically the same things. Beware of claims that sound great but are really ludicrous.

Beauty Note: Benzoyl peroxide has been a major player in the fight against acne in both prescription and over-the-counter acne products. It is a good disinfectant and can be helpful for some types of acne, even though it is potentially quite irritating. A few years ago, several studies suggested that benzoyl peroxide is a possible carcinogen, but significant research indicates it is not. Most dermatologists still recommend benzoyl peroxide and contend that the evidence is on the side of its being safe. However, a small number of dermatologists instead recommend 3% hydrogen peroxide. As you know, I also encourage the latter.

Acne-Statin

I am extremely skeptical about cosmetics products that claim to get rid of acne, eliminate blackheads, or dry up oil. What I know from personal experience, and from the thousands of letters I receive each year from women the world over (not to mention interviews with cosmetic chemists and dermatologists), is that these over-the-counter products don't work nearly as well as they would like you to believe. The truth is, you can't cure acne or dry up oil with over-the-counter, nonprescription medications. Over-the-counter products can help only about 40 percent of a given population (some suggest it is even less than that), and by "help" I mean they reduce flare-ups, rather than curing them. What about the 60 percent who don't benefit? Well, they jump from one product to the next, hoping to find something that works.

How does **Acne-Statin** *($34.90 for 4 ounces)*, a face wash and moisturizer all-in-one product, fit in? Well, to be perfectly honest, I'm not sure. Because Acne-Statin doesn't list ingredients on its label, much of what is inside is a mystery and hard to evaluate. Due to a grandfather clause in the FDA's mandatory ingredient listing rules, Acne-Statin doesn't have to list any of its nonactive ingredients. They do have to list the active ingredients, though, so what isn't a mystery is that Acne-Statin contains 0.5% triclosan, a standard disinfectant found in many acne products. The other 99.5% of the product is composed of standard cosmetics ingredients that hold no hope for acne sufferers.

Acne-Statin's claims sound sweeping and impressive. But as consumers, we are given only advertising and hype to help us make a decision. The ingredient list, the only verifiable truth on any cosmetics label, is kept a secret. If the Acne-Statin products could cure acne, as the ads and infomercial claim, who would have acne? Bottom line: The active ingredients listed can't do what the product claims it can do.

Acne-Product Reviews

Below are reviews of an assortment of acne products, mostly available at the drugstore. By far these are not all the products available, but this selection will help familiarize you with what is available and with how shockingly similar these products are. **Note:** My rating system of the small faces that appear next to each product are explained in the beginning of Chapter 7.

☹ **Aapri Apricot Facial Scrub, Gentle Formula** *($4.29 for 2 ounces)* contains walnut shell powder as an agent, which would be OK if the product did not also contain a very drying detergent cleanser as well as apricot oil and lanolin oil, both of which can cause breakouts and allergic reactions.

☹ **Aapri Apricot Facial Scrub Original Formula** *($4.29 for 2 ounces)* has almost the same ingredients as the scrub above, minus the oils but with the same detergent cleansing agent, which is too drying and irritating for most skin types.

☹ **Acne-Aid Cleansing Bar** *($3.49 for 4 ounces)* can't aid acne, at least not any better than any other bar soap made of tallow and a detergent cleansing agent. It is a good bar of soap, as far as soap goes; it's just not anything special or unique. Tallow can cause breakouts.

☹ **Acnomel Acne Medication Cream** *($8.29 for 1 ounce)* contains 2% resorcinol, 8% sulfur, and 11% alcohol, plus clay. Both resorcinol and sulfur are potent disinfectants that can be extremely irritating to the skin. In 1992, resorcinol lost its FDA approval rating for claims about disinfecting and preventing acne.

☹ **Aveeno Natural Colloidal Oatmeal Cleansing Bar for Combination Skin** *($2.99 for 3 ounces)* contains about 50% oatmeal, which can be a soothing agent. It also contains glycerin, lactic acid (about 5%), petrolatum (like Vaseline), and thickeners. The petrolatum makes it questionable for combination skin, and the AHA ingredient could be too irritating if you use another AHA product afterwards.

☹ **Aveeno Natural Collodial Oatmeal Cleansing Bar for Dry Skin** *($2.99 for 3 ounces)* contains about 50% oatmeal, which can be a soothing agent. It also contains a detergent cleanser, vegetable oil, vegetable shortening, glycerin, lactic acid (about 4%), mineral oil, and preservatives. Although it could be a good bar soap if you have dry skin, the AHA ingredient could be too irritating if you use another AHA product afterwards.

☹ **Aveeno Natural Colloidal Oatmeal Cleansing Bar for Acne Prone Skin** *($2.99 for 3 ounces)* contains about 50% oatmeal, which can be a soothing agent. It also contains lactic acid (about 5%), thickeners, salicylic acid (about 1%), and preservatives. Although it could be a good bar soap if you have dry skin, the AHAs and BHAs could be too irritating if you use another AHA product afterwards.

☹ **Basis Soap for Combination Skin** *($2.69 for 3 ounces)* is a standard tallow-based soap. Tallow can cause blackheads.

☹ **Benoxyl 10 Lotion Acne Treatment Lotion** *($7.29 for 1 ounce)* contains 10% benzoyl peroxide, thickeners, and preservatives. Benzoyl peroxide can disinfect, but it can also be a skin irritant; additionally, one of the lotion's thickening agents is isopropyl palmitate, which can cause breakouts.

☹ **Brasivol Base Facial Cleanser for Oily Skin** *($6.75 for 3.8 ounces)* contains a detergent cleansing agent, thickeners, and preservatives The cleansing agent is sodium lauryl sulfate, which can be a strong irritant and drying for most skin types.

☹ **Brasivol Medium Facial Cleanser and Conditioner** *($8.19 for 6 ounces)* contains aluminum oxide (scrubbing particles), water, a detergent cleansing agent, thickeners, and preservatives. The cleansing agent is sodium lauryl sulfate, which can be a strong irritant and drying for most skin types.

☺ **Buf-Puf Singles Skin Conditioning Cleanser** *($4.69 for 40 sponges)* contains soft fabric sponges soaked in a solution of detergent cleansers, thickeners, preservative, and coloring agents. It is a standard detergent cleanser, although it tends to be drying and the pads are a waste of money. If "conditioning" means good for dry skin, it isn't.

☺ **Buf-Puf Singles Oil-Free Cleanser** *($4.69 for 40 sponges)* is virtually identical to the Skin Conditioning Cleanser above, and the same review applies.

☺ **Buf-Puf Singles Cleanser for Normal to Oily Skin** *($3.66 for 40 sponges)* is virtually identical to the Skin Conditioning Cleanser above, and the same review applies.

☺ **Buf-Puf Singles Cleanser for Normal to Dry Skin** *($3.41 for 40 sponges)* is virtually identical to the Skin Conditioning Cleanser above, and the same review applies.

☹ **Clean & Clear Blemish Fighting Pads** *($3.69 for 50 pads)* contains salicylic acid (skin irritant and peeling agent); preservative; camphor, clove oil, eucalyptus oil, and peppermint oil (all skin irritants); alcohol; and water. This won't fight anything, but it will cause irritation.

☹ **Clean & Clear Blemish Fighting Stick** *($3.99 for 1 ounce)* contains the same ingredients as the pads, and the same warning applies.

☹ **Clean & Clear Bar & Buff** *($2.69 for 3 ounces)* contains sodium tallowate (can cause blackheads and irritation), water, glycerin, alcohol, thickeners, detergent cleansers, slip agent, preservatives, and coloring agents. It's a standard bar soap, although the alcohol can make it particularly drying.

☹ **Clean & Clear Bar, Regular** *($2.19 for 3.75 ounces)* contains ingredients similar to those in the Bar & Buff, but it has a mild antiseptic and no alcohol. It is drying to the skin.

☹ **Clean & Clear Deep Action Cream Cleanser** *($3.85 for 6.5 ounces)* contains mostly thickeners, salicylic acid, fragrance, menthol, and preservatives. The menthol can be a skin irritant, and salicylic acid in a cleanser is a problem for the eyes. Also, because it contains a BHA ingredient (salicylic acid), it could be too irritating if you use another BHA or AHA product afterwards.

☹ **Clean & Clear Foaming Facial Cleanser** *($2.65 for 8 ounces)* is a standard detergent-based, water-soluble cleanser. The cleansing agent is sodium lauryl sulfate, which can be drying and irritating for most skin types.

☺ **Clean & Clear Sensitive Skin Foaming Facial Cleanser** *($3.79 for 8 ounces)* may be a good detergent-based, water-soluble cleanser for someone with normal to oily skin. It is definitely more gentle than the cleanser above.

☹ **Clean & Clear Sensitive Skin, Invisible Blemish Treatment** *($3.85 for 0.75 ounce)* is a 5% salicylic acid product that also contains thickener and alcohol. The combination of alcohol and salicylic acid makes this product too irritating for most skin types.

☹ **Clean & Clear Oil Controlling Astringent** *($3.79 for 8 ounces)* contains water, alcohol, eucalyptus oil, camphor, peppermint oil, clove oil, and salicylic acid. If you don't have red, dry, irritated skin before using this product, you will after. This product cannot control oil; in fact, the irritation it causes can make oily skin more oily.

☹ **Clean & Clear Sensitive Skin, Oil Controlling Astringent** *($3.79 for 8 ounces)* is almost identical to the astringent above, but with slightly less alcohol. It could be a disaster for someone with sensitive skin.

☺ **Clean & Clear Dr. Prescribed Acne Medicine, Extra Strength** *($4.99 for 1 ounce)* is a 5% benzoyl peroxide liquid. If you want to try a benzoyl peroxide product, this one would be just fine.

☺ **Clean & Clear Dr. Prescribed Acne Medication, Maximum Strength** (*$4.99 for 1 ounce*) is a 10% benzoyl peroxide liquid. If you want to try a stronger benzoyl peroxide product, this one would be just fine.

☺ **Clean & Clear Sensitive Skin Skin Balancing Moisturizer** (*$3.79 for 4 ounces*) contains mostly water, thickeners, silicone oil, more thickeners, salicylic acid (5%), and preservatives. This amount of salicylic acid renders the product useless for someone with sensitive skin, but it could be an option for someone looking for a minimally moisturizer-based BHA product.

☺ **Clean & Clear Skin Balancing Moisturizer** (*$3.79 for 4 ounces*) is virtually identical to the moisturizer above, and the same review applies.

☹ **Clearasil Adult Care Acne Medication Cream** (*$3.69 for 0.6 ounce*) contains mostly water, alcohol, clay, sulfur, resorcinol, thickeners, silicone oil, and preservatives. Both resorcinol and sulfur are potent disinfectants that can be extremely irritating. Resorcinol is no longer approved by the FDA for disinfecting and preventing acne. Also, one of the thickeners is isopropyl myristate, which can cause breakouts. Aside from being very drying and irritating, this product may also clog pores.

☹ **Clearasil Antibacterial Soap** (*$1.91 for 3.25 ounces*) is a standard tallow-based soap with a detergent cleansing agent. It contains the disinfectant triclosan, but its effects are washed away in a soap, and the tallow can cause blackheads.

☺ **Clearasil Daily Face Wash** (*$4.99 for 6.5 ounces*) is a standard detergent-based, water-soluble cleanser that may be OK for someone with oily skin, though it can be drying. It contains the disinfectant triclosan, but its effects are washed away in a soap.

☹ **Clearasil Medicated Deep Cleanser** (*$7.50 for 7.75 ounces*) is misnamed. There's nothing deep about this cleanser, and it can be irritating. It contains mostly water, aloe, menthol, soothing agent, thickeners, fragrance, water-binding agents, and preservatives. The amount of water-binding agents is too small to be significant. In addition, menthol is a skin irritant, and salicylic acid is wasted in a cleanser and increases the risk of irritation if you use other BHA products afterwards.

☹ **Clearasil Double Textured Pads Maximum Strength** (*$4.19 for 40 pads*) is mostly alcohol and salicylic acid. This product would be too drying and irritating for most skin types.

☹ **Clearasil Double Textured Pads Regular Strength with Skin Soothers** (*$4.19 for 40 pads*) contains a small amount of aloe vera, but it won't counteract the irritation of the alcohol and salicylic acid.

☺ **Clearasil Moisturizer** *($6 for 3 ounces)* contains mostly water, thickeners, water-binding agent, more thickeners, mineral oil, silicone oil, salicylic acid (2%), and preservatives. This could be an option if you want a moisturizer-based BHA product, but mineral oil and silicone oil can cause problems for oily skin.

☹ **Clearasil Tinted Cream Maximum Strength** *($6 for 1 ounce)* is a 10% benzoyl peroxide product with a tint, but few people have skin the color of this tint. You can find similar products without tints that won't look strange on your skin.

☹ **Clearasil Vanishing Cream Maximum Strength** *($6 for 1 ounce)* is unlikely to cause anything to vanish. It is a 10% benzoyl peroxide product that also contains clay and thickeners. One of the thickeners is isopropyl myristate, which can cause breakouts.

☺ **Clearasil Vanishing Lotion Maximum Strength** *($5.69 for 1 ounce)* is similar to the cream above, minus the isopropyl myristate. It could be an option for someone looking for a minimally moisturizer-based benzoyl peroxide product.

☹ **Clearasil Clearstick Maximum Strength** *($5.19 for 1.2 ounces)* is mostly alcohol, aloe, menthol, and salicylic acid. Menthol is a skin irritant, and you already know about salicylic acid. No one needs the alcohol or menthol.

☹ **Clearasil Clearstick Regular Strength** *($5.79 for 1.2 ounces)* is almost identical to the Clearstick above, and the same review applies.

☹ **Clearasil Clearstick Sensitive Skin Maximum Strength** *($6 for 1.2 ounces)* is the same as the maximum-strength Clearstick above, minus the menthol, and the same review applies.

☹ **Cuticura Medicated Antibacterial Bar Fragrance-Free Formula for Sensitive Skin** *($2.04 for 3 ounces)* is a standard tallow-based bar soap with petrolatum and thickeners. It contains the disinfectant triclosan, but its effects are washed away in a soap, and the tallow can cause blackheads.

☹ **Cuticura Medicated Antibacterial Bar Original Formula for Blemish-Prone Skin** *($2.44 for 5.25 ounces)* is virtually identical to the soap above, and the same review applies.

☹ **Exact Deep Cleaning Acne Treatment** *($4.58 for 4 ounces)* contains 2% salicylic acid, which is a problem in a cleanser because most of its effects are washed away, it can cause irritation if it gets in the eyes, and it increases the potential for irritation if you use other salicylic acid products afterwards.

☹ **Exact Acne Medication Tinted Cream** *($3.25 for 0.65 ounce)*, a 5% benzoyl peroxide product, is unlikely to be helpful; few people have skin the color of this tint. You can find similar products that don't have tints and won't look strange on your skin.

☺ **Exact Acne Medication Vanishing Cream** *($3.25 for 1 ounce)* won't cause anything to vanish. This 5% benzoyl peroxide product can be effective for some skin types, but it contains thickening agents that may clog pores.

☹ **Fostex Acne Medication Cleansing Bar** *($3.62 for 3.75 ounces)* is a detergent-based cleansing bar that contains boric acid, which can cause irritation if it gets in the eyes. It also contains 2% salicylic acid, which has minimal effect on the face because it is washed away, but could be a problem if you use other salicylic acid products afterwards.

☹ **Fostex Acne Medication Cleansing Cream** *($6.56 for 4 ounces)* is a detergent cleanser that contains 2% salicylic acid, which has minimal effect on the face because it is washed away but can be an irritant if it gets in the eyes.

☹ **Fostex 10% Benzoyl Peroxide Acne Medication** *($4.72 for 3.75 ounces)* is a 10% benzoyl peroxide liquid that also contains boric acid, which, according to the FDA and the American Medical Association, is not safe in cosmetics.

☺ **Fostex 10% Benzoyl Peroxide Vanishing Gel** *($7.69 for 1.5 ounces)* is a 10% benzoyl peroxide lightweight gel. If you want to try a strong benzoyl peroxide product, this is a good option.

☹ **Hibiclens Antiseptic Antimicrobial Skin Cleanser** *($4.69 for 4 ounces)* contains a mild antiseptic, fragrance, alcohol, water, and coloring agent. The antiseptic might be an option, but the fragrance, coloring agent, and alcohol are too irritating or unnecessary.

☺ **Mudd Spa Treatment Original Masque** *($4.99 for 4 ounces)* is a standard clay mask that also contains thickeners and preservatives. This basic clay mask is as good as any on the market. It does contain a disinfectant, but not one recommended for acne.

☺ **Mudd Spa Treatment Aloe Masque** *($4.99 for 4 ounces)* is similar to the mask above, but with plant extracts. Nice natural touch, but useless for acne.

☺ **Mudd Spa Treatment Sea Masque** *($4.99 for 4 ounces)* is similar to the Original Masque above, but with marine extracts. Nice natural touch, but useless for acne.

☹ **Noxzema 2-1 Pads Regular Strength** *($3.49 for 50 pads)* contains mostly alcohol, salicylic acid, water, thickener, clove oil, camphor, eucalyptus oil, and menthol. This product contains several skin sensitizers and is also very drying and irritating for almost all skin types.

☹ **Noxzema 2-1 Pads Maximum Strength** *($4.29 for 75 pads)* is not recommended. "Maximum Strength," in this case, means maximum irritation and dryness.

☹ **Noxzema Astringent for Normal Skin** *($2.78 for 8 ounces)* contains mostly alcohol and menthol. This astringent is extremely drying and irritating for almost all skin types.

☹ **Noxzema Sensitive Toner** *($2.78 for 8 ounces)* contains mostly water, alcohol, soothing agents, water-binding agents, and preservatives. The soothing agents and water-binding ingredients are nice, but they won't prevent the irritation and dryness caused by the alcohol. No one with sensitive skin would want to use this product for very long.

☹ **Noxzema Astringent for Oily Skin** *($3.79 for 8 ounces)* contains mostly water, alcohol, fragrance, and menthol. The only thing this product can do is irritate the skin; alcohol and menthol can't improve or help oily skin.

☹ **Noxzema Medicated Deep Cleanser** *($5.35 for 3.5 ounces)* contains salicylic acid, alcohol, water, witch hazel, aloe, menthol, soothing agent, fragrance, thickener, water-binding agent, more thickener, and preservative. This isn't much of a cleanser; it can irritate the skin and should be kept away from the eyes.

☹ **Oxy Acne Medication for Sensitive Skin** *($3.99 for 50 pads)* contains less than 1% salicylic acid, but it has a lot of alcohol and menthol, which makes it inappropriate for most skin types.

☹ **Oxy Acne Medication, Maximum Strength** *($3.99 for 50 pads)* is similar to the medication above, but with 2% salicylic acid. The same review applies.

☹ **Oxy Acne Medication Regular Strength** *($3.99 for 50 pads)* contains no salicylic acid, but has a good amount of menthol and alcohol. It would be drying and irritating for most skin types.

☹ **Oxy Acne Medicated Cleanser** *($2.59 for 4 ounces)* contains less than 1% salicylic acid, but has a lot of alcohol and menthol, which makes it a problem for most skin types.

☹ **Oxy Acne Medicated Soap** *($2 for 3.25 ounces)* is a standard tallow-based bar soap that also contains the disinfectant triclosan. Disinfectants are wasted in soap because they are washed away before they can have an effect. Also, tallow can clog pores.

☺ **Oxy Night Watch Maximum Strength** *($5.69 for 2 ounces)* contains mostly salicylic acid, thickener, and preservatives. How many salicylic acid products can one person use? It's OK as a mild exfoliant but can be irritating for some skin types.

☺ **Oxy Night Watch for Sensitive Skin** *($4.55 for 2 ounces)* contains almost the same ingredients as the product above, and the same review applies.

☺ **Oxy Residon't Medicated Face Wash** *($4.99 for 8 ounces)* is a standard detergent-based, water-soluble cleanser that can be good for someone with oily skin. May be drying.

☹ **Oxy 10 Benzoyl Peroxide Acne Wash** *($5.49 for 4 ounces)* is a standard detergent-based, water-soluble cleanser that also contains 10% benzoyl peroxide. Benzoyl peroxide is wasted in a cleanser because most of it gets washed away, and it can cause problems if it gets in the eyes.

☺ **Oxy 10 Maximum Strength Vanishing Acne Medication** *($5.16 for 1 ounce)* is a 10% benzoyl peroxide gel and a fine option for someone who wants to try this type of product.

☺ **Oxy 10 Sensitive Vanishing Acne Medication** *($4.98 for 1 ounce)* is almost identical to the medication above, but contains 2.5% benzoyl peroxide. The same review applies.

☹ **Oxy 10 Tinted Acne Medication Maximum Strength** *($4.98 for 1 ounce)*, a 10% benzoyl peroxide product, is unlikely to be helpful; few people have skin the color of this tint. You can find similar products that don't have tints and won't look strange on your skin.

☹ **Pan Oxyl Bar 10% Benzoyl Peroxide** *($6.79 for 4 ounces)* contains 10% benzoyl peroxide as well as detergent cleansers. Benzoyl peroxide is wasted In a cleanser because most of it is washed away before it has a chance to disinfect the skin.

☹ **ProActiv Renewing Cleanser** *($49 for all four ProActiv products)* contains mostly 2.5% benzoyl peroxide, detergent cleansing agents, thickeners, silicone oil, and preservatives. It is not oil-free, and I can't imagine why anyone would stick benzoyl peroxide in a water-soluble cleanser that might get in the eyes and is mostly rinsed off.

☺ **ProActiv Revitalizing Toner** *($49 for all four ProActiv products)* contains mostly water, glycolic acid, slip agents, plant extract, witch hazel, thickener, water-binding agents, and preservatives. This is a potentially good AHA liquid, but if you combine it with the two benzoyl peroxide products in the ProActiv line and the sulfur-based mask, your skin will definitely swell up and become red.

☺ **ProActiv Repairing Lotion** *($49 for all four ProActiv products)* contains 2.5% benzoyl peroxide, water, slip agents, soothing agent, and preservatives. This is a fine benzoyl peroxide product, but it won't repair anything in the skin; it only disinfects.

☹ **ProActiv Mask** *($49 for all four ProActiv products)* is a clay mask that contains sulfur. Sulfur is a disinfectant but also a strong skin irritant.

☹ **PropapH Acne Medication Cleansing Lotion for Sensitive Skin** *($2.47 for 6 ounces)* contains 5% salicylic acid, alcohol, detergent cleansing agent, preservative, menthol, and fragrance. The salicylic acid, alcohol, and menthol make this inappropriate for most skin types.

☹ **PropapH Acne Medication Cleansing Lotion for Normal to Combination Skin** *($2.49 for 6 ounces)* is almost identical to the lotion above, and the same review applies.

☹ **PropapH Astringent Cleanser Acne Medication and Moisturizer for Normal to Sensitive Skin** *($3.79 for 6 ounces)* is very similar to the lotions above, except it also contains peppermint oil and an AHA ingredient. The AHA ingredient used isn't a very effective one, and there is no research about the effect of BHAs (salicylic acid) and AHAs when used together.

☹ **PropapH Foaming Face Wash, Acne Medication and Moisturizer** *($5.49 for 10 ounces)* is similar to the Acne Medication Cleansing Lotion for Sensitive Skin, but with 2% salicylic acid; the same review applies.

☹ **SalAc Acne Medicated Cleanser** *($8.79 for 6 ounces)* contains 2% salicylic acid, benzoyl alcohol, detergent cleansers, thickener, water, and more thickener. One of the cleansing agents is sodium C14-16 olefin sulfate, which can be quite drying. Also, salicylic acid is a problem in a cleanser because most of its effectiveness is washed away, and it can cause irritation if it gets in the eyes.

☹ **Sayman Soap Cleansing Bar with Witch Hazel for Oily Skin** *($1.89 for 3.5 ounces)* is a standard tallow-based bar soap. Tallow can cause breakouts, and this product also contains lanolin and sesame oil, which should be avoided by anyone with oily skin.

☹ **Sea Breeze Facial Cleansing Bar for Normal to Oily Skin** *($2 for 3.3 ounces)* is a standard tallow-based bar soap with detergent cleansing agents. Tallow can cause breakouts.

☺ **Sea Breeze Foaming Face Wash for Normal to Oily Skin** *($3.64 for 6 ounces)* is a standard detergent-based, water-soluble cleanser that could be good for someone with oily skin. It may be drying for some skin types.

☺ **Sea Breeze Foaming Face Wash for Sensitive Skin** *($3.58 for 6 ounces)* is almost identical to the face wash above, and the same review applies.

☺ **Sea Breeze Whipped Facial Cleanser** *($4.99 for 6 ounces)* is similar to the face washes above, but with more gentle cleansing agents.

☺ **Sea Breeze Exfoliating Facial Scrub** *($3.64 for 4 ounces)* contains a synthetic scrub agent, thickeners, and preservatives. It is an OK lightweight, relatively nonirritating scrub for some skin types.

☹ **Sea Breeze Astringent for Sensitive Skin** *($2.49 or 4 ounces)* contains mostly water, alcohol, glycerin, camphor, clove oil, eucalyptus oil, fragrance, and coloring agents. Sensitive skin would not do well using this product, since it contains almost exclusively irritating and sensitizing ingredients.

☹ **Sea Breeze Astringent for Oily Skin** *($2.49 for 4 ounces)* is almost identical to the astringent above, except that it contains more alcohol and peppermint oil, which makes it even more irritating.

☹ **Sea Breeze Towelettes** *($4.19 for 20 towelettes)* is almost identical to the Astringent for Sensitive Skin above, and the same review applies.

☺ **Stridex Clear Antibacterial Face Wash, Maximum Strength** *($4.88 for 8 ounces)* is a standard detergent-based, water soluble cleanser that can be OK for someone with oily skin. The face wash contains the disinfectant triclosan, but that would be washed away before it could have any positive effect on the skin.

☹ **Stridex Antibacterial Cleansing Bar with Glycerin** *($1.85 for 3.5 ounces)* is a standard tallow-based bar cleanser. Tallow can cause breakouts.

☹ **Stridex Antibacterial Cleansing Bar with Triclosan** *($1.85 for 3.5 ounces)* is a standard tallow-based bar cleanser. Tallow can cause breakouts. It does contain the disinfectant triclosan, but in a cleanser the potential benefit of a disinfectant is washed away.

☹ **Stridex Dual Textured Pads, Maximum Strength** *($3.16 for 32 pads)* contains mostly 2% salicylic acid, alcohol, detergent cleansing agent, fragrance, menthol, and silicone oil. Alcohol dries the skin, and this is just one more salicylic acid product.

☹ **Stridex Super Size Pads Super Scrub Oil Fighting Formula** *($3.36 for 55 pads)* is virtually identical to the pads above, and the same review applies.

☹ **Stridex Super Size Pads Regular Strength** *($3.36 for 55 pads)* is similar to the Dual Textured Pads above, except with 0.5% salicylic acid. The same review applies.

☹ **Stridex Super Size Pads for Sensitive Skin** *($3.36 for 55 pads)* is similar to the Dual Textured Pads above, but without alcohol. It is indeed better for someone with sensitive skin.

☺ **Stridex Invisible Clear Gel Maximum Strength** *($4.76 for 1 ounce)* is a 2% salicylic acid product (there's a surprise). It can exfoliate skin but also be a skin irritant.

Seeing a Dermatologist

Although at times I disagree with dermatologists on the subject of daily skin care, when it comes to chronic acne or serious skin problems, there is absolutely no other option but to see a dermatologist. If you have minor skin problems, such as occasional breakouts, daily skin care is best handled with cosmetic cleansing routines and possibly Retin-A (which must be prescribed by a dermatologist). But if you have acne that is chronic, causing scarring or disfigurement, make an appointment immediately to see a dermatologist.

I also advise seeking a dermatologist if you are fair-skinned and have spent a great deal of time in the sun getting a tan; the chances are fairly high that signs of skin cancer could appear sooner than you think. (I know several women in their early 30s who are sun worshippers and already have uneven brown patches on their skin.) In general, you should never try to handle chronic or serious skin problems only by visits to the cosmetics counters or the drugstore. In these cases, it is essential to consult a dermatologist.

Accutane—A Cure for Acne?

Have you patiently waited for your skin to clear up? Spent untold dollars on dermatologists and followed their instructions, diligently wiping antibiotic lotions over your face and taking oral antibiotics for years? Chances are that for most of that time your skin may have improved, but it probably never really stopped breaking out. In spite of the improvement from using antibiotics, you probably don't want to stay on them permanently. You may not be willing to live with the negative side effects, such as chronic low-grade stomach problems. Who knows how long your skin will continue breaking out? But with Accutane, this persistent cycle can be over in four months. Sounds unbelievable, doesn't it? Well, it isn't.

Most dermatologists will tell you that it is possible—in fact, highly probable—that Accutane can cure acne. Accutane, which has been around for more than ten years, is a synthetic drug made to resemble the molecules in vitamin A, and it is taken orally. It essentially stops the oil production in your sebaceous glands (the oil-producing structures of the skin) and literally shrinks these glands to the size of a baby's. This prevents sebum (oil) from clogging the hair follicle, mixing with dead skin cells, rupturing the follicle wall, and creating pimples or cysts. Oil production resumes when treatment is completed and the sebaceous glands slowly begin to grow larger again, but they never (or at least rarely) grow as large as they were before treatment.

Are you ready for this? In 85 percent of patients who complete a four-month treatment with Accutane, acne is no longer considered to be clinically significant. In other words, for all intents and purposes, their acne is cured! Does this mean you'll never break out again? No, you will once in a while, but an occasional pimple here and there is hardly anyone's definition of acne—especially anyone who has had, on a daily basis, multiple breakouts on her face and body.

What about the remaining 15 percent of patients who do experience serious recurrences? When the breakouts return, three to six months after treatment, they are typically milder, easier to treat, and can generally be cured with a second treatment. Yes, cured. I have to keep repeating that to myself just to comprehend the significance of this drug. To no longer have oily, acned skin is a miracle for anyone who has suffered with problem skin.

By the way, dosage and duration depend on the severity of the patient's acne, but treatments generally last 16 weeks. If a second treatment is necessary, an eight-week rest period is required in between. Interestingly, acne continues to improve even after the course of treatment is completed, although doctors do not know exactly why this happens.

So what's the catch with this "miracle" drug, and why don't doctors prescribe it to everyone? Why hasn't anyone told you about it before? If you've been seeing a dermatologist for acne, the prescriptions are always the same: everything but Accutane, and the acne never really goes away.

Accutane is a controversial drug for many reasons, principally because of its most insidious side effect: it causes severe birth defects in nearly 90 percent of the babies born to women who were pregnant while taking it. Before physicians knew about this alarming hazard, when it was first prescribed in France back in the 1970s, more than 800 babies out of 1,000 births were born seriously deformed.

Roche Dermatologics, the company that produces Accutane, has launched a fervent campaign to inform doctors and patients about the risks involved for pregnant women. Female patients of childbearing age are required to use effective birth control (which includes abstinence) for one month before, all during, and one month after treatment, in addition to having regular pregnancy tests during treatment.

If you aren't pregnant, are there still risks? Yes, but for many reasons they are only somewhat more serious than the risks of taking antibiotics for 10, 20, or 30 years, which for many women is how long their acne lasts.

Other commonly reported, although temporary, side effects are dry skin and lips, mild nosebleeds (your nose can get really dry for the first few days), aches and pains, itching, rashes, skin fragility, increased sensitivity to the sun, and peeling of palms and hands. More serious, although much less common, side effects can include headaches, nausea, vomiting, blurred vision, changes in mood, depression, severe stomach pain, diarrhea, decreased night vision, bowel problems, persistent dryness of eyes, calcium deposits in tendons (doctors don't know yet whether this is a potentially serious problem or a temporary condition, but all indications point to it being temporary), increased cholesterol level, and yellowing of the skin. However, as scary as all that sounds, most patients tolerate Accutane very well. One dermatologist reported that over the past 15 years he has prescribed Accutane to thousands of patients, and only five have had to stop because of negative side effects.

Understandably, most people, doctors included, are scared off by the side effects. Most dermatologists recommend Accutane only to patients with chronic acne (large, recurring cysts or blemishes that can permanently distort the shape and appearance of the skin), or sometimes to people with less severe acne that has not responded successfully to other forms of treatment. Doctors are hesitant to prescribe Accutane liberally, largely because they fear malpractice suits in cases where a patient does experience serious negative side effects or accidentally becomes pregnant. Many doctors won't prescribe Accutane at all.

Although the high risk of birth defects and the other side effects should be taken seriously, it seems a shame that Accutane has been kept secret from many acne patients. It is the most effective drug for acne available today. The public is largely misinformed about its potential dangers as well as its potential benefits. Many doctors believe that if it weren't for proven birth defects, Accutane would be prescribed almost as frequently as antibiotics. Not surprisingly, it is prescribed much more frequently for men.

I wish somebody had told me about Accutane ten years ago! It would have saved me a lot of time, money, and heartache. Although oral and topical antibiotics can work successfully for people who eventually outgrow their acne, the question remains, When are you going to outgrow it? How do you know if you're ever going to? People who don't are looking at years of antibiotics and topical solutions that sometimes work and sometimes don't. Plus, antibiotics can negatively affect the digestive system and create further complications over long periods of time. Accutane seems to be a practical option. (Although some dermatologists might not agree with that assessment, there are many who do.)

Is Accutane for You?

How do you determine whether your acne is short-term or long-term, or, better yet, whether your acne is severe enough to merit taking Accutane? Men often have more severe acne as adolescents, but also have a better chance of outgrowing their acne in adulthood. Many women never outgrow it, while others develop adult-onset acne that can last for years. If you have had acne for five or more years, or if you have acne on your face, chest, and back, it is likely your acne will continue to be a problem. Even if you won't have acne forever, it could continue for another three to ten years. If your skin is manageable or breakouts are infrequent and minimal, Accutane is probably not necessary for you. Assess how much of a problem acne is in your life, what kind of treatment it presently requires, whether the treatment is working to your satisfaction, and whether you are willing to put up with the potential side effects of Accutane. If you have been on antibiotics for several years and don't foresee that changing, if your acne is not responding to current treatments, or if your acne is severe cystic acne, you might want to ask your doctor about Accutane. Doctors, like everyone else, have their biases, so try not to be swayed by one doctor's opinion. I spoke with several dermatologists about Accutane, and their opinions varied. Some felt strongly that Accutane should be taken off the market, while others felt that it was a safe and valuable drug that should be recommended for use more often.

Acne Rosacea

When is acne not acne? Many women and men suffer from a skin condition that closely resembles acne but isn't. The condition is called acne rosacea, but using the word "acne" to describe it is actually quite misleading, because it isn't acne, nor is it treated like acne. Acne rosacea is no fun. This stubborn skin disorder is frustrating and extremely difficult to treat. It is not clear exactly what causes this problem (either bacteria or some other microscopic critter that affects the skin), and there are few, if any, answers or solutions. Rosacea is distinguished by redness and inflammation over the nose and cheek area. The redness is often ignored by women as being just a skin-color problem and not a disease. Another problem with identifying rosacea is that pustules and papules (pimples) that resemble acne are often present. Perhaps one of the most distinguishing characteristics is that rosacea is rarely, if ever, associated with blackheads. The skin is almost always extremely sensitive, however, and both dry, flaky skin as well as severely oily skin can be present at the same time.

Several factors can make rosacea worse. These catalysts include hot liquids, spicy foods, exposure to extreme temperatures (including cooking over a hot stove), alcohol consumption, sunlight, stress, saunas, and hot tubs.

Because blemishes can make rosacea look like acne, many doctors misdiagnose it, prescribing everything but the one course of treatment that can cure it. Only three drugs on the market can successfully treat rosacea: topical drugs called MetroGel and MetroCream, and oral tetracycline. Using the topical cream or gel with the oral antibiotic can often be effective. But first, you and your doctor need to know what you are dealing with. Knowing the difference between acne and acne rosacea can make a definite difference in the health of your skin.

APPLYING MAKEUP BEAUTIFULLY

Step-by-Step Makeup Application

All those foundations that are meant to create the illusion of smooth, flawless skin, and the vast assortment of luscious colors to shape the eyes and add color to the face and lips, enliven the cosmetics counters and displays. The dazzling promise of beauty is yours if you choose the right ones. What you buy and how you put it on are the most important questions for women who choose to wear makeup (and it *is* a choice).

There is an order to dressing your face, just as there is an order to dressing your body. Getting your body dressed involves a certain progression and an array of options, and so does wearing makeup. When you get dressed in the morning, even though it seems automatic, there are a series of choices you make so that you can leave the house feeling and looking great. No one choice is necessarily any more important than any other, but the ones you make definitely affect the way you look: bra and underpants first, then nylons, pants, shirt, and jacket; or no bra and underpants, just nylons, pants, shirt, and no jacket; or bra, underpants, no nylons, skirt, blouse, jacket, scarf, and belt; and the variations go on and on from there. The same sorts of decisions apply to wearing makeup.

For example, I prefer to apply the foundation first (powder is optional, and I often don't use it at all), then the concealer, contour, blush, and finally the eye design. Or sometimes I put on the contour after the eyeshadows are applied. Some makeup artists start with the foundation only over the eye area, follow with the eye design, then apply the rest of the foundation, concealer, powder, blush, and contour. This way any drips from the eyeshadow won't become a permanent part of the makeup. Although I think this approach is too time-consuming, it can work. Experiment to see which order works best for you. Throughout this chapter I will proceed in the order I customarily use, pointing out exceptions and options along the way.

The following list describes possible steps for applying makeup. Which ones you choose are up to you. I think the nuances and permutations are intriguing and part of what makes wearing makeup so much fun. The other part is the fashionable looks you can achieve when it all goes on the way it is supposed to. More in-depth descriptions and explanations can be found in the third edition of my book *Blue Eyeshadow Should Absolutely Be Illegal*.

Step 1—Foundation

As the name implies, foundation is the base for the rest of your makeup. It actually involves two options: foundation and concealer. (Concealer is sometimes called under-eye highlighter or corrector, depending on the company.) The order in which you put on the concealer and the foundation is up to you. The main rule is that the foundation should never be obviously pink, green, orange, peach, rose, ash, or true yellow. Whether you have the lightest shade of Caucasian skin or the deepest shade of African-American skin, your foundation should always be a neutral shade of beige to tan to dark brown to ebony, with no overtones of the aforementioned colors. Please carefully follow my recommendations regarding color in Chapter 7. There are a lot of pink-, peach-, orange-, rose-, and ash-colored foundations out there in many cosmetics lines, both expensive and inexpensive. Don't get this one wrong. Your face is a central focus point, and wearing a color that doesn't match your skin will make you look overly made-up no matter how sheer the foundation is.

Foundation is supposed to match exactly. If you see a color difference between your neck and the foundation, it is the wrong color. A foundation that is a different color than your neck will look like a mask on your face.

Almost every cosmetics line has several styles of foundation for you to choose from. Whether you prefer a liquid (can be formulated for many different skin types), cream (usually for dry skin types), or powder (best for normal to oily or combination skin types), the rule is to choose a lightweight foundation that provides even coverage but that absolutely never looks like foundation. Avoid heavy-duty foundations at all costs. There is almost never a reason to hide your skin under a thick layer of makeup. It always looks artificial. If you have serious facial discolorations or scars to cover, that is another issue, but that is the exception to the rule.

Finding good oil-free foundations is a problem for many women. It's not that you can't find a wide selection of lightweight oil-free foundations, but none of them will stop your oily skin from being oily. Don't be lured by claims of oil control. As I mentioned earlier, many products claiming to be oil-free contain silicone oil. That can be a problem for women with oily skin.

Once you've narrowed down the color and coverage, the only way to tell whether a foundation is the right one for you is to wear it, see how it feels, and check the color frequently in the daylight (along the jawline) to be sure it is an exact match. Texture preference is very subjective. It has to feel comfortable on your skin. Only you can make that decision. Choose carefully; if you get the foundation color wrong, the chances are that all other aspects of the makeup will be wrong too. For this reason I always recommend purchasing a foundation that you can try on before buying it. That makes shopping at the drugstore for foundation almost impossible. If you can't test a foundation, it is probably best not to buy it.

Beauty Note: I never recommend color correctors under foundation. I'm sure you've seen those pink, yellow, mauve, or green concealers that are supposed to go on under your foundation to change the color of your skin before you apply foundation. If your skin is red, you're supposed to put on yellow or green; if your skin is yellow, you're supposed to put on mauve. This step is unnecessary because it doesn't change the skin tone all that well and it can be very tricky to use. You can also end up feeling as if you have too much makeup on the skin. The foundation should be enough if it is the right color. If you insist on checking out color correctors, apply the corrector to one side of your face and then apply foundation all over; if you don't see an improvement, it isn't worth it.

Step 2—Concealer

Apply the concealer next to the inside corner of the eye and gently blend it out along the lower lashes, avoiding the top of the cheek. The goal here is to not see where the concealer stops and starts. Blending is the best way to prevent lines of demarcation. Use your foundation to help soften obvious edges. To help prevent the concealer from slipping into the lines around the eyes, avoid greasy or thick products and apply only a thin layer; it also helps to refrain from using heavy, greasy, or very emollient moisturizers around the eyes. A light (and I mean light) dusting of powder over the face after you apply your foundation will also make a difference, but don't overdo it.

Considering the array of concealers and highlighters on the market, you might think that none of us would have to worry about dark circles again. Unfortunately, in spite of the whopping selection of shades and consistencies, many of the products are either too dark, too orange, too peach, too yellow, too rose, too pink, too greasy (filling in the lines around the eye), too dry, too thick, or too thin. I can understand the different textures—something for every preference—but the strange assortment of shades is beyond me. There is no way a concealer that is darker than your foundation, darker than your skin tone, or tinted peach or pink can make any dark area lighter. If you want to lighten a dark area, you must put a light color on it—something that matches the foundation or, at the very least, doesn't darken it. Concealers in non-neutral tones will alter the shade of the foundation around the eye; the result is an odd color wherever the concealer and the foundation merge, and they must merge in order to look blended. I recommend concealers in neutral tones that are at least one or two shades lighter than the foundation, and there are plenty of those on the market.

I think it is fairly safe to shop for a concealer at the drugstore. The color choices offered there are about the same as at the cosmetics counters, with a good range of consistencies in a handful of shades. Follow my color and texture suggestions, because there are some strange colors out there.

Although I use concealers only under the eye, most cosmetics companies also recommend using concealers to cover blemishes. Covering a blemish with an extra product in addition to the foundation usually builds up too much makeup over the blemish and actually makes it more obvious.

Step 3—Powder

After your foundation and concealer are blended on evenly, with no lines or edges anywhere on the face, you can apply your loose or pressed powder. I generally do not use this step first thing in the morning; instead, I save it for touching up as the day goes by. I prefer the dewy look foundation leaves on the face to the matte, opaque look of powder, but this choice is completely up to you. Powder one side of your face and leave the foundation alone on the other, and see which you prefer.

Some makeup artists work only with loose powder, and some work only with pressed powder. Because loose powder is lighter and doesn't contain waxes, it is considered a better choice than pressed powder, but loose powder is also messy. Pressed powder is easier to use. Whichever you choose, be sure to apply it only with a full brush and never a sponge or puff (that technique is reserved for television or stage). Never build up too much powder, and always knock the excess off the brush before applying it to your face. Too much powder can make the face look chalky, so be careful not to overpowder. For the most part, you can only get away with powdering two or three times a day before the face starts looking thick and heavy.

I guess it isn't surprising that a product as simple and basic as pressed or loose powder can end up with as much marketing hype as any wrinkle cream or skin treatment. The best thing about "setting" or "finishing" powders is that they come in a wider range of colors than ever, in consistencies ranging from silky to sheer. (The more expensive powders do tend to have a silkier feel, but not always.) No matter how silky it is, if you build up too much powder on the skin it will look caked. Many of the expensive cosmetics lines have replaced talc with a range of other absorbent powders, but none of them is any more effective than talc, and some people feel talc is better. There is absolutely no reason to spend a lot of money on pressed or loose powders. This is one area where it is best to shop at the drugstore or in-home sales.

Step 4—Eyeshadow

Eyeshadow application is probably the most challenging facet of wearing makeup, and the one where you can display the most creativity. Eyeshadow offers almost unlimited choices, more than I care to count or can summarize here. Lids can be any color (well, not any, according to me, but the options do exist) in a spectrum of shades from light to medium to dark; underbrow color can be light, medium, or dark; crease color can be medium to dark; and shading at the back corner of the eye can be any rich color or basic black. To fully discuss all these options would take a separate book, and it just so happens that I have written extensively about this very subject in my book *Blue Eyeshadow Should Absolutely Be Illegal.* What I will summarize here are some of the basic rules to be aware of when shopping for and applying eyeshadow.

While color placement is almost completely optional, as a general rule the lighter color goes all over the eyelid, a deeper color follows the crease and back corner of the eye, and a third, lighter color (or the lid color) highlights under the eyebrow.

Avoid shiny eyeshadows. They are still around, but the cosmetics companies have finally caught on, and now it is almost impossible to find a cosmetics line that doesn't have at least a few matte eyeshadows. Sometimes they throw in a little shine, which I still suggest you avoid, but it isn't as bad as it used to be. Just to remind you, the major reasons to avoid shiny eyeshadows are that they make the skin on the lid look wrinkly, and they are as inappropriate for daytime wear as a sequined evening gown. Unless you are wearing a specific evening look, you should also avoid pastel or vibrant-colored eyeshadows. Stick to neutral shades such as tan, beige, brown, sable, chestnut, camel, mahogany, hazel, gray, charcoal, slate, mauve, plum, navy, and so forth. The variations on the neutral theme are endless. Keep in mind that the purpose of eyeshadow is to shade the eye, not color it. Color is provided by the blush and lipstick. You do not want to overcolor the face. Colored eyeshadow is too obvious and doesn't define the eye. Neutral colors can be worn with just about everything and look extremely sophisticated. Greens, blues, lavenders, and bright pinks are best left out of your eye design.

Finally, never use sponge-tip applicators; use only eyeshadow brushes. Sponge-tip applicators pack the makeup on in a layer and tend to drag along the skin, making the powder streak. Brushes pick up a lighter layer of powder and glide over the skin.

Step 5—Eyeliner

You might think that selecting an eyeliner is easy—just choose a brown or black pencil or liquid. But if you want to get creative, the number of options for lining the eye can be astounding: liquid liners in a tube, thin eye pencils, fat eye pencils, automatic eye pencils, eye pencils designed like felt-tip pens, pencils that don't have to be sharpened because the material around the tip peels away, pencils with sponges at one end, pencils with a powder eyeshadow and applicator at one end, waterproof pencils for those who want their eyes to stay lined while they jog in the rain. The different textures produce a wide assortment of looks, from subtle to exotic. Liquid liners and felt-tip-pen eyeliners create a more dramatic, obvious line, while thin pencils or automatic pencils can look either soft or obvious. Many pencils come packaged with a sponge tip at one end for blending (to soften the line) or for shading at the back corner of the eye. How do you choose? It depends on the look you want. Experimentation is the only way to know which ones you prefer.

Beauty Note: Many eye pencils come from the same manufacturing company in Germany, so spending more dollars on eye pencils will not improve the look of your eyes. Regardless of brand, consider using only automatic pencils. They sometimes cost more than regular pencils, but they don't require sharpening, which is extremely convenient.

Additional Beauty Note: I prefer lining with eyeshadows instead of pencils. All I do is use a dark shade of eyeshadow and a tiny eyeliner brush to line my eyes. This can be done either wet or dry. The line can be made to look soft or dark, and it stays particularly well under the lower lashes. This look is also less expensive, because all of your eyeshadows can double as eyeliners and you won't need to buy an additional product. I usually use various shades of brown or black eyeshadow to do my eye lining. It always works great.

Step 6—Eyebrows

Filling in eyebrows is tricky because nothing can make a face look more artificial or dated than "drawn-on" brows. An eyebrow pencil has been the standard choice for decades. If you know how to feather it on so it doesn't look heavy or like a line above the eye it can be just fine to use. Some brow pencils come with a brush at one end, thus encouraging the user to comb through the line and soften it. Although alternatives like eyebrow powders or using an eyeshadow that matches your brow color can look soft and natural, for some reason they have never really replaced brow pencils. If you've been using eyebrow pencil I strongly recommend you try a powder just to see how it works for you. You just may like it and kick the eyebrow pencil habit for good.

My favorite products for the brows are brow gels, both with or without color. These mascara-like products are brushed on through the brow much the way mascara is brushed on through the eyelashes, making the existing brow look fuller, thicker, and darker. It is tricky to get used to using gels, but they do a remarkable job and can even be used in addition to a brow powder. Using the gel and powder together can create a very full, thick brow and, if done carefully, can give a remarkably natural look. Most lines don't include brow gels, but the few that do—Chanel, Borghese, and Lancome—are worth testing for yourself. I prefer Borghese's Brow Milano, but the others aren't bad either.

Step 7—Blush

We all know where our cheeks are, and we all want a soft blush after we apply what was once called rouge, but why does it so often look like stripes, smudges, or patches of color? Applying blush correctly is even trickier than choosing the right color. One of the first mistakes most women make is using a brush that is not full enough. The brushes that come with most blushes are garbage and should not be used. You must purchase a good blush brush in order to do this step correctly. Brush down as you proceed straight back; do not brush in a straight line or it will look like a line. If you follow these instructions, your cheeks will look blushed and not striped or smudged. The way to choose the right blush color is to coordinate it with the color of your lipstick. If your lipstick is plum, your blush should be plum or a mauve-pink. The other consideration is to always choose a color that provides the softest application. Stay away from obvious blush colors.

Almost every cosmetics line now carries several types of blush: standard powder blush, gel blush, and cream-to-powder blush. The cream-to-powder blushes are an interesting alternative for most skin types. They tend to blend easily and merge well with the skin.

Beauty Note: Many makeup artists choose blushes in the peach, tan, or almost beige color families. To me this is not blush, and the results look a little too pale and blanched. I prefer blush in a soft pastel color such as rose, pink, mauve, coral, or plum. All skin types look more alive and tasteful with a blush that is neither too vivid nor too pale. However, the brown blushes are an excellent choice for contouring. For more explanation about this step, refer to my book *Blue Eyeshadow Should Absolutely Be Illegal.*

Step 8—Lipstick

The colossal range of lipstick colors is nothing less than outstanding, and the textures are, for the most part, sublime. Choosing the color is actually more difficult than choosing the cosmetics line you want to buy it from. I often hear women say that one particular company or another has the best lipsticks on the market. The truth is that most cosmetics companies get this one right. The worst assumption a woman can make is that expensive lipsticks are somehow superior to inexpensive lipsticks. That just isn't the case.

Lipstick texture can be creamy, greasy, matte, ultra-matte, and everything in between. Some lipsticks are tinted, which makes the color hang around longer after the creamy part is gone. Avoid shiny, luminous, luster, and pearl lipsticks; they tend to look whitish and even dry as they wear off. Creamy lipstick has enough shine on its own— you don't need to add any more. You should also avoid greasy lipsticks. These are OK for teens, but they simply don't last long enough or have enough color for someone who wants a more sophisticated look.

Most makeup artists will tell you that lip lining is an essential part of getting your lipstick on correctly. I won't argue that lip lining is helpful; I just wouldn't call it indispensable. Unless you have difficulty putting lipstick on evenly, it is only an option—a good option, but nothing more. There are a handful of lip-lining products around, including waterproof lip pencils (if having red lips while swimming is important to you), lip pencils that incorporate a lip brush at one end of the pencil, and automatic lip pencils that conveniently eliminate the need for sharpening. All of these pencils, regardless of their price tag, do essentially the same job. There is little to no difference between a $3 lip pencil and a $22 lip pencil. Most lip pencils come from the same manufacturing company in Germany, so spending more on lip pencils will not improve the look of your mouth.

Step 9—Mascara

If I wear no other makeup, I wear mascara. A good mascara goes on quickly and easily and doesn't flake, smudge, wear off, or clump. If one thing has changed dramatically in the world of cosmetics, it is the quality of mascaras. There are many available in all price ranges that go on beautifully, without clumping or smearing. Buying an expensive mascara simply does not make sense.

Speaking of mascaras, waterproof mascaras do not stay on any better than water-soluble mascaras. Both will smudge and smear if your eye area tends to get oily during the day or if you wear a very emollient eye cream or a moisture-rich foundation or concealer. Oils break up both waterproof and water-soluble mascara.

Waterproof mascaras are also hard on the lashes because they can be removed only with a greasy cleanser that is wiped off. Such wiping can easily pull out delicate lashes.

Step 10—Brushes

Excellent professional makeup brushes are available at most department stores. Please make this a priority. You can buy the most exceptional products in the world, but they won't look right without the right applicators. Many pressed powders, particularly at the drugstore, come packaged with powder puffs. Throw these away and use a brush. Puffs lay too much powder on the skin, making it look thick and overly made-up.

Makeup Fashion

Is blue eyeshadow coming back? Should I tweeze my eyebrows thin like the women on the cover of *Harper's Bazaar* or leave them thick? What about Madonna's latest look—should I try that?

This is where the subject of makeup gets tricky and I get very conservative. There is every reason in the world to be both circumspect and knowledgeable about what is going on in the world of fashion. Mind you, I'm not talking about what is trendy or chic, I am talking about what is currently fashionable. Fortunately, "fashionable" is no longer as narrowly defined as it once was. Actually, in some regards that makes getting dressed that much harder. Deciding what to wear used to be rather straightforward. When bell-bottom pants were "in," that's what you wore. Now every length and width is fashionable, so what do you choose?

Well, you could opt for the good old standby, "I wear only what looks good on me, and damn the fashion world." But to suggest in the same breath that false eyelashes, bright blue eyeshadow, dark brown lipstick, or peach-colored foundation looks good on you is missing the point. I would be the last person to suggest that we should be controlled by the dictates of Madison Avenue and the subsequent pronouncements of the fashion magazines, yet I'm not going to work in go-go boots or a Nehru jacket.

There is a difference between using fashion and being a slave to it. I do want to be fashionable—after all, that's part of being attractive—but when fashion starts working against me, that's where fashion stops and I start. Fashion works against women when it takes away their power, when it makes them little more than made-up dolls with four-inch high heels that are harmful to the back and feet. This book is about having both beauty and power at the same time. Any fashion statement that looks exaggerated, contrived, or overdone, or that wears you instead of the other way around, is not a reliable or even a healthy option for most women. It's not that you can't do what you want, but you should think about what it's doing to your opinion of yourself.

So should you overly tweeze your eyebrows, or wear blue eyeshadow because it is supposedly coming back into fashion, or imitate Madonna or whoever is currently hot? The answer is decidedly no. Many fads in the fashion and entertainment world are better ignored or left to rock stars and wannabes who have nothing better to do.

I always assumed no one really takes seriously many of the fashion statements in the fashion magazines. But then a friend of mine plucked her beautiful, full, expressive eyebrows down to one line of hair across her brow bone. It looked dreadful. Her face seemed constantly surprised, not to mention the after-five shadow and irritation spots from all that plucking. When I asked her what had provoked her to make such a rash decision, she said, "But that's all they're showing in the fashion magazines now." I said, "Yes, it's true, but they show a lot of things in the fashion magazines, like five-inch platform shoes, see-through blouses sans bras, and $2,000 blazers. You can't do everything the fashion magazines consider important—particularly when it hurts, takes too much time, and is blatantly a trend that won't last."

Please, no overly tweezed eyebrows: natural growth with a slight arch only. Why go back to all that tweezing and pain? The grow-back alone makes it too time consuming to even consider.

How do you choose what to follow and what to ignore? Great question, hard answer. Frequently, it is just a gut feeling, a sense that trendy isn't the direction you want to go. Another good guideline is to ask whether something will make you look elegant and sophisticated or showy and conspicuous. True style isn't about blending into a crowd, nor is it about standing out because you look strange. Finding a compromise between those two extremes isn't easy, but it is the essence of combining power and glamour for every woman.

Choosing What Looks Good on You

Unfortunately, this is the hardest thing to write about. I can't evaluate how something looks on you without seeing you. If you're blonde and fair-skinned, a soft bronze lipstick might look beautiful on you, but if your blonde hair comes from a bottle and your skin is sallow, bronze lipstick could make you look sick. If you have vibrant red hair and classic white skin, magenta lipstick or pink eyeshadow could make your face look inflamed and swollen. Once you've established what colors look best on you, you must also consider your lifestyle, the colors in your wardrobe, the look you want to achieve at work and at play, how much makeup you feel comfortable wearing, and the appropriate amount of makeup for each occasion. All of these factors should influence what makeup shades you choose to wear.

There is also the question of taste, individuality, and the effort you're willing to expend on your looks. Besides, you probably have a very specific notion of what makes you look good and what works for you, and there is almost nothing anyone can do to change that opinion. Women have a hard time being objective about themselves. One of the most entertaining portrayals of this challenge was shown in the movie *Working Girl*, with Melanie Griffith and Sigourney Weaver. Weaver plays a successful businesswoman and Griffith is her overly made-up, rather gauche assistant who desperately wants to move ahead in her career. Part of the assistant's game plan involves acquiring a more sophisticated hairdo and wardrobe and more subtle, less obvious makeup. With these changes, along with her natural drive and brains, she makes it to the top. Could she have done the same thing looking the way she did at the beginning of the movie? Highly unlikely. How we look affects the way others see us, and that affects what we achieve in life.

Choosing what looks good when it comes to makeup colors is just like shopping for clothes. It requires patience and trial and error. Find a look in a fashion magazine that you are attracted to, and try it on for size at the makeup counters. This is when getting your makeup done can be so wonderful. The makeup artist might get it wrong, but remember that you are just experimenting, just trying things on to see what looks good.

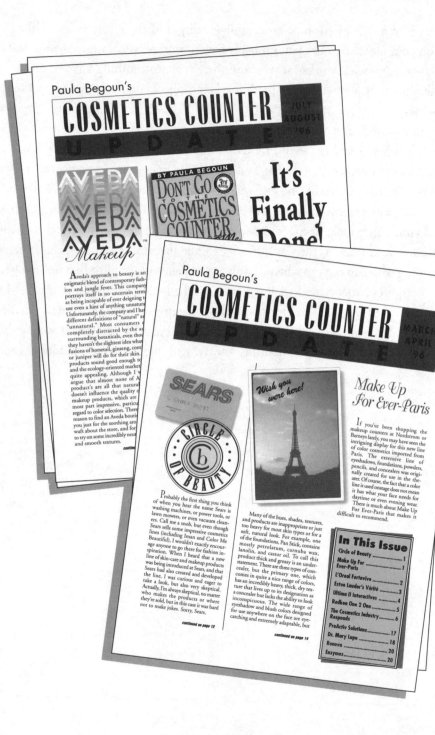

Paula Begoun's
COSMETICS COUNTER
UPDATE
JULY AUGUST '96

Aveda Makeup

Aveda's approach to beauty is an enigmatic blend of contemporary fashion and jungle fever. This company portrays itself in no uncertain terms as being incapable of ever deigning to use even a hint of anything unnatural. Unfortunately, the company and I have different definitions of "natural" and "unnatural." Most consumers are completely distracted by the aura surrounding botanicals, even though they haven't the slightest idea what infusions of horsetail, ginseng, comfrey or juniper will do for their skin. These products sound good enough to eat and the ecology-oriented marketing is quite appealing. Although I would argue that almost none of Aveda's product's are all that natural it doesn't influence the quality of their makeup products, which are for the most part impressive, particularly in regard to color selection. There is good reason to find an Aveda boutique near you just for the soothing aromas that waft about the store, and for the chance to try on some incredibly neutral colors and smooth textures.

continued...

It's Finally Done!

Paula Begoun's
COSMETICS COUNTER
UPDATE
MARCH APRIL '96

Circle of Beauty

Probably the first thing you think of when you hear the name Sears is washing machines, or power tools, or lawn mowers, or even vacuum cleaners. Call me a snob, but even though Sears sells some impressive cosmetics lines (including Iman and Color Me Beautiful), I wouldn't exactly encourage anyone to go there for fashion inspiration. When I heard that a new line of skin-care and makeup products was being introduced at Sears, and that Sears had also created and developed the line, I was curious and eager to take a look, but also very skeptical. Actually, I'm always skeptical, no matter who makes the products or where they're sold, but in this case it was hard not to make jokes. Sorry, Sears.

continued on page 12

Make Up For Ever-Paris

If you've been shopping the makeup counters at Nordstrom or Barneys lately, you may have seen the intriguing display for this new line of color cosmetics imported from Paris. The extensive line of eyeshadows, foundations, powders, pencils, and concealers was originally created for use in the theater. Of course, the fact that a color line is used onstage does not mean it has what your face needs for daytime or even evening wear. There is much about Make Up For Ever-Paris that makes it difficult to recommend.

Many of the hues, shades, textures, and products are inappropriate or just too heavy for most skin types or for a soft, natural look. For example, one of the foundations, Pan Stick, contains mostly petrolatum, carnuba wax, lanolin, and castor oil. To call this product thick and greasy is an understatement. There are three types of concealer, but the primary one, which comes in quite a nice range of colors, has an incredibly heavy, thick, dry texture that lives up to its designation as a concealer but lacks the ability to look inconspicuous. The wide range of eyeshadow and blush colors designed for use anywhere on the face are eye-catching and extremely adaptable, but

continued on page 14

NEWSLETTER HIGHLIGHTS

Cosmetics Counter Update

I began writing and publishing *Cosmetics Counter Update*, a bimonthly subscription newsletter, about five years ago, shortly after the first edition of *Don't Go To The Cosmetics Counter Without Me* was published. Although I had reviewed more than 80 cosmetics lines and thousands of products in the book, some lines were left out, new products were being introduced, an abundance of just-completed cosmetics research was being published, additional information about ingredients was becoming available, and reliable new sources were willing to grant me interviews. Meanwhile, the fashion magazines were still publishing their brand of cosmetics "information" every month, information that was almost always totally one-sided and that supported the cosmetics industry's absurdities.

So I began *Cosmetics Counter Update*. Every issue continues my efforts to bring as objective a voice as I can to the insane world of beauty and fashion, with reviews that evaluate new products and lines, reports on new facts my research has uncovered, straightforward information about skin care and makeup lines, and editorials about the fashion industry's latest dictates. I also devote several pages to answering questions posed by readers.

This effort has been really exciting. It keeps me on top of what is happening in the world of cosmetics and gives the consumer an alternative source of information besides fashion magazines. If you want to see for yourself what the stories and reviews are all about, ordering information is located at the front of this book. To request a one-time introductory copy of *Cosmetics Counter Update*, simply send $1 with your name and address to: **Beginning Press**, 5418 S. Brandon St., Seattle, WA 98118.

In the meantime, here are some of my favorite excerpts from recent newsletters and my newspaper column.

A Change of Testing

As a result of consumer boycotts of cosmetics that are tested on animals, many cosmetics companies have stopped this practice. Now you can add L'Oreal and Lancome to that list. According to James Nixon, executive vice president for Cosmair, Inc. (Cosmair, Inc. is the exclusive U.S. licensee for Lancome and L'Oreal), Lancome and L'Oreal stopped testing their products on animals more than three years ago. The reason they waited to announce that fact publicly last month was their desire to be sure that safety standards were still being met.

Mr. Nixon said that Cosmair has developed in vitro methodologies that can successfully replace animal testing, and the company also has access to an enormous computer bank that provides detailed information about already-existing ingredients that have been tested and how they behave on the skin.

Another Season, Another Show

Did my eyes deceive me, or did the fashion designers stick their collective heads in the sand and produce one more season of clothing embarrassment? Baby-doll dresses, bared stomachs, see-through blouses, and skirts with barely enough fabric to merit the name flowed across runways in mock sincerity. And what fashion season for women looking to spend thousands of dollars on a wardrobe would be complete without body-cinching dresses and double-breast-revealing jackets? Surely the women who buy these frocks don't work at an office, because who would hire (or continue to employ) someone dressed this way?

It's perfectly sensible to stare aghast at these creations, because many designers fabricate them more for the spectacle (and the under-25 market) than for anything else. Attention-grabbing headlines are essential for most fashion houses, and outrageous costumes are the best way to get them. Why the need for this kind of spotlight? Get your name in the media, and a major licensing business can be yours. Popular monikers such as Yves St. Laurent, Bill Blass, Perry Ellis, and Anne Klein grace more products than their namesakes have probably ever seen. Today, the fashion business (at least the part that gets noticed) isn't about ability or genuine design talent, it's about building name recognition.

Toluene-Free Zone

Many women are becoming mindful of the fact that nail polishes containing toluene are a possible health concern (a handful of studies suggest that toluene may cause birth defects). Slowly but surely, nail products are now coming to market without toluene and declaring that fact boldly on their labels. Maybelline, Christian Dior, Elizabeth Arden, and more than a dozen other cosmetics companies have agreed to remove toluene from their nail products, at least in California, a state that has been a leader in cosmetic health concerns for the past several years. Many of these companies also keep toluene out of products distributed to the rest of the country, but you, the consumer, will have to check the ingredient list to be sure. Companies such as Cover Girl, Max Factor, Sally Hansen, L'Oreal, and Lancome have yet to comply.

The Cosmetics Industry Responds

Dear Ms. Begoun,

I have several comments about Murad's Age Spot Gel, Murad's Dry Skin Formula, and the use of alcohol in cosmetics.

Your comparison of the drug Retin-A to the cosmetic properties of alpha hydroxy acids (AHAs) needs clarification. Retin-A and AHAs both encourage exfoliation, but the similarity stops there. Retin-A is an FDA-approved drug indicated for acne and is pending approval for the treatment of photo-aging (under the name Renova Cream). AHAs—specifically, partially neutralized (pH 3.5 to 5.5) glycolic acid in concentrations from 1% to 15%—strictly elicit cosmetic benefits (i.e., smoothness, refinement, and clarity). Since Retin-A causes changes to the dermis and epidermis, it's unlikely that a glycolic acid user would experience any reaction close to the type experienced by a Retin-A user (i.e., dermatitis, photosensitivity, and acute skin dryness). It is unlikely that Murad's Skin Smoothing Lotion or Cream would cause drying. Some individuals experience a mild dryness and/or tautness while the skin begins to [exfoliate].

As you know, there are various types of alcohol used in cosmetic formulations. When SD alcohol is mixed with water and other emollient ingredients, [it is] a highly effective delivery system for other ingredients such as the hydroquinone in Murad's Age Spot & Pigment Lightening Gel. Contrary to what you wrote, the efficacy of our Age Spot Gel doesn't hinge on the amount of AHAs in it. Hydroquinone (2%) is the [lightening] agent.

> Paul Scott Premo
> Director of Education,
> Murad Skin Research Labs

Dear Mr. Premo,

Your information regarding hydroquinone is appreciated. I apologize if the article you read implied that the AHA ingredient in the product worked or enhanced the effectiveness of the hydroquinone. It indeed only exfoliates, which slightly improves the appearance of brown spots (not age spots, as your product indicates, but sun spots, because that's what causes the discoloration). Two percent hydroquinone is the ingredient used in all skin-lightening products and has been for years, and not all that successfully. There is no benefit to mixing hydroquinone with AHAs. Exfoliation helps improve the smoothness of the skin, and the peeling can slightly enhance the lighter appearance of the spots, but the hydroquinone won't work any better than it does by itself.

We disagree about the effect of AHAs in comparison to Retin-A. There seems to be some evidence that Retin-A can rebuild collagen and elastin in the skin, but how much, and whether it is significant in terms of how it affects the long-term appearance of the skin, is yet to be established. Plus, it is clear from the existing research that the skin returns to the way it was, once Retin-A or Renova is stopped. If collagen and elastin was increased it couldn't have been very much as it definitely wasn't stable. Because AHAs are cosmetic ingredients, none of the studies required for Retin-A are being done on them. Who would want to spend the money on AHA research when AHA products are selling so well without it? Without any consequential research, there is no real way to know how AHAs compare to Retin-A. Although you state that it is unlikely that AHA users would experience any of the side effects associated with some strengths of Retin-A (especially the alcohol-based Retin-A gels), much is unknown.

These unknowns benefit companies that make AHA products, such as Murad, because of the money saved on otherwise necessary drug-status research. This is the catch-22 of the cosmetics world—as a cosmetic ingredient, AHAs don't require any research; if it is discovered that AHAs cause changes in the skin, they become a drug and extensive expensive research is mandatory. Therefore, it is best for AHA companies to sit back and be quiet about any possible drug-related benefits so they don't risk having their product taken off the market. Without the research everything is a guess in the world of cosmetics, for both good and bad ingredients.

Finally, SD alcohol in a cosmetic, particularly a liquid, is always a potential irritant, as the alcohol properties are never entirely eliminated. Because of the possible irritation caused by AHAs, the additional irritation caused by SD alcohol is something I never recommend. Some AHA companies have become sensitive to that issue and are producing liquid (or toner-type) AHA products without SD alcohol or other irritants. They might know something you don't (or at least they seem to agree with me).

Dear Paula,

Thank you for taking the time to visit with me yesterday about glycolic acid products. As I mentioned on the phone, Dr. Melvin Elson [who has a long list of accomplishments, including dermatologic surgery and founding the Cosmeceutical Research Institute] attended our Beauty For All Seasons convention in Las Vegas in January 1995. He advised our group that 84 companies were currently using glycolic acid in skin care products, but Beauty For All Seasons and Dr. Elson's brand, AlphaComplex, were among the few companies he was aware of that were using glycolic acid derived from sugarcane.

Dr. Elson spoke for two hours, showing the effects of using sugarcane glycolic acid versus the technical or cosmetic grade of glycolic acid. He explained that the technical or cosmetic grade is made by bubbling carbon monoxide through formaldehyde, thereby getting a cloudy, milky liquid that has a 70% purity and is fairly harsh to the skin. [The pharmaceutical grade, in its pure crystal form called Glypure from Dupont,] is from sugarcane [and is the preferred ingredient].

Paula, I appreciate your openness and frankness and would welcome any further questions you might have regarding glycolic acid or Beauty For All Seasons in particular.

John V. Galazin, President/CEO
Beauty For All Seasons

Dear Mr. Galazin,

You need to check on your sources of information. I called Dupont to check on your assertions about Glypure. After talking to the head of the cosmetic ingredient department, I found out that almost 99 percent of the cosmetics industry, including your company and practically every other company that lists glycolic acid on the ingredient label, is using Glypure from Dupont, and it is not sugarcane-derived as you stated. Rather, it is, as Dr. Elson described, synthesized from formaldehyde and monoxide. Yes, all the glycolic acid Dupont manufactures is chemically synthesized from monoxide (not carbon monoxide) and formaldehyde. That includes their cosmetic or pure-grade form of glycolic acid, which they call Glypure. Dupont does not make any glycolic acid extracted from sugarcane. There are only a few companies in Europe that extract glycolic acid from sugarcane, but that process isn't any prettier a picture than synthesizing glycolic acid from monoxide and formaldehyde. Sugarcane contains only 5% glycolic acid, which is extracted by using such ingredients as formaldehyde, phenol, and other highly corrosive acids. Solvent extraction is no more "pure" or "natural" than chemical synthesis.

By the way, using monoxide and formaldehyde to create glycolic acid is not as lethal or noxious as it sounds. Remember, good old-fashioned table salt is chemically comprised of pure sodium (which can eat through a car) and pure chloride (which can do the same thing), but when combined they create table salt.

Dr. Elson may be a good speaker, but either you misunderstood him or he misled you. You should have called Dupont before teaching your salespeople to say something about your product that just isn't true.

Dear Ms. Begoun,

I felt compelled to respond to your column of October 1995 on acne breakouts referencing the Almay Clear Complexion products. It is a fact that products sold in the United States that purport to treat acne all contain similar active ingredients as defined by the FDA Over-the-Counter Monograph [formal statement of regulation] on acne. Although these ingredients may not cure severe acne, numerous studies show that they are helpful in mild to moderate acne as experienced by most individuals. They will make acne worse only if improperly formulated.

The Almay Clear Complexion Light and Perfect Makeup does have something new to offer. For the first time, the active ingredient salicylic acid has been formulated in a foundation makeup allowing daily wear and coverage as a stable formulation. The end benefit to the consumer is a real treatment makeup that can help clogged pores and inflammatory lesions.

By a pure chemical definition, these formulas may not be oil-free, since they do contain silicone oils. However, the silicone oil is not penetrating and in fact evaporates from the skin, allowing for an easy application without [clogging pores].

Both the scientific literature and a survey of dermatologists would all confirm that sulfur and salicylic acid are helpful ingredients to the acne sufferer. They can be associated with some irritation, but this is a function of the final formula and how frequently [the product is] used. The Almay products have been formulated to minimize their irritation potential.

Please feel free to contact me if you would like to discuss this further or if I can provide further information on this or related topics.

Stanley B. Levy, M.D.
Director, Medical Affairs, Almay

Dear Dr. Levy,

In a brief newspaper column I do not have the space to adequately state how I reached my conclusions regarding over-the-counter acne preparations. However, in both of my cosmetics books I explain at length my disagreement over the years with many dermatologists concerning the use of salicylic acid, alcohol, sulfur, menthol, and camphor in any skin care products, let alone acne products. I have seen and reported on studies that indicate these products have less than a 40 percent improvement rate, but improvement is a very subjective concept. After years and years of personally struggling with acne, and after receiving thousands of letters from women in similar situations, I felt that no company was paying attention to the fact that improvement is not an operative term when the skin is irritated, turns red, dries out, and becomes more oily because of the potential for a rebound effect when you overstimulate oil production. Plus, at the end of the discomfort, you still have acne and blackheads, because, as you state, these ingredients do not represent a cure. Because hardly any acne products containing these ingredients state the potential for irritation, the tendency is for an overeager consumer to buy several acne products, all containing similar ingredients, as well as scrubs, more exfoliants, and drying soaps, which only exacerbate the problem.

It is also important to note that although many dermatologists disagree with me on this point, there are also many who agree with me completely, including cosmetic chemists. Even Procter & Gamble has pulled its salicylic acid products from the market, and many cosmetics companies no longer use alcohol in their toners or astringents. With the advent of AHAs, extensive research on the prescription medication Retin-A, the use of 3% hydrogen peroxide solution or 2.5% benzoyl peroxide, and the availability of nonirritating cleansers, there is no reason to use products that contain potentially irritating ingredients. Actually, nowadays it's a rare dermatologist who encourages the use of sulfur or salicylic acid for acne patients.

In the past I have presented both sides of the coin and will continue to do so when space permits, but I stand by my research and subsequent reviews. If you have any questions regarding my comments, please feel to free to contact me at your convenience.

Invasion of the Thigh Creams

You've seen the products all over the place by now. Remember the headlines? "Swimming in cellulite? Fear no more, researchers have found a cure." A study published in October 1994 claimed that a cream for the thighs containing 2% aminophylline, an oral asthma medication, could trim off inches and reduce the unsightly bumps and lumps of cellulite. Hysteria set in. Hundreds of thousands of women rushed to buy the cream. The companies that were first on the scene racked up sales of over $50,000 a day, and from all accounts are still doing well. Literally overnight, competitors hammered out their own versions of aminophylline cream. Talk shows broadcast stories about the new "dream cream" for weeks. Although the wallets of the companies churning out these creams got bigger and bigger, there was not one little bit of proof that anyone lost an ounce of cellulite by using these creams, according to many scientists, consumer advocates, and health writers.

According to investigative reporting done by Kathy Jones, editor of *Shop!* magazine, a new consumer periodical, the thigh-cream study that triggered the media blitz was riddled with problems that should have sent red flags up the pole and kept consumers' money in their pockets.

Jones discovered that when researchers Dr. Frank Greenway (a private practitioner in Marina del Rey, California, who directed the research) and Dr. George Bray (executive director of Louisiana State University's Pennington Biomedical Research Center, who was not present when the study was conducted) announced their findings at a conference held by the North American Association for the Study of Obesity (NAASO), they did not disclose that six months earlier they had sold the legal right to use their thigh cream to Herbalife International, a maker of weight-loss products that had paid $850,000 in 1986 to settle a lawsuit concerning false claims that its products eliminated cellulite. Revelation of the doctors' deal, first published in the *Tufts University Diet and Nutrition Letter*, prompted NAASO president William Dietz to urge his organization to adopt stricter disclosure rules "to guard against the possibility that some in our society may use their membership to market or endorse their program of treatment."

Another issue not dealt with by the media was Greenway and Bray's research technique. Only 11 women were in the study, which Greenway performed at his Marina del Rey office. Bray was not even present when the study was conducted.

The 11-woman trial hardly amounted to a comprehensive survey. ("Trivial," says Dr. Ahmed Kissebah, chief of endocrinology at the Medical College of Wisconsin and the organizer of the obesity conference.) Greenway told Jones that the women lost an average of 1.5 centimeters after six weeks of using the cream, a difference the Tufts newsletter said would be impossible to detect.

Rather than using sophisticated measuring equipment to confirm fat loss, Dr. Greenway had one of his assistants (a community college student who had never conducted research of any kind before) use only a tape measure, a method that Kissebah called "highly subjective." (Given the fact that there was a thigh cream in the making, there was a strong conflict of interest as well.) Equally suspicious is that many of the 11 women were Greenway's own office workers, which another expert said "poses a potential conflict."

There have been no follow-up studies to the original. Greenway and Bray said a second study exists that had even more impressive results—an average loss of 3 centimeters—but Greenway refused to release any written details. "I'm not going to publish my findings through you," Greenway told Jones. A critical eye is not something Bray or Greenway seems to want right now.

One of the hallmarks of valid scientific research is something called peer review. Published studies are almost always made available to other scientists for their input, feedback, duplication, corroboration, or possible detraction. Thus far, Greenway and Bray have refused to make their data available to anyone, a step experts say is critical in determining whether the fat-melting claims have merit. "If scientists have a product to sell, they have an absolute ethical obligation to make the research available," said Gail Zyla, the Tufts newsletter's senior editor, who reported on the thigh cream.

The only piece of written data on the 11-woman study is a four-paragraph abstract published in the October issue of NAASO's scientific journal, *Obesity Research*.

That bit of information doesn't impress Dr. Richard Dobson, editor of the *Journal of the American Academy of Dermatology*, or Dr. John Renner, head of the Consumer Health Information Research Institute of Kansas City, Missouri. The study "wouldn't get through my purview for a high-school biology class," Renner said. Dobson reported that "there was insufficient data to even evaluate it."

When asked about the second study that Greenway and Bray won't release, Dobson said, "I'd pay no more attention to it than to an office rumor."

After the October conference, sales of Herbalife's thigh cream containing aminophylline, Thermojectics Body Toning Cream, soared. In response to a deluge of requests for the cream and for media interviews, Bray and Greenway issued a press release saying, "To the best of our knowledge . . . there is no product currently on the market using our patented study formula, and there will not be such a product in the near future."

The press release didn't explain why Herbalife was already selling what seemed to be such a product—at $35 for 4 ounces—but Greenway defended his statement, explaining that Herbalife had bought only the "concept" of an aminophylline cream, not the doctors' actual formula—a technicality that upheld the press release, but definitely didn't change the doctors' bottom line.

When it came to appeasing the appetite of women weary of battling their cellulite, competition was the name of the game. A Utah-based company, Neways Inc., rolled out its own version of a thigh cream containing aminophylline, called Skinny Dip. Sales of Skinny Dip began taking a significant bite out of Greenway and Bray's wallets as well as those of their business partner, Dr. Bruce Frome, who had helped them sell their thigh-cream "concept" to Herbalife and was now helping them create a plan to market their own formula. Not to be upstaged, the doctors took Neways to court for false advertising and unfair competition. But they took no action against Herbalife, which also claimed to be the thigh-cream formula "featured in national news."

Instead of doing more research to "confirm the cream's safety and efficacy," as the doctors had stated they planned to do in their aforementioned press release, they sold the license for their formula to Heico, Inc., which owns Nutri/System—a company disciplined by the Federal Trade Commission in December 1993 for making false claims about its weight-loss programs. Heico introduced its Smooth Contours version of the thigh cream in January at $39.95 for 4 ounces and is selling it through Nutri/System diet centers and an 800 number.

Although Smooth Contours avoids making fat-trimming claims, Greenway apparently doesn't. He told Jones that Smooth Contours contains 0.5% aminophylline—the same percentage used in the unpublished second study, in which Greenway claims women's thighs were reduced "an average of 3 centimeters."

A different story was told by attorney and publicist Laurelle LeVine, who is Dr. Frome's wife and now a spokesperson for Smooth Contours. "The studies that Dr. Greenway did [with the 2% cream] showed a reduction in thigh girth," while Greenway's 0.5% solution merely "smoothed thighs," LeVine said. When told that Greenway was still claiming that his 0.5% cream thinned thighs by 3 centimeters, LeVine said, "I'm not familiar with that study."

The FDA's official position, according to spokesperson Mike Shaeffer, is that "the fact that there might be exaggerated claims is not enough for the FDA to get worried about it. The FDA can't jump on every marketing strategy that comes along [for cosmetics]."

Was everyone fooled? "I rejected the story within five minutes," said *New York Times* science writer Gina Kolata. Both the *Times* and *The Wall Street Journal* refused to do stories based on Greenway's research.

Although the financial picture for the thigh-cream companies seems rosy, according to publicist LeVine, the doctors themselves haven't even "recouped the costs of their initial investment" due to high legal fees for pursuing copycat cream makers.

But the doctors aren't taking this lying down (or should I say they are not resting on their dimpled laurels). LeVine told Jones that they are now working on a breast-firming cream. The new offering will use "the same technology as the thigh cream," according to LeVine. When will it come to market? Neither LeVine nor Greenway would disclose the date.

What about scientific studies and research for the new breast-lifter?

"We have to wait until the manufacturer gears up," Greenway said, and then "the publicity can go ahead."

Obviously, what the doctors have learned is that marketing is more important than research when it comes to women's products.

Weird Science?

One of the most frequently asked questions in the entire world of cosmetics is, Which anti-wrinkle products really work? Every month I receive dozens of letters asking me to examine one recently advertised skin care miracle or another. You should see the pile of newspaper and magazine articles and ads for products that claim to stop, reduce, or alter the signs and effects of aging. Over the past few weeks alone I have received 45 letters asking about a wide assortment of products that promise to build elastin, increase collagen, boost cell renewal, enhance the firmness of skin tissue, and on and on. To add credibility to these assertions, the ads feature before-and-after pictures so amazing they would knock the wrinkles off an elephant; in fact, some seem to show just that (I'm not referring to the folks in the ads, just the amazing difference in their appearance). But I'm sure you've heard this all before—and perhaps you've even bought a few wrinkle creams yourself, just in case the startling results were true.

In spite of what you've previously seen and heard, what is particularly insidious about the recent influx of miracle anti-aging products is that not only do the claims and descriptions of these potions sound alluring, but many of the products have been either created or endorsed by extremely reputable chemists, dermatologists, medical researchers, and pharmacists with exceedingly distinguished credentials. How can you argue with that? If a medical researcher at the University of California at Los Angeles (UCLA) claims he has discovered an ingredient—ethocyn, to be specific—that erases wrinkles by building elastin, who wouldn't want to pay whatever it costs to be in on that discovery? If credibility was lacking before, it is now abundantly available, and money is flowing in for the apparently well-documented fountain of youth.

But wait! Duke University reportedly has a study that shows a certain form of vitamin C can prevent skin damage and rebuild skin. That ingredient is used in the product Cellex-C, so wouldn't your money be better spent on this skin-rejuvenating wonder? In the same vein, there's Dr. Albert Kligman's promise of wrinkle-free skin if you use his acne-drug discovery, Retin-A, to stop wrinkles. Shouldn't you run out and get a prescription to stop the inevitable from being inevitable (everybody else has, haven't they)? And let's not forget Dr. Murad, a well-known dermatologist, and his now equally well-known infomercial promising instantly younger skin if you use his products. Isn't that the direction to go? These sources all have loads of credibility. That's exactly what makes them so hard to ignore or shrug off as another cosmetics industry ruse.

Not to be outdone, another UCLA researcher, this one a dermatologist, has supposedly proven that a new product line called Face Life System can do everything possible to stop skin from aging. Yet another age-stopping product, tantalizingly named Envious, has been developed by a Dr. Barry Sears, a former researcher at the Massachusetts Institute of Technology (MIT). How can you go wrong with that? And there are other products too, promoted or invented by other distinguished authorities; but after a while the names and claims start to merge, and the entire subject is blurred by a distorted, almost perverse aura of scientific expertise.

What makes all this so skewed is that besides the research conducted by the doctors who own these products, there are no independent corroborating studies. Every one of the researchers mentioned in this article has a licensed product on the market that retails for between $30 and $75 for a few ounces. When the people who stand to gain monetarily from specific research are the selfsame people who conduct the research and there is no other substantiating research, the findings are at the very least suspect and by most standards completely unacceptable.

According to Dr. Robin Ashinoff, chief of dermatology and laser surgery at New York University, "[Except for Retin-A], when there are no independent researchers substantiating that any of these products can do what they claim, then it remains unproven. By the very definition of scientific research, if the results cannot be duplicated by other researchers, it isn't considered valid."

From a more pragmatic point of view, it is just not possible that every one of these experts has found the secret of reversing aging. If that were the case, drugstore shelves would have a hard time keeping anti-wrinkle products in stock, and plastic surgeons would be closing their doors right and left.

On a technical level, these products don't resemble one another even vaguely. The ingredient lists are as different as night and day, and the specific claims are also diametrically opposed. Except for Retin-A, they are not considered drugs, meaning review and examination by the FDA is almost nonexistent. A $4 bottle of aspirin has to be backed by vast scientific data to support claims of efficacy, while cosmetics require none—not one iota.

What happens when scientists become entrepreneurs? If you take a good look at several of the products mentioned above and below, it becomes clear that the results aren't what they always appear to be.

Chantal Ethocyn

In the May 1995 issue of my newsletter I reviewed a pricey little line of skin care products called Chantal Ethocyn (that review is also included in Chapter 7). Ethocyn supposedly increases elastin by leaps and bounds. It's certainly helped the company's stock price increase by leaps and bounds: it went from $1.25 in December 1994 to $25 one year later.

I'm sure many of you have watched the Chantal Ethocyn infomercial or seen the magazine and newspaper advertisements. Dr. John Bailey, director of the FDA's Office of Cosmetics and Colors, says, "The intense marketing campaign for this product reminds me of what happened with thigh creams two years ago." The Cosmetic, Toiletry, and Fragrance Association lists ethocyn as nothing more than a "skin-conditioning agent." Nonetheless, the product line is being endorsed by a Dr. Richard Strick, a medical doctor from the UCLA School of Medicine.

On the surface, that endorsement is extremely impressive. However, I interviewed several dermatologists and medical researchers, including two doctors who had worked with Dr. Strick at UCLA, and not one was familiar with his work on ethocyn (work that he has been involved with since at least 1986), nor were any of them willing to say that he had discovered anything significant or worthwhile.

Dr. Ashinoff was adamant in her assertion that "because data on ethocyn has never been published in any medical journal and has also not been subject to peer review, it isn't anything I would be interested in." Only one doctor I spoke to was interested in checking out the information I had received on the product; after she did, she was unconvinced but would not go on record with her comments. However, what I was told repeatedly was that building elastin might be helpful for the skin, but without building collagen, which is the major support structure of the skin, at the same time, it may look interesting in the laboratory under a microscope, but it won't help remove a wrinkle. (According to the ethocyn patent, Dr. Strick is in fact claiming that his product builds elastin but decreases collagen.)

My intense skepticism regarding ethocyn was boosted by a personal letter from Strick that accompanied the package of information I received from the Chantal Pharmaceutical Corporation (formerly called Chantal Cosmetics, but that doesn't sound quite so scientific, does it?). The letter states that "[ethocyn] has been around for about 15 years or so from the time it was first discovered . . . [but] this is the company's first product to actually be sold to the general public." That simply isn't true. Chantal Ethocyn, under the name Elasyn, was retailed to the public at Saks and Bloomingdale's back in 1986, while the patent was still pending. It was also advertised in *Vogue, Harper's Bazaar,* and *Elle* magazines. It failed and was removed from the market.

Cellex-C

I also reviewed Cellex-C Serum in a previous newsletter (March 1994) and also for this book in Chapter 7. What makes it relevant to this discussion is the marketing claim that this product is based on research performed by Dr. Sheldon Pinnell, chief of dermatology at Duke University, and Dr. Lorraine Faxon Meisner, professor of preventive medicine at the University of Wisconsin.

The brochure implies that these two esteemed researchers found a way to produce collagen. Their rationale is based on evidence that vitamin C maintains collagen and prevents free-radical damage. According to Meisner, "You can do the same thing for the skin, except more directly, by applying vitamin C directly on the skin." Cellex-C is presumably a unique form of vitamin C that is readily usable by the skin.

As enticing as that sounds, once again there is no way to corroborate their results. Given that Meisner and Pinnell have licensed Cellex-C to Anti-Aging International in Toronto, they have a vested interest in their research. Worse, Dr. Meisner based her findings on empirical evidence (visual analysis only, as opposed to skin biopsies), which means this might be a good moisturizer, but there's no way to know if it produces more collagen.

Meisner explains that in a 30-day double-blind study, two cosmeticians looked at the effects of two products, Cellex-C and a placebo, on 50 subjects, and the Cellex-C side won. Meisner even admits that the double-blind study wasn't truly blind, since by the end of the 30-day trial period the cosmeticians knew which cream was Cellex-C. No other comparison to any other product was done, and no other clinical studies were conducted.

That means all we know about Cellex-C is that it made skin look somewhat better than a single unknown cream—not exactly conclusive evidence. Another claim the researchers for Cellex-C make has to do with its effectiveness over other forms of vitamin C. They insist their form of vitamin C is more biologically available to the skin then others. That might be all fine and good, but, according to Dr. Blumberg Chief of Antioxidant Research Laboratory at Tufts University, "How absorbent or biologically available the vitamin C is, isn't important when it comes to free-radical damage. If you have a vitamin C that absorbs five or even ten minutes faster than another form of vitamin C, that is insignificant when you are discussing a life long chronic problem [sun damage or exposure to air] that occurs every second of every day." Even if Cellex-C does work faster it isn't going to make any observable difference on the skin. Furthermore, Dr. Blumberg added, "there are thousands of antioxidants, vitamin C is only one, there isn't enough research to indicate which antioxidant is the best or in what amount it is needed to be effective for humans."

Without deeper investigation or more comparisons, the research for Cellex-C isn't the kind that should make anyone run out and spend $75 for 1 ounce of product.

Face Lift

Face Lift is a new product line that stands out among the rest, but only for its pretense. According to the literature I received from the company, a Dr. Nicholas Lowe, another dermatologist from UCLA, has been researching this product, which is made by a company called University Medical Products. Although this name sounds as if it is associated with a prominent university, it is not. (Did it have you fooled? It had me going for a while. How cunning to give your company a name that leads consumers to believe something that isn't true.)

Similarly, every claim made for these products leads you to believe you will never have another wrinkle in your life: Face Lift is supposed to prevent free-radical damage, improve oxygenation of the skin cells, and reverse skin damage. Sound unbelievable? Well, it even sounded unbelievable to Lowe. Shockinly, when I called Lowe to ask him about these products and his research, he said, "I never heard of this product and am not conducting any research concerning these products whatsoever."

So what are Face Lift products all about? Basically, Face Lift is a kit with three skin care products that sells for $39.95 (not a bad price for the fountain of youth). The three products are **Prima Hydroxy Cleanser** *(4 ounces),* **Luxury Moisturizer with SPF 15** *(4 ounces),* **and Cell Regeneration Cream** *(1.5 ounces).* Prima Hydroxy Cleanser contains mostly water, plant extracts, thickener, water-binding agents, fruit extract, and more thickener. This is a mediocre cleanser that doesn't remove makeup very well without wiping it off. The fruit extracts are not AHAs, although the name of the product suggests they are. Luxury Moisturizer with SPF 15 is actually a good standard sunscreen for someone with normal to somewhat dry skin. Cell Regeneration Cream contains mostly water, liposomes, a weak cortisone, an antioxidant, thickeners, plant oils, vitamin E, water-binding agents, and preservatives. Although the antioxidants and anti-inflammatory agents are nice, they won't stimulate cell production any more than any other moisturizer with antioxidants. This is a good moisturizer for someone with normal to dry skin, but buying it in hopes of eliminating wrinkles will leave you looking for another wrinkle cream in a few months.

Envious

Another new product that has been showing up in magazines is **Envious Facial Lotion** *($49.95 for 2 ounces)*. Its claim to fame is the use of a special fatty acid that has supposedly been researched and proven effective in fighting wrinkles by Dr. Barry Sears, a biochemist who used to be affiliated with MIT and Boston University but now owns his own company (called Surfactant Technologies). According to Sears, the skin needs "active fatty acids" to maintain moisture and encourage skin renewal. Surprise! Envious Facial Lotion contains just such a fatty acid.

Once again, there is no independent research confirming Sears' findings. Several of the dermatologists I spoke to said that fatty acids are good moisturizing ingredients, but that isn't exactly an amazing claim. Envious contains mostly water, several thickeners, fatty acid, more thickeners, plant oil, vitamin E, water-binding agents, and preservatives. It's a good moisturizer, but there is no objective or corroborating data that indicates it is anything else.

It isn't easy to be skeptical of the work scientists and physicians do, but when the bottom line is money, objectivity is hard to find, at least in the world of cosmetics. As always, even if the packaging and credentials seem to promise scientific proof, if the product sounds too good to be true, it probably is. If any of these claims were even remotely true, these products would be classified as drugs, not cosmetics. As consumers we need to be very skeptical about unsubstantiated research. When there is truly a new wrinkle in the world of skin care, I will let you all in on it, and we can all go out and buy the product and the stock, because it will be worth billions.

By the way, all of the independent researchers I talked to who were doing clinical studies of skin care products that can temporarily smooth wrinkles mentioned the same ones over and over: Retin-A and AHAs. They also all agreed that using sunscreen is the only way to stop wrinkles. See, I told you so.

Ducking Sales Techniques

If women were better prepared to handle the persuasive language they run into when they are buying cosmetics, saving money would be easy. There are many ways to accomplish this, but the best is to know what you need, what you don't, what is optional if you want to splurge, and what you should ignore when a product is being described.

The sales pressure and advertising promises haven't changed since I wrote the first edition of this book. If anything, they have gotten worse and are likely to continue in that direction. Step up to any counter or talk to any cosmetics salesperson anywhere, and you are likely to hear sagas of cleansers that deep-clean, creams that diminish wrinkles, masks that close pores, lotions that feed the skin, and scrubs that rejuvenate the face. Perhaps I would be more forgiving if I felt that women were purchasing products that were really worth the money, but that is rarely the case. There is no reason to spend more than $15 on any skin care product (and even that's high) and if you only splurge on foundations, concealers, and a handful of specialty products, your skin and your pocketbooks would both be happy.

Aside from the sheer waste and expense, I am also unhappy that in so many cases, women are being sold the wrong products. Women with dry skin are told to use toners that contain alcohol or cleansers that dry the skin; women with oily skin are sold moisturizers or oil-free moisturizers, even though their skin isn't dry; and women with normal skin end up with an armload of products in hopes of warding off the inevitable damaging effects of age, sun, and environment.

One of the best ways to equip yourself when shopping for makeup or skin care products is to be aware of what you do and don't need. That isn't as difficult as it sounds. Although everyone's skin is different, some basics are universal. For example, everyone has to clean their face and protect their skin from the sun; however, not everyone needs a moisturizer. A toner may feel good on the skin, but it is not an essential product that will change your skin. The following list outlines what products are necessary, unnecessary, and optional for most skin types.

Necessary: Cleanser, irritant-free toner (really optional, but many women find it an important part of their skin care routine), a sunscreen of SPF 15 in either your foundation or your moisturizer (but not both), an exfoliant (that includes AHA products), moisturizer if your skin is dry, and, for breakouts, a topical disinfectant.

Unnecessary: Eye-makeup remover, wipe-off cleanser, a nighttime moisturizer if you have oily skin, two or more products that contain a sunscreen, facial masks, eye creams (unless the skin around the eyes has different needs that the "face" moisturizer can't address, such as being more dry than the face), throat cream, cellulite cream, emergency skin treatments that are supposed to "repair" your skin in a week or two, and premoisturizer that is supposed to be worn under a moisturizer.

Optional: Bath gel, foot cream (only those that contain salicylic acid or AHAs, because these ingredients can peel calluses; other foot creams are just moisturizers and aren't worth the expense of buying an extra product), Retin-A (not a cosmetic), cuticle cream, and facial masks (only those that do not contain irritants).

Follow this list closely and you can survive most sales pitches because you will know when you should simply say, "No, I don't need that." If all this seems glaringly simple, it is meant to be just that: simple. The cosmetics industry makes things too complicated and involved, and it doesn't have to be that way. I can tell you that using an eye cream or an expensive moisturizer isn't the least bit necessary, but when the attractively dressed sales representative is telling you that it can smooth, refine, restore elasticity, protect, reduce stress, soothe, plump, revive, improve cell turnover, increase moisture, reduce visible signs of aging, firm, repair, hydrate, and diminish wrinkles, and is dermatologist- and ophthalmologist-tested, designed by makeup artists, designed by dermatologists, or designed by pharmacists; and won't cause breakouts, it isn't so easy to remember my warnings. If a you can deflect these come-ons by ignoring them or realizing that they have little meaning, you will be way ahead of the game.

Besides, what it really boils down to is that every product label and every cosmetics salesperson at every cosmetics company in the world says the same thing: that their line is the indisputable, most beautiful best. Now here's the tricky question. How can you tell which of the 300-plus cosmetics lines is telling the truth? Which one really does have a wrinkle cream that smoothes, refines, plumps, and diminishes wrinkles? Can it be that 299 of these lines are deceitful and only one is telling the truth? It gets even more absurd when I inform you that if you wanted to go out today and buy a moisturizer for normal to dry skin, you could choose from among well over 5,000 products. Astounding. I can help narrow the field, but you have to be the one to keep the cosmetics industry in perspective. Remember the following caveats when you consider your next cosmetics purchase.

Beware of hyperbole. Regardless of the product, practically every salesperson earnestly declares that every item in her line is the best available and that it can vastly improve your skin if you use it. The formulations, regardless of the line, are all described as superior—nothing less than phenomenal. There are no phenomenal skin care products; there are only good products. I have yet to see a woman use a skin care product and be cured of acne or lose a wrinkle (and I've been in this field for almost 20 years).

Beware of the authority claim. Every product is promoted as having been tested and certified by the proper scientific authorities, including dermatologists, pharmacists, and ophthalmologists. But physicians do not formulate cosmetics. That is not what they are trained to do. When we called many of the lines that make these kinds of claims, such as Clinique and Physicians Formula, there were no doctors to be found. There were cosmetic chemists, but no physicians. (Actually, I am much more comfortable knowing cosmetic chemists are formulating cosmetics.)

Beware of universal approval. The salesperson assures you that she and all the other people who shop the line can't live without the product(s). Recently, a dignified saleswoman at the Estee Lauder counter told me, "You would be making a big mistake if you don't try Fruition. It's 5 percent of our total line sales. It is the biggest thing to ever come out of Estee Lauder. Everyone loves it. It is perfect for everyone's skin, really." Very convincing. I can understand how easy it must be for consumers to believe what is told them. As it turns out, Fruition is an OK product, but it does not alter the skin or do anything that isn't done even better by less expensive drugstore products such as Alpha Hydrox or Pond's Age Defying Cream.

Beware of special ingredients. A product can contain one or even several novel or unusual ingredients and still not take care of your skin care needs. If you are dead set on finding a product that contains vitamins A, C, and E because they are good antioxidants, you might forget to also look for a high SPF number in your daytime moisturizer or good emollients such as oils and water-binding agents in your nighttime moisturizer. One ingredient does not make a product. Vitamin A (retinol or retinyl palmitate), the other vitamins, thymus extract, yeast, placental extract, herbs, proteins, and amino acids are the least important ingredients, yet they are the ones that attract the most attention. If you disagree with me on this point, that's fine, but please notice that often these "exclusive" ingredients are listed at the end of the ingredient list or after the fragrance and preservatives, which means you are getting a negligible amount of the so-called good stuff. If you really want these ingredients, don't get sold short. They should be in the first half of the ingredient list.

Night Repair

The notion that skin can be "repaired" by a moisturizer is nonsense. Even if the skin did age or get damaged on a daily basis, it could not be mended by any moisturizer, regardless of the exotic-sounding ingredients. Moisturizers cannot reconstruct elastin or collagen, create new cells, or firm the skin. If they could, plastic surgeons would soon be out of a job. Besides, the skin does not break during the day and need fixing at night.

There is no evidence that pollution and stress age the skin; if they did, women in Montana would have far fewer wrinkles than women who live in New York City, and that is not the case. If anything, living in a big city where the sun is blocked by tall buildings, shielding skin on a daily basis, might be a better guarantee of having firm, less wrinkled skin than living in the most unpopulated tropical paradise. Anyway, sun damage, which we know ages the skin, is not immediate but cumulative.

What moisturizers can do, beautifully, is take care of dry skin. Skin cells that dry up can be softened with moisturizer any time of the day. Of course, almost all moisturizers serve that function; that's why they're called moisturizers.

The notion that the skin is more receptive at night has no validity or proof I've ever seen. The same air is around at night, as is dry heat or air conditioning, and that is what does a number on the skin. The only thing missing at night is the sun, but the sun does not prevent the skin from getting the benefits of a moisturizer.

Animal Testing

The new, eighth edition of *Personal Care for People Who Care* is now on my reference shelf, and it's a must-read source for any consumer interested in purchasing products that have not been tested on animals. Published by the National Anti-Vivisection Society (NAVS), this comprehensive guide lists which companies do and do not test their products on animals. According to the book, "Frequently cosmetic companies purchase ingredients for their products from outside sources. With or without the company's knowledge, these ingredients may be subject to animal testing. As a result, it [is] only fair to distinguish 'cruelty-free' companies from those unsure of ingredient and supplier testing status." Companies that do not test their final products on animals, do not use ingredients from suppliers who test on animals, and do not contract for such testing are indicated by a red heart. You can obtain the book by calling NAVS at (800) 888-NAVS; by communicating via e-mail at navs@navs.org; or by writing them at P.O. Box 94020, Palatine, IL 60094-9834. The publication costs about $4.95, but an extra donation is good karma and helps NAVS to continue their work. NAVS even has a World Wide Web site at *http://www.navs.org.*

I was also pleased to read, in an article in *The Wall Street Journal*'s "Marketplace" on October 23, 1995, that a Dr. Marque Todd's work to find alternatives to animal testing is being funded by Mary Kay Cosmetics Inc. (Dr. Todd is one of many researchers working in this field in the United States and abroad as a result of pressure from animal-rights groups.) Even more consequential is an upcoming ban in Europe, starting in 1998, on the sale of any cosmetic tested on animals. Another incentive that encourages cosmetics companies to find other methods of safety testing is the cost and time involved in animal testing. In vitro tests are much less expensive to perform, and the results are often more accurate and quicker to ascertain.

Of course, the sticking point of all this is the FDA's continued contention that the best model for proving cosmetics safety is still animal testing. According to Dr. John Bailey, head of the FDA's Office of Cosmetics and Colors, "Though animal testing isn't perfect, it is the best we have right now." That makes it legally difficult for companies that know animal testing will be required to prove reliability if the FDA calls a product's safety into question. Whether or not the FDA changes its mind on this one won't stop the trend. Consumers all over the world care about the issue of animal testing, and consumer demand drives the marketplace. More often than not, especially in this case, it is a good thing it does.

Cosmetics Cop On-Line

Surfing the Internet is much like floating around in the middle of the ocean. The water is refreshing but there is so much of it that you're not sure you will ever reach shore. Floating around in cyberspace, surfing from location to location, is amazing. Cyberspace is truly a universe unto itself, with a language, protocol, and navigating systems (Yahoo and Web Crawler, to name just two) that are complex and frustrating, yet simple and convenient. Frustration occurs when the computer crashes in the midst of a search, or it takes 15 minutes to find a particular Web page and then, when you get there, the page proves to be an utter waste of time. But what bliss you feel when you finally find what you are looking for, or get information in the blink of an eye that otherwise might have required all day at the library or a local shopping mall or two.

Why am I telling you all this? What can this possibly have to do with cosmetics, skin care, and hair care? Everything. If you think cosmetics counters, drugstores, specialty boutiques, television, and fashion magazines are filled with choices, wait until you see the Internet. A recent search for the words "skin care" brought up over 1,800 selections or possible Web pages.

A Web page, or home page, is a location on the Internet. A Web page might be maintained by just about anyone, from a small business to a major corporation to a university or government agency to a computer-savvy kid who wants her own Web site, or to even someone like me. In addition, there are newsgroups (served by Usenet) that provide continuing discussions on over 12,000 different subjects, including one in particular that is dedicated to issues of fashion.

As someone who owns a publishing company, writes books, and does extensive research, I find the information superhighway completely fascinating (and "fascinating" is a lot better than "intimidating," which is how I regarded it when I first got started). I frequently post to a newsgroup called alt.fashion. Although I am only moderately computer-literate, I have found it to be a wonderful forum for sharing information that women wouldn't necessarily find anywhere else. I have been answering questions and adding my input to ongoing discussions.

I have also developed my own Web page. For those of you who surf the Net, my URL address is *http://www.cosmeticscop.com.* One of the features I'm particularly excited about is offering complete ingredient lists to women in countries where ingredient lists aren't mandatory, which is every country but the United States and Australia. For a small fee per cosmetics line, I can download my database and reviews. Obviously women who are interested must understand English, but if they do they no longer have to be in the dark about what they are putting of their faces and bodies.

If you happen to be looking around the Web, you also might want to check out the FDA's Web page at http://www.FDA.gov. Their information is objective and relatively thorough. I wish they had more, but what they do have is interesting for consumers of cosmetics or any other products the FDA regulates.

> # Look for Paula's web page at
> ## *http://www.cosmeticscop.com.*

CHAPTER

S • E • V • E • N

PRODUCT-BY-PRODUCT REVIEWS

The Process

For the most part, my evaluation process for this edition was the same as for previous editions of this book. I reviewed each cosmetics line for several different elements. The first consideration was overall presentation and how user-friendly the displays were. Many display units had convenient color groupings that divided a majority of the makeup products into yellow and blue tones; this was always considered an asset. Skin care products that were convenient to sample without the help of a salesperson were also rated high. I also applied specific criteria for each of the individual product categories—everything from blushes, to eyeshadows, concealers, foundations, cleansers, toners, scrubs, moisturizers, facial masks, AHA products, brushes and wrinkle creams.

Makeup products were assessed mostly on texture (was it silky smooth or grainy and hard?), color (was a large range of colors available, and was there an adequate selection for women of color?), application (could it be applied easily or was it difficult to spread or blend?), ease of use (was the container poorly designed: were colors placed too close together in an eyeshadow set; was foundation put in a pump container that squirted too much product or didn't reach to the bottom of the jar?); and price (which speaks for itself). Almost every product was rereviewed for this edition.

Skin care products were evaluated almost exclusively on the basis of content versus claim. If a product said it was good for sensitive skin, it couldn't contain irritants, skin sensitizers, or drying ingredients. Almost every product was rereviewed for this edition.

I also asked the following questions: (1) Given the ingredient list, could the product do what it promised? (2) How did the product differ from other products? (3) If a special ingredient or ingredients were showcased how much of it was actually in the product? (4) Did the product contain problematic preservatives or other ingredients?

(5) How far-fetched were the product's claims? (6) Would I use or recommend this product?

I wish I had the space to challenge and explain every single exaggerated claim and lofty explanation that accompanies the products listed in this chapter, but there is just not enough room (or time) to tackle that prodigious task. A book that big would be impossible to lift, let alone read. My goal is to provide you with all the information you need to overcome the sales and advertising pitches so you can focus on a product's quality and feel.

Beauty Note: For a further explanation of specific ingredients, please refer to the Chapter 2, "Skin Care Update" section on "Understanding the Ingredients."

Evaluation of Makeup Products

FOUNDATION: My fundamental expectation for any foundation is that it not be any shade or tone of orange, peach, pink, rose, green, or ash. Consistency, coverage, and feel are also important. All foundations, regardless of texture, need to go on smoothly and evenly, not separate or turn color, and be easy to blend. Foundations that claimed to be matte had to be truly matte, and foundations that claimed to moisturize had to contain ingredients that could do that. Many foundations that claim to be oil-free contain silicone oil, which means they are absolutely not oil-free. That may not be a problem for women with oily skin, particularly if the silicone oil being used is cyclomethicone or phenyl trimethicone, but other silicone oils can feel slippery on the skin.

CONCEALER: Concealers should never be any shade of orange, peach, pink, rose, green, or ash, and they should not slip into the lines around the eye. I looked for creamy smooth textures that went on easily without pulling the skin, didn't look dry and pasty, and, perhaps most important, did not crease into lines. I generally do not recommend using concealers over blemishes, but there is rarely a problem with using most concealers on other parts of the face if they match the skin.

POWDER: Finishing powders come in two basic forms: pressed and loose. I evaluated them on the basis of whether they went on sheer, chalky, or heavy, and whether they were too pink, peach, ash, or rose. I consistently gave higher marks to powders that went on sheer and had a silky soft texture with a natural beige, tan, or rich brown finish. Talc is the most frequently used ingredient in powders in all price ranges, and it is probably one of the best ingredients for absorbing oil and giving a smooth finish to the face. Other minerals are used to this end, but they are not better for the skin.

When it comes to bronzing powders, I generally suggest using them as a contour color and not an all-over face color. Darkening the face almost always looks overdone. After all, if a foundation is supposed to match the skin, how can the use of a powder that darkens the skin be rationalized? The face will be a decidedly different color than the neck, and there will be a line of demarcation where the color starts and stops. Also, most bronzing powders are iridescent. Dusting a color over the face that is darker than your skin tone is one bad enough, but why make it more obvious with particles of shine all over, particularly in daylight?

BLUSH: I considered it essential for blushes to have a smooth texture and blend on easily, and the silkier the feel, the better the rating. I don't recommend shiny blushes. Although they don't make cheeks look as crepey or wrinkly as shiny eyeshadows do the eyes, sparkling cheeks look out of place during the day. Blushes that went on with a sheen or shine but did not sparkle are described with a warning, and are not rated as highly as matte blushes. This is more a matter of personal preference than a problem; you simply should know exactly what you are buying and what you can and cannot expect.

EYESHADOW: It won't surprise you to find out that I don't recommend shiny eyeshadows of any shade or vivid shades of blue, violet, green, or red whether they shine or not. Intense hues may be a personal preference, but I don't encourage anyone to use them. Texture and ease of application played the largest part in determining my eyeshadow preferences. I point out which colors have heavy, grainy textures, because they can be hard to blend and can easily crease. Eyeshadows that are too sheer are also a problem because the color tends to fade as the day wears on. I am also leery of eyeshadow sets that include difficult-to-use color combinations. Many lines have duo, trio, and quad sets of eyeshadows with the most bizarre colors imaginable. Sets of colors must be usable as a set, coordinated in complementary colors; they should never paint a rainbow or kaleidoscope of color across the eye. Generally, it is best to buy eyeshadow colors singly, not in sets. That way you can be assured of liking all the colors you buy, not just two out of three or four.

EYE AND BROW SHAPER: Basically, all pencils, regardless of brand, have more similarities than differences. Most eye pencils, lip pencils, and eyebrow pencils are manufactured by the same company, and whether they cost $20 from Chanel or $4 from Almay, they are likely to be exactly the same. Some pencils are greasier or drier than others, but for the most part there are not marked differences among them. Eye pencils that smudge and smear and eyebrow pencils that go on like a crayon are all rated as ineffective. (Keep in mind that whether an eye pencil smears along the lower eyelashes depends to a large extent on the number of lines around your eye, how much moisturizer you use around the eye area, the type of under-eye concealer you use, and how greasy the pencil is. The greasier the moisturizer or the under-eye concealer, the more likely any pencil will smear, and you can't blame that on the pencil.)

As a general rule, I do not recommend pencils for filling in the brow. I use only powder, and I encourage you to do the same. Any eyeshadow color that matches your eyebrow color *exactly* can do the trick, applied with a tiny eyeliner or angle brush. Brow gel and eyeshadow or brow shadow work superbly together to fill in the brow. A handful of companies make a clear brow gel meant to keep eyebrows in place without adding color or thickness. This works well, but no better than hairspray brushed through the brow on a toothbrush.

LIPSTICK AND LIP PENCIL: Every woman has her own needs and preferences when it comes to lipsticks. Some women like sheer applications; others prefer glossy or matte finishes. Colors are also difficult to recommend because of the wide variation in taste. Given those limitations, I primarily reviewed the range of colors and textures available. The general groupings are gloss, creamy, creamy with shine or iridescence, matte, and ultra-matte. I gave highest marks to creamy or semi-matte lipsticks that go on evenly and aren't glossy, sticky, thick, or drying. The ultra-matte lipsticks (introduced first by Ultima II with their LipSexxxy, and then made overwhelmingly popular by Revlon's Color Stay, which is virtually identical to the former) are unique because of their dry, flat finish and because they don't easily come off on coffee cups or teeth. I evaluated them for how dry their finish is and how well they stay on. Please note that ultra-matte lipsticks can dry out the lips and peel off during the day. I usually don't recommend lip glosses, because they don't stay on longer than an hour or two, while most women want long-lasting lip makeup. I evaluated lip pencils according to whether they go on smoothly without being greasy or dry.

MASCARA: Mascaras should go on easily and quickly while building length and thickness. Brush shape has improved drastically over the years. A brush can be awkward to use if it is too big or too small. Mascara should never smear or flake, regardless of price. A $4 mascara is no bargain if it doesn't go on well. However, no mascara can hold up to a heavy layer of moisturizer around the eyes. If you pile on any kind of moisturizer, whether it be oil-free, a gel, or a product designed especially for the eyes, your mascara will be affected.

Except for swimming and special occasions that may produce tears, I don't recommend waterproof mascaras. Trying to remove waterproof mascara is awful for the eyes and worse for the lashes. All that pulling and wiping isn't good for the skin and tends to pull out lashes. There are dozens of waterproof mascaras out there, but only a handful are truly reliable. I've included those that passed my dunk test in Chapter 8, "The Products I Liked Best."

BRUSHES: Brushes are essential to applying makeup correctly and beautifully. Blush and eyeshadow brushes are offered by some of the major cosmetics lines, and most department stores sell brush sets of some kind. Brushes were rated on overall shape and function as well as the softness and density of the bristles. An eyeshadow or blush brush with scratchy, stiff, or loose bristles was not recommended. Also, let me warn you against buying brush sets. They almost always include brushes you don't need or can't use. It is best to buy brushes individually so you can select the best ones for your needs and for the shape of your face and eyes.

Evaluation of Skin Care Products

While I want to emphasize the extent of the misleading portrayals of skin care products by the cosmetics industry, I also want to underscore what great products *do* exist for all skin types. However, it is difficult for me to describe my elation or enthusiasm about any product without always being careful to let you know what can really be expected and how out of line the price often is for what you are getting.

Every skin care product was evaluated on the basis of what it contains. The ingredients are the basis for whether a claim can be verified. **For every product, I summarize what the ingredients are in the order they appear on the ingredient list (ingredients listed first are the primary constituents of the product) and then what the product can and can't do, based on that prominently displayed but hard-to-decipher data.** This way I can, with a certain degree of accuracy, tell you whether a product will be good for your skin, a potential problem, or a big mistake. I can also let you know how it compares to similar products that cost much less. Of course, you will have to test for yourself how any specific product feels on your skin and how you react to its fragrance or lack thereof.

In the product reviews, I frequently use the phrase "contains mostly," often followed by one or all of the following terms: **thickener** or **thickening agent; slip agent; water-binding agent; film former; detergent cleansing agent** or **standard detergent cleanser; preservative; fragrance; plant extract** or **plant oil; vitamin; antioxidant; soothing agent;** and **anti-irritant.** It was easiest to summarize groups of ingredients by using these general terms, but they need more explanation before you read the reviews.

Beauty Note: When reading ingredient lists, remember that the closer a specific ingredient is to a preservative (such as methylparaben, propylparaben, ethylparaben, imidazolidinyl urea, or quaternium-15) or a fragrance, or the closer it is to the end of the ingredient list, the less likely it is that any significant amount is present in the product.

Thickeners add texture, thickness, viscosity, spreadability, and stability to a product. Thickeners are also vital for helping keep other ingredients mixed together. **Thickening agents** often have a wax-like texture or a creamy, emollient feel, and can be great lubricants. There are literally thousands of ingredients in this category, and they are the staples of every skin care product out there, regardless of the products' price or claims about "natural" ingredients.

Slip agents help other ingredients spread over or penetrate the skin. These include propylene glycol, butylene glycol, polysorbates, and polypropylene glycol.

Water-binding agents are known for their ability to help the skin retain water. These ingredients range from mundane glycerin to the more exotic hyaluronic acid, mucopolysaccharides, sodium PCA, NaPCA, collagen, elastin, proteins, amino acids, and on and on. They all work equally well. Looking for a specific one is a waste of your time and energy. They are what they are: good water-binding ingredients.

Film formers are ingredients such as PVP, methylacrylate, and polyglycerylacrylates presently being used in a vast number of moisturizers, wrinkle creams, and eye gels to help the skin look smoother. Film formers are usually found in hairspray because they place a thin, transparent, plastic-like layer over the hair and keep it in place. They form a similar thin, transparent layer over the skin, and thus help smooth it out. These film-forming ingredients do a good job, but they can be irritants, although they are generally used in small amounts and so are unlikely to be a problem for most skin types.

In products in which an ingredient is included primarily for its sudsing or degreasing ability, such as skin cleansers, I use the term **detergent cleansing agent** or **standard detergent cleanser**. Ingredients in this category include sodium lauryl sulfate, sodium laureth sulfate, TEA-lauryl sulfate, cocamide DEA, ammonium laureth sulfate, and ammonium lauryl sulfate. Because sodium lauryl sulfate, TEA-lauryl sulfate, and sodium C14-16 olefin sulfate are very strong detergent cleansing agents that can dry and irritate skin, I warn against using a product that contains these ingredients in the first part of its ingredient list.

When **preservatives** or **fragrances** are listed in the ingredients I indicate this by simply stating it as such. I have not included specific warnings for preservatives I have mentioned in the past, such as quaternium-15, 2-bromo-2-nitropane-1,3-diol, and phenoxyethanol. At one time research seemed to show that these ingredients posed a higher potential for irritation than other preservatives. More recent data, however, strongly dispute that conclusion. After discussing this matter with several cosmetic chemists, I have concluded that all preservatives can be a problem for many different types of skin, so it would be unfair to pinpoint one specific preservative as a problem. If you are concerned, you can easily avoid any of these ingredients, however, as several cosmetic chemists warned me, a reliable preservative system is better for the skin because microbial contamination of a product causes more problems for the eyes, lips, and skin than the risk of a reaction to a preservative.

On a related matter, some of you may be familiar with research that warns against using cosmetics that contain triethanolamine or TEA-lauryl sulfate along with formaldehyde-releasing preservatives such as imidazolidinyl urea, quaternium-15, 2-bromo-2-nitropane-3,1-diol, or dmdm hydantoin. There is evidence that suggests these combinations can form nitrosamines in a cosmetic, creating a potential carcinogen. There is substantial disagreement among the cosmetic chemists I spoke to as to how significant a problem this is for the skin (or even if it is a problem). They suggested that going out of the house without a sunscreen or sitting in a bar exposed to second-hand cigarette smoke poses more risk to the skin than any combination of skin care ingredients could ever be.

It is impossible to list all the individual **plant extracts** and **plant oils** used in cosmetics. According to the various cosmetics companies, each has its own amazing merits. When a product uses a truly significant plant extract with a known benefit to skin, I point it out; otherwise, I mention these ingredients only under the generic category of plant extracts. Plant oils are almost always beneficial as emollients and lubricants. Some plant oils can be irritants or photosensitizers, and I indicate when this is the case.

I usually list the exact name of any **vitamin** included in a product. Vitamins in skin care products can't feed the skin, but they can work as antioxidants when the product contains enough, and theoretically that can benefit the skin. When specific antioxidant ingredients such as superoxide dismutase, selenium, and glutathione are included, I refer to these specifically as **antioxidants**.

Soothing agents are known for their ability to soothe the skin. A unique but also small group of ingredients function as **anti-irritants**. When either of these types of ingredients are present in a product, such as bisabol, allantoin, or green tea, I refer to them by these terms.

Many products use an assortment of exclusive-sounding adjectives—deionized, purified, triple-purified, demineralized—to describe what is actually just plain water. These terms indicate that the water has gone through some kind of purification process, which is standard for cosmetics. You will also find phrases such as "infusions of" or "aqueous extracts of," followed by the name of one or more plants. That means you're getting plant tea, or plant juice and water. Such products are basically 99% water, but they sound pure and natural, so we think they'll make our skin do better (they won't)

Water is water. The kind of water used does not affect the skin or the final product. After the water is combined with other ingredients, its original status is unimportant.

My reviews of skin care products in each line are, with a few exceptions, organized in the following categories: cleanser, eye makeup remover, exfoliant (scrub), toner, moisturizer (of all kinds), sunscreen, eye cream, specialty products, acne products, and facial masks.

CLEANSER: In reviewing facial cleansers, I was primarily interested in how genuinely water-soluble they are. Facial cleansers should rinse off easily, without the aid of a washcloth, and be able to remove all traces of makeup, including eye makeup. Once a water-soluble cleanser is rinsed off, it should not leave skin feeling either dry or greasy or filmy. And it should never burn the eyes or irritate the skin. Removing makeup with a greasy cleanser is an option for some women but not one I recommend. Wiping at the skin pulls at it and causes the skin to sag. Plus wiping at the skin with a washcloth or Kleenex is irritating.

EYE MAKEUP REMOVER: Virtually all eye makeup removers are almost completely unnecessary. An effective but gentle water-soluble cleanser should take off all your makeup, including eye makeup, without irritating the eyes. Moreover, wiping off eye makeup stretches the skin, which causes the skin to sag faster than it would otherwise. I can't think of any reason to recommend this step unless you are wearing waterproof mascara or can't get the knack of removing your eye makeup with a water-soluble cleanser.

EXFOLIANT: When it came to scrubs I looked for products with the smallest amount of irritants, as well as scrub particles that were uniform in size. You can exfoliate only so much before you start ripping off skin and causing irritation.

My major consideration for alpha hydroxy acid (AHA) and beta hydroxy acid (BHA) products was the percentage of AHAs or BHAs used in the product, with 5% or greater being optimal for exfoliation. As I explained earlier in this book, I prefer AHA products to BHA products; BHA products for the face rarely contain a percentage considered optimal for exfoliation. I am very suspicious of products that claim an association with AHAs but contain ingredients such as fruit extracts or sugarcane extracts, which sound like AHAs but do not necessarily exfoliate the skin. If you want an AHA product that can exfoliate the skin, choose one that lists glycolic acid or lactic acid as the second or third ingredient. That way you can be fairly assured of getting a product with independently researched AHA ingredients and an appropriate pH.

TONER: Toners, astringents, fresheners, tonics, and other liquids meant to refresh the skin after a cleanser is rinsed off should not contain any irritants whatsoever. I evaluated these products on that basis alone. Claims that toners can close pores or refine the skin are not realistic, so I ignored such language and looked primarily for toners that left a smooth, soft feeling on the face and did not irritate it.

MOISTURIZER: In spite of all the fuss surrounding wrinkle creams and moisturizers, this category was actually quite easy to review. Wrinkle creams and moisturizers all do the same thing, so I expected the same thing from all of them: they had to contain ingredients that could smooth and soothe dry skin. Most other claims are exaggerated and misleading. My reviews indicate which products contain unique water-binding agents and antioxidants. I also list the ingredients I think are more hype than help, such as brewer's yeast, bee pollen, placental extract, and many plant extracts. Additionally, I was interested in what order the "good" or "hyped" ingredients were listed on the container. Often the percentage of the most interesting or the most extolled ingredients are so negligible that those ingredients are practically nonexistent. Just because an ingredient is in there doesn't mean there's enough to make a difference.

EYE CREAM: Eye creams are altogether extraneous. For the most part their ingredient lists and formulations are identical to the face creams and lotions sold by the same line. That doesn't mean there aren't some great products out there for dry skin, but why buy a second moisturizer when the one you are already using on the rest of your face is virtually identical? Even more bothersome, most cosmetics companies give you a tiny amount of eye cream but charge you much more for it, despite the similarities.

SUNSCREEN: SPF 8 to SPF 12 is OK for limited daily sun exposure. If you are only going from your car to the office and then to the store, and then driving in your car pool, you will probably be just fine in terms of sun protection. Nevertheless, I still strongly recommend using SPF 15 on a daily basis because you never know how much sun you're really going to get on any given day. Sunscreen ingredients can be irritating no matter what a product's label says, because the way these ingredients work can cause a reaction on the skin. You just have to experiment to find the one that works best for you. Although nonchemical sunscreens use titanium dioxide as the active ingredient and it is considered completely non-irritating, it can clog pores and aggravate breakouts and acne. My main consideration when looking at each sunscreen was to determine which skin type it was best for and whether it contained potentially irritating ingredients.

ACNE PRODUCTS: See Chapter Four, "Clearing the Air on Acne," for an explanation of what I do and don't expect from acne products.

FACIAL MASKS: Most facial masks contain clay-like ingredients, which absorb oil and, to some degree, exfoliate the skin. The problem with many masks is that they contain additional irritating ingredients or ingredients that can clog pores. Although your face may feel smooth when the mask is first rinsed off, after a short period of time problems may be created by the mask's drying effect. As a rule I don't recommend most facial masks. The few clay masks that contain emollients and moisturizing ingredients can still be too drying for dry skin and can cause oily skin to break out. Despite this, for those who are interested, I've pointed out the ones that do not contain any additional irritating ingredients except for the clay.

Beauty Note: I have received many requests from readers asking me to devise a rating system for products. Although I was reluctant at first, it eventually became clear that it would be a useful tool for someone reading quickly through the book or using it as a reference. I came up with the following simple but succinct (and cute) symbols to depict my impression of a specific product:

☺   A great product that I recommend highly, definitely worth checking into or buying.

☺   A possibly OK but unimpressive product, or an OK product that can cause problems for certain skin types. Depending on your personal preferences, it may be worth checking out.

☹   A bad product from almost every consideration, including price.

☺   **$$$** A great product that I would recommend without a doubt were it not absurdly overpriced, either in comparison to similar products or in relation to what you get for your money.

☺   **$$$** An average product whose excessive price makes it not worth consideration.

Because the cost of drugstore cosmetics often fluctuates from store to store, and because cosmetics companies often change prices every six months, the prices listed in this chapter may not be completely accurate. Use the prices as a basis for comparison, but realize that they may not precisely reflect what you will find when you go shopping. Cosmetics companies also change or reformulate their product lines, sometimes in a minor way and sometimes extensively. I report changes of this nature in my newsletter, *Cosmetics Counter Update.*

For the most part, I give only the English names of foreign-produced products. The French and Italian names are pretty, but they don't tell you anything about the product if you don't speak the language.

You Don't Have to Agree

As you read my comments, you may find yourself disagreeing with me. That is perfectly understandable and as it should be, because the criteria you use to evaluate cosmetics may differ from mine. Or, for any one of a dozen reasons, a product I dislike may work well for you. What I present are merely guidelines, based on my experience as well as on extensive research, about what works and what doesn't. If you decide to follow any of my suggestions, be aware that my recommendation is not a guarantee. But I hope I can help you narrow down a very crowded field so you can make the best choices possible.

I want to make a few more points about these reviews. Neither the information nor the evaluations are endorsements, nor do they represent a particular company's sponsorship. None of the cosmetics companies paid me for my remarks or critiques.

The cosmetics are listed alphabetically by brand names, so the order in which they appear does not represent my preference. There is no implied winner among any of the cosmetics companies included; no one line has all the answers or the majority of great products (even my own). Almost every line has its strong and weak points.

I encourage you to take this book with you on shopping trips to the cosmetics counters or the drugstore. Then you will have all the information you'll need readily at hand. There is no way you can remember the details of each product, color, and brand. Do try to be discreet at the department-store cosmetics counters—don't be surprised if you find that using the book in clear view of the salespeople makes them defensive or irritated. There are always risks when a consumer comes prepared with information. I urge you to persevere. Nothing will change at the cosmetics counters if you don't change first.

Beauty Note: Color suggestions were often based on tester units available at the cosmetics counter, samples (including gifts with a purchase or discounted promotions), or products that were purchased. The color, shade, or tone of a particular product can fluctuate for a number of reasons. If I refer to a particular foundation as being "too peach" and you find that it's just right, it may be that we simply disagree, or it may be that the product I tested is different from the one you used. For those women who have read previous editions of this book, you may notice that my reviews for some products have changed. There are four basic reasons why this happens: either I was wrong the first time I checked the product; I have acquired new research that supports a different evaluation; the company changed the product since I last tested it or looked at the ingredient listing; or based on new information I've changed my criteria to include a different perspective then I did when I last updated this book. Whatever the reason, I can assure you the product reviews are all current and that practically every single product was looked at anew for this edition.

Adrien Arpel

Adrien Arpel has been very busy on the QVC channel selling her skin care products, especially her instant face-lift kits. What Ms. Arpel might have overlooked is that the products her company sells at the cosmetics counters are in need of a face-lift, and have been for some time. But from what I've been able to find out, that doesn't seem likely to happen anytime soon. Very little has changed since I first reviewed this line more than four years ago. Skin care seems to be the company's main focus, and they are continually adding some new wrinkle eraser or moisturizer with a colorful-sounding name. Many of the products are too thick and heavy, out of date, or don't work well. For example, all the foundations in this line are supposed to be applied over a mauve "primer" called Porcelain Coverbase, which goes on rather lavender-white. That extra layer can feel uncomfortable. Two of the foundations have no colors I can recommend, and their consistencies are not the best. (Even the salespeople at the Adrien Arpel counters confided that the color choices are poor.) The eyeshadows in this line are almost all too shiny, which is unfortunate, since you can choose any two or three colors for the duo or trio containers (a nice concept because, in theory, you don't end up buying a color you won't use). The blushes are all rather dull shades of mauve, which might be all right for some skin tones, but not for those who want a soft, pastel look. Overall, the color line is sparse and stagnant. The lipsticks are good, but the selection is also small. With all the emphasis on selling the Arpel line on television, the counter service has declined dramatically, and several stores have let go of the line altogether.

Adrien Arpel Skin Care

☺ **Aromafleur Petal Daily Cleanser** *($21 for 4.5 ounces)* is a detergent-based, water-soluble cleanser that would work well for someone with normal to oily skin. It has its share of plant extracts, which are at the end of the ingredient list, but even if they could benefit the skin (they can't) it wouldn't matter, since they all get washed down the drain.

☹ **Foam Cleanser** *($20 for 8 ounces)* is a plant oil–based cleanser that doesn't quite take off all the makeup and can leave a greasy film on the face. It has its share of interesting plant extracts and water-binding agents, but in a cleanser any benefit from these is washed away.

☹ **Freeze-Dried Embryonic Collagen Protein Cleanser, Super Dry Skin Formula** *($20 for 4 ounces)* contains mostly water, a long list of thickeners, animal protein, detergent cleanser, standard water-binding agent, more thickener, and preservatives. This product has several problems: two of the thickening agents are known for causing breakouts, and the detergent cleansing agent is particularly drying and one I don't recommend when found high up on the ingredient list, as it is in this product. The showcase ingredient, embryonic collagen, is calf skin, and although it may be a good water-binding agent, in a cleanser any benefit is washed down the drain.

☹ **Sea Kelp Cleanser** *($20 for 4 ounces)* contains mostly water, mineral oil, thickeners, petrolatum, thickeners, kelp, pumice (scrub agent), more thickeners, algae, and preservatives. This cleanser is really a fairly greasy scrub that uses a rather formidable abrasive (pumice). Despite the name, there's only a small amount of sea kelp, and the mineral oil and petrolatum can leave a greasy residue on the skin.

☹ **Coconut Cleanser** *($19 for 4 ounces)* contains mostly water, safflower oil, propylene glycol, some lanolin, and very little coconut (oil). It will not rinse off without the aid of a washcloth, and all the oils and lanolin can leave a very greasy film on the skin.

☺ **Honey and Almond Scrub** *($32.50 for 5 ounces)* contains mostly glycerin, almonds, thickeners, lemon oil (possible skin irritant), more thickeners, water-binding agents, plant oils, and preservatives. The almonds will help slough skin, although baking soda mixed with a little water will do the same thing for a lot less. Water-binding agents serve little purpose in a cleanser, and almonds can be unevenly ground and rougher on the skin than you may think.

☹ **Lemon & Lime Freshener** *($18.50 for 8 ounces)* is an alcohol-free freshener containing mostly water, slip agents, antioxidants, fragrance, plant extracts, and preservatives. Several of the ingredients are potential skin irritants, including one of the antioxidants and plant extracts such as balm mint, lemon peel, and lime extract.

☹ **Herbal Astringent** *($18.50 for 8 ounces)* contains mostly slip agent, arnica extract, other plant extracts, more slip agents, and preservatives. Arnica is a plant extract that is sometimes used externally for bruises and sprains. It has astringent properties, but for the face, which doesn't get bruised or sprained very often, it can be a potent skin irritant, especially when used every day.

☺ **Bio Cellular Night Cream with AHA** *($35 for 1.25 ounces)* contains mostly water, silicone oil, honey, thickeners, AHAs, more thickeners, several water-binding agents, more AHAs, linseed extract (can be an irritant), RNA, DNA, and preservative. This cream contains about 4% AHAs and an entire arsenal of water-binding agents. It is a better moisturizer than it is an AHA product. The RNA and DNA are almost at the end of the ingredient list, which means the product contains only a negligible amount, but in any case they can't affect skin cells in any significant way, even though they sound very impressive.

☹ **Skin Correction Complex Four Cremes in One with Alpha Hydroxy** *($24.95 for 4 ounces)* calls itself "the only creme you will ever need." What about a sunscreen? You can't do anything about preventing wrinkles until you protect your face from the sun. Now if the topic is exfoliation and smoothing the skin, specifically with AHAs; this cream is only mediocre, with minimal, and I mean *minimal,* AHA content. It contains mostly water, a rather long list of standard thickening agents, malic and tartaric acid, a pH balancer, water-binding agent, plant oil, and preservatives. This product is less than 2% AHA, and the AHAs used are not considered the best for the skin (glycolic and lactic acid are generally considered state-of-the-art AHAs).

☺ **$$$ Swiss Formula Day Cream #12 with Collagen** *($32 for 1 ounce)* is a very emollient, rich moisturizer for someone with very dry skin. It contains water, mineral oil, slip agent, water-binding agent, lanolin, thickeners, plant oils, brewer's yeast, and preservatives. It claims to be nongreasy, but that doesn't jive with the inclusion of mineral oil and lanolin, both fairly greasy ingredients. Brewer's yeast has no effect on wrinkles.

☺ **$$$ Swiss Formula Day Eye Creme, with Vitamin A Palmitate and Collagen** *($27.50 for 0.5 ounce)* contains mostly water, mineral oil, thickener, plant oil, petrolatum, more thickeners, water-binding agents, vitamin A, plant extracts, and preservatives. Vitamin A can be a good antioxidant, but there isn't enough in this cream to do much for the skin. Other than that, this is a good emollient moisturizer for someone with dry skin.

☺ **Vital Velvet Moisturizer** *($22.50 for 2 ounces)* contains mostly water, standard water-binding agent, lanolin, thickeners, mineral oil, more thickeners, oils, collagen, and preservatives. This is a fairly emollient moisturizer and would work well for extremely dry skin only.

☺ **Moisturizing Blotting Lotion** *($23.50 for 2 ounces)* contains water, mineral oil, slip agent, thickeners, lanolin, water-binding agents, lard, more thickeners, soothing agent, and preservatives. This is a very rich moisturizer, best for someone with extremely dry skin.

☺ **$$$ Freeze-Dried Collagen Protein Night Creme and Freeze-Dried Collagen Protein Eye Creme** *($65 for 1 container with each product in a separate compartment)* offers two products. The Eye Creme contains petrolatum, plant oil, thickener, lanolin oil, more thickeners, water-binding agent, and preservatives. The Night Creme is almost identical. These are both incredibly emollient moisturizers, best for someone with extremely dry skin. However, collagen is nothing more than a water-binding agent, and a fairly ordinary one at that.

☹ **Eyelastic Lift** *($40 for capsules and creme)* is a two-part product: you're supposed to mix the **Extra Strength Puff Deflator Capsules** *(45 0.5-ounce capsules)* with the **Eyelastic Lift and Firm Creme** *(0.5 ounce)*. It won't lift the eye anywhere. The Puff Deflator (do you believe that name?) contains mostly silicone oil, water-binding agents, placenta extract (doesn't say whose), and preservatives. The rather common ingredients make for a good moisturizer, but that's about it. Placenta extract can't make your skin one hour younger, no matter where it comes from. The Lift and Firm Creme contains mostly water, water-binding agent, silicone oil, mineral oil, oat flour, plant extract, a long list of thickeners, and preservatives. It works as a paste and contains some moisturizing ingredients. It may have a temporary but OK effect on the skin.

☺ **$$$ Skinlastic Lift** *($40 for 1.7 ounces—18 vials)* contains mostly water, water-binding agent, plant extract, slip agent, more water-binding agents, and preservatives. This is a good, although absurdly expensive, lightweight moisturizer for someone with normal to somewhat dry skin. If you believe it will lift your skin, though, I have a bridge I'd like to sell you.

☺ **Aromafleur Flower Petal and Botanical Extract Masque** *($24 for 4 ounces)* contains water, slip agents, a long list of plant extracts, thickeners, fragrance, and preservatives. There are definitely plenty of plants in here, so if you have allergies this mask could be a problem. Other than that, it is an OK lightweight mask for someone with normal to slightly dry skin.

☺ **Aromafleur Flower Petal Mini-Facial in a Jar** *($29.50 for 4.5 ounces)* contains mostly water, silicone oil, a long list of thickeners, flower petals, water-binding agents, plant extracts, more thickeners, and preservatives. Again, there are definitely plenty of plants in here, so if you have allergies this mask could be a problem. Other than that, it is an OK lightweight mask for someone with normal to slightly dry skin.

☺ **Sea Mud Mask** *($24.50 for 4 ounces)* contains water, clay, alcohol, thickeners, slip agent, talc, more thickeners, soothing agent, and preservatives. There's no sea mud in here. Bentonite, the second ingredient, is clay from the southwestern United States. This is just an ordinary clay mask, and the alcohol and one of the thickeners (PVP, a fixative found in hairsprays) can be irritants.

☹ **Freeze-Dried Collagen Protein Moisture Lock Masque, Super Dry Skin Formula** *($25 for 4 ounces)* contains mostly water, a long list of thickeners, water-binding agent, more water-binding agent, and preservatives. This could be a good mask for someone with normal to dry skin, but don't expect the collagen to do more for the skin than any other water-binding agent. One of the first thickening agents on the ingredient list can cause breakouts.

☺ **$$$ Freeze-Dried Protein Lip Peel and Salve** *($39.50 for 1 ounce of peel and 0.25 ounce of salve)* is a two-part system. The peel contains mostly water, wax, thickeners, soothing agent, water-binding agent, and preservatives. The salve ingredient list reads much like one for an emollient lipstick, with castor oil, petrolatum, lanolin, water-binding agents, and preservatives. This won't get rid of laugh lines and it isn't vaguely worth the steep price tag, but it can feel good over the lips, and the peel will help rub off dead skin.

☹ **Bio-Cellular Lip Line Cream with Alpha Hydroxy Complex** *($22 for 0.5 ounce)* is a mystery. Why would anyone need a specialty AHA product just for around the lips? This one contains mostly water, plant oil, thickeners, water-binding agent, petrolatum, more plant oils, more thickeners, more water-binding agents, AHAs, and preservatives. This is a very emollient moisturizer for any part of the face, but it contains only 1% to 2% AHAs, which means it doesn't have the exfoliating properties of a 5% or higher AHA product.

☹ **Bio-Cellular Night Eye Gelee with AHA Complex** *($26 for 0.4 ounce)* contains mostly mineral oil, lanolin, plant oil, petrolatum, thickeners, plant extract, AHAs, water-binding agents, and preservatives. This is the "greasy kid stuff." If you have extremely dry skin, this product would be just fine, but the small amount of AHAs means they'll work only as water-binding agents, not as exfoliants.

☹ **Underglow Line Minimizing Moisturizer** *($35 for 1.25 ounces)* contains mostly water; thickeners; water-binding agents; aloe; more thickeners; vitamins E, A, and D; plant oil; and preservatives. The vitamins work as antioxidants, which can be good, but other than that, this is a lightweight moisturizer for someone with normal to slightly dry skin.

☹ **Vegetable Peel Off** *($20 for 2 ounces)* contains mostly water, waxes, thickeners, lanolin, plant extracts, and preservatives. It is mostly wax and lanolin, which will peel off skin when you remove it. The plant extracts are almost nonexistent; besides, alfalfa and parsley would have no benefit for the skin even if there were more in the product.

☹ **Wrinkle Peeling Gel** *($32.50 for 3.25 ounces)* contains mostly water, alcohol, film former, slip agents, aloe, plant extracts, antioxidant, and preservatives. The film former leaves a plastic-like layer over the face that, when peeled off, does exfoliate a layer of skin. However, the plants and antioxidant are token, and have little effect at these amounts.

☺ **Oil Control Moisturizer, SPF 15** *($32.50 for 3 ounces)* won't control oil in the least, but it is a good sunscreen. It contains mostly water, slip agent, thickeners, several water-binding agents, soothing agent, and preservatives. The thickening agents and water-binding agents can be a problem for someone with oily skin.

☺ **$$$ Morning After Moisturizer, SPF 20** *($30 for 1 ounce)* seems misnamed— I would put it on *before* going out in the morning. This is a good, basic, lightweight sunscreen/moisturizer. The collagen, the elastin, and the good water-binding ingredients are far down on the ingredient list, though.

Adrien Arpel Makeup

☹ **FOUNDATION: Sheer Souffle** *($24)* is hardly sheer; rather, it can go on heavy and greasy unless you really know how to blend. It would be good only for someone with extremely dry skin, except that the colors are all too peach for most skin tones.

☹ **Glycerin Liquid** *($24)* has an unusual slippery texture, gives light to medium coverage, is tricky to blend, and might take a bit of getting used to. Arpel recommends it for oily or combination skin, but most of the colors are just awful and unsuitable for any skin tone.

☺ **Powdery Creme Foundation** *($25)* has a wonderful consistency and goes on smoothly; it comes packaged with an under-eye concealer, which would be more impressive if the concealer weren't so dark and yellow. **All of these colors are great:** Naturelle (slightly peach), Flesh, Nude, Bare, and Buff.

☺ **SPF 15 Total Sunblock Creme Makeup** *($30)* has a rich creamy texture and provides medium to almost thick coverage. The SPF is great, but there are only four colors, leaving a lot of women out in the cold. **All of these colors are great:** Bisque, Beige Silk, Tawny Beige, and Midnight Suntan.

⊗ **Color Tint Sport Moisturizer** *($20.50)* comes in Light, Medium, Dark, and Bronzer. **They are all too peach**. The bronzer is too shiny, but may be OK for darker skin tones for evening wear.

⊗ **CONCEALER:** Adrien Arpel has a unique concealer system called **Moisturizing Undereye Concealer** *($17)*. The yellow-orange color is too dark for most fair, light, and medium skin tones, and it tends to crease under the eye. It is not meant to be worn alone; rather, it is supposed to be blended over a product called **Coveraway** *($17)*. Coveraway is blue, but goes on kind of whitish blue. (Arpel claims that blue deflects shadows better than white or light beige. I disagree; it just looks off-white under the eye.) **Moisturizing Shadow Undercoat** *($15)* for the eyelid is unnecessary because foundation and powder essentially do the same thing. One of the inherent problems with this line, and many other lines, is the ludicrous number of products the company wants you to use. Case in point: If you use the Shadow Undercoat, the **Porcelain Coverbase** *($23)*, the Coveraway, the Undereye Concealer, *and* foundation, it's quite likely that your face will feel weighed down with makeup, because it is.

☺ **POWDER:** **Real Silk Powder** *($20)* is a pressed powder that comes in three good shades. You aren't getting any serious amount of real silk, although this product does have a soft texture.

⊗ The **Silk Bronzing Powder** *($22.50)* products are all shiny, and I don't recommend them either.

☺ **BLUSH:** I like Arpel's **Mix & Match Cheek Color** *($21.50 for two shades plus compact; $7 per color for refills)*, which offers the consumer an empty container with two sections for individually packaged tins of blush and contour color. It is a cost-effective idea that doesn't require you to buy a color you won't use in order to get a shade you will. Unfortunately, the selection is limited to darker blush colors, many of them intensely shiny. (You can also choose from a selection of pressed powders that come in a nice array of colors, but it isn't very convenient to buy a compact with two pressed powder colors.) **All of these colors are OK:** Contour, Ginger, Apricot, Azalea, Natural Pink (more mauve than pink), Pink Mauve, and Strawberry. The **Powdery Creme Blush** *($21.50)* also comes in a limited range of colors, but the shades are softer and brighter. **All of these colors are good:** Aubergine, Pink, Chocolate (good contour color), and Rouge.

⊗ **EYESHADOW:** Like the blush, **Mix & Match Eyeshadows** *($20.50 for two shades plus compact; $7 per color for refills)* are a great idea, but again the color selection is poor—they're all too shiny. The **Powdery Creme Eyeshadow** *($15)* stays well, but is difficult to recommend because it is difficult to blend evenly. The colors are all matte, but they go on dry and have a tendency to crease.

☹ **EYE AND BROW SHAPER:** Two-Tone Brow Pencil *($12.50)* goes on very dry and hard across the brow, and two colors are not necessary. **Kohl Eye Rimmer Pencils** *($11.50)* comes in four shades, each with a slick, almost greasy texture that smears. **Eye Trimmers** *($11)* are fat eye pencils that are difficult to sharpen and can smear during the day. The **Brow Thickener** *($17)* comes in only one shade, and obviously that color isn't going to suit everyone, but it does thicken the brows and holds them in place.

☹ **LIPSTICK AND LIP PENCIL:** Arpel makes a product called Arpel offers three types of lipstick. **Matte Powder Creme** *($15.50)*, which contains kaolin (clay), goes on almost like a powder, and has a tendency to dry out the lips. **Creme Lipstick** *($15.50)* has a nice consistency but a small selection of colors. **Sheer Lipstick** *($10.50)* is really a lip gloss in a tube. **Lipstick Lock** *($12.50)* is supposed to prevent lipstick from bleeding into the lines around the mouth and keep the color the same all day. It does neither.

☺ **Lip Liner Pencils** *($12.50)* come with a lipstick brush on one end—a nice idea and somewhat convenient, but a decent pencil with a separate lipstick brush would be just as effective and less expensive. This is a lot of money for an ordinary pencil.

☹ **MASCARA:** **Super Brush Mascara** *($14)* isn't all that super. It had smudged and flaked off by the end of a long day and didn't build very thick lashes. **Every Other Layer Lash Thickener and Conditioner & Separating Creme** *($16)* can't "condition" the lashes, but if used before you apply the mascara, it can help make thicker lashes. Of course, the mascara should do that on its own, without the need for an additional product.

Alexandra de Markoff

Alexandra de Markoff was recently bought by a small company called Parlex (it was previously owned by Revlon), and things are up in the air. The salespeople have indicated that the products may be changing soon, but as this book went to press the products listed in this section were current.

Alexandra de Markoff is without question a prestige line of cosmetics. It offers the same illusion of affluence as does Chanel or Borghese. Marketers aim high-end products like these at a certain type of clientele, namely older women with money to spare. The Alexandra de Markoff line has been designed to appeal to women with dry skin. This is most apparent in the foundations, which are either very greasy or very emollient. Even the matte-finish foundation is not all that matte, but it feels very moisturizing, and the ingredient list supports my contention. In general, the line is limited and, for the money, relatively unimpressive.

Alexandra de Markoff Skin Care

☹ **Comfort Cleanser** *($40 for 4 ounces)* is a standard mineral oil–based wipe-off cleanser. This is a lot of money for oil and standard waxy thickeners. The cleanser also contains protein and elastin, but they are only emollients and are useless in a cleanser because they are wiped away.

☺ **$$$ Complete Foaming Cleanser** *($28.50 for 6 ounces)* is a standard detergent-based wash-off cleanser. It is overpriced for what you get, but it cleans the face without leaving it feeling greasy or dry, although it can be too drying for some skin types. At the end of the ingredient list are plant oils and plant extracts, which sound nice but have no function in cleaning the skin; some of them are potential allergens.

☺ **Balancing Cleanser** *($28.50 for 6 ounces)* is a mineral oil–based cleanser that also contains a detergent cleansing agent, thickeners, and a tiny amount of plant oils. This can be a good cleanser for someone with very dry skin, but it may leave skin feeling greasy. An incredibly long lineup of water-binding agents appears at the end of the ingredient list, which means they are barely present, and in a cleanser they don't serve much function anyway.

☺ **$$$ Triple Effect Gentle Eye Makeup Remover** *($22.50 for 4 ounces)* is a gentle but standard eye makeup remover. It is extremely similar to many others that cost a lot less.

☺ **Skin Refining Gel Exfoliator with Comfrey and Lemon Grass** *($28 for 3.8 ounces)*, like many exfoliators, uses synthetic particles that can work as a gentle scrub. There are plenty of plant extracts and oils in this product, including a few that can be fairly irritating to the skin, such as lemongrass and clove oil. It may be OK for some skin types.

☹ **Fresh Solution with Sage and Witch Hazel** *($26 for 7.5 ounces)* contains mostly water, water-binding agent, calamine, clay, witch hazel, plant extracts, more water-binding agents, vitamin B, mineral salts, thickeners, plant oils, and preservatives. This is a lot of money for what is essentially calamine lotion. Several ingredients in here—clove oil, witch hazel, and sandalwood oil—are potential irritants, although the amounts may be too small to be significant. However, calamine has a very strong potential for irritation.

☺ **$$$ Compensation Skin Serum** *($65 for 2 ounces)* contains mostly water, silicone oil, plant extracts (tea water), mineral oil, thickener, plant oils, vitamin A, water-binding agents, and preservatives. This is a good emollient oil for someone with very dry skin, and it contains a small amount of antioxidant.

☹ **Daytime Moisturizer** *($32 for 2 ounces)* contains isopropyl myristate, notorious for causing breakouts; in fact, it's the first ingredient on the list. Otherwise, it contains mostly water, glycerin, thickeners, and preservatives. This is a fairly ordinary moisturizer that would be OK for someone with dry skin who has never had a blemish in her life. However, it isn't best for daytime use unless your foundation is rated SPF 15.

☹ **Fresh Eye Cream** *($45 for 1 ounce)* contains mostly water, thickeners, plant extracts, barium sulfate (a whitening agent that can cause skin irritation), petrolatum, silicone oil, glycerin, several thickeners, vitamins A and E (antioxidants), more thickeners, and preservatives. This product is very expensive, the risk of irritation is significant, and the ingredients are extremely standard.

☺ **$$$ Fresh Moisture Lotion** *($48 for 4 ounces)* contains mostly water, plant extracts, glycerin, several thickeners, vitamin A, plant oils (several that are potential irritants), vitamin E, water-binding agents, silicone oil, and preservatives. This is an OK lightweight moisturizer for someone with normal to slightly dry skin, and it contains a small amount of antioxidants.

☺ **$$$ Moisture Reserve Cream** *($55 for 2.25 ounces)* contains mostly water, plant extracts, several thickeners, silicone oil, water-binding agents, plant oils (several are potential irritants), plant extracts (including balm mint, which can be a skin irritant), vitamins A and E, more thickeners, and preservatives. This is an OK lightweight moisturizer for someone with normal to slightly dry skin, and it contains a small amount of antioxidants.

☹ **Oil-Free Matte Moisture** *($38 for 4 ounces)* contains mostly water, witch hazel, several thickeners, vitamin E, water-binding agents, vitamin A, plant extracts, acrylates, and preservatives. It is definitely oil-free, but it contains several potential skin irritants, including witch hazel and an acrylate like that found in hairspray. Using this moisturizer can cause more problems than it can help.

☺ **Skin Refining Gel Exfoliator** *($28.50 for 3.8 ounces)* can indeed exfoliate the skin, and relatively gently. It does contain several plant extracts and oils, including lemongrass, clove oil, and sandalwood, that can cause the skin to flake or cause irritation.

☺ **$$$ Enriched Night Care** *($45 for 2 ounces)* is definitely rich. It contains mostly water, thickeners, petrolatum, more thickeners, slip agent, and preservatives. This is an incredibly ordinary moisturizer for someone with very dry skin. The second ingredient is isopropyl myristate, which can cause breakouts.

☺ **$$$ Skin Renewal Therapy Restorative Eye Cream** *($42 for 0.5 ounce)* won't renew anything, but it can be a good, though absurdly expensive, moisturizer. It contains mostly water, thickeners, plant oil, more thickeners, water-binding agents, silicone oil, anti-irritants, and preservatives.

☺ **$$$ Sleep Tight Firming Night Cream with Comfrey** *($60 for 1.7 ounces)* boasts one of the most amazing lists of ingredients I've ever seen. It contains mostly water, a very long list of thickeners, slip agent, silicone oil, water-binding agents, vitamin E, more thickeners, more water-binding agents, more thickeners, plant oils (many are potential skin irritants), and preservatives. There isn't enough comfrey in this product to warrant a mention, much less title billing. This won't firm the skin, but it is an OK moisturizer for someone with normal to somewhat dry skin, and it does contain a small amount of antioxidant vitamins.

☺ **$$$ Skin Tight Firming Eye Cream** *($50 for 0.35 ounce)* won't firm skin, but it is very emollient—good for someone with dry skin. It contains mostly water, thickeners, slip agents, shea butter, a long list of additional thickeners, film former, antioxidants, several water-binding agents, plant oil, silicone oil, and preservatives.

☹ **Vital 10 New Age Skin Complex with Marigold, SPF 6** *($65 for 2 ounces)* isn't vital, it's pointless. SPF 6 isn't adequate to protect the skin from sun, and that what's really needed to fight wrinkles.

☹ **Extra Help Gel for Lips** *($20 for 1 ounce)* contains mostly water, slip agent, thickener, film former, thickener, water-binding agent, and preservatives. This offers minimal help for dry lips. It has almost no emollients or skin softening ingredients. It can put a film over the lips to make them look temporarily smooth but it won't feel very good, particularly in the winter.

Alexandra de Markoff Makeup

☹ **FOUNDATION: Countess Isserlyn Makeup** *($45)* is a mineral oil–based foundation in which the mineral oil floats on the top and the color lies at the bottom. You have to shake this product really hard to get it to mix together, and even then it tends to separate on the skin. Some of the colors are OK, but several are very peach and shouldn't be worn by anyone. If you have seriously dry skin you may want to consider this, but it is a greasy mess more than anything else. **Colors to consider:** 81 1/2, 82 1/2, and 92 1/2. **Colors to avoid because they are too pink or peach:** 71 1/2, 72 1/2, 76 1/2, 86 1/2, 98 1/2, and 99 1/2.

☹ **Countess Isserlyn Moisturizing Matte Makeup** *($45)* is identical to the makeup above except it uses silicone oil instead of mineral oil. Although it feels less greasy, it is hardly matte. The oil in this foundation still rises to the top, and the color sits at the bottom of the bottle. Chances are pretty good the color will streak or separate on the skin when blending. **Colors to consider:** 72 1/2, 81 1/2, 82 1/2, 86 1/2, and 92 1/2. **Colors to avoid:** 76 1/2, 91 1/2, and 96 1/2.

☺ **$$$ Countess Isserlyn Creme Makeup** *($45)* is more than creamy—it is very rich and emollient. The third ingredient is lanolin oil, which makes it appropriate only for someone with extremely dry skin. It has a rich texture and provides medium coverage. **Colors to consider:** 72 1/2, 81 1/2, 82 1/2, and 92 1/2. **Colors to avoid because they are absurdly peach or pink:** 76 1/2, 86 1/2, 89 1/2, 96 1/2, and 99 1/2.

☺ **$$$ Countess Isserlyn Soft Velvet Makeup Oil-Free** *($42.50)* isn't oil-free—it contains silicone oil—but at least this product is completely up-front about that; it indicates as much on the back of the label. This very emollient foundation provides medium coverage that feels quite soft and relatively velvety. Soft Velvet Makeup is the best of the line's foundations, although the color choices are pretty limited. **Colors to consider:** 82 1/2, 88 1/2, and 92 1/2. **Colors to avoid because they are too pink or peach:** 71 1/2, 72 1/2, 86 1/2, 91 1/2, and 96 1/2.

☺ **$$$ Countess Isserlyn Powder Creme Finish Makeup** *($32.50)* is a very soft cream-to-powder makeup that has a wonderful feel on the skin. This foundation has the best colors in the entire line. **Avoid these colors:** 76 1/2, 96 1/2, and 98 1/2. **The other colors are beautifully neutral**.

☺ **Sheer Advantage** *($25)* is a tinted moisturizer with SPF 8, which is OK for limited sun exposure, but the tint may not be good for most skin tones.

☹ **CONCEALER:** The **Concealer** *($18.50)* comes in three very good colors and has a good consistency, but it can crease into the lines around the eyes.

☺ **$$$ POWDER: Moisturizing Pressed Powder** *($30)* is a standard powder that comes in four very good colors and has a wonderful soft, silky texture, but it is far more drying than emollient.

☹ **Moisturizing Loose Powder** *($35)* has a soft texture but is on the dry side, and the colors aren't impressive.

☺ **$$$ <u>BLUSH:</u> Cheek Chic** *($30)* is a cream-to-powder blusher with a good soft texture and an attractive selection of soft colors. Chic Spice is a good contour color, while Chic Bronze has more shine than anyone needs.

☹ **Moisturizing Powder Blush** *($30)* isn't even slightly moisturizing; all the colors are shiny, and I do not recommend any of them.

☹ **<u>EYESHADOW:</u>** The line offers a small selection of duo eyeshadow sets called **EyeShapers** *($27)* and trio sets called **Professional Palette Eyeshadow Trio** *($34)*. The duo sets have one basic problem: one of the colors in each set is either shiny or strange. The trio sets contain only shiny, iridescent colors. Preselected eyeshadow sets are a waste of money.

☺ **$$$ Professional Palette Eyeshadow Singles** *($27)* are expensive, but a handful are matte and come in soft neutral shades. **Colors to consider:** Buff, Chamois, Beige, Taupe, and Caviar. **Colors to avoid because they are too shiny:** Smoke, Beaujolais, Tea Leaf, Pink, Peach, Celadon, and Night Light.

☺ **$$$ <u>EYE AND BROW SHAPER:</u> Eye Definer** *($18.50)* is a standard eye pencil similar to dozens of other pencils on the market. You guessed it: overpriced and nothing to write home about. **Soft Effect Brow Pencil** *($18.50)* is essentially identical to the Eye Definer, except that both sides have color. I imagine that's so you can stroke on multiple colors. Not a bad idea, but complicated and unnecessary, and pencils aren't the best way to fill in brows.

☺ **$$$ <u>LIPSTICK:</u>** It was easy to predict that Alexandra de Markoff would have a lipstick similar to Revlon's ColorStay. It's called **Lips Like Hers** *($17.50)*, probably because Revlon used to own de Markoff. It is nothing more than a knockoff with a higher price tag and less impressive colors. **Lasting Luxury Lipsticks** *($16.50)* are shiny and somewhat creamy, with a slight tint, so they have some staying power. I don't prefer iridescent lipsticks, but these aren't bad, just not interesting enough for the money. **Under Color for Lips** *($25)* comes in two colors: Clear and Neutral. It is designed to keep lipstick from bleeding, which it does, but it also tends to peel and feel dry. **Lip Definer** *($18.50)* is a standard pencil. One side has the color and the other a lipstick brush. Nice touch, but Max Factor's lip pencil is similar and costs only one-fourth as much.

☹ **<u>MASCARA:</u> Professional Finish Mascara** *($18.50)* builds surprisingly long lashes but, strangely enough, it doesn't build any thickness. If you already have thick lashes, this may be an option, but is there a woman alive who thinks her lashes are thick enough?

☹ **Lash Amplifier** *($18.50)* is a clear mascara that is supposed to enhance the lashes, but it's no better than an extra coat of mascara. Besides, if the regular mascara is any good, why would it need an amplifier in the first place?

Almay

Almay has a long-standing reputation for being one of the few lines that is 100% hypoallergenic. (Given that the FDA has never issued specific guidelines about which ingredients are less likely to cause allergic reactions, this is an admirable marketing feat.) For the most part, Almay does a good job of eliminating well-known irritants such as fragrance, formaldehyde compounds, lanolin, and lauryl sulfate compounds. But those may not be the ingredients that cause your particular skin problems.

There are several areas in which Almay excels. It makes some of the best mascaras, blushes, and lipsticks I've tested, and it also has a superior under-eye concealer that comes in a tube and has a creamy, soft texture. The line also has some excellent skin care products and one of the largest selections of moisturizers I've ever seen. On the other hand, Almay's color selection is a bit sparse.

Almay Skin Care

☹ **Anti-Bacterial Foaming Cleanser** *($3.50 for 7.75 ounces)* is a standard detergent-based water-soluble cleanser that contains menthol, which can burn the eyes and irritate the skin. It does contain the antibacterial agent triclosan (the same one found in Acne-Statin products), but the effects of any disinfectant are lost in a cleanser because it is so quickly washed away.

☺ **Deep Cleansing Cold Cream** *($3.50 for 4 ounces)* is a traditional mineral oil–based cold cream that needs to be wiped off and will leave the skin feeling greasy. I don't recommend wipe-off cleansers, although if you're looking for cold cream, this is a good one.

☺ **Deep Cleansing Cold Cream Pump (Water Rinseable Formula)** *($2.72 for 8 ounces)* isn't all that rinseable. It contains mineral oil, and that's hard to rinse off with water. It may be good for someone with very dry skin.

☹ **Cold Cream Cleansing Bar** *($2.25 for two 4-ounce bars)* is a standard bar soap that contains mineral oil to help cut the irritation from the soap. However, the soap is still irritating.

☺ **Moisture Balance Cleansing Lotion for Normal Skin** *($5.25 for 7.25 ounces)* is a mineral oil–based cleanser that does not rinse off well without the aid of a washcloth, and it leaves some makeup behind. If you have normal skin you will find this cleanser somewhat greasy, but if you have extremely dry skin and use a washcloth (which I don't recommend because of irritation), it is passable.

☺ **Moisture Renew Cleansing Cream for Dry Skin** *($4.50 for 4.75 ounces)* is similar to the lotion above, and the same review applies.

☺ **Sensitive Care Cleansing Cream for Super Sensitive Skin** *($4.48 for 3.75 ounces)* is almost identical to the cream above, and the same review applies.

☹ **Sensitive Skin Foaming Cleanser** *($2.79 for 7.75 ounces)* is a detergent-based water-soluble cleanser that isn't all that special for sensitive skin, except that it does contain anti-irritants. This would be good for someone with oily skin, but it could be drying and irritating.

☹ **Time-Off Age Smoothing Cleansing Lotion** *($7.99 for 7.25 ounces)* is a standard mineral oil–based cleanser that contains methoxypropylgluconamide (the ingredient found in Revlon's Alpha Recap), a good water-binding agent that doesn't have much purpose in a cleansing lotion. This cleanser doesn't rinse off all that well, and it tends to leave a greasy film on the skin.

☹ **Moisture Renew Facial Soap for Dry Skin** *($2.09 for 3.5 ounces)* is soap with some mineral oil. Soap dries the skin and causes irritation, and mineral oil can't change that.

☹ **Oil Control Cleansing Gel for Oily Skin** *($5.49 for 7.25 ounces)* is a detergent-based water-soluble cleanser that can be good for someone with oily skin, but it is only a cleanser. There is nothing in it that will control or stop oil. It does contain a small amount of menthol, which can irritate the eyes.

☹ **Oil Control Complexion Scrub** *($6.50 for 4 ounces)* is a detergent-based water-soluble cleanser with abrasive scrub particles. It can be irritating to some skin types, and it won't stop or control oil.

☹ **Moisturizing Eye Makeup Remover Lotion** *($3.75 for 2 ounces)* and **Moisturizing Eye Makeup Remover Pads** *($2.80 for 35 pads)* are just mineral oil and some slip agents. They will wipe off eye makeup, but they also make a greasy mess.

☹ **Moisturizing Gentle Gel Eye Makeup Remover** *($4.03 for 1.5 ounces)* is similar to the lotion above, only in gel form. It's still mineral oil, and it's still fairly greasy.

☹ **Non-Oily Eye Makeup Remover Lotion** *($3.75 for 2 ounces)* and **Non-Oily Eye Makeup Remover Pads** *($2.80 for 35 pads)* are indeed non-oily; they are just lightweight detergent cleansing agents that cut through makeup. They are OK, but the numerous cleansers in this line should be fine for removing eye makeup.

☺ **Non-Oily Eye Makeup Remover Gel** *($4.03 for 1.5 ounces)* is similar to the lotion above, and the same review applies.

☹ **Moisture Renew Balance Toner for Dry Skin** *($5.25 for 7.25 ounces)* contains mostly water and alcohol, and can irritate the skin.

☹ **Moisture Balance Toner for Normal Skin** *($5.25 for 7.25 ounces)* contains ingredients almost identical to those in the toner above, and it too can irritate the skin.

☹ **Oil Control Astringent for Oily Skin** *($5.49 for 7.25 ounces)* contains mostly alcohol and salicylic acid. When will someone get the hint that this combination doesn't control oily skin, it makes it worse?

☹ **Time-Off Age Smoothing Toner** *($7.99 for 7.25 ounces)* would be a rather soothing toner with methoxypropylgluconamide (among several other good water-binding agents), but the second ingredient is witch hazel, and that can be a skin irritant.

☹ **Sensitive Care Toner for Super Sensitive Skin** *($5.49 for 7.25 ounces)* is similar to the toner above, and the same review applies.

☺ **Moisture Balance Moisture Lotion for Normal/Combination Skin** *($7 for 4 ounces)* lists mineral oil as the second ingredient, and also contains several thickeners, film former, plant oil, and even a tiny amount of Vaseline. Now, who in the world with combination skin would be happy with this formula? It could be good for someone with dry skin, though.

☺ **Moisture Renew Moisture Lotion for Dry Skin** *($7 for 4 ounces)* is almost identical to the lotion above, and the same review applies, which means it is just fine for someone with dry skin.

☺ **Moisture Balance Moisture Lotion SPF 15 for Normal/Combination Skin** *($7.39 for 4 ounces)* is similar to Moisture Balance Moisture Lotion above, only with sunscreen. The same review applies.

☺ **Moisture Renew Cream for Dry Skin** *($5.27 for 2 ounces)* contains mostly water, mineral oil, thickeners, slip agent, water-binding agent, film former, vitamin A, plant oil, and preservatives. This would be a good moisturizer for someone with dry skin, but the label suggests that it is greaseless, which is a stretch, and the tiny amount of vitamin A is insignificant for the skin.

☺ **Moisture Renew Firmasome with Ceramide Liposomes for Dry Skin** *($7.14 for 1 ounce)* contains mostly water, glycerin, thickeners, slip agent, several water-binding agents, and preservatives. "Firmasome" is a silly made-up word, but this is a good, very interesting moisturizer for someone with dry skin.

☺ **Moisture Renew Moisture Lotion for Dry Skin SPF 15** *($7.39 for 4 ounces)* contains mostly water; slip agent; glycerin; silicone oil; vitamins E, A, and C; film former; several thickeners; and preservatives. This is a very good sunscreen for someone with dry skin, and it contains antioxidants.

☺ **Moisture Renew Night Cream for Dry Skin** *($7 for 2 ounces)* contains mostly water, thickeners, mineral oil, slip agent, glycerin, more thickeners, petrolatum, plant oil, vitamins A and E, and preservatives. This is a good but ordinary moisturizer with antioxidants for someone with dry skin.

☺ **Moisture Balance Eye Cream for Normal Skin** *($5 for 0.5 ounce)* is a very rich cream that would work better for extremely dry skin than it would for normal skin. It contains petrolatum, lanolin oil, mineral oil, propylene glycol, water, and paraffin.

☺ **Moisture Renew Eye Cream for Dry Skin** *($5.70 for 0.5 ounce)* contains mostly water, thickener, mineral oil, glycerin, slip agent, plant oil, more thickeners, petrolatum, water-binding agents, soothing agent, vitamin A, film former, and preservatives. This is a good moisturizer for dry skin, with a minuscule amount of antioxidant, but it is not as good for dry skin as the cream for normal skin above.

☹ **Oil Control Lotion for Oily Skin** *($7 for 4 ounces)* contains two types of silicone oil, which will not help control oil. In fact, other than talc, there is nothing in it that will control oil.

☺ **Oil Control Lotion for Oily Skin SPF 15** *($7.39 for 4 ounces)* is similar to the lotion above, only with sunscreen. It may be an option for someone with oily skin, but it won't control oil.

☹ **Oil Control Overnight Treatment for Oily Skin** *($5.32 for 4 ounces)* has many problem ingredients, including alcohol, silicone oil, and film former. It does contain anti-irritants, which are helpful, but nothing in the product will stop oil.

☹ **Oil Control Anti-Blemish Gel for Oily Skin** *($4.75 for 2.3 ounces)* contains a surprise: salicylic acid in an acne product (that's my attempt at serious sarcasm). It also contains silicone oil and oil-absorbing agents. It's OK but potentially irritating, and some of the thickening agents can be a problem for oily skin.

☺ **Clear Complexion Moisture Lotion 100% Oil-Free SPF 8** *($8.64 for 1.7 ounces)* contains mostly water, slip agent, silicone oil, glycerin, more slip agents, thickeners, salicylic acid, vitamins, water-binding agents, more thickeners, and preservatives.

This product is not 100% oil-free in the least. It is just a basic salicylic acid-based exfoliant that has some good moisturizing properties. This one is quite similar to Clinique's Turnaround Cream, only it's much less expensive and has an SPF 8, which is OK for limited sun exposure.

☹ **Clear Complexion Moisture Cream 100% Oil-Free SPF 8** *($8.64 for 1.7 ounces)* is almost identical to the one above, only the consistency is thicker; the same review applies.

☺ **Perfect Moisture** *($4.79 for 4 ounces)* causes me to ask, If this one is perfect, what are all the other Almay moisturizers for? This one contains water, slip agent, glycerin, silicone oil, thickeners, petrolatum, vitamins A and E, more thickeners, and preservatives. This is a good simple moisturizer for someone with dry skin, with a small amount of antioxidants, but it isn't perfect or all that different from several other products in this line.

☺ **Sensitive Care Cream for Super Sensitive Skin** *($5.32 for 2 ounces)* contains nothing to ensure that it is good for sensitive skin. It contains mostly water, slip agent, petrolatum, glycerin, several thickeners, vitamins E and C, film former, and preservatives. It is a good ordinary moisturizer for someone with dry skin, and it contains a small amount of antioxidants.

☺ **Time-Off Age Smoothing Moisture Lotion** *($8.69 for 2 ounces)* is a rather good moisturizer for someone with dry skin, and it has antioxidants. It contains mostly water, water-binding agents, several thickeners, vegetable oil, vitamins E and A, soothing agent, more thickeners, and preservatives.

☺ **Time-Off Age Smoothing Night Cream** *($9.69 for 2 ounces)* is similar to the lotion above, with the addition of a few fancy water-binding agents. This would be a very good moisturizer for someone with dry skin.

☺ **Time-Off Age Smoothing Moisture Cream** *($8.69 for 2 ounces)* is similar to the cream above, and the same review applies.

☺ **Time-Off Age Smoothing Moisture Lotion SPF 15** *($7.39 for 4 ounces)* is similar to the Time-Off moisturizers above, but with sunscreen, and the same review applies.

☺ **Time-Off Age Smoothing Eye Cream** *($6.49 for 0.5 ounce)* is almost identical to the moisturizers above, only somewhat more emollient. An eye cream isn't necessary, but this is still a good moisturizer.

☺ **Time-Off Wrinkle Defense Capsules with Micro-Fillers** *($8.23 for 0.29 ounce)* contain mostly silicone oils, slip agent, water, water-binding agents, vitamins E and

A, more water-binding agents, and preservatives. If you're looking for a substitute for Elizabeth Arden's Ceramide Capsules, this is a convincing alternative for far less money.

☺ **Time-Off Wrinkle Defense Cream with Micro-Fillers** *($8.30 for 2 ounces)* is similar to the capsules above, but with sunscreen, and the same review applies.

☺ **Stress Cream** *($10 for 1.9 ounces)* contains mostly water, slip agent, thickeners, mineral oil, plant oil, water-binding agents, vitamins E and A, film former, soothing agent, and preservatives. Like many of the moisturizers in this lineup, it is good for dry skin. It can't counteract stress, as its name implies, but it will improve dry skin and contains a small amount of antioxidants.

☺ **Stress Eye Gel** *($7.50 for 0.5 ounce)* contains mostly water, film former, slip agent, water-binding agents, and preservatives. Like many products that contain film-forming agents, it can temporarily make skin look smooth. It is a good lightweight moisturizer.

☺ **Anti-Irritant** *($1.25 for 0.3 ounce)* contains mostly water; petrolatum; thickeners; aloe; anti-irritants; vitamins A, C, and E; film former; and preservatives. It is a good moisturizer for dry skin, with several anti-irritants and antioxidants.

☺ **Replenishing Lotion** *($6 for 1.8 ounces)* is a lightweight moisturizer for normal to slightly dry skin, with a small amount of antioxidants. It contains mostly water; standard water-binding agents; thickeners; water-binding agent; vitamin A, C, and E; soothing agent; thickeners; and preservatives.

☹ **Moisture Balance Cleansing Mask for Normal Skin** *($4.50 for 2.5 ounces)* is a standard clay mask that contains mostly water, clay, alcohol, more clay, thickeners, and preservatives. This won't balance the skin, and it can be quite drying for most skin types.

☹ **Oil Control Clay Mask for Oily Skin** *($4.50 for 2.5 ounces)* contains water, clay, preservative, detergent cleanser, slip agents, more clay, and more preservatives. It won't control oil, and it is potentially irritating.

Almay Makeup

☹ **FOUNDATION:** Almay's foundations include **Moisture Renew Foundation for Dry Skin** *($4.51)*, **Moisture Balance Foundation for Normal to Combination Skin** *($4.51)*, **Moisture Oil-Control Foundation for Oily Skin** *($4.51)*, **Time-Off Age Smoothing Makeup** *($5.52)*, **Sensitive Care Formula SPF 15 Cream to Powder Foundation** *($4.89)*, **Sensitive Care Formula SPF 8 Liquid Makeup** *($4.70)*, **PowderWear Pressed Powder Foundation** *($5.71)*, and **Liquid to Powder**

Makeup *($5.64)*. Unfortunately, testers are not available for any of them. That's regrettable, because some have excellent textures and very good color selections. But no matter how good the foundation, if you get the color wrong, it looks bad.

☹ **Clear Complexion Light and Perfect Makeup** *($4.50)* claims to be oil-free and nonirritating, and to contain proven anti-acne ingredients. None of these claims are true. The second ingredient is silicone oil; the "anti-acne" ingredients have not been proven to be all that effective; and they are not nonirritating. The foundation contains salicylic acid, which peels the skin to some extent but is also a skin irritant, and irritating the skin can make it more oily. **Clear Complexion Compact Makeup and Powder In One Step** *($6.92)* is a good cream-to-powder makeup but, like the Light and Perfect Makeup, it contains salicylic acid, which can be a problem for the face. **Moisture Tint Sports Foundation** *($4.11)* is supposed to be waterproof, but it's not.

☺ **CONCEALER: Cover-Up Stick** *($3.43)* is a good concealer that comes in three workable shades: Light, Medium, and Dark. The lipstick-like applicator helps it go on creamy, but not greasy, and it tends not to crease in the lines around the eyes. This one is definitely worth looking into, although the consistency may be too moist for someone with oily skin. **Extra Moisturizing Undereye Cover Cream** *($3.43)* comes in three excellent shades: Light, Medium, and Dark. It goes on somewhat greasy, though it is anything but extra-moisturizing. It dries to a matte, almost powdery finish. It isn't best if you have lines around the eyes or dry skin, but it doesn't crease in the lines around the eyes, and that's great. **Time-Off Age Smoothing Concealer** *($4.38)* doesn't erase wrinkles, but it goes on smooth and doesn't crease. The color selection, though small, is terrific.

☹ **Clear Complexion Acne Blemish Concealer** *($3.43)* contains sulfur, which is drying and irritating and can cause problems for someone with acne-prone skin.

☺ **POWDER: Moisture Renew Pressed Powder for Dry Skin** *($4.70)*, **Moisture Renew Pressed Powder for Normal to Combination Skin** *($4.70)*, **Moisture Renew Oil-Control Pressed Powder for Oily Skin** *($4.70)*, **Time-Off Age Smoothing Pressed Powder** *($5.52)*, **Clear Complexion Light and Perfect Pressed Powder** *($4.51)* are all good possibilities except that each is packaged in a box that prevents you from getting a peek at the real color.

☺ **BLUSH: Cheek Color** *($3.95)* and **Brush-On Blush** *($6.50)* are very similar and both are excellent; the latter comes with an attractive mirrored compact. Most of the colors are matte. **These colors should be avoided:** Blush, Mid Pink, Soft Rose, Soft Bronze, and Peach.

☺ **EYESHADOW:** Long Lasting Eyecolor Singles *($2.40)*, **Duos** *($2.82)*, and **Quads** *($4.19)* come in a small but good color selection; they go on soft and blend nicely. The shades labeled matte actually have a slight amount of shine, but not enough to show up. The shades labeled shiny are indeed shiny, though, and should be avoided. **Amazing Lasting Eyecolor** *($4.50)* comes in a lipstick-like applicator, goes on very smooth and creamy, and dries to a powdery finish. It comes in a small but exceptionally neutral group of colors. It is supposed to last up to 12 hours, but most eyeshadows last that long and then some. I don't prefer this type of eyeshadow because blending or layering can be tricky, but it is an option for a one-shadow look.

☹ **EYE AND BROW SHAPER:** **Eye Defining Liquid Liner** *($4.79)* is a standard liquid liner that can create a very dramatic line. It doesn't budge once it dries, but it does dry matte. **I-Liner** *($4.36)* is a good liquid liner that goes on smoothly and easily, creating a thick, dramatic line without flaking or looking crinkled. There's nothing soft and subtle about this product. **Amazing Lasting Eye Pencil** *($3.79)* is a standard pencil in a twist-up, no-sharpen pen applicator. It's nice but not amazing.

☹ **Kohl-Formula Eye Pencil** *($4.75)* is an incredibly greasy pencil that smudges and smears easily. **Wetproof Shadow Liner** *($3.57)* is another greasy pencil. It isn't all that waterproof, and it wipes off easily and tends to smear and smudge. **Soft Brow Color** *($3.51)* is a standard pencil that tends to be greasy rather than soft, with a brow brush on the cap.

☺ **LIPSTICK AND LIP PENCIL:** **Color Basic Lipstick (with or without SPF 4)** *($4.46)* goes on fairly greasy for a basic lipstick, but the color selection is quite nice. **Demi Sheer SPF 15 Lip Color** *($4.14)* is more of a sheer gloss and doesn't stay on very well, although SPF 15 provides good protection from the sun. **Lip Opaque Lip Color** *($4.40)* goes on fairly matte rather thick. It can easily feather into the lines around the lips, contrary to the claim on the package. **Glossy Lip Shine** *($3.20)* is a basic gloss, but a good one. The automatic **Lipcolor Pencils** *($4.95)* are excellent, with a dry but smooth texture.

☺ **MASCARA:** **One Coat Mascara** *($4.95)* and **Mascara Plus** *($4.95)* create beautiful lashes without clumping or smearing, and the price is right! However, the term One-Coat isn't true in the least; it takes several applications to get the length and thickness you want. **Triple Thick Mascara** *($3.99)* builds long, thick lashes and has good staying power.

☹ **Amazing Lash** *($3.99)* goes on almost too fast and thick. It builds incredible length and definition, but it also tends to clump. If you're looking for thick and long, this product delivers, but you will have to keep a small toothbrush or lash comb nearby to work through the clumps. **Longest Lashes Mascara** *($4.75)* is a good mascara, but not in comparison to those reviewed above.

☹ **Perfect Definition Mascara** *($4.79)* is slow going; it takes forever to get even a little thickness.

Alpha Hydrox by Neoteric (Skin Care Only)

Alpha Hydrox Lotion and Alpha Hydrox Face Creme were two of the more reasonably priced and effective alpha hydroxy acid products that first appeared on the market when the AHA craze was launched four years ago. While other companies often hedge when telling you how much AHA their product contains, Alpha Hydrox is more than forthcoming. The AHA in its products is glycolic acid, which is considered one of the best, and the pH of the products is at an effective level. If you are interested in trying an AHA moisturizing or cream-type product, I encourage you to start here. The prices and the product quality are excellent. One word of caution: To capitalize on the success of its two showcase products, Alpha Hydrox has introduced an additional 12-plus products to its line, including several that have no AHA content. The non-AHA products are nowhere near as impressive, but there are some interesting and reasonably priced products to check out.

☺ **Foaming Face Wash** *($5.50 for 6 ounces)* is a standard detergent-based water-soluble cleanser that does not contain AHAs. It can be good for someone with normal to oily skin, but may be too drying for other skin types.

☹ **Toner-Astringent for Normal to Oily Skin** *($5.50 for 8 ounces)* contains mostly water, alcohol, witch hazel, slip agent, glycolic acid, chamomile extract, menthol, pH balancer, and preservatives. The chamomile can't counterbalance the irritation caused by the alcohol and menthol.

☺ **Oil-Free Lotion for Normal to Oily Skin** *($8 for 4 ounces)* contains mostly water, thickeners, silicone oil, more thickeners, anti-irritant, vitamin E, preservatives, and film former. It isn't oil-free, but it may be OK over dry patches for someone with normal to oily skin.

☺ **Hydrating Eye Gel** *($9.50 for 0.5 ounce)* is an average lightweight gel that contains mostly water, slip agent, water-binding agent, aloe, thickener, and preservatives.

☺ **Daily Lotion for Normal Skin** *($8 for 4 ounces)* contains mostly water, thickeners, glycerin, more thickeners, silicone oil, vitamin E, water-binding agents, and preservatives. This would be a good moisturizer for someone with dry skin only. One of the thickening agents can cause breakouts.

☺ **Night Replenishing Creme for Normal to Dry Skin** *($8.50 for 2 ounces)* contains mostly water, mineral oil, thickener, glycerin, plant oil, more thickeners, silicone oil, vitamin E, water-binding agents, and preservatives. This would be a very good, though standard, moisturizer for someone with dry skin (but not normal skin). It contains a tiny amount of antioxidants.

☹ **Oil-Free Facial Gel for Partly Oily and Oily Skin** *($8 for 4 ounces)* contains water, alcohol, slip agent, glycolic acid, pH balancer, thickener, and preservative. Alcohol serves no purpose but to further irritate and dry out the skin. That makes the skin more likely to react negatively to the AHAs.

☺ **Enhanced Creme All Skin Types 10% AHA** *($9.50 for 2 ounces)* contains mostly water, glycolic acid, pH balancer, slip agent, thickeners, silicone oil, more thickeners, and preservatives. This is a good high-percentage AHA product, but it is not appropriate for all skin types. The thickening agents could be a problem for someone with normal to combination skin.

☺ **Sensitive Skin Creme 5% AHA** *($7.89 for 2 ounces)* contains mostly water, slip agent, thickener, glycolic acid, more thickeners, pH balancer, silicone oil, and preservatives. It's a simple but emollient base for someone with dry, sensitive skin who wants a less intense concentration of AHAs.

☺ **Lotion for Normal to Dry Skin 8% AHA** *($8.64 for 6 ounces)* contains mostly water, glycolic acid, pH balancer, water-binding agent, thickeners, petrolatum, more thickeners, and preservatives. This is a very good 8% AHA moisturizer, but it is best for someone with normal to slightly dry skin.

☺ **Hand and Body Lotion 8% AHA** *($8 for 6 ounces)* is a very good AHA product for the face and the body that is quite similar to the lotion above, and the same review applies.

☺ **Creme 8% AHA for Normal Skin** *($8.64 for 2 ounces)* contains mostly water, glycolic acid, slip agent, thickeners, pH balancer, more thickeners, silicone oil, and preservatives. This is a very good AHA moisturizer for normal to dry skin types.

☺ **SPF 15 Moisturizing Daily Lotion** *($7.58 for 4 ounces)* contains mostly water, pH balancer, thickeners, glycerin, more thickeners, vitamin E, water-binding agents, silicone oil, and preservatives. This is a good sunscreen for someone with normal to dry skin, but the pH balancing ingredient, triethanolamine, is listed second, which means there is a significant amount in there, and that can be irritating for many skin types.

Amway

There are a lot of people selling Amway products throughout the world, and unless you have been living in a shell or on a mountaintop, someone by now has likely approached you with the opportunity to either share in the theoretical wealth or at least become a customer. One of the more notorious aspects of multilevel selling (really a pyramid hierarchy with an automatic cut-off point, but the people involved hate the term "pyramid") is that besides being encouraged to buy the products, you are likely to be asked (or converted) to start a small, part-time business of your own. I have written before about my extreme skepticism regarding what I perceive to be the in-home sales line Pledge of Allegiance. It goes something like this: "I do hereby pledge that all the products my company sells are perfect and wondrous, they are the best thing(s) ever made, and the customers, including myself, are lucky to have the opportunity to use them as well as sell them." That just gets to me.

Surely you can be a good salesperson without being a "believer." If you believe all your products are perfect, then a customer's objections have no value. There is little room for earnest consumer awareness with this attitude. As one Amway sales representative said to me, "Why would the company make anything that wasn't wonderful?" I responded by saying, "I don't know, but it happens all the time. No one's perfect. Sometimes executives make mistakes. Companies aren't God, they're just businesses. Moreover, if Amway cosmetics were so perfect, why was it necessary to revamp the entire line [which Amway did this past January]?"

Obviously, no cosmetics line is perfect, although Amway did do a pretty good job of revamping its products. If you want to shop in the privacy of your own home and enjoy being able to test the products, I encourage you to consider taking a look at Amway's skin care and makeup lines. I hope this doesn't mean I've unleashed a monster on any of you who have an Amway representative in your area. Make it clear from the beginning that you are interested only in buying. If you *are* interested in selling, try hard not to be converted to the in-home selling religion; just be a very good, consumer-compassionate salesperson.

I had to get that off my chest, but what is more important is the number of agreeable items in the Artistry by Amway line: the skin care routine is simple enough (if you don't get waylaid by the extra specialty products), and some of the moisturizers are impressive; the foundations are excellent, and the colors are very workable for many skin types; and there are several matte eyeshadow shades, some beautiful blush colors, and a nice range of under-eye concealers. These are the line's strongest points. Unfortunately, the weak points are really weak: the concealer pencil is on the dry side and would be appropriate only for oily skin types; the lipsticks are on the greasy side and easily bleed into the lines around the mouth; there are too many shiny eyeshadows and blue eyeshadows (which is just unforgivable); the facial cleansers aren't the best; and the specialty skin care products make an otherwise simple cleansing system complicated.

Artistry by Amway Skin Care

☺ **Moisture Rich Cleansing Creme for Normal to Dry Skin** *($15.45 for 4.2 ounces)* is a standard mineral oil–based cleanser that needs to be wiped off and can leave a greasy residue on the skin. It also contains isopropyl palmitate, which can cause breakouts in some skin types.

☺ **Moisture Rich Toner for Normal to Dry Skin** *($16.45 for 8.1 ounces)* is a very good irritant-free toner that contains mostly water, glycerin, aloe, plant extracts, water-binding agents, and preservatives. Ignore the avocado and rose extracts; they are window dressing and have little impact on the skin. The same is true of the essential oils at the end of the ingredient list.

☺ **Moisture Rich Moisturizer for Normal to Dry Skin** *($17.35 for 2.5 ounces)* contains mostly water, glycerin, several thickeners, aloe, several water-binding agents, plant extracts, more water-binding agents, and preservatives. There is a negligible amount of plant oils at the end of the ingredient list. This would be a very good daytime moisturizer for someone with dry skin, but its SPF is only 8, which is good for only limited sun exposure.

☺ **Clarifying Cleansing Gel for Normal to Oily Skin** *($15.45 for 4.2 ounces)* is a very good facial cleanser that cleans well without drying out the skin or irritating the eyes, and can remove all of your makeup.

☹ **Clarifying Astringent Toner for Normal to Oily Skin** *($16.45 for 8.1 ounces)* is a standard alcohol-based toner with some plant extracts thrown in for good measure. The alcohol is too irritating for most skin types and can cause a rebound effect, making oily skin oilier.

☺ **Clarifying Moisturizer for Normal to Oily Skin** *($17.35 for 2.5 ounces)* contains mostly water, glycerin, several thickeners, several water-binding agents, plant extracts, more thickeners, and preservatives. This would be a good moisturizer for someone with normal to slightly dry skin. The SPF 8 is good for only limited sun exposure. I would never recommend this moisturizer for people with oily skin, although they might need it if they are drying out their skin with the Clarifying Astringent Toner.

☺ **Delicate Care Cleanser for Sensitive Skin Types** *($15.45 for 4.2 ounces)* is an OK cleanser that won't do a great job of removing makeup (it doesn't have enough cleansing agents), and it can leave a greasy film on the skin.

☺ **Eye Makeup Remover Gel** *($7.95 for 0.9 ounce)* is mostly mineral oil, thickeners, and a tiny amount of plant oils. It will take off eye makeup, but I never recommend wiping off eye makeup. Essentially, this is a fairly pricey standard mineral oil–based cleanser that could easily be replaced for pennies with a bottle of pure mineral oil.

☺ **Exfoliating Scrub** *($18.95 for 3.4 ounces)* is a mineral oil–based cleanser that contains some scrub particles. It will exfoliate the skin gently, but it can leave a greasy film on the skin.

☹ **Delicate Care Toner for Sensitive Skin Types** *($16.45 for 8.1 ounces)* would be an OK toner except that the third ingredient is benzyl alcohol, which is a skin irritant and not something I would recommend for someone with sensitive skin. Back to the drawing board on this one, Amway.

☺ **Delicate Care Hydrating Fluid for Sensitive Skin Types** *($17.35 for 2.3 ounces)* contains mostly water, plant oil, thickener, several water-binding agents, plant extracts, more thickeners, and preservatives. It would be a very good moisturizer for someone with dry skin. The plant extracts can make it a problem for someone with sensitive skin.

☺ **Eye Balm** *($14.20 for 0.5 ounce)* is one more moisturizer that contains a film-forming ingredient similar to those found in hairsprays. These acrylates form a nice film on the skin that can smooth it out, but they can also cause skin irritation.

☹ **Deep Cleansing Masque** *($14.55 for 3.3 ounces)* is a standard clay mask that also contains alcohol. Clay masks can be irritating enough as it is; the alcohol makes the potential for irritation that much greater.

☺ **Hydrating Masque** *($14.55 for 2.6 ounces)* would be an emollient face mask for someone with dry skin. It contains mostly water, glycerin, petrolatum, several thickeners, plant oil, and preservatives.

☺ **Revitalizing Night Treatment** *($27.50 for 2.5 ounces)* contains mostly water, petrolatum, glycerin, several thickeners, aloe, several water-binding agents, plant oil, vitamins A and E (antioxidants), more thickeners, and preservatives. This would be a very good moisturizer for someone with dry skin, although it is very overpriced.

☺ **$$$ Progressive Emollient** *($27.50 for 2.5 ounces)* is almost identical to the moisturizer above, and the same review applies.

☺ **$$$ Moisture Essence Serum with Alpha Hydroxy Acids** *($26 for 1 ounce)* is Amway's entry in the AHA sweepstakes. It contains about 7% AHAs with a mixture of lactic, citric, and malic acids. This liquid/gel also contains some good water-binding agents and a handful of exotic-sounding plant extracts thrown in for effect. This would be a very good AHA product for all skin types, although someone with sensitive skin is likely to have problems with the plant extracts and possibly the AHA concentration.

Artistry by Amway Makeup

☺ FOUNDATION: **Liquid Foundation** *($14)* has a sheer light texture and is good for normal to dry skin. **All of these colors are excellent:** Natural, Fawn Beige, Deep Beige, Honey Creme, Light Golden Tan, Soft Olive, Cappuccino, Mocha, and Cocoa. **Avoid these colors because they are too peach, pink, or rose:** True Beige, Shell Beige, and Sand Beige.

☹ **Creme Foundation** *($17.60)* may be good for someone with dry skin, but it tends to be greasy. **All of these colors are excellent:** Natural, Soft Olive, True Beige, Deep Beige, Cappuccino, and Mocha. **Avoid these colors because they are too peach, pink, or rose:** Honey Creme, Shell Bisque, and Sand Beige.

☺ **Oil-Free Foundation** *($15.75)* is a very good foundation for someone with normal to oily skin, without being too heavy or drying. **All of these colors are excellent:** Honey Creme, Natural, Soft Olive, True Beige, Deep Beige Cappuccino, and Mocha. **Avoid these colors because they are too peach, pink, or rose:** Bisque and Sand Beige.

☺ **Powder Foundation** *($14.30)* is really a standard talc-based pressed powder with silicone oil; it can be used either all over by itself or over the other foundations, which is pretty standard for most pressed powders. **Most of the colors are very good; colors to avoid are:** Sand Beige and Shell Bisque.

☹ **Base Controllers** *($15.75)* are standard lavender and green under-makeup color correctors that are supposed to camouflage yellow or red skin tones. It shouldn't take an extra product to do that; if the foundation is a good neutral color, it should be able to even out skin tones. If you apply too many products—moisturizers, concealers, skin-tone correctors, and then a foundation—your skin can't handle it for very long without either breaking out or feeling heavy and uncomfortable.

☹ **Eye Foundation** *($12.10)* is OK, but basically contains just talc and waxes. It comes in only one color, which is not the best for darker skin tones. Foundation with powder over it does the same thing as this product.

☹ <u>CONCEALER:</u> **Amway's Concealer Pencil** *($11.30)* comes in four great colors (the Tan shade can be slightly coppery for some skin tones). It is an interesting way to cover up dark circles, but the pencil idea wears thin quickly when sharpening becomes an issue or if you have dry or mature skin (meaning any amount of sagging). The pencil goes on rather dry; a moisturizer can help with the application, but even then the concealer would be easier to blend if it were creamier or came in a more liquid formula.

☺ <u>POWDER:</u> The **Loose Powder** *($15.75)* is a standard talc-based powder with mineral oil; it comes in three fairly reliable colors.

☺ <u>EYESHADOW AND BLUSH:</u> Amway's eyeshadows and blushes come in individual tins that are placed into a compact you purchase separately, either a **Two Pan Compact** *($9.65)* or a **Four Pan Compact** *($11)*. That means you can create your own makeup-collection compact that includes blushes and eyeshadows. It's a nice idea. The prices given below for the Powder Blush and Eye Colour are for the tins only, without a compact.

☺ The handful of wonderful **Powder Blush** *($9.90)* colors have a silky texture that goes on soft and evenly.

☺ The **Eye Colour** *($6.60)* eyeshadows also have a beautiful soft texture and go on smoothly and evenly. Some of the colors are ridiculously out of date, but as one Amway sales representative explained to me, there are some really out-of-date people out there. The more neutral, matte shades are very usable and attractive. **All of these colors are definite possibilities:** Premier Rose, Crushed Berry, Iris, Masquerade, Pewter, Misty, Graphite, Ash Black, Sand, Peach Blossom, Pacific Coral, Fawn, and Chocolate. **Avoid these colors because they are too shiny or too blue or green:** Dusty Plum, Morning Sky, Cabernet, Smoking Amethyst, Wedgwood, Moonstone, Jamaica Blue, Real Teal, Box Office Gold, Olympic Bronze, Sierra, Tahitian Sunset, Sage, and Critic's Choice Green.

☺ <u>EYE AND BROW SHAPER:</u> **Softstick for Eyes** *($10.20)* pencils have eight colors to choose from and are just fine. A brow pencil called **Softstick for Brows** *($7.60)* is available in five colors. These are standard pencils, as good as those of any other line.

☺ <u>LIPSTICK AND LIP PENCIL:</u> Standard lip pencils called **Softstick for Lips** *($9.90)* come in only six colors, but they are all good possibilities.

☹ **MASCARA:** **Smudgeproof Mascara** *($11.55)* is indeed fairly smudgeproof, but it doesn't build much length or thickness; the tube I purchased felt as if it were already used up and dry when I got it.

☹ **BRUSHES:** The **Cosmetic Brush Set** *($19)* is disappointing. It comes with six brushes, of which three are OK; the other three are not worth the money. The powder brush is fine, but the bristles are a little too loose, so the powder can be hard to control on the face. The eyeshadow and angle brushes are also OK and usable. The eyebrow/eyelash comb is like those found everywhere; an old toothbrush would work equally well. The lipstick brush is a good six inches long and wouldn't fit easily in most makeup bags; the smaller, retractable lipstick brushes are much better. The blush brush is too small to be suited to anyone's cheeks.

Aqua Glycolic (Skin Care Only)

Herald Pharmacal has a line of drugstore AHA products called Aqua Glyde and Aqua Glycolic (for information on availability in your area, call (800) 253-9499). The same company also makes M.D. Formulations products, sold only by physicians and aestheticians. If it seems confusing that both aestheticians (who receive minimal skin care education—usually only six months to a year of questionable training) and physicians sell the same AHA products, that's because it is. So-called professional products, whether sold by a dermatologist or an aesthetician, are just cosmetics. They are formulated and regulated the same way. Aqua Glycolic products have fairly strong concentrations of AHAs, and they are not for everyone.

☹ **Facial Cleanser, Advanced Cleansing Care, 12% Glycolic Compound** *($12.50 for 8 ounces)* is sort of like Cetaphil Lotion but with a strong concentration of AHAs. I do not recommend washing the face with an AHA product because of the risk it poses for the eyes. Additionally, most of the potential effectiveness is washed away.

☹ **Astringent, Advanced Oily Skin Therapy, 11% Glycolic Compound** *($9.95 for 8 ounces)* is an alcohol-based AHA product; the alcohol compounds the irritation of the glycolic acid. It also contains eucalyptus oil, another skin irritant.

☺ **Face Cream, Advanced Smoothing Therapy, 10% Glycolic Compound** *($15.95 for 2 ounces)* is a good basic AHA in a lightweight moisturizing base. It would be suitable for someone with normal to somewhat dry skin.

Arbonne (Skin Care Only)

Arbonne in many ways sounds like a Nu Skin clone. Both of these companies boast more about what their products do not contain than about what they do. That isn't necessarily good or bad, but I happen to like some of the ingredients Arbonne warns against. Much of its literature states that things such as mineral oil, lanolin, collagen, artificial fragrances, and artificial colors are *not* used in any Arbonne products. I disagree strongly with Arbonne's argument that mineral oil, petrolatum, and collagen are inherently bad for the skin because their molecular structure is too large to be absorbed into the skin, and therefore they can clog pores, cause blemishes, and interfere with skin respiration. Many other cosmetic ingredients are too large to be absorbed into the skin, including elastin, mucopolysaccharides, waxes, and other thickeners. One of the best ways to prevent dehydration is to keep air off the face, and one of the best ways to do that is with a cosmetic ingredient that works as a barrier between your skin and the air. If everything were absorbed into the skin, what would be left on top to keep air off the face? Mineral oil, petrolatum, and collagen are not so totally occlusive that the skin suffocates; they just protect it from the air. Besides, just because a cosmetic ingredient is absorbed into the skin doesn't mean it won't clog pores. Quite the contrary: once inside the pore, the ingredient is trapped and can't easily be washed or wiped away. Also, this idea of the skin breathing is very strange, even though it sounds credible; it has little to do with the moisturizing process. Anyway, Arbonne uses dimethicone, a silicone oil that is just as occlusive as petrolatum and mineral oil.

Arbonne also doesn't like beeswax. The company's theory is that because beeswax is sticky, bacteria and dirt will stick to the skin. But like many waxes in cosmetics, beeswax is just another thickener, and there is rarely very much of it in a product. Beeswax isn't all that different from the synthetic waxes used in cosmetics to keep the product blended. Arbonne's products contain ingredients such as myristyl myristate and cetyl alcohol, which are quite similar to beeswax.

Arbonne also takes exception to lanolin. The worry here, which I'm sure you've heard before, is that lanolin is a potential allergen. My view is that although some people have problems with lanolin, most experience no negative effects. Lanolin also happens to be an excellent emollient for dry skin. Avoiding this ingredient would be a mistake for someone with extremely dry skin.

My final area of disagreement with Arbonne concerns artificial coloring agents and artificial fragrances. Just because a coloring agent or fragrance is natural does not mean you are less likely to have problems with it. Many natural fragrances and natural coloring agents can cause problems for the skin. To suggest that natural colors and fragrances are somehow better for the skin is misleading. What I really recommend are products that are fragrance-free and have no coloring agents. The chances of an allergic reaction are decreased when these ingredients are not present, whether natural or synthetic. Arbonne's products have some coloring agents, and they do contain a small amount of fragrance.

I do agree totally with Arbonne's recommendation against alcohol because of its drying and irritating effect on the skin. If only the company excluded all other irritants, such as witch hazel and certain plant extracts, the line would be even better.

As you would expect, Arbonne also has a list of the ingredients it does use and considers critical for good skin care. One is a "bio-hydria" complex that contains a bunch of plant extracts—essentially, a tea. Arbonne claims that these plant extracts can rehydrate the skin. They can't. All the plant water in the world won't prevent dehydration. Besides, the plants are often so far down on the ingredient list as to be almost inconsequential.

Allantoin and aloe vera are two other supposed big pluses in these products, but many cosmetics also contain these ingredients, and they are fairly far down on the ingredient lists of Arbonne's products. Biotin (a B-complex vitamin) is promoted as affecting oil production and increasing skin tissue growth. It can't. If something really could accelerate skin tissue growth, it would be a drug and not a cosmetic.

None of that means I don't like some of these products, and I am glad that Arbonne does not use animal products or perform animal testing. But the marketing language is not convincing and seems to be rather misleading. All of the natural-sounding ingredients in the world can't keep you from reacting to an irritating preservative or fragrance or from breaking out due to cosmetic waxes such as stearic acid or myristyl myristate.

To call Arbonne International and find a representative in your area or to order products, call (800) ARBONNE.

☹ **Cleansing Lotion** *($12.50 for 3.25 ounces)* is supposed to be a water-soluble cleanser, but oils are listed among the first ingredients and it will leave a greasy film on your face.

☺ **Cleansing Cream** *($13.50 for 2 ounces)* contains mostly water, plant oil, thickener, more plant oil, a long list of additional thickeners, plant extracts, and preservatives. It is a fairly greasy cleanser that leaves an oily film on the skin and doesn't take off all the makeup without the aid of a washcloth.

☺ **Freshener for Normal to Dry Skin** *($16.50 for 8 ounces)* contains mostly water, witch hazel, water-binding agents, aloe vera, preservatives, and plant extracts. Witch hazel is an irritant.

☹ **Toner** *($16.50 for 8 ounces)* contains water; witch hazel; glycerin; peppermint, lemon, and papaya extracts; and preservatives. Witch hazel, peppermint, and lemon are very irritating and drying, and they won't change the amount of oil your skin produces.

☺ **Facial Scrub** *($15 for 2 ounces)* contains mostly water, thickeners, ground nuts, more thickener, plant oil, slip agents, and preservatives. The plants and vitamin E come well after the preservatives and are barely present. This is an OK scrub, but ground nuts are not the best way to exfoliate and can scratch the skin.

☺ **$$$ Bio Hydria Gentle Exfoliant** *($22.50 for 4 ounces)* is a bit too oily to be considered a good cleanser, but it does contain a scrub agent, so it can be used as an exfoliant. It is probably best only for someone with very dry skin.

☺ **$$$ Facial Lotion** *($13.50 for 4 ounces)* contains mostly water, standard water-binding agent, safflower oil, thickeners, sunflower oil, more thickeners, and preservatives. There are more ingredients following the preservatives, but their position so far down on the ingredient list makes them insignificant. This is a good emollient moisturizer, but the label suggests it for someone with oily skin, and that would be a big mistake. The oils and thickeners in this product make it good only for someone with dry skin.

☺ **Moisture Cream for Normal to Dry Skin** *($16.50 for 2 ounces)* contains mostly water, safflower oil, thickeners, water-binding agent, apricot oil, more thickeners, plant oils, vitamins A and E (antioxidants), plant extracts, and preservatives. This is an excellent emollient moisturizer for dry skin. I would not recommend a product this rich for someone with normal skin.

☹ **Moisture Cream for Normal to Oily Skin** *($16.50 for 2 ounces)* contains mostly water, almond oil, standard water-binding agents, thickeners, several plant oils, more thickeners, and preservatives. There are more ingredients following the preservatives, but their position so far down on the ingredient list makes them insignificant. Arbonne recommends this cream for someone with normal to oily skin. Why they think that someone with oily skin would be interested in putting more oil on her skin is beyond me.

☺ **Night Cream for Normal to Dry Skin** *($19.50 for 2 ounces)* contains mostly water, sunflower oil, water-binding agent, thickeners, almond oil, more thickeners, jojoba oil, vitamins A and E (antioxidants), plant oils, plant extracts, yeast, soothing agents, and preservatives. The plants do nothing for the skin, but all the other ingredients make this an excellent moisturizer for dry skin. I would not recommend a product this rich for someone with normal skin.

☹ **Night Cream for Normal to Oily Skin** *($16.50 for 2 ounces)* has almost the same ingredients as the Moisture Cream for Normal to Oily Skin, and the same review applies.

☺ **Rejuvenating Cream for All Skin Types** *($27.50 for 2 ounces)* won't rejuvenate anything. It is a good moisturizer for someone with normal to dry skin (but definitely not for all skin types). It contains mostly water, plant oils, standard water-binding agents, thickeners, more plant oils, vitamins A and E (antioxidants), aloe vera, plant extracts, amino acids, more thickeners, and preservatives.

☺ **Skin Conditioning Oil** *($15 for 1 ounce)* is a blend of several plant oils, aloe vera, vitamin E (an antioxidant), and some plant extracts. For someone with very dry skin, this would be a nice extra for problem areas.

☺ **$$$ Bio Hydria Night Energizing Cream** *($55 for 2 ounces)* contains mostly water, several plant extracts, thickeners, sesame oil, more thickeners, several plant oils, aloe vera, soothing agents, more thickeners, more plant oils, vitamins A and E, and preservatives. This is a good emollient moisturizer for someone with dry skin, but it won't energize the skin or "retard the formation of wrinkles," as the label claims. And the price tag is completely ludicrous for what you get.

☺ **$$$ Bio Hydria Eye Cream** *($22.50 for 0.75 ounce)* is very similar to the cream above, and the same review applies.

☺ **Mild Masque** *($15 for 5 ounces)* contains mostly water, clay, glycerin, soothing agent, plant oil, vitamin E, and preservatives. For a clay mask, this is indeed fairly mild, but it is still just a clay mask. It can leave the skin feeling soft, but it can make extremely dry skin feel even drier.

☹ **Extra Strength Masque** *($15 for 5 ounces)* is a fairly standard clay mask that contains mostly water, clays, glycerin, scrub agent, witch hazel, jojoba oil, cornmeal, ginseng, vitamin E, soothing agents, and preservatives. Someone with oily skin won't be pleased with the oil in this product, and the grains can be rough on the skin. The ginseng and soothing agents sound good, but they won't protect your skin from the irritation caused by the other ingredients.

Aveda

When it comes to "natural" skin care and makeup products, the Aveda line has enough herbs, vegetables, fruits, and flowers to satisfy any plant lover's dreams and enough enlightened philosophies to satisfy anyone on a spiritual journey. The company even has an entire line of products, the Chakra line, meant to help get your body's spiritual chemistry into alignment. I wonder how the company could possibly substantiate that claim, but I suspect that if you have to ask, you shouldn't be buying those products.

Aveda's approach to beauty is an enigmatic blend of contemporary fashion and jungle fever. This company portrays itself in no uncertain terms as being incapable of ever deigning to use even a hint of anything unnatural. Unfortunately, the company and I have different definitions of "natural" and "unnatural." What an advertising campaign! Most consumers are completely distracted by the aura surrounding botanicals, even though they haven't the slightest idea what infusions of horsetail, ginseng, comfrey, and juniper will do for their skin. The products sound good enough to eat, and the ecology-oriented marketing is quite appealing. Taking care of the environment and using "natural and pure" ingredients seem like the right things to do. Of course, when they are charging $18 for 4 ounces of skin lotion, companies often forget to mention that the lotion mainly consists of standard cosmetic ingredients. Furthermore, when mixed into cosmetics, plants retain little if any of their original form or purpose; that's assuming they had a purpose in the first place.

More often than not, when you see a long list of herbs and plants on the ingredient list, what you are really purchasing is a rather expensive tea. Helpful for the skin? After these herbs have been cooked and preserved in a cosmetic, they don't contain much of whatever constituted their original promised benefit. And there is absolutely no independent evidence that proves any of the exaggerated claims on the labels. But "natural" products are very seductive, and it is hard not to conclude that you will have "natural," perfect skin if you use them. To make its products even more seductive, Aveda publishes an impressive little booklet (on recycled paper) that describes at length some of the benefits allegedly bestowed by the plants used in its products. The descriptions are exquisite, bordering on hypnotic. After reading the claims, you will want to cover yourself in these "ancient" potions and elixirs. Aveda's boast is "2,500 years of research," but there are no Romans or ancient Egyptians around to show us their test results.

The labels further state, "Only distributors, salons, and licensed professionals who or which have received essential education may sell Aveda products." Very impressive. But exactly what is "essential education"? I have received letters from several salon owners who sell Aveda and are unsure of what these products can and can't do. The marketing is designed to appear exclusive, but the reality is just the opposite.

Some of these products are definitely worth your attention, though. And if you are interested in plants, this line is the king (or queen) of the hill.

Aveda Skin Care

☺ **$$$ Purifying Cream Cleanser** *($18 for 5.5 ounces)* is supposed to be a water-soluble cleanser, but it leaves a film on the face, requiring a washcloth to get it all off. This product contains primarily a tea of white oak bark and witch hazel (which can be irritating), thickeners, glycerin, plant oils, detergent cleansers, oil, fragrance, more oils, vitamin E, and preservatives. It may be OK for someone with dry skin.

☺ **$$$ Purifying Gel Cleanser** *($16.50 for 5.5 ounces)* is a fairly typical detergent-based, water-soluble sudsing cleanser that contains plant water and, way down on the ingredient list, some plant oils. It may be good for someone with oily skin, but the plant oils can be a problem for sensitive skin.

☺ **$$$ Pure Gel Eye Makeup Remover** *($14.50 for 4 ounces)* contains mostly plant water, detergent cleansing agents, and preservatives. It will take off eye makeup, but some of the plant extracts may irritate the eyes.

☹ **Exfoliant** *($14 for 5.5 ounces)* is a liquid toner that contains lavender water (which can be an antiseptic), chamomile, lemon balm (which has antiseptic properties), witch hazel and alcohol (both can be quite irritating), and salicylic acid (which peels the skin and can be an irritant). For most skin types, this product can be quite irritating.

☹ **Toning Mist** *($13.50 for 5.5 ounces)* is a fairly irritating product that contains primarily a tea of white oak bark, witch hazel, aloe, and peppermint, as well as rose water, alcohol, grapefruit extract, and glycerin. The glycerin won't soothe the irritation caused by the witch hazel, white oak bark, peppermint, alcohol, and grapefruit extract.

☺ **$$$ Skin Firming/Toning Agent** *($16.50 for 5.5 ounces)* contains rose water, an herb called echinacea (which can soothe the skin, but how much of its original properties are still present in a cosmetic is highly questionable), soothing agent, slip agent, and preservative. This is a good irritant-free toner, but it won't firm anything.

☺ **$$$ Beautifying Formula** *($17 for 2 ounces)* contains jojoba, rosemary, lavender, and bergamot oils. Bergamot and lavender oil are possible irritants when skin is exposed to sunlight. The oils are soothing on the skin if you stay out of the sun.

☺ **$$$ Miraculous Beauty Replenisher** *($17.50 for 1 ounce)* is basically a blend of several oils, including jojoba, rose, sour orange, lavender, fennel, geranium, chamomile, borage, and vitamin E. Some of these ingredients can be soothing, but some are potential skin sensitizers. This is a relatively overpriced blend of oils, since you can apply any one of these oils alone, in its pure form, and get the same effect much more cheaply. For normal to dry skin only.

☺ **$$$ Hydrating Lotion** *($24 for 5.5 ounces)* contains a tea of chamomile, lavender, rosemary, and comfrey, as well as glycerin, thickeners, rice oil, and jojoba oil. Several of the thickeners are possible irritants. This lotion can be good for normal to slightly dry skin that isn't sensitive.

☺ **$$$ Calming Nutrients** *($17 for 2 ounces)* contains jojoba, rose, borage, and vitamin E oils. If you buy this, you're paying a lot of money for oils that can't calm the skin. These are just oils, good for dry skin, but a problem for your wallet.

☺ **$$$ Energizing Nutrients** *($17 for 2 ounces)* contains jojoba oil, herb oils, borage oil, and vitamins E and A (antioxidants). You can't feed the skin from the outside in. These are just oils that can feel good on dry skin, nothing more.

☹ **$$$ Bio-Molecular Recovery Treatment** *($28 for 1 ounce)* contains mostly plant water, lactic acid, glycerin, salicylic acid, vitamins E and A, thickeners, fragrance, and preservatives. This is about a 5% AHA and BHA product combined. I don't recommend salicylic acid, but if you prefer it, this product seems to be an OK exfoliant for normal to oily skin. However, the price is out of line for a fairly average AHA and BHA product.

☺ **$$$ Pure Vital Moisture Eye Creme** *($26 for 0.5 ounce)* contains mostly plant water, thickeners, glycerin, more thickeners, several water-binding agents, vitamin E, silicone oil, and preservatives. This is a good moisturizer for someone with dry skin, but most of the really interesting ingredients are at the end of the ingredient list and don't add up to much.

☹ **$$$ Deep Cleansing Herbal Clay Masque** *($20 for 4.5 ounces)* is, for the most part, just a standard clay mask that contains kaolin as its primary ingredient. White oak bark, witch hazel, and aloe comprise the tea water, and there are also some oils, standard thickeners, and a detergent cleanser. As a clay mask it may be more gentle than most, but it can still prove irritating for sensitive skin and too greasy for oily skin.

☹ **$$$ Intensive Hydrating Masque** *($29 for 5.5 ounces)* contains mostly a tea of aloe, kelp, lavender, and rose water, as well as glycerin, thickener, water-binding agent, soothing agent, protein, and preservatives. It also contains a "tissue respiratory factor," described on the label as biofermentation of corn. Fermentation in this instance means the action of bacteria on corn. The bacteria breaks down the corn, resulting in the release of gases such as hydrogen sulfide and carbon dioxide. It sounds better when you don't know what it really is, doesn't it?

☺ **$$$ Daily Light Guard SPF 15** *($16.50 for 5 ounces)* contains mostly plant water, several thickeners, fragrance (including lavender oil), anti-irritants, silicone oil, vitamin E, plant oil, and preservatives. This would be a good sunscreen, but the inclusion of lavender oil is very confusing because it is a known photosensitizer, meaning when it can cause allergic reactions on the skin when worn in sunlight.

Aveda Makeup

☺ <u>FOUNDATION:</u> **Equilibrium Fluide Foundation** *($20.50)* is a silicone oil-based foundation with a rather thick matte finish. The coverage isn't what I would call natural, so be careful how you blend this one on. **Most of the colors are wonderful, with no overtones of peach or pink. This color is too ashy green for most skin tones:** Olive.

☺ **Dual Performance Creme Powder** *($19.50)* is a fairly standard cream-to-powder foundation with an incredible color selection.

☹ <u>CONCEALER:</u> **Protective Creme Concealer** *($12.50)* goes on rather thick and somewhat greasy, and dries to a matte finish. It tends to crease and can make any lines under your eyes look worse. The first ingredient is isopropyl myristate, which can cause breakouts.

☺ **$$$** <u>POWDER:</u> **Pure Finish Pressed Powder** *($17.50)* and **Pure Finish Loose Powder** *($17.50)* are standard talc-based powders with a silky dry finish. The color selection is beautiful and the application sheer and soft.

☺ <u>BLUSH:</u> **Silk Powder Blush** *($11)* comes in a beautiful selection of subtle matte shades, blends on easily, and has a smooth, dry finish.

☺ <u>EYESHADOW:</u> **Velvet Powder Eye Shadow** *($10)* comes in a lovely assortment of neutral matte shades that go on even and soft. **These colors are too shiny:** Olivine, Dawn Aube, Tiger Eye, Moon Lune, Opal, and Wisteria.

☺ <u>EYE AND BROW SHAPER:</u> **Definitive Eye Pencil** ($9) is a standard pencil that comes in an attractive group of colors.

☺ <u>LIPSTICK AND LIP PENCIL:</u> **Fresh Essence Lip Matte** *($13)* is a creamy opaque lipstick with a smooth semi-matte finish. **Fresh Essence Lip Colour** *($11.50)* is similar to the Lip Matte, but slightly more creamy. **Uruku Lip Colour** ($13) makes a big fuss about using annatto, a natural coloring agent, in these slightly glossy lipsticks. Of course, they also contain good old synthetically derived iron oxides to help create a variety of colors.

☹ **MASCARA:** **Maximum Lash Mascara** *($14.50)* tends to smear, and no matter how long you keep applying it, the lashes never get very long and thick.

☺ **BRUSHES:** Aveda has a wonderful collection of brushes *($6.95 to $23.50)*; only a few should be avoided. The **Powder Brush** *($23.50)* is too loosely packed and the bristles are rather long for good control. The **Eye Liner Brush** ($8.50) is too thick to create a controlled line along the lashes. The handle of the **Lip Brush** *($19.50)* is too long to be convenient; the **Retractable Lip Brush** *($6.95)* is cheaper and works better. All the other brushes are worth checking out, particularly the eyeshadow brushes.

Avon

One of the major complaints I have about Avon is their sales force. Although these women try hard, most of them are little more than order takers. In fact, most of the representatives I talked to were quite honest about how much they didn't know about makeup or skin care, or specifics about the products they were selling. Avon has an amazing number of products. I doubt any salesperson could keep track of them all. (Avon's catalog, which comes out every other week, is one of their major sales tools. These slick, rather voluminous compendiums make for some intense consumer browsing. Jewelry, fragrances, clothing, knickknacks, date books, video tapes, gift items, shampoos, men's grooming products, bath accessories, and toys are within the diverse range of merchandise that fills these mini-books.) In addition, most of the women who work for Avon do it part-time, to earn extra money, not as a major source of income. (The average sales representative earns about $5,000 a year, top sellers earn about $10,000, and the rare exceptions earn more than $20,000 a year.) That constitutes a sales force whose main interest is not necessarily Avon. For me this meant many failed attempts to find reliable information or sales representatives who had enough (or any) samples so I could make a complete evaluation without having to buy every single product. That means you, the consumer, must go by the pictures in the product book and guess about the products you are ordering. (Avon does guarantee 100% satisfaction, and they are true to that policy.) But if you know what you want, there are some incredible bargains, particularly the lip and eye pencils, mascara, concealers, and lipsticks, and some very good skin care products, particularly the water-soluble cleansers and AHA products.

Avon's Anew moisturizer was one of the first alpha hydroxy acid products on the market, and it's still one of the few that lets you know how much AHA it contains. Anew is now an entire group of products, some with and some without AHAs, helping Avon's bottom line immensely.

I must praise Avon's commitment to consumer information. The operators at their ordering number—(800) 233-2866—and their consumer information center number—(800) 445-2866—were quite helpful. No matter how many products I requested ingredient lists for, they provided them without hesitation or question. Thank you, Avon, for great customer service.

Beauty Note: In Canada some of Avon's products have different names. In particular, Anew is called Nova.

Avon Skin Care

☺ **Avon Anew Perfect Cleanser** *($10.50 for 3.4 ounces)* is a standard detergent-based water-soluble cleanser that can be good for someone with normal to oily/combination skin. It does contains a small amount of orange oil, which can be a skin irritant.

☺ **Anew Perfect Moisturizer SPF 15** *($13.50 for 3.4 ounces)* is a good emollient sunscreen for someone with dry skin. It contains mostly water, slip agent, thickeners, petrolatum, aloe, vitamins A and E, water-binding agents, anti-irritants, plant oil, more thickeners, and preservatives. The antioxidants are good, but some plant oils may be skin irritants.

☺ **Anew Perfecting Complex for the Face** *($15.50 for 3.4 ounces)* is an AHA moisturizer that contains about 4% glycolic acid. The ingredients are water, thickeners, slip agent, emollient, AHA, thickener, AHA, more thickeners, vitamins A and E (antioxidants), standard water-binding agent, herb extracts, oils, and preservatives. It will indeed slough skin, and works well as a mild AHA product.

☺ **Anew Intensive Treatment for Face** *($17.50 for 1.7 ounces)* has about 7% AHA in an emollient base that would be very good for someone with dry skin. It contains mostly water, thickeners, AHA, more thickeners, vitamins A and E, anti-irritants, water-binding agents, plant extracts, more thickeners, silicone oil, and preservatives.

☹ **Anew Perfecting Lotion for Problem Skin** *($15.50 for 1.7 ounces)* is a fairly standard salicylic acid–based lotion that also contains about 4% AHA. It won't perfect problem skin, and the salicylic acid may cause irritation.

☹ **Anew Alpha Peel Off Facial Mask** *($12.50 for 2.53 ounces)* contains a film former that hardens and then is peeled off. It also contains about 4% AHA. A face needs only one AHA product at a time: too much risks irritation and dryness, instead of simple exfoliation.

☺ **Anew Perfect Eye Care Cream with SPF 15** *($12.50 for 0.53 ounces)* contains mostly water; slip agent; silicone oil; thickeners; plant oil; more thickeners; more plant oil; AHAs; vitamin E and C; water-binding agents; plant extracts, soothing agent, and preservatives. This is a very good emollient moisturizing sunscreen that is partially nonchemical. The amount of AHAs in this product is about 2% which makes them good water-binding agents, not good exfoliants.

☺ **Sun Seekers Sunblock Lotion SPF 15** *($4.08 for 8 ounces)* contains mostly water, thickeners, aloe, more thickeners, vitamin E, plant oil, preservatives, and fragrance. This can be a very good emollient moisturizing sunscreen for someone with dry skin.

☺ **Skin Refiner and Gentle Action Scrub** *($8 for 2 ounces)* contains mostly water, plant oil, mineral oil, thickener, more thickeners, and preservatives. This product uses a standard synthetic scrub agent like many other scrub products. The oils make it fairly greasy, but it may be passable for someone with very dry skin.

☺ **Hydrofirming Cream Night Treatment** *($12.50 for 2.1 ounces)* contains mostly water; glycerin; petrolatum; thickeners; slip agents; plant oil; plant extracts; vitamins A, E, and C (antioxidants); preservatives; several water-binding agents; plant oils; more water-binding agents; silicone oil; and preservatives. This is a good emollient moisturizer for someone with dry skin. It contains many interesting water-binding agents, but unfortunately they come after the preservative, which means there isn't much.

☹ **Collagen Booster** *($10 for 0.85 ounce)* is a very misleading name. First, you can't boost collagen from the outside in with any cosmetic; second, the main ingredient is alcohol, which makes this product quite irritating and drying; and third, collagen is the last ingredient, which means there isn't that much in here. This product is a waste of money.

☺ **Dramatic Firming Cream for Face and Throat** *($11.50 for 1.5 ounces)* won't firm anything, but it is a good moisturizer for dry skin. It contains mostly water, thickeners, plant oils (one is arnica, which can be an irritant and is probably what makes the skin look firm), more thickeners, plant oil, more thickeners, anti-irritant, and preservatives. At the very end of the ingredient list are some interesting water-binding agents, but not enough to have any real effect.

☹ **Maximum Moisture Super Hydrating Complex** *($10 for 2 ounces)* is not a great moisturizer. Calling it super hydrating is misleading. It contains a strange list of ingredients, including a tiny amount of sunscreen; cornstarch, which can be drying;

lots of thickeners; and a preservative listed near the top of a long list of ingredients, which means the more important ingredients that follow are present in such tiny amounts they can't be much help to the skin.

☹ **Visible Advantage Skin Reviving Liquid** *($10 for 1 ounce)* is supposed to enliven tired, dull-looking skin. It contains mostly water; slip agents; alcohol; film former; thickener; minerals; anti-irritant; water-binding agents; vitamins E, B, and K; plant extracts; thickeners; and preservatives. The alcohol negates all the positive components of this product. What a shame! It could have been a very good lightweight moisturizer with antioxidants, but the alcohol makes it potentially drying and irritating.

☺ **BioAdvance 2000 Skin Lotion and Fortifier** *($20 for 0.85 ounce of the skin lotion and 0.12 ounce of the fortifier)* are two separate components of one product that you mix together. Who knows why it doesn't come premixed: there is nothing about the ingredients that can't work together, although the instructions suggest you should purchase a new supply every month. Obviously you're supposed to believe the miraculous properties of this line minimizer are destroyed over time. The ingredients don't bear this out—there's enough preservative in here to make it last quite a while. The lotion contains water, film former, silicone oil, petrolatum, preservative, more thickeners, and preservatives. The fortifier contains mostly silicone oil, alcohol, thickener, vitamin A, plant oil, and preservatives. The vitamin A is nice, but it can't change a wrinkle, and the alcohol can irritate the skin.

☹ **Nurtura Replenishing Cream** *($7 for 2 ounces)* contains mostly water, thickener, plant oils, glycerin, a small amount of sunscreen, more thickeners, and preservatives. There isn't enough sunscreen in here to protect skin even a little, and the sunscreen used is PABA, which can cause skin irritation.

☺ **Moisture Shield SPF 15** *($9.50 for 1.5 ounces)* contains mostly water, slip agent, petrolatum, thickeners, mineral oil, more thickeners, and preservatives. This is an OK to mediocre moisturizer, but the SPF 15 can protect from sun damage.

☺ **Eye Perfector with Liposomes** *($8.50 for 0.6 ounce)* contains mostly water; witch hazel; slip agent; plant extracts; water-binding agents; more plant extracts; thickeners; vitamins A, E, and C; and preservatives. The witch hazel can be a skin irritant, particularly around the eyes; otherwise, this would be a good lightweight moisturizer for dry skin.

☹ **Pore Reducer Beauty Treatment Mask** *($8.50 for 3 ounces)* is basically a clay mask (bentonite) that contains alcohol and rice starch with some glycerin. It won't reduce pores (there isn't a clay mask on earth that can), but it can dry out and irritate the skin.

☹ **V.I.P. Intensive Facial Hydrator Peel-Off Mask** *($8.50 for 4 ounces)* contains mostly water; film former; alcohol; glycerin; thickener; vitamins A, E, and C; water-binding agents; thickeners, plant oil, fragrance, and preservatives. Peeling a plastic-like film off the face can make it feel smoother, but the alcohol is a skin irritant, and the other ingredients, though interesting, can't change that.

☹ **Banishing Cream Skin Lightener with Sunscreen** *($7 for 3 ounces)* is an emollient but ordinary moisturizer that contains mostly water, thickeners, petrolatum, more thickeners, hydroquinone (a standard skin-lightening agent), sunscreen, silicone oil, and preservatives. The sunscreen is PABA, which is rarely used anymore because of the high risk of skin irritation. Also, the second ingredient is isopropyl myristate, which can cause breakouts.

☺ **Daily Revival Moisturizing Cleanser for Dry Skin** *($6.50 for 6.75 ounces)* contains mostly water, mineral oil, petrolatum, thickeners, preservative, more thickeners, preservative, another thickener, preservative, and fragrance. The remaining ingredients are herb extracts and aloe vera gel, which are inconsequential considering their placement after the preservatives. This is really a wipe-off cleanser that is too greasy to rinse off. It would be appropriate for someone with extremely dry skin, but it doesn't really clean that well.

☺ **Daily Revival Oil-Clearing Cleanser Oily Skin** *($6 for 6.75 ounces)* contains water, slip agent, glycerin, detergent cleanser, herb extracts, thickener, detergent cleanser, preservatives, and fragrance. This can be a good cleanser for someone with normal to oily skin, but it won't stop skin from being oily.

☺ **Daily Revival Gentle Cleanser for Normal/Combination Skin** *($6.50 for 6.75 ounces)* contains water, glycerin, detergent cleansers, thickeners, water-binding agents, fragrance, and preservatives. This can indeed be a gentle water-soluble cleanser for normal to somewhat dry or oily skin types.

☺ **Daily Revival Alcohol-Free Toner for Normal/Combination Skin** *($7.50 for 6.75 ounces)* contains water, lightweight detergent cleanser, and preservatives. It's a very boring toner, with little benefit for the skin other than an extra cleansing step, and it is indeed alcohol-free.

☹ **Daily Revival Deep Cleansing Toner** *($7.50 for 6.75 ounces)* is an alcohol-based toner that also contains other irritants such as eucalyptus and lemon extracts. I do not recommend this product.

☹ **Daily Revival Moisture Lotion for Normal/Combination Skin SPF 6** *($7.50 for 3 ounces)* is mostly water, glycerin, thickeners, mineral oil, thickener, petrolatum, preservatives, more thickeners, and a long list of additional ingredients such as herb extracts and water-binding ingredients that are really inconsequential, since they come after the preservatives. The mineral oil would not make someone with combination skin very happy, and SPF 6 is not enough to protect from sun damage.

☹ **Daily Revival Oil-Free Moisture Lotion SPF 6** *($7.50 for 3.4 ounces)* is indeed oil-free, but it contains alcohol (the second ingredient), which is very drying and irritating, as well as aluminum starch (the fourth ingredient), which is very irritating and can cause breakouts. I do not recommend this product. I should mention the poor SPF number, but after all this it doesn't even matter.

☹ **Daily Revival Moisture Creme for Dry Skin SPF 6** *($7.50 for 2.5 ounces)* does not contain enough sunscreen to make it a viable moisturizer for regular daytime use.

☹ **Daily Revival Eye Creme with SPF 6** *($6.50 for 0.5 ounce)* would be a very good moisturizer for normal to dry skin, but SPF 6 is not enough to protect from sun damage.

☺ **Daily Revival Moisturizing Night Treatment** *($9.50 for 2.5 ounces)* contains mostly water, glycerin, slip agent, thickener, plant oil, more thickeners, water-binding agents, vitamins E and A (antioxidants), plant oil, more water-binding agents, more plant oils, and preservatives. This would be a very good moisturizer for someone with dry skin.

☺ **Daily Revival Warming Facial Treatment Mask** *($8 for 2.53 ounces)* contains mostly water, thickener, lanolin oil, several thickeners, vitamin E, water-binding agents, and preservatives. Aluminum starch is the fifth ingredient and it can cause breakouts and skin sensitivities. It may be good for someone with dry skin but I doubt it.

☺ **Hydrafirming Cream Night Treatment** *($12.50 for 2.1 ounces)* contains mostly water; glycerin; petrolatum; thickeners; plant oil; plant extracts; vitamins A, B, C, and E; several water-binding agents; more plant oils; silicone oil; thickeners; and preservatives. This cream won't firm anything, but it is an excellent emollient moisturizer for someone with seriously dry skin.

☹ **Nurtura Replenishing Cream** *($7 for 2 ounces)* would be a very good moisturizer for dry skin but it contains a small amount of PABA, a sunscreen that can be a skin irritant. It also doesn't contain enough sunscreen to protect from sun damage.

☹ **Clearskin Maximum Strength Cleansing Pads** *($3.49 for 42 pads)* contains salicylic acid (skin irritant and peeling agent), water, alcohol, witch hazel (skin irritant), an antiseptic, preservative, fragrance, menthol (skin irritant), aloe, and vitamin E. It is too strong and drying for most skin types, particularly in association with any of the other Clearskin products.

☺ **Clearskin Foaming Facial Cleanser** *($3.29 for 4 ounces)* contains water, detergent cleansers, coloring agent, preservatives, and menthol (skin irritant). Can be irritating for most skin types, but may be an OK water-soluble cleanser for younger skin.

☹ **Clearskin Antibacterial Cleansing Scrub** *($2.99 for 2.5 ounces)* contains mostly water, slip agent, vegetable oil, mineral oil, thickener, glycerin, more thickener, alcohol, detergent cleanser, menthol, and a blue salt coloring agent. As a scrub it is OK, but the oils are not great for anyone with oily skin, and the menthol and alcohol are irritating.

☹ **Clearskin Antibacterial Astringent Cleansing Lotion** *($3.49 for 8 ounces)* contains alcohol, antiseptic (can be irritating), water, slip agents, antiseptic (can be irritating), isopropyl myristate (can cause breakouts), and coloring agent. This lotion is too drying and irritating for most skin types; the reasoning behind the inclusion of isopropyl myristate is a mystery.

☹ **Clearskin Astringent Cleansing Lotion for Sensitive Skin** *($3.49 for 8 ounces)* is mostly water, glycerin, and alcohol. This isn't appropriate for any skin type, especially not for someone with sensitive skin.

☹ **Clearskin Clearbreeze Astringent** *($3.49 for 8 ounces)* contains mostly water, alcohol, peppermint oil, eucalyptus oil, and camphor. The number of irritating ingredients in this product is astounding and none of them are beneficial for the skin.

☺ **Clearskin 10% Benzoyl Peroxide Vanishing Cream** *($3.39 for 0.75 ounce)* contains water, slip agent, thickener, preservative, sodium hydroxide, and benzoyl peroxide. It can be an OK, but strong, benzoyl peroxide disinfectant, although the sodium hydroxide can be irritating for most skin types.

☺ **Clearskin Overnight Acne Treatment** *($3.49 for 2 ounces)* contains salicylic acid (skin irritant and peeling agent), water, alcohol, and thickeners. It will peel the skin and dry it out terribly—not a great thing to wake up to in the morning.

Avon Makeup

☺ <u>FOUNDATION:</u> **Oil-Free Foundation** *($5)* provides lightweight coverage and a very smooth matte finish. It is good for someone with normal to oily skin, and there is a good range of colors for light to very dark skin tones. **These colors are very good:** Creamy Beige, Porcelain Beige, Almond Beige, Warm Bronze, Rich Honey, Toasted Brown, Deepest Brown, and Mahogany. **These colors are too peach, pink, orange, or rose:** Ivory Beige, True Beige, Soft Bisque, Blush Beige, Rosetint Beige, Honey Beige, Warmest Beige, Cool Copper, Toasted Tan, Rich Copper, and Copper.

☺ **Liquid-to-Powder Foundation** *($7.95)* has a greasy feel at first but blends to a dry powder finish. The second ingredient is aluminum starch, which can be a skin irritant and can cause breakouts. It tends to go on thick, so be careful blending it. **These colors are very good:** Porcelain Beige, Creamy Beige, Warmest Beige, Honey Beige, Almond Beige, Rosetint Beige, Rich Honey, Warm Bronze, Cool Copper, Deepest Brown, Toasted Brown, Cocoa, and Mahogany. **These colors are too pink, peach, or orange:** Rich Copper, Toasted Tan, Blush Beige, True Beige, Soft Bisque, and Ivory Beige.

☺ **Face Lifting Foundation** *($7.95)* has a rich consistency and glides over the face, providing light to medium coverage and a semi-matte finish. (Of course, this foundation won't lift the face anywhere; it does have a smattering of good water-binding agents, but those don't lift the skin.) This is a terrific product for normal to dry skin. **These colors are exceptional:** Ivory Beige, Porcelain Beige, Soft Bisque, Creamy Beige, True Beige, Warmest Beige, Honey Beige, Almond Beige, Warm Bronze, Toasted Tan, Toasted Brown, Rich Honey, Cool Copper, Cocoa, Deepest Brown, and Mahogany. **These colors are too peach or pink:** Blush Beige, Rosetint Beige, and Rich Copper.

☺ **Hydrating Foundation** *($5)* isn't the least bit hydrating, but it is a good lightweight, matte-finish foundation that provides smooth, even coverage. Sad to say, most of the colors are just awful. **These colors are very good:** Almond Beige, Warm Beige, Creamy Beige, and Porcelain Beige. **These colors are too peach, pink, or orange:** Soft Bisque, Ivory Beige, True Beige, Honey Beige, Rosetint Beige, Blush Beige, and Toasted Tan.

☺ **Self Adjusting Foundation** *($5)* doesn't self-adjust, but it is a very creamy, smooth foundation that blends on sheer and soft with a dry matte finish. **These colors are beautiful:** Porcelain Beige, Soft Bisque, Warmest Beige, Creamy Beige, Almond

Beige, Toasted Tan, Cocoa, Toasted Brown, Cool Copper, Warm Bronze, Deepest Brown, Rich Honey, and Mahogany. **These colors are too peach, pink, or orange:** True Beige, Rosetint Beige, Rich Copper, and Ivory Beige.

☺ **Anew Perfect Foundation** *($9.95)* is far from perfect, but it is a very good moist foundation that blends on silky and light and has a matte finish. It is very good for someone with normal to dry skin who wants medium coverage. The colors are limited; there is nothing for lighter skin tones, but a stunning variety for medium to very dark skin tones. **These colors are great:** Light Beige, Golden Beige, Golden Honey, Pecan, Soft Brown, Sable, and Ebony. **These colors are too peach or pink:** Soft Ivory, Buff, and, Deep Beige.

☺ **Perfect Match Wet/Dry Powder** *($7.95)* is a standard talc-based powder that goes on very smooth and soft and has a great but small selection of colors.

CONCEALER: Face Lifting Moisture Firm Concealer with SPF 8 *($4.19)* won't lift or firm, but it is a very good under-eye concealer, with little to no slippage into the lines around the eyes. By the way, it isn't all that moisturizing; it has a rather dry, fairly matte finish. It's best if dry skin isn't an issue for you.

☹ **Concealing Stick** *($3.50)* goes on quite smooth and soft, but has a dry finish. It blends OK, provides good coverage, but creases into the lines around the eyes and can look dry and thick. **Pure Care Concealer** *($3.50)* has a poor color selection and can crease into the lines around the eyes.

☺ **POWDER: Translucent Pressed Powder** *($6.50)* is a standard talc-based powder with a soft, sheer finish and good color selection. **Oil-Control Pressed Powder** *($6.50)* is also talc-based and contains no oil. It has a dry, smooth texture and good color selection.

☹ **Anew Pressed Powder** *($9.95)* is supposed to protect against free-radical damage and control oil, but it is nothing more than a standard powder with shine. It will make oily skin look oilier because of the shine, and the amount antioxidant vitamins is at best insignificant. **Translucent Loose Powder** *($6.50)* also has shine.

☺ **BLUSH: True Color Powder Blush** *($6.75)* has a moist smooth texture, and most of the colors are wonderfully matte. It blends on easily and holds up well during the day.

☺ **Natural Radiance Blush Stick** *($4.75)* comes in a twist-up stick with a convenient applicator, and the colors are nice enough, but it isn't the easiest product to work with.

☹ **EYESHADOW:** Avon's **Silk Finish** eyeshadow collection is quite extensive. The **Silk Finish Singles** *($2.75)*, **Duos** *($3.75)*, and **Quads** *($4.75)* are conveniently broken up into cool and warm tones, and there are some attractive, soft neutrals. (I recommend buying single shades, because with quads you usually end up using only one or two, so the other two are wasted.) Another apparent convenience is that the label states whether a color is shiny or matte. Yet almost all of the colors designated matte turned out to be shiny—very disappointing, since shiny eyeshadow makes skin look wrinkly. **These Singles colors are truly matte and wonderful:** True Taupe, Honey Brown, and Sweet Dreams.

☹ **Perfect Wear Eye Color** *($5.50)* goes on like a cream and dries to a powder. Eye colors like these are hard to control when you blend them because they have too much movement, and once the colors dry, it is difficult to adjust your blending. Worse, all of the colors are slightly iridescent.

☺ **EYE AND BROW SHAPER:** Luxury Eye Lining Pencil *($2.75)*, **Glimmerstick Brow Definer** *($4)*, and **Glimmerstick Eye Liner** *($4)* are standard pencils with a soft, smooth texture; they're so much alike that it's hard to tell them apart (the Glimmersticks have no-sharpen, twist-up containers). Stay away from the blue, green, and shiny shades. **Fine Eye Line Pen** *($5.75)* is a liquid eyeliner with a pen-tip applicator. It creates a line that is dramatic, but softer than most.

☺ **LIPSTICK AND LIP PENCIL:** Color Rich Lipstick *($4.50)*, **Maximum Color** *($4.50)*, **Beyond Color with SPF 12** *($4.25)*, and **Color Release** *($4.50)* are all very emollient, mostly glossy cream lipsticks in an extensive collection of highly reflective colors; **Moisture 15 Satin Smooth Lipstick with SPF 15** *($4.50)* is more gloss than lipstick. Except for the Satin Smooth Lipstick, they have a slight tint, which helps keep the color around a little longer than normal.

☺ **Perfect Wear Lip Color** *($5.50)* is Avon's version of Revlon's ColorStay. It goes on fairly creamy and greasy, and takes about a minute to dry into a truly dry, ultra-matte finish. **Luxury Lip Lining Pencil** *($2.75)* is a standard pencil that goes on slightly drier than most, so it can help prevent bleeding. **Glimmerstick Lip Liner** *($4)* goes on much thicker and creamier than the Luxury Lip Lining Pencil, but is very rich and moist.

☺ **MASCARA:** Voluptuous Full-Figured Mascara *($2.59)* is excellent; it builds thick long lashes quickly and easily, and doesn't smear. **Incredible Lengths** *($4.25)* almost lives up to its name. It builds long, thick lashes and tends not to smear. **Pure Care Mascara** *($4)* claims to have been designed for contact wearers, but seems no different from most other mascaras in how it goes on, wears, and washes off. It's not great, but it's good.

☺ **Wash-Off Waterproof Mascara** *($4)* has a most confusing name! Although it does wash off just fine, it's just OK as a mascara.

☹ **BRUSHES:** Avon often sells a small collection of brushes *($19.95)*. The set comes with a blush and powder brush, a lip or eyeliner brush, a small eyeshadow brush, and an eyebrow or lash comb. The blush and powder brush is quite good, but the eyeliner brush is too thick and the eyeshadow brush is too flimsy. The set looks like a good deal, but you would be better off buying brushes individually elsewhere.

Basis (Skin Care Only)

☺ **Facial Cleanser for Normal to Dry Skin** *($7 for 8 ounces)* is a standard detergent-based water-soluble cleanser that may be good for someone with oily skin.

☺ **Extra Gentle Facial Cleanser for Sensitive Skin** *($7 for 8 ounces)* is a standard detergent-based water-soluble cleanser that may be good for someone with oily skin. It can be drying for some skin types.

☺ **Hydrating Cleansing Lotion for Extra Dry Skin** *($7 for 8 ounces)* contains mostly water, thickener, glycerin, mineral oil, more thickeners, and preservatives. It could be suited for someone with normal to dry skin. It can leave a greasy residue on the skin.

☹ **Facial Bar for Combination Skin** *($2.79 for 3 ounces)* is a detergent/tallow-based bar soap. Tallow can cause breakouts, and the detergent cleansing agents are quite drying. This bar also contains lanolin, which can cause problems for someone with combination skin.

☹ **Facial Bar for Extra Dry Skin** *($2.39 for 3 ounces)* is identical to the soap above except that it also contains almond oil and petrolatum, which won't undo the irritation and dryness caused by the other ingredients.

☹ **Facial Bar for Normal to Dry Skin** *($2.79 for 3 ounces)* is identical to the soap above except that it does not have almond oil, and the same review applies.

☹ **Facial Bar for Sensitive Skin** *($2.79 for 3 ounces)* is almost identical to the soap above, and nothing about it makes it particularly appropriate for someone with sensitive skin.

☺ **Overnight Recovery Creme** *($8 for 1.6 ounces)* contains mostly water, mineral oil, petrolatum, thickeners, AHAs, more thickeners, and preservatives. This is about a 3% AHA product, which makes it a good moisturizer but not a good exfoliant.

☺ **Protective Facial Moisturizer for Sensitive Skin, SPF 15** *($8 for 4 ounces)* contains mostly water, thickeners, silicone oil, slip agent, mineral oil, more thickeners, and preservatives. This is a good sunscreen for someone with dry skin, but nothing about it makes it particularly appropriate for someone with sensitive skin.

BeautiControl

BeautiControl tries very hard to be all things to all women. The company not only gives you information about skin care and makeup application when you book a free consultation with one of its sales representatives, but they also analyze your wardrobe and tell you which colors look best on you and which clothing styles complement your body shape Unfortunately, as always, you must depend on the expertise of the salesperson, and several of the sales representatives I met seemed to be in dire need of wardrobe counseling themselves. The color information is helpful, but it takes skill and training to translate it into a total look.

BeautiControl has attempted to update its skin care and color line, but it should take another look at how it went about its overhaul. For example, of the three types of foundation, none is appropriate for someone with dry skin; one is oil-free, the second is a very thick cream-to-powder, and the third is a powder meant to be used as a foundation. That isn't a bad selection, but it's limited.

All of the colors are divided into warm and cool groups, which is helpful, but there are almost twice as many cool colors as warm. If I were an Autumn or Summer, that would be a serious shortcoming. On the other hand, a Winter or Spring might be quite pleased—though she will probably wish for a better selection.

Several of the skin care products are rather impressive, and the average price for many of these products is under $12. As you would expect, the wrinkle products are all absurdly expensive (and unnecessary), but if you stay away from them you won't get soaked. One word of caution: The company claims that your skin type and product needs are determined by a "precise, scientific...dermatologist-tested, proven Skin Condition Analysis." There is nothing precise or necessarily scientific about it. Little pieces of sticky paper the company calls "sensors" are stuck on different cleansed areas of your face. What comes off on these strips determines the products you are to use. Depending on the time of day I had the test done, I received different evaluations. Also, the sensors ripped off skin and left irritation and rough spots. The results aren't surprising and are often wrong. Skin isn't static: it changes with the seasons, your menstrual cycle, stress, and your environment. The idea is cute, but I wouldn't choose skin care products based on this analysis alone.

Hey, BeautiControl, you've got a great idea; update your makeup line again and keep working on your training program for sales representatives. It could only help your image—and the image of the women buying your products.

BeautiControl Skin Care

☺ **Mild Rosemary Cleansing Fluide** *($12 for 8 ounces)* is a fairly standard mineral oil–based cleanser that must be wiped off. It also contains lanolin oil, which means this cleanser can leave a greasy film that can make dry skin look dull.

☺ **Chamomile Balancing Cleansing Lotion** *($12 for 8 ounces)* is a mineral oil–based cleanser that also contains some detergent cleansing agents. It can leave a greasy film but could be good for someone with dry skin.

☺ **Purifying Cleansing Gel** *($12 for 8 ounces)* is a standard detergent cleanser that can be good for normal to oily skin.

☹ **Renewing Botanical Peel** *($12.50 for 3 ounces)* is an alcohol-based plastic-like peel-off mask that places a plastic-like ingredient over the face that then dries. Both the alcohol and the film-forming ingredient can dry and irritate the skin.

☺ **Almond Clarifying Scrub/Masque** *($12.50 for 3 ounces)* is a standard clay mask that also contains apricot seeds and almond meal. It is also a scrub, but it can be drying for most skin types.

☹ **Perfectly Balanced Duo Scrub/Masque and Peel** *($15.50 for two 2-ounce products)* consists of the Almond Masque and Renewing Peel. They aren't all that balanced, and can be irritating and drying for most skin types.

☺ **Quick and Mild Eye Makeup Remover** *($8 for 4 ounces)* is a standard detergent-based wipe-off eye-makeup remover. Wiping off eye makeup on a regular basis can cause the skin to sag.

☺ **Soothing Chamomile Tonic** *($12.50 for 8 ounces)* contains mostly water, slip agent, water-binding agent, witch hazel, more slip agent, plant extracts, more water-binding agents, and preservatives. Although this toner doesn't contain alcohol, it does contain witch hazel, a skin irritant that is part alcohol.

☹ **Balancing Tonic** *($12.50 for 8 ounces)* is an alcohol-based toner that can be irritating and drying for most skin types.

☹ **Clarifying Mallow Tonic** *($12.50 for 8 ounces)* is an alcohol-based toner that can be quite irritating and drying for most skin types.

☺ **Essential Moisture Lotion AM/PM** *($14 for 4.5 ounces)* is a very good emollient moisturizer for normal to dry skin. It contains mostly water, plant oil, thickener, mineral oil, more thickeners, more plant oil, vitamins, plant extracts, and preservatives. Because it doesn't contain a sunscreen, this moisturizer is best used at night. There aren't enough vitamins in it to have any effect as antioxidants.

☺ **Balancing Moisturizer AM/PM** *($14 for 4.5 ounces)* contains mostly water, thickener, plant oils, slip agent, more thickeners, water-binding agents, plant extracts, silicone oil, mineral oil, and preservatives. This is a good emollient moisturizer for normal to dry skin, but because it doesn't contain sunscreen it is only appropriate for use at night. The company recommends this moisturizer for someone with combination skin, but the oils in it aren't good for that skin type.

☹ **Oil-Free Moisture Supplement AM/PM** *($14 for 4.5 ounces)* is supposed to be oil-absorbing, but it won't absorb oil very well and it isn't even oil-free. It contains mostly water, silicone oil, thickeners, glycerin, more thickener, plant extract, vitamin E, water-binding agents, plant extracts, and preservatives. This is a good moisturizer for someone with normal to dry skin, but it is way too emollient for someone with oily skin. Moreover, without sunscreen, this product is appropriate only for nighttime.

☺ **Oil Controller Oil Absorbing Formula** *($14 for 4.5 ounces)* contains mostly water, thickener, silicone oil, more thickeners, and preservatives. There is very little in this product that can control oil, and the thickening agents can clog pores.

☺ **$$$ Regeneration Face and Neck Complex** *($30 for 2 ounces)* is BeautiControl's attempt at an AHA product. It uses lactic, citric, and tartaric acid. The company won't reveal the AHA content of the product, but the sales reps will tell you everything from 10% to 15%. One even said it was 95% AHAs. The truth is probably closer to less than 4%. It is a good moisturizer and a mild AHA product, but it won't produce miracles. The brochure suggests that a 50-year-old woman can expect her skin become like that of a woman of 35! All that from about 4% AHAs, a percentage that can be found in a hundred different products. This is a good AHA product in an ordinary but good moisturizing base.

☺ **$$$ Regeneration Face and Neck Complex 2** *($30 for 2 ounces)* is identical to the product above, but with about 6% AHAs, and the same review applies.

☺ **$$$ Regeneration for Oily Skin** *($30 for 2 ounces)* contains about 6% AHAs and is similar to the product above, which means it is too emollient for someone with oily skin. However, it could be good for someone with normal to dry skin who wants to try a stronger AHA product.

☺ **$$$ Regeneration for Oily Skin 2** *($30 for 2 ounces)* is identical to the product above except that it contains about 7% AHAs, and the same review applies.

☹ **Regeneration Blemish Duo** *($14.50 for 0.11 ounce of Blemish Gel and 0.12 ounce of Blemish Cover-Up)* is a tube with **Oil-Free Blemish Cover-Up**, which is nothing more than foundation (it comes in two colors, neither of which match most skin tones) at one end, and **Blemish Gel**, which is mostly alcohol and salicylic acid, at the other. The gel contains about 1% AHA, too little for the AHAs to be much more than water-binding agents.

☺ **$$$ Regeneration Extreme Repair** *($30 for 4 ounces)* is similar to Regeneration for Oily Skin, but with about 4% AHA. It's completely unnecessary.

☺ **$$$ Microderm Oxygenating Nighttime Line Control** *($25 for 0.81 ounce)* is a good basic moisturizer for someone with normal to dry skin. It contains mostly water, silicone oil, thickeners, slip agent, antioxidant, more thickeners, vitamin E, water-binding agent, and preservatives. The antioxidants are nice, but they won't change or prevent a wrinkle on your face, and they certainly aren't oxygenating.

☺ **$$$ Microderm Oxygenating Firming Gel** *($18 for 0.75 ounce)* is identical to the product above except without silicone oil, and the same review applies.

☺ **$$$ Microderm Eye-X-Cel Daily Therapy Creme** *($28.50 for 2 ounces)* contains mostly water, glycerin, a long list of thickeners, anti-irritant, plant extracts, silicone oil, and preservatives. This is a good, but extremely ordinary, moisturizer for someone with dry skin.

☺ **$$$ Lip Apeel** *($16 for 1.25 ounces)* is a two-part product (peel and balm) that helps peel dry skin off the lips. The peel is a bit of wax, clay, and silicate that can indeed peel off dead skin. The balm is simply a very emollient lip gloss of castor oil, petrolatum, and lanolin. It does the trick and is one of my favorite winter products for lips, but the price tag is absurd.

BeautiControl Makeup

☺ **FOUNDATION:** **Oil-Free Liquid Sheer Foundation** *($10.50)* is a lightweight foundation that provides light to medium coverage and has a matte dry finish. All of the shades are divided into cool and warm tones, but most are too pink or peach. Someone with warm skin tones should not wear a vivid peach foundation, nor should someone with cool skin tones wear a vivid pink foundation. **These are the only colors to consider:** Nude, Natural, Alabaster, Buff, Porcelain Beige, Dark, Tawny, and Mahogany. **These colors are too pink or peach:** Ivory, Bisque, Beige, Golden Honey, Peaches & Cream, Sunglow, Bronze, Desert Tan, Caramel, Nutmeg, Toffee, and Mocha.

☹ **Perfecting Creme to Powder Finish Foundation** *($11.50)* is a very thick, greasy foundation that does have a powder finish but never loses its greasy feel. Its claim to be waterproof is pretty accurate, but it is almost cleanser-proof too. It can easily clog pores if you're not careful.

☺ **Perfecting Wet/Dry Finish Foundation** *($18.50)* is a standard talc-based pressed powder that has a decent color selection and covers softly and smoothly. The texture and finish are great. It's supposed to be able to diffuse light in order to minimize lines, but it can't do that. Most of the large color selection is reliable and neutral. **The only colors to avoid are:** Peaches & Cream, Bisque, Golden Honey, Sunglow, and Bronze.

☺ **CONCEALER: Extra-Help Concealer** *($5.50)* blends on easily and provides good medium coverage, but it has a slight tendency to crease into the lines around the eyes moments after being applied.

☹ **Color Protectors** *($9.50)* are standard skin-color correctors that come in three shades: Mint, Mauve, and Lilac. They can't change skin tone convincingly, cause havoc when you choose a foundation, and layer on more makeup than any woman needs.

☺ **POWDER: Loose Perfecting Powder** *($10.50)* is a standard talc-based powder that has a soft, silky texture and comes in three good colors. **Oil-Free Translucent Pressed Powder** *($10.50)* has a soft, somewhat dry texture. The colors are very neutral and would work well for someone with normal to oily/combination skin.

☹ **Face Feminizer Pressed Powder** *($10.50)* is a compact of either shiny pink or peach powder. Enough said.

☺ **BLUSH:** The **Unbelievable Blushes** *($12)* all have some amount of shine, but not enough to be a problem for most skin types. (Someone with oily skin may not be happy.) The colors are beautiful and the texture is soft and smooth.

☹ **EYESHADOW: Sensuous Shadows** *($11.50)* come in compacts of three shades, but some of the combinations are poor and the colors range from somewhat shiny to very shiny; if you have any lines on your eyelids, shine will make them look worse. **Tinted Shadow Control Creme** *($6.50)* helps to keep your eyeshadow on, without creasing, for the entire day. There are four colors, but, like the eyeshadows, they are all shiny.

☺ **EYE AND BROW SHAPER:** Eye Defining Pencils and Brow Defining Pencils *($6.50)* are standard pencils that come in a nice range of colors. They tend to be on the dry side, which makes them a little harder to apply, but they also tend to last longer. **Brow Control Creme** *($6.50)* comes in a squeeze tube that you apply to a mascara-like wand and then roll through the brow. I like this way of making brows look fuller, but this is a messy option. Similar products come with the brush inside, so the color is evenly distributed.

☺ **LIPSTICK AND LIP PENCIL:** Lasting Lip Color *($6.50)* is a very creamy, slightly greasy lipstick that doesn't last all that long, but the color selection is very attractive. The colors are divided into cremes and frosts, which helps prevent the accidental purchase of an iridescent lip color. **Lip Control Creme** *($6.50)* is excellent. It prevents even greasy lipstick from feathering into the lines around the mouth, however, it would be better if it came in an easier to use applicator then having to spread it with your finger or a lipstick brush. **Lip Shaping Pencils** *($6.50)* are just standard pencils in a nice array of colors.

MASCARA: Water-Resistant Mascara *($6.50)* comes off easily with water and cleanser, and it doesn't smear after a long day. It would be a great mascara if it could build long, thick lashes, but it can't. It's just OK.

Beauty Without Cruelty (Skin Care Only)

Many companies proudly boast that they do not test their products on animals. However, it isn't always clear whether the products contain animal-derived ingredients or whether individual ingredients were ever tested on animals. Some companies, including The Body Shop, have a self-imposed five-year "grandfather clause," which means they use ingredients previously tested on animals as long as the testing took place five years prior to the date the raw ingredient was purchased. Beauty Without Cruelty is one of the few companies with a strict, rigorously defined position concerning animal testing. Its products are not tested on animals, none of its products contain animal by-products, and not one of the ingredients it uses has been tested on animals since 1965. The ethics of this company in this regard are admirable.

Beauty Without Cruelty recently revamped their entire skin care line. Of course, the company makes elaborate claims about the benefits of their plant ext cts, but if you ignore that and look for the ingredients that really make a differenc , you can find some very good products. They are typically distributed in health food stores and in drugstores such as PayLess and Drug Emporium. You can also order direct by calling (707) 769-5120.

Beauty Note: Almost all of these products contain an assortment of vitamins at the end of the ingredient list, which means there isn't enough to have an effect on the skin.

☺ **Alpha Hydroxy Facial Cleanser** *($7.50 for 8.5 ounces)* is a standard detergent-based water-soluble cleanser that can be very good for someone with normal to oily skin. There isn't much AHA in here and the type isn't even delineated, so it isn't significant one way or the other.

☺ **Herbal Cream Facial Cleanser** *($7.50 for 8.5 ounces)* is a detergent-based water-soluble cleanser that also contains some plant oils. This can be a very good cleanser for someone with dry skin.

☺ **Extra Gentle Facial Cleansing Milk** *($9.50 for 8.5 ounces)* contains mostly plant water, glycerin, plant oils, thickeners, aloe, more thickeners, plant oils, soothing agent, and preservatives. This is a fairly standard wipe-off cleanser that can leave a greasy film on the skin.

☺ **Extra Gentle Facial Smoother** *($7.50 for 4 ounces)* contains mostly plant water, glycerin, thickeners, plant extracts, more thickeners, oatmeal, almond meal, and preservatives. This can be an OK facial scrub for someone with normal to dry skin, but it isn't easy to rinse off.

☺ **Extra Gentle Eye Makeup Remover** *($5.95 for 4 ounces)* contains mostly plant water, glycerin, detergent cleansing agents, and preservatives. This is a fairly standard eye makeup remover, but the other cleansers in this line work well and don't irritate the eyes, so why bother with this product?

☺ **Balancing Facial Toner** *($7.50 for 8.5 ounces)* is a good, almost irritant-free, toner that contains mostly plant water, aloe, water-binding agents, plant extracts, glycerin, plant oils, and preservatives. The plant oils can be a problem for some skin types.

☺ **Refreshing Floral Mist** *($7.50 for 8.5 ounces)* is similar to the toner above, and the same basic review applies. This one contains jasmine, which can be a skin irritant.

☺ **Oil-Free Facial Moisturizer** *($12.50 for 2 ounces)* contains mostly plant water, glycerin, aloe, thickeners, silicone oil, more thickeners, soothing agent, plant oils, and preservatives. Did anyone at this company read the ingredient list before naming this product? It isn't the least bit oil-free, but it would still be a good moisturizer for someone with normal to slightly dry skin.

☺ **All Day Moisturizer** *($12.50 for 2 ounces)* doesn't contain a sunscreen, which makes it a poor choice for all day, but it can be a very good, emollient nighttime moisturizer for someone with dry skin. It contains mostly plant water, plant oil, thickener, glycerin, more thickeners, more plant oil, water-binding agents, vitamins A and E (antioxidants), soothing agents, anti-irritant, and preservatives.

☺ **Nutrient Rich Maximum Moisture Cream** *($14.50 for 2 ounces)* is similar to the moisturizer above, and the same review applies.

☹ **Renewal Moisture Cream Alpha Hydroxy Complex** *($13.50 for 4 ounces)* doesn't contain much AHA (possibly 2% to 3%) and the type of AHA isn't even listed, so it isn't significant one way or the other. This could be a good moisturizer, but it isn't a good AHA product.

☺ **SPF 12 Daily Facial Lotion** *($9.50 for 4 ounces)* is a very good, emollient, nonchemical sunscreen for someone with dry skin. SPF 15 would be better, but 12 isn't bad. It contains mostly plant water, glycerin, thickener, plant oils, more thickener, more plant oils, water-binding agent, and preservatives.

☺ **Green Tea Nourishing Eye Gel** *($14.50 for 1 ounce)* is a very good lightweight moisturizer that can be used on the entire face. It contains mostly plant water, thickener, water-binding agents, thickener, more water-binding agents, and preservatives.

☺ **Purifying Facial Mask** *($8.50 for 4 ounces)* is a standard clay mask that also contains plant water, glycerin, thickeners, water-binding agent, and preservatives. This is as good an irritant-free clay mask as any you will find.

BeneFit

Can you benefit from BeneFit? What can I say about a cosmetics line that has a self-tanning product called Aruba in a Tuba; blemish products called Boo-Boo Stick and Boo-Boo Zap; eyeshadows with names like Roadkill, Guess Again, and Striptease; lipsticks called Buck Naked, Misunderstood, and Lane Change; and a wrinkle cream called Mrs. Robinson (only those of us over 40 will understand that one)? The only thing I can think of is "Cute, very cute." But what about quality? That's another story, one that takes much longer to tell.

BeneFit was developed by twins Jean Danielson and Jane Blackford, whose brief claim to fame was a stint as the Calgon twins back in the 1960s. They opened their first cosmetics store in San Francisco, circa 1976. Although they eventually branched out to three Face Place stores, they decided a little less than two years ago to establish their products as a national line. With an infusion of investment capital and a new name (one of the twins had just returned from Italy, where everything was *bene, bene*), they established their product line as BeneFit. The cleverness didn't stop with the name.

Beauty can be fun, and possibly kinky, but assuredly successful, according to the two entrepreneurs, who are now in their late 40s. With appearances on the Home Shopping Network and mentions in fashion magazines, this line is hard to ignore, and that has helped sales soar into the millions.

Essentially, this line is a kicky version of M.A.C., with several gimmicks thrown in to grab attention. Does anyone really need seven products to take care of the lips, or Boo-Boo Sticks that contain standard acne ingredients also found in drugstore products? Hardly, but on the serious side, BeneFit has some great foundations and a beautiful brush collection, and some (but not all) of its lip products are interesting.

BeneFit's skin care line is relatively straightforward, with standard products and exaggerated claims. None of the acne products contain a single ingredient or formula that isn't available a thousand times over in drugstore acne products and every cosmetics line imaginable.

BeneFit's makeup line is a little more cumbersome to describe, but it has some interesting products, including great brushes, two truly matte foundations with wonderful neutral colors, and some specialty products that are surprisingly special, or at least unique, such as Lip Smoo…ch and D'eye'namite. Shortcomings on the makeup end of things are numerous. Both foundations are matte, which leaves someone with normal to dry skin out in the cold. In contrast, almost all of the eyeshadows are shiny, so despite the fact that there are so many to choose from, with some pretty bizarre colors for those with eccentric tastes, very few are matte. Regardless of taste, shiny eyeshadow can make the eyelid look wrinkly.

BeneFit has a lot of personality going for it, as well as prices that are almost cheap in comparison to its neighbors at Saks Fifth Avenue, where it is presently being sold. Fun is a refreshing change of pace when it comes to makeup and skin care, but no matter how you slice it, wasting money on products that don't work, can't live up to their claims, or can be found cheaper and better elsewhere isn't really any fun at all. If you want to consider this line, call (800) 781-2336 for a catalog or the retail location nearest you.

BeneFit Skin Care

☺ **All Types Skin Wash** (*$13 for 4 ounces*) is about as close a knockoff of Cetaphil Lotion as I've seen, except perhaps Trish McEvoy's or Cher's (now-defunct) versions. At least they're on the right track for a sensitive skin cleanser, but they're charging two to three times as much as Cetaphil.

☹ **Mint Souffle, Facial Cleanser for Normal to Oily and Combination Skin** *($22 for 4 ounces)* is a standard wipe-off cleanser that contains spearmint oil, which can be a skin irritant. It also contains many ingredients that would not make someone with oily skin happy, such as shea butter (an emollient) and other plant oils.

☺ **Squeaky Clean** *($13 for 4 ounces)* is a standard detergent-based water-soluble cleanser. It can be fairly drying for some skin types, and the spearmint oil can burn the eyes and irritate the skin.

☹ **Alpha Clean** *($17 for 5.56 ounces)* is a gentle cleanser that contains a small amount of clay. It also contains plant oils. The oils are OK for someone with dry skin, but the clay is better for someone with oily skin; this product is a bit confused. It also claims to contain 5% AHA—which it might, but it doesn't say which one, which tells us nothing about its effectiveness. Besides, AHAs are wasted in a cleanser and can irritate the eyes.

☺ **Honey Almond Wake-Up** *($13 for 4 ounces)* is a standard honey and almond-meal scrub that contains mostly water, honey, almond meal, clay, glycerin, thickeners, and preservatives. This is the old-fashioned way to exfoliate the skin. For less money and equal or greater effectiveness, using Cetaphil Lotion and baking soda is still the only way to go for a mechanical scrub.

☺ **Clean Sweep** *($13 for 4 ounces)* is a detergent-based eye makeup remover. It will indeed wipe off your eye makeup, but why bother if cleansers can do the job?

☺ **Alpha Smooth** *($17 for 5.56 ounces)* could be a good 5% liquid AHA product that contains no additional irritants. However, the type of AHA used isn't listed, which means there is no way to know how effective it really is.

☺ **Azulene Tonic** *($13 for 4 ounces)* contains mostly water, witch hazel, slip agent, citric acid (to adjust pH), plant oil, plant extracts, and preservatives. This is a fairly standard witch hazel–based toner, and witch hazel can be an irritant for sensitive skin types. The plant oils and extracts can be irritants as well, but the amounts are so insignificant they will probably have no effect on the skin.

☺ **Rosewater Tonic** *($13 for 4 ounces)* is mostly water, witch hazel, water-binding agent, glycerin, soothing agents, and preservatives. The witch hazel can be a skin irritant, but other than that, this is an OK skin toner for some skin types.

☺ **$$$ Peel and Polish** *($20 for 1 ounce)* contains mostly aloe vera, wax, petrolatum, and thickeners. Using any kind of wax on the skin can exfoliate it, and this product is no exception.

☹ **$$$ Seven % Fine Wrinkle Line Remover** *($35 for 1 ounce)* doesn't list the type of AHAs it contains, so it's impossible to tell whether they might be acids that aren't as good as lactic or glycolic acid. The product contains mostly water, some kind of AHA, thickeners, plant oil, vitamin E, silicone oil, water-binding agents, and preservatives. If only I knew what kind of AHAs it contains, this could be a very good product to recommend.

☺ **$$$ Benevitale** *($21 for 1.75 ounces)* contains mostly water, seaweed extract, water-binding extract, thickeners, plant oil, silicone oil, more water-binding agents, vitamin E (an antioxidant), more thickeners, spleen extract, and preservatives. Spleen extract: Does anyone really believe this stuff has a function in cosmetics anymore? Nevertheless, this is a good, emollient, moisturizing toner for someone with dry skin.

☺ **$$$ Mrs. Robinson** *($22 for 2 ounces)* contains mostly water, slip agent, plant oils, plant extracts, water-binding agents, soothing agent, and preservatives. This would be a good moisturizer for someone with dry skin, regardless of whether you are old enough to know who Mrs. Robinson is.

☹ **$$$ Envy** *($22 for 2 ounces)* contains mostly water, several thickeners, water-binding agents, and preservatives. The amount of collagen and elastin is at best minuscule. It is a very ordinary, plain moisturizer that would be OK for someone with normal to slightly dry skin. I wouldn't envy anyone who uses it, though.

☺ **$$$ Hyaluronic Creme** *($20 for 2 ounces)* contains mostly water, plant oil, thickeners, water-binding agents, preservatives, vitamin E, and pollen extract. The amount of vitamin E and pollen extract in this product is at best a dusting; however, it is still a good emollient cream for someone with dry skin. Hyaluronic acid is a good water-binding agent, but no better than dozens of others such as collagen, elastin, and mucopolysaccharides.

☺ **$$$ Vita Hydrating Creme** *($20 for 2 ounces)* contains mostly water; vitamins E, D, and A; plant oil; slip agent; thickeners; water-binding agents; and preservatives. This is a good moisturizer for someone with dry skin, and if you want antioxidants, they're in here.

☹ **Oasis Mist** *($15 for 4 ounces)* contains mostly water, aloe vera, water-binding agent, plant extracts, and preservatives. This product is mostly water, with some plant water. It is an OK toner-like water spray.

☹ **Azulene Oasis Mist** *($15 for 4 ounces)* is almost identical to the product above, and the same review applies.

☺ **$$$ Bio Brite Eye Balm** *($23 for 1 ounce)* contains mostly water, plant oil (carrot fat), water-binding agent, and plant extracts. Nothing in this product will diminish dark circles any better than any other moisturizer. Skin simply looks less dark when it isn't dry, and most moisturizers can take care of that problem.

☺ **$$$ Eye Lift** *($24 for 1 ounce)* contains mostly water, silicone oil, glycerin, plant extracts, water-binding agents, vitamins A and E, and preservatives. This is a good, emollient moisturizer, but nothing about it will lift the eye, although at this price it should.

☹ **Mint Firming Mask** *($19 for 2 ounces)* contains mostly water, silica (like sand), glycerin, clay, thickener, aloe, water-binding agents, preservatives, spearmint oil, and peppermint oil. Like hundreds of other clay masks, this one won't firm the skin. The mint oils can irritate the skin.

☺ **$$$ Soothing Gel Mask** *($19 for 2 ounces)* contains mostly water, water-binding agents, plant extracts, and preservatives. This is a good lightweight mask if you aren't sensitive to the plant extracts used. It supposedly contains "plant tissue complex," whatever that is. This product is just a water-binding agent; it doesn't replace or add to your own skin tissue.

☺ **$$$ Seaweed Mud Mask** *($19 for 2 ounces)* contains mostly water; plant oil; glycerin; lanolin; thickeners; seaweed; water-binding agents; vitamins E, A, and D; and preservatives. There isn't any mud in it, but if you have dry skin, this would be a good emollient mask to leave on your face for a while.

☹ **$$$ Boo-Boo Zap** *($15 for 0.25 ounce)* contains mostly water, two types of alcohol, salicylic acid, camphor, witch hazel, styrene (a resin), and preservative. Alcohol, salicylic acid, camphor, and witch hazel have no effect on blemishes other than causing more irritation. The number of drugstore acne products that contain the same ingredients as this product, and also do nothing to stop blemishes, is overwhelming. If you want to see how these ingredients might work on your skin, there are dozens upon dozens of other products you can try, although I wouldn't recommend them either.

☹ **European Acne Creme** *($45 for 1 ounce)* contains water, plant oil, thickeners, sulfur, and menthol. It's supposed to heal acne, but nothing in it has any proven effect on acne. In addition, the sulfur and menthol can cause skin irritation. There is nothing European about this product; it is like a hundred other acne products that contain the same stuff. Also, why would someone with acne want to put oil on her skin?

☺ **$$$ Balance Control Lotion** *($16 for 1 ounce)* contains mostly water, thickener, slip agent, water-binding agents, silica (like sand), more thickeners, and preservatives. Silica is a white powder that has some ability to absorb oil, but a thin layer of Phillips' Milk of Magnesia mixed with an equal amount of water would absorb oil better and be a lot cheaper.

☺ **$$$ Dayscreen 15** *($23 for 2 ounces)* isn't anything fancy, containing mostly thickeners and a few water-binding agents. It would be a good sunscreen for someone with normal to somewhat dry skin.

☺ **"Aruba in a Tuba" Ultra Sunless Tan** *($22 for 5 ounces)* is a sunless tanner that uses the exact same active ingredient to turn the skin brown that all other sunless tanners use: dihydroxyacetone. It was not my intention to include self-tanning agents for this edition of the book because they are all so markedly alike, however the name of this one was just too good to ignore. It is a good, but markedly ordinary, self-tanner, the clever name notwithstanding.

BeneFit Makeup

☺ <u>**FOUNDATION:**</u> If you are looking for truly matte foundations in **all beautiful neutral colors,** BeneFit has two of them. Creamy **matte makeup** *($18)* is incredibly matte, despite how emollient it looks in the jar, and liquid **matte tint** *($18)* has a slightly lighter but similar finish. Another strong point is the selection of light skin-tone colors in both of these foundations. If you have very white skin, there is a color here for you, but only if you have oily skin. These matte foundations are quite drying and not for everyone. Surely, this is a shortcoming that BeneFit will take care of soon; given the expansive nature of its line, it is almost shocking that it doesn't include a foundation for women with normal to dry skin. One word of warning: The matte tint's second ingredient is isopropyl myristate, which is known to cause breakouts. If you have a problem with blemishes, you will want to approach this foundation with trepidation. All the colors for both of these foundations are excellent.

☺ **Sheer genius** *($25)* is a standard talc-based powder meant to be used as a foundation. It comes in only four colors, which is extremely limiting. It does have a light silky texture, but it is better used as a regular powder than as a foundation.

☹ **Chartreuse** *($18)* is a standard green "color corrector." A lot of cosmetics lines have tried to sell green (or lavender and red) color correctors; these products don't work well, but they still come around and here is another one. I don't recommend this product; it just looks green, puts yet another layer of makeup on the face, and doesn't really hide any redness.

☺ **CONCEALER: Ooh La Lift** *($15)* is a pink highlighting concealer/foundation in a tube. It is supposed to contain skin-tightening botanicals, but the amount of plant extracts in this product isn't enough to tighten one skin cell. (There aren't any plants that can tighten the skin, though, so the amount is actually irrelevant.) Nevertheless, this is a good highlighter and a fun makeup boost if you have time to bother with an extra step.

☹ **Boi-ing** *($15)* is a concealer that comes in limited shades of Light, Medium, and Dark. It is rather thick and has a nasty habit of creasing into the lines around the eyes.

☹ **POWDER: Powder tint** *($20)* is a very drying, almost chalk-like face powder that comes in seven colors. **Colors to avoid:** Ivory Coast, which is white; Chamois, which is yellow (it is meant to even out redness, but it just looks yellow on the skin); and White Lavender (you can figure that one out for yourself). **The other four are excellent neutral shades** and very good for someone with exceptionally oily skin.

☺ **$$$ BLUSH: Benetint** *($24)* is just what it says it is: a red tint for the cheeks. If you have smooth skin, meaning no pores, this gives a very natural color that just melds with the skin. However, if you have pores or dry skin, you may not be happy with the results.

☺ **EYESHADOW: Lemon aid** *($15)* is an eyeshadow base that is supposed to correct lid discoloration but actually works no better than a little foundation over the lid. **Eye bright** *($13)* is a pink stick concealer that turns white when you apply it. It does brighten the eye lid, but any light concealer would do the same. **Show girls** *($12)* are little pots of iridescent eyeshadow; if you want a Las Vegas look, this will do the job.

☹ **Jumbo matte eye shadow** *($10)* comes in a huge selection of colors, but, lamentably, even though they are priced to compete with M.A.C. (they even look the same), most of the shades are slightly shiny to very shiny (while M.A.C. has an extensive range of matte colors). Moreover, BeneFit's eyeshadow colors range from the soft and beautiful to the strange and downright ugly (M.A.C. is known for its large selection of neutrals and offers few or no bizarre colors).

☺ **EYE AND BROW SHAPER:** Some things you just can't explain, and **d'eye'namite** *($14)* is one of them. This thick, heavy, white, waxy powder is supposed to go just above the lash line to enhance the eyes. Along with thick black eyeliner, it creates a very retro-'50s look. **Brow zings** *($14)* are brow colors that are a cross between a pencil and a powder: a thick waxy powder that you apply with a stiff brush. They are meant to tame brows, but they can make the brow look overdone and matted, so be sure you like the effect before you decide to go for it. **Eye pencils** *($9.50)* come in a nice assortment of colors and go on smoothly. They are fairly standard but not badly priced. **Babe cake** *($13)* is a pot of eyeliner you use wet, for the dramatic eyeliner look some of us used to wear in the '70s. **She laq** *($13)* is little more than hairspray for the brows in a bottle. Not bad, but any hairspray used with a toothbrush will do the same thing for less. BeneFit also recommends that you use this product over eyeliner, but the ingredients are way too irritating to put that close to the eyes.

☺ **LIPSTICK AND LIP PENCIL:** The number of lip products BeneFit offers is nothing less than amazing. Does anyone really think she needs such a makeup arsenal for her lips? Makeup addicts will think they have found heaven; I hope the rest of us will recognize some serious cosmetics puffery and foolishness when we see it. **Smoo...ch** *($14)* is a lip moisturizer/gloss in a tube. It is a good emollient, but nothing out of the ordinary; lip balms by Almay and Physicians Formula (among others) are just as good and much less expensive. **Lip plump** *($15)* is supposed to make your lips look large, pouty, and smooth. It has a concealer-like texture, only more waxy. I didn't see a difference when I tested this product, but it did slightly smooth out my lips. I can't imagine using it on a regular basis every time I apply my lipstick, though. If you have lipsticks you want to make lighter or darker, that's what **depth charge** *($14)* and **light switch** *($14)* are for. Basically, they are light and dark lipsticks just to the greasy side of creamy. **Matte transformation** *($14)* is a base coat that flattens out creamy lipsticks and helps keep them from moving or sliding around. If you're thinking what I'm thinking, you might wonder, Why not just buy a matte lipstick in the first place? **De-groovie** *($24)* is supposed to prevent lipstick from feathering. It does an OK job, but you can buy much better products for a lot less money, such as Ultima II The Base or Coty's Stop It and Hold It.

☺ **Lipstick** *($11)* comes in creams, mattes, and sheers. The creams are fairly greasy and moist, the sheers are similar to the creams but shiny, and the mattes are fairly matte but still tend to feather. **Glosses** *($11)* come in both tubes and pots; both are exceptionally greasy and emollient, reminiscent of the '70s. **Lip liners** *($9.50)* come in an attractive range of colors and, although they are quite standard, go on easily and wear well.

☺ **MASCARA:** **Masca...rah** *($11)* is just an OK mascara. It goes on nicely and tends not to smear, but it doesn't build well; if you're looking for thick lashes, this mascara is not for you.

☺ **BRUSHES:** It is always a welcome sight when a cosmetics line offers a selection of usable soft brushes. BeneFit does just that, and the 14 brushes *($7 to $21)* are impressive and not priced to blow your budget. This is a decided strong point, and by itself is worth a visit or a look through BeneFit's catalog if you need to augment your brush supply. The eyeliner and eyeshadow brushes are especially great.

Black Opal

Several cosmetics lines are courting the African-American consumer, and some are doing so with aplomb and style. Black Opal is one such line, along with Iman and Posner. (Black Opal and Posner are both sold at drugstores, and Iman is sold at J.C. Penney and Sears.) Black Opal, to its credit, has some remarkably matte, velvety deep shades of eyeshadow, blush, and lipstick, as well as beautiful foundation colors for a small range of darker skin tones. Actually, its color line is where Black Opal excels— what a shame there aren't more color choices. The skin care products, although reasonably priced, have some problems. They were supposedly designed by a dermatologist, but either the dermatologist didn't do all the chemistry homework necessary to design a skin care line or there were inadvertent oversights. When a skin care line boasts about its plant extracts, I wonder exactly what a dermatologist could be thinking, given the potential for allergic reaction and the lack of evidence that these types of ingredients provide a benefit for the skin. The skin care products also contain combinations of preservatives that most dermatologists would consider fairly irritating, such as quaternium-15 and dmdm hydantoin. Lastly, the designer of the skin care line seems to think that women of color have only oily or combination skin; that makes it limiting. Still, Black Opal offers some great products, and should not be overlooked by anyone with medium to very dark skin.

Black Opal Skin Care

☹ **Lemon and Sage Cleansing Emulsion** *($6.44 for 8 ounces)* contains mostly water, aloe, plant oil, thickeners, slip agent, more thickeners, plant extracts, soothing agents, vitamins E and D, more plant extracts, and preservatives. This is pretty much a wipe-off cleanser that can leave skin feeling greasy. Vitamins are wasted in a cleanser because their antioxidant benefit is wiped away.

☺ **Oil Free Cleansing Gel** *($3.99 for 6 ounces)* is a standard detergent-based water-soluble cleanser that can be good for someone with oily skin. It can be drying for some skin types.

☺ **Purifying Astringent** *($3.99 for 6 ounces)* won't purify anything, but it is a good irritant-free toner that contains mostly water, glycerin, slip agent, plant water, soothing agent, more plant extracts, aloe, and preservatives.

☺ **Skin Retexturizing Complex with Alpha-Hydroxy Acids** *($6.69 for 1 ounce)* contains mostly water, silicone oil, glycolic acid, pH balancer, film former, thickeners, plant extracts, anti-irritants, vitamin E, water-binding agents, and preservatives. This would be a very good 7% AHA product for most skin types.

☺ **Oil Free Moisturizing Lotion** *($3.99 for 1.75 ounces)* contains mostly water, glycerin, thickeners, silicone oil, water-binding agent, plant extracts, and preservatives. It isn't oil-free, and some of the thickening agents aren't good for oily skin. Still, this could be a good moisturizer for someone with normal to somewhat dry skin.

☹ **SPF 15 Daily Protection for Photosensitive Skin** *($3.99 for 2.25 ounces)* is a decent sunscreen for someone with normal to dry skin, but it contains aluminum starch, which could be a skin irritant, rather high up on the ingredient list.

☺ **Advanced Dual Complex Fade Gel** *($7.99 for 0.75 ounce)* is a standard hydroquinone product that also contains about 7% glycolic acid. Hydroquinone with a good percentage of AHA, like that contained in this product, can minimally help fade dark, ashy areas of the skin. But don't expect a radical difference, just a slight fading.

☹ **Blemish Control Gel** *($3.99 for 0.35 ounce)* contains mostly water, slip agent, resorcinol (disinfectant), camphor, menthol, eucalyptus oil, and peppermint oil. These standard acne ingredients can cause many more problems than they can help. Because they can dry and irritate skin, they can cause ashy skin-tone problems for women of color.

☹ **Knees and Elbows Target Treatment, New Breakthrough Formula with Vitamin C and Alpha-Hydroxy Acids, for Ash-Free, Soft, and Supple Skin** *($3.99 for 2 ounces)* contains mostly water; thickener; plant oil; glycerin; plant extracts; more thickeners; silicone oil; water-binding agents; plant oils; vitamins E, A, and D; and preservatives. This product lists its AHA as plant extracts. That doesn't tell you what kind of extracts, but it does at least tell you it's not an acid extract, and that's the kind you need to exfoliate the skin. The product is a good moisturizer, however; you just have to get around the other claims before you can understand what you are actually getting.

☺ **Skin Refining Peel** *($3.99 for 1.75 ounces)* is a standard clay mask with some wax, thickeners, glycerin, silicone oil, and preservatives. It would be a good clay mask for someone who likes this skin care step.

Black Opal Makeup

☹ **FOUNDATION:** **True Color Cream Stick Foundation SPF 8** *($5.95)* comes in a stick form and looks like it will go on quite greasy, but just the opposite is the case. It goes on smooth and then dries to a soft, matte finish. It tends to stay in place once it's on, so blending can be tricky. There are only five colors that are quite good for the most part, but some are too orange. Without testers, as is true for most all drugstore foundations, it's impossible to recommend the Black Opal foundations. **True Color Liquid Foundation Oil-free** *($5.95)* has just a tiny bit of silicone oil, so it isn't really oil-free, but it goes on quite smooth and sheer, drying to a matte finish. It can feel very dry on the skin.

☺ **POWDER:** **Oil Absorbing Pressed Powder** *($5.95)* is a standard talc-based powder that comes in a small assortment of colors. It has a soft silky texture and blends easily.

BLUSH: **Natural Color Blush** *($2.85)* comes in eight beautiful matte shades that go on silky and impart rich, lasting color. These are a real find for darker skin tones.

☺ **EYESHADOW:** **Color Rich Eyeshadows** *($2.85)* have an exceptional matte finish and come in a small but wonderful array of colors. The shadows blend on evenly and show up well on darker skin tones.

☺ **EYE AND BROW SHAPER:** **Precision Eye Definer** *($2.85)* is a standard eye pencil with a small but good selection of colors. At this price, if you're into pencils, buy them all.

☺ **LIPSTICK AND LIP PENCIL:** **Matte Plus Moisture Lipstick** *($3.75)* isn't all that matte, but it is somewhat creamy and has a small but terrific color selection. **True Tone Vitamin Rich Lipstick** *($3.97)* is more emollient than matte, but not in the least bit greasy. This is a very good moist lipstick. **Simply Sheer Lipstick with SPF 15** *($4.05)* is, as the name implies, a sheer, more glossy lipstick with a good sunscreen. **Precision Lip Definer** *($2.85)* is a standard lip pencil with a small but good selection of colors. At this price, if you're into pencils, buy them all.

☹ **MASCARA:** **Lash Defining Mascara** *($4.59)* doesn't build well and tends to clump.

Bobbi Brown Essentials

Bobbi Brown is a well-known New York City makeup artist who commands a consultation fee of $200, and that's just for the first hour. She has been one of the most quoted and referred-to makeup artists in fashion magazines for several years now, and her handiwork has graced the faces of countless models and celebrities. I was not surprised when she finally came out with her own cosmetics line a few years ago. What did astound me was the clamor for these products. The limited color selection and very yellow foundation choices (when the line was first launched, it included only one type of foundation that was appropriate for normal to dry skin only) didn't faze the eager women lined up at the counters when I went shopping at Bergdorf Goodman (the only store then carrying the line) in New York City. *Vogue* and *Glamour* had recently mentioned that a few of Bobbi Brown's products were the hottest thing in town, and the reaction of Manhattan's fashion police was quick and decisive. New York women were finally getting the neutral, flat look they wanted, the pale Manhattan look of the Upper East Side crowd. Women wanted those products, even though many of the eyeshadows and blushes looked suspiciously like those in the M.A.C. line.

Although I still think Brown's line is just a M.A.C. clone with better foundations, it seems to be filling a niche. The eyeshadows are incredibly neutral and dark, but thankfully all matte. The lipsticks are also fairly neutral and brown-toned; this line is not about pastels or vivids. Foundations now include an excellent oil-free version, and the overly yellow tones are yielding to more neutral shades. I know some of you may recall my complaining that foundations are supposed to be yellow-toned, and they are, but there's yellow-toned and then there's yellow. Some of Brown's foundations tend to make a person look jaundiced, so be careful.

At first, Brown's line sported only makeup products, but recently skin care products were added. Although many of the products are absurdly overpriced, there are some good options. However, a glaring problem with this line is the lack of a sunscreen of any kind. Whoever was consulting on this project must have been brain-dead during the past few years. Not only does the lack of a good sunscreen promote wrinkles, it can be deadly due to skin cancer.

Nevertheless, you just aren't truly fashionable if you haven't checked out this line, so stop by and see if your tastes match those of "the ladies who lunch."

Bobbi Brown Skin Care

☺ **$$$ Face Cleanser** *($27 for 6 ounces)* contains mostly water, thickener, glycerin, detergent cleanser, plant oil, plant extracts, and preservatives. There are some fairly irritating plant extracts in this product, which can be a problem for the eyes and for sensitive skin. If you don't have sensitive skin, this could be a good water-soluble face cleanser.

☺ **$$$ Gel Cleanser** *($27 for 6 ounces)* is a standard detergent-based water-soluble cleanser that can be good for someone with normal to oily skin; some skin types may find it drying. There are some fairly irritating plant extracts in this product, which can be a problem for sensitive skin.

☺ **$$$ Eye Makeup Remover** *($16.50 for 4 ounces)* is a fairly standard eye makeup remover, like hundreds of others. It works as well as any.

☺ **$$$ Face Cream** *($38 for 2.2 ounces)* contains mostly water, thickener, glycerin, more thickeners, silicone oil, water-binding agents, anti-irritant, vitamins E and A, and preservatives. This is a fairly ordinary as well as overpriced moisturizer that would be good for someone with normal to dry skin. The interesting ingredients and vitamins are too far down on the ingredient list to be more than just a dusting. By the way, the anti-irritant in here is nice, but it comes right after an irritating ingredient, lemon oil.

☺ **$$$ Face Lotion** *($38 for 2 ounces)* contains mostly water; thickener; silicone oil; slip agent; glycolic acid; more thickeners; plant extracts; anti-irritant; silicone oil; water-binding agents; vitamins E, A, and C; and preservatives. This is about a 6% AHA product, which would be fine for someone with normal to dry skin. However, for the money, it can't hold a candle to Pond's or Alpha Hydrox.

☺ **$$$ Eye Cream** *($32.50 for 0.65 ounce)* contains mostly water; plant oil; silicone oil; thickeners; slip agent; more plant oil; water-binding agents; vitamins E, A, and C; and preservatives. This would be a good moisturizer for someone with dry skin, but the vitamins and some of the water-binding agents barely amount to anything.

Bobbi Brown Makeup

☺ **$$$ <u>FOUNDATION:</u>** I have to admit I was particularly surprised at the strange (and rather small) array of foundation colors Brown first came out with. They were not just yellow, they were *extremely* yellow, and the foundation colors for darker skin tones and women of color were on the coppery side. The saleswoman I spoke to at the Bobbi Brown counter told me that the reason the foundations were so yellow was to complement a woman's underlying skin color, which is almost exclusively more yellow than any other color. In theory I agree, but these shades push the theory to the extreme. Foundation should be a neutral color toward the warm side of the color spectrum, without a tinge of pink or orange, but a true shade of yellow is going too far in the other direction. The one type of foundation first offered was **The Foundation** *($35)*, a stick that goes on slightly greasy but very sheer, and is good for someone with normal to dry skin, a definite limitation. **These colors are great for many Caucasian skin tones:** Warm and Sand. **These colors are quite yellow:** Beige, Natural, and Honey. **These colors can turn copper:** Almond, Walnut, Chestnut, and Espresso; they might work for some darker skin tones.

☺ **$$$ Oil-Free Foundation** *($37.50)* is a rather impressive, truly matte foundation. The texture is just great and the colors, though limited, are all wonderfully neutral. It's worth checking out if you want to try something different. One minor cautionary word: The coverage tends to be on the medium side, which isn't great if you want a sheer and natural look.

CONCEALER: This line doesn't have a specific under-eye concealer. Instead, you are supposed to use a lighter-colored foundation under the eye. Unfortunately, because of the consistency of the foundations, you are almost guaranteed slippage into the lines around the eyes.

☹ **$$$ POWDER:** Both the **Loose Face Powder** *($27.50)* and **Pressed Powder** *($22.50)* are standard talc-based powders that go on sheer and soft. The colors are once again extremely sallow; Sunny Beige, Golden Orange, and Pale Yellow are all very yellow. Basic Brown, however, is a great shade for darker skin tones.

☹ **$$$ BLUSH:** The **Blush** *($17.50)* comes in six soft shades. Nothing exciting, but they are nice colors.

☹ **$$$ EYESHADOW:** With only 14 **Eye Shadow** *($15)* colors to choose from, the selection seems a bit sparse, but there are some great matte neutral colors.

☹ **$$$ EYE AND BROW SHAPER:** The **Eye Pencils** *($12.50)* are standard pencils with a small selection of colors. They go on like almost every other pencil I've ever tested.

☹ **$$$ LIPSTICK AND LIP PENCIL:** The standard **Lipstick** *($15)* has a creamy texture tending slightly toward the greasy side. The **Lip Stains** *($15)* don't really stain the lips; they're just lip glosses in stick form. The **Shimmer Lipsticks** *($17.50)* offer soft colors with a small amount of shine. These are OK lip products, but nothing special or unique. The **Lip Pencils** *($12.50)* are standard pencils with a small selection of colors. They go on like almost every other pencil I've ever tested.

☺ **$$$ BRUSHES:** Forgive the comparison once again to the M.A.C. line, but this is one of the only other lines at the cosmetics counters to offer a truly great selection of brushes. Most are very soft and workable. The only ones I would avoiding are the **Eye Shader** *($25)*, which is too big for most women to use on their eyes, and the **Eyeliner Brush** *($17.50)*, which is too thick to create a controlled fine line.

The Body Shop

The Body Shop seems very interested in redeeming itself from a lot of bad press lately and reversing the resulting depressed stock prices, and it is doing a superlative job. Stories in the mainstream press (not fashion magazines, of course) about the minuscule amounts of natural ingredients and the presence of very unnatural ingredients in its products, its misleading statements about its use of animal testing, and its ad copy touting ingredients that aren't even in the products have caused problems for the popular British-based corporation and founder Anita Roddick. For example, one Body Shop hair gel was described as being based on plant mixtures used by "South Ethiopian [women who] traditionally styled their hair with ochre, butter, and acacia gum." Yet not one of those ingredients is in the product. Of course, that information isn't shocking to those of you who read my newsletter and books, but it caused a sensation in the mainstream press.

Further shock resulted when The Body Shop unsuccessfully tried to block an exposé of some of its other so-called natural products. By putting legal pressure on *Vanity Fair,* the company was able to get the embarrassing story dropped. The irate reporter wanted revenge and made it his mission to get the story published anyway; to The Body Shop's woe, he did. The result was that The Body Shop received an enormous amount of unflattering news coverage, not only for using ingredients that were indeed tested on animals as recently as 1992, but also for trying to restrain freedom of the press, and as a result its stock price plummeted.

To my own amazement, I have found myself *defending* The Body Shop regarding its ingredients. Although I concur with all the stories I've read about The Body Shop and have reported as much myself, The Body Shop is no more at fault for misleading the public about the natural content or the effectiveness of its products than any other company I've reviewed. It's what the entire cosmetics industry does, so why pick on The Body Shop? That doesn't mean The Body Shop's story shouldn't be told, and the company's attempt to keep the story out of the press is deplorable. But I wish the mainstream press would get as shocked about Clarins, Borghese, Aveda, and on and on and on. And of course, all these companies suppress negative stories about themselves as well; ever read a negative story about a cosmetics company in a fashion magazine?

As a result of The Body Shop's efforts to regain its standing it is worthwhile to visit one of their stores. Upon entering you are greeted by an enthusiastic sales staff wearing jeans and T-shirts that say "Cruelty-Free." Brochures describing the horrors of animal testing, the efforts of Amnesty International, the educational impact of The Body Shop in Harlem, and the beauty philosophy of the Woodabe tribe of Africa are more prominent than any information about makeup and skin care. I even got a long explanation about how one of The Body Shop's products was being discontinued because they found out the manufacturer used an ingredient from a company that tested on animals (the display for this product even had a noticeable warning sticker attached to it). Yet this is indeed a makeup and skin care boutique, imported directly from England. Starting with only one small storefront in London, it has grown to hundreds of shops all over America, Europe, and Australia. (Recently, The Body Shop has experienced additional financial problems as a result of overexpansion and increased competition from an amazing number of Body Shop clones.)

What a unique experience it is to visit these affectionate, unassuming shops. Sad to say, as was true when I first reviewed The Body Shop, I wish I could say only wonderful things about this company because of its impressive social and humane philosophy (of course, how they handle the press is another issue altogether). But although many of its products are good, they aren't as exceptional as the company's outlook, and The Body Shop has its share of cleansers that dry the skin and toners that can irritate the skin. The products boast a great deal of food, herbs, and vitamins, which is great for those who are interested in that sort of thing (a lot of people are), and the prices aren't bad. The skin care products are available in small trial sizes, so if you want to explore on your own, you can try them for a minimal amount of money.

Colourings is the name of The Body Shop's color line; it has expanded considerably over the years and there are some very interesting products to consider, such as foundation, lip products, blushes, brushes, and face powders. However, most of the powder eyeshadows are shiny, the foundation colors are limited, and the mascaras just average. The cosmetics display area in the stores is quite accessible and you are free to play with the demos all you want, which is nice, but there isn't any convenient shelving where you can put your things down, and the mirrors aren't the best. There is no sales pressure here, and the personnel is much better trained about the products than they have been in the past.

The Body Shop Skin Care

☺ **Balancing Cleansing Gel for Normal to Oily Skin** *($9 for 6.76 ounces)* is a standard detergent-based water-soluble cleanser that could be good for someone with normal to oily skin. It does contain witch hazel, which may irritate the eyes.

☺ **Oil-Free Cleansing Wash for Oily Skin** *($9 for 6.76 ounces)* is similar to the cleanser above, and the same review applies.

☺ **Foaming Cleansing Cream for Normal to Dry Skin** *($9 for 6.7 ounces)* is a standard detergent-based water-soluble cleanser that may be good for someone with normal to slightly dry skin; it may be too drying for someone with extremely dry skin.

☹ **Rich Cleansing Cream for Dry Skin** *($9 for 6.7 ounces)* is basically a cold cream–type wipe-off cleanser that can leave a greasy film on the skin.

☹ **Conditioning Cream Scrub for Normal to Dry & Dry Skin** *($12 for 3.7 ounces)* contains mostly water, plant oil, aloe, cornstarch, lentils (as the scrub agent), thickeners, plant oils, and preservatives. It's not much of a conditioner, it can leave a greasy residue on the skin, and cornstarch can be a skin irritant, even when it's called maize.

☺ **Foaming Gel Scrub for Normal to Oily & Oily Skin** *($12 for 3.7 ounces)* is basically a detergent-based water-soluble cleanser that contains walnut shells as the scrub agent. It can be a good scrub for normal to oily skin, but it would be a problem for someone with very oily skin. It does contain a small amount of witch hazel, which can be a skin irritant.

☹ **Equalizing Freshener for Normal to Oily & Oily Skin** *($8 for 6.76 ounces)* is just your average water–and–witch hazel toner. Witch hazel can be a skin irritant, and the peppermint and mint extracts in this product can be additional irritants.

☹ **Exfoliating Lotion for All Skin Types** *($9 for 6.76 ounces)* contains about 3% AHA, but it also contains alcohol and witch hazel, which irritate and redden the skin. There are better, more effective, and more gentle AHA products to be found.

☺ **Hydrating Freshener for Normal to Dry & Dry Skin** *($8 for 6.76 ounces)* is a very good irritant-free toner for most skin types. It contains mostly water, water-binding agent, slip agent, and preservatives.

☺ **Hydrating Moisture Lotion, for Normal to Dry Skin** *($16 for 3.38 ounces)* contains mostly water, plant oil, plant extract, thickeners, silicone oil, more thickeners, water-binding agent, and preservatives. This would be a very good moisturizer for someone with dry skin. There are tiny amounts of vitamins at the end of the ingredient list, but not enough to have any effect.

☺ **Light Moisture Lotion for Normal to Oily Skin** *($16 for 3.38 ounces)* contains mostly water, silicone oil, plant extract, thickeners, and preservatives. It is indeed light, but someone with oily skin isn't going to be crazy about some of the thickening agents. There are tiny amounts of vitamins at the end of the ingredient list, but not enough to have any effect.

☹ **Oil-Free Moisture Gel for Oily Skin** *($16 for 3.38 ounces)* contains mostly water, film former, plant extract, glycerin, witch hazel, thickeners, preservatives, and small amounts of peppermint and mint extracts. The witch hazel and the mint extracts can be irritants, but otherwise this is an OK, extremely lightweight moisturizer for someone with normal to slightly dry skin; it is completely unnecessary for someone with oily skin. There are tiny amounts of vitamins at the end of the ingredient list, but not enough to have any effect.

☺ **Rich Moisture Cream, for Dry Skin** *($16 for 3.52 ounces)* contains mostly water, glycerin, thickener, plant oil, water-binding agent, more thickeners, silicone oil, and preservatives. This is indeed an emollient moisturizer for someone with dry skin. There are tiny amounts of vitamins at the end of the ingredient list, but not enough to have any effect.

☺ **Eye Supplement for All Skin Types** *($12 for 0.5 ounce)* contains mostly water, silicone oil, plant extracts, glycerin, thickeners, film former, and preservatives. It's a good lightweight moisturizer, but it doesn't add much of anything to the skin.

☺ **Intense Moisture Mask for All Skin Types** *($12 for 3.38 ounces)* contains mostly water, glycerin, film former, water-binding agent, soothing agent, and preservative. I wouldn't call this intense, but it is an OK mask for someone with normal to slightly dry skin. The film former can be a skin irritant.

☹ **Warming Mineral Mask, for All Skin Types** *($12 for 5.1 ounces)* really seems warm on the skin because of the cinnamon and ginger oil, sort of like the way Red Hot candies heat up your mouth. They can be skin irritants, and they don't do much for the skin. This is just a standard clay mask with a twist.

☺ **Tea Tree Oil Facial Wash** *($3 for 2 ounces)* is a standard detergent-based water-soluble cleanser with a small amount of tea tree oil. Tea tree oil has attained quite the reputation for being a wonder for the skin, when all it really turns out to be is a form of urea. That doesn't make it bad for the skin, just not a miracle. It can be a soothing agent when there isn't much of it in a product, but if there's too much it can be a skin irritant.

☹ **Tea Tree Oil Soap** (*$3.70 for 3.5 ounces*) is a standard soap with tea tree oil. Soap is drying, and tea tree oil can't change that. Best used from the neck down.

☹ **Wheatgerm Oil Soap** (*$3.70 for 3.5 ounces*) is similar to the soap above, but with a minute amount of wheat germ oil instead of tea tree oil, and the same review applies.

☹ **Wheatscrub Soap** (*$4.95 for 3.5 ounces*) is identical to the soap above, except that it contains wheat germ, and the same review applies.

☹ **Aloe Face Soap** (*$3.70 for 3.5 ounces*) is a standard soap that also contains aloe, but aloe can't undo the drying and irritating effect of the soap. Best used from the neck down.

☺ **Honeyed Beeswax, Almond and Jojoba Oil Cleanser** (*$7.75 for 1.6 ounces*) is, as the name implies, mostly almond oil, water, wax, jojoba oil, and preservatives. If you want to wipe your makeup off with oil, this will do it, but pure almond oil from the health food store, which costs a lot less, would work just as well.

☺ **Pineapple Facial Wash** (*$9.70 for 3.5 ounces*) is an OK detergent-based water-soluble cleanser that can take off all the makeup, but because it contains some plant oils, it can leave a slightly greasy film on the face.

☹ **Viennese Chalk Facial Wash** (*$5.75 for 2.5 ounces*) contains calcium carbonate (chalk), thickener, water, lanolin, and fragrance. The chalk is supposed to exfoliate, but it doesn't rinse off very well, nor does the lanolin. This could really clog pores in many skin types, and it doesn't remove makeup very well at all.

☺ **Cucumber Cleansing Milk** (*$4.90 for 4.2 ounces*) contains mostly water, glycerin, mineral oil, thickeners, cucumber extract, and lanolin. It must be wiped off with either a washcloth or a tissue, and it definitely leaves a greasy residue on the skin.

☺ **Passion Fruit Cleansing Gel** (*$4.90 for 4.2 ounces*) is an OK water-soluble cleanser that can be slightly irritating to sensitive or dry skin types.

☺ **Orchid Oil Cleansing Milk** (*$4.90 for 4.2 ounces*) contains mostly water, rose water, sweet almond oil, and oil of orchid. This cleanser must be wiped off with a washcloth or tissue, and it leaves a greasy residue on the skin.

☹ **Glycerin & Oatmeal Facial Lather** (*$7.75 for 1.7 ounces*) is a potassium hydroxide–based cleanser that can be fairly drying for most skin types.

☺ **Blue Corn Cleansing Cream** (*$9.95 for 3.5 ounces*) is an oil-based cleanser that is not water-soluble. It leaves a film on the skin, and you'll need a washcloth to remove all traces of makeup. It does contain blue corn tea, but that won't help clean the face. (The blue corn is purchased from Santa Ana, Mexico, in a trade agreement that helped the town buy a new grinding mill. The arrangement is commendable, but nothing about blue corn improves a cosmetic or makes it better for the skin.)

☺ **Chamomile Eye Make-up Remover** *($3.85 for 2 ounces)* is about as standard an eye makeup remover as they come. When chamomile extract is as high up on the ingredient list as it is in this product, it can be a skin irritant and a problem for the eyes.

☹ **Blue Corn Water** *($5 for 4.2 ounces)* is an alcohol-based toner that contains mostly water, alcohol, blue corn tea, watermelon extract, slip agent, and preservative. As intriguing as the other ingredients sound, the alcohol makes it too drying and irritating for most skin types.

☹ **Elderflower Water** *($5 for 4.2 ounces)* is an alcohol-based toner containing mostly water, alcohol, slip agent, and elderflower extract. The alcohol makes it too drying and irritating for most skin types.

☺ **Cucumber Water** *($5 for 4.2 ounces)* is an irritant-free toner that contains mostly water, rose water, plant extracts, water-binding agents, and preservatives. Rose water is a pretty standard ingredient—basically, it's just scented glycerin—but it would be good for someone with normal to dry skin. Don't ask me why lettuce and tomato extracts are in here—it's a mystery to everyone I've talked to at The Body Shop. Maybe it has something to do with a BLT craving?

☺ **Honey Water** *($5 for 4.2 ounces)* is an irritant-free toner that contains mostly rose water—that's scented glycerin—and preservatives. Pretty standard, and fine for most skin types.

☺ **Tea Tree Oil Freshener** *($13.50 for 8.4 ounces)* contains mostly water, aloe, slip agents, film former, tea tree oil, and preservatives. This product is supposed to be for acne, and tea tree oil is somehow supposed to reduce blemishes. I've seen no independent research supporting that conclusion, but it shouldn't hurt anything either.

☺ **Tea Tree Oil Moisturizing Gel** *($13.50 for 8.4 ounces)* is identical to the product above except that it is in gel form, and the same review applies.

☺ **Aloe Vera Moisture Cream** *($8.15 for 1.7 ounces)* is a rich cream containing mostly water, almond oil, glycerin, cocoa butter, thickeners, and aloe vera extract. It should take good care of very dry skin.

☺ **Blue Corn Moisture Cream** *($11.95 for 3.5 ounces)* contains mostly water, plant extract, slip agents, thickeners, plant oil, more thickeners, silicone oil, preservatives, and fragrance. This would be an OK, if uninspired, moisturizer for someone with normal to dry skin.

☺ **Carrot Moisture Cream** *($9.40 for 1.8 ounces)* is only for skin types that do not break out. The second ingredient in this cream is isopropyl myristate, which can cause blackheads. Otherwise, this is an emollient moisturizer, suitable for someone with dry skin, that contains water, almond oil, glycerin, thickeners, and carrot oil.

☺ **Jojoba Moisture Cream** *($12.10 for 1.6 ounces)* is only for skin types that do not break out. The second ingredient in this cream is isopropyl myristate, which can cause blackheads. Other than that, this is a rich cream that contains water, jojoba oil, wheat germ oil, thickener, and glycerin, and would be good for dry skin.

☺ **Moisture Cream with Vitamin E** *($9.20 for 1.6 ounces)* contains mostly water, thickeners, lanolin, more thickeners, vitamin E, and preservatives. The amount of vitamin E in this cream is hardly worth mentioning, but it is a very emollient moisturizer for someone with very dry skin who doesn't have a problem with breakouts.

☺ **Rich Night Cream with Vitamin E** *($9.20 for 1.4 ounces)* contains mostly water, petrolatum, mineral oil, lanolin, thickeners, preservatives, vitamin E, and fragrance. The amount of vitamin E in the cream is hardly worth mentioning, but it is a very emollient moisturizer for someone with very dry skin who doesn't have a problem with breakouts.

☹ **Elderflower Eye Gel** *($5.95 for 0.4 ounce)* contains mostly plant water, witch hazel, glycerin, alcohol, and preservatives. Witch hazel is a skin irritant, and so is the alcohol. This is one of the last products I would consider putting around the eye area.

☺ **Under Eye Cream** *($6.05 for 0.5 ounce)* contains mostly water, wax, plant oil, emollients, thickeners, and preservatives. This is a very emollient moisturizer for extremely dry skin.

☹ **Tea Tree Oil Blemish Stick** *($4.50)* won't help anything. Even if the tea tree oil could help breakouts, the alcohol in this product would just make a mess of things.

☹ **Sage & Comfrey Blemish Gel** *($7.75 for 1.7 ounces)* contains mostly alcohol (need I say more?), witch hazel, plant extracts, thickeners, and preservatives. Great—just what we need, another alcohol-based acne product.

☹ **Sage & Comfrey Open Pore Cream** *($7.75 for 1.7 ounces)* contains mostly water, alcohol, witch hazel, and comfrey and sage extract. The alcohol and witch hazel make it too irritating for most skin types.

☹ **Parsley & Mint Face Mask** *($9.95 for 3.5 ounces)* contains mostly water, slip agent, alcohol, burdock root (a possible irritant), thickeners, plant water, soothing agent, parsley, mint, and preservatives. There's not much parsley or mint in here, but there is alcohol, and that is drying and irritating.

☺ **Blue Corn Scrub Mask** *($9.95 for 4.3 ounces)* contains mostly water, clay, blue corn powder, thickener, glycerin, alcohol, preservatives, and plant oils. This is a fairly standard clay mask. The blue corn powder provides minimal abrasiveness.

☺ **Honey & Oatmeal Scrub Mask** *($11.25 for 2.5 ounces)* is similar to the mask above, but with oatmeal instead of corn powder, and the same review applies.

☺ **Peanut & Rosehip Face Mask** *($9.95 for 3.4 ounces)* contains mostly water, peanut oil, thickeners, glycerin, more thickeners, rose hip pulp, more thickeners, and preservatives. This would be a comfortable facial mask for someone with dry skin.

☹ **LipScruff** *($5.95)* is inexpensive and claims to rid the lips of unwanted flaky skin. To my amazement, LipScruff burned my lips immediately after I applied it, and the burning sensation lasted for some time afterwards. To my chagrin, it was then I noticed the plastic wrapping around the product that warned, "Not recommended for use on sore or chapped lips." But the salesperson had assured me that it would be perfect for my winter-dry lips, which happened to be sore and chapped. As natural and wonderful as the products from The Body Shop sound, this experience once again proved to me that "natural" and "good" are not the same thing (read my tingling, irritated lips). Even though my lips got rubbed the wrong way, the exfoliant action of this product is minimal.

☺ **Watermelon Facial Sun Block SPF 20 (Stick)** *($5.95 for 0.6 ounce)* is an emollient sunscreen for someone with dry skin, but the price is incredibly steep given the need to use a lot of sunscreen. The watermelon is useless, not to mention far down on the ingredient list.

☺ **Watermelon Sun Block SPF 20** *($8.95 for 4.2 ounces)* is a good emollient sunscreen (part titanium dioxide) for someone with dry skin. The watermelon is cute but has no real purpose; however, there are plenty of emollients and plant oils. It does contain a small amount of PVP (commonly found in hairspray), which can be a skin irritant. The tiny amounts of antioxidants at the end of the ingredient list don't count for much.

The Body Shop Makeup

☺ **FOUNDATION:** The Body Shop has several types of foundation. Most have excellent textures and colors; sadly, the color choices are quite limited, with little to nothing for darker skin tones. What they do have is worth checking out if you have light skin. **All-in-One Face Treat SPF 15** *($14.95)* is a very good cream-to-powder foundation that has a soft finish and a nonchemical SPF of 15. Like all foundations of this type, it doesn't work well on dry skin or on skin with large pores. Also, it is difficult to wash off. There are only four shades, which is absurdly limited, although those four are very good.

☺ **All-in-One Face Base** *($14.95)* can go on either wet or dry. It goes on smooth, with a slightly powdery finish. It is better used dry and is fine for some skin types. Again, there are only four colors; although they're all very neutral and good, that's still almost no choice at all.

☺ **Every Day Foundation** *($6.95)* goes on very creamy and light, with a smooth, soft texture. The quality is excellent, but the limited number of colors is a problem. **All of the colors are excellent**; 1604 may be slightly peach for some skin tones.

☹ **Adjustable Coverage Foundation** *($7.50)* has a very thick texture that blends out drier than you would think from first impressions. **The colors are all too pink, peach, or rose for most skin tones.**

😐 **Tinted Moisturizer SPF 12** *($6.95)* comes in two shades: Fair to Medium (which is fairly pink) and Medium to Dark. These go on very sheer, but can give the skin a strange color.

😐 **Cover & Bronze** *($8.95)* comes in three shades, but none are what I would call bronzers. **These colors are good:** 01 and 02, which go on more like a sheer moisturizing foundation than anything else. **This color is too orange for most skin tones:** 03.

☹ **Corrective Prebase** *($5.95)* is a fairly standard assortment of under-makeup colors of peach, lavender, white, and pink. I never recommend this unnecessary step; it colors the skin strangely, and affects the color of the foundation you put over it.

☹ <u>**CONCEALER:**</u> **Every Day Concealer** *($4.50)* comes in a stick and goes on smooth, with a dry but somewhat smooth texture, but it tends to crease into the lines around the eye. **The colors are OK but not the best:** 001 is good, but 01 and 02 are too yellow for most skin tones, and 03 is fairly peach. **Extra Cover Concealer** *($6.95)* is very heavy and greasy. It comes in two colors that are both too yellow for most skin types, and it can crease into the lines around the eyes. **Emergency Cover** *($5.95)* is little more than a foundation. Its two colors don't represent much of a choice, and it doesn't work well because it stands out from your foundation as a separate color. **Lightening Touch** *($9.95)* is like a tube of gloss, but the color is shiny pink and it dries to a powder. It's an OK highlighter if you're into shiny pink, but it isn't a look I recommend.

☺ <u>POWDER:</u> Soft Pressed Face Powder *($8.95)* and **Color Balance Loose Powder** *($8.95)* have a soft, silky texture and come in three very good colors. **Tinted Bronzing Powder** *($6.95)* is a great color, but that is the only color, so it isn't for everyone.

☺ <u>BLUSH:</u> **Cream Blush** *($5.95)* comes in only two colors, but it does have a nice texture for a cream blush. **Powder Blush** *($6.95)* has a smooth, even texture and eight very good soft shades. **Brush-On Rose** *($9.95)* and **Brush-On Bronze** *($12.95)* are beaded, colored powders with a slight amount of shine. I find this a messy and inconvenient way to apply a product that is nothing more than blush, but it's eye-catching and fun. Speaking of fun, test the **Twist & Bronze** *($13.95)* and **Twist & Blush** *($9.95)*. These truly unique products are a two-in-one blush and brush set. The brush twists up into a layer of pressed color that you then apply to the face. It goes on rather soft and slightly shiny. It isn't my style of makeup, but it's one of those fun splurge items I rarely encourage women to bother with.

☹ <u>EYESHADOW:</u> Almost all of the regular **Eyeshadows** *($6.50)* are too shiny and not worth the money. How disappointing, because some of the shades are exceptional. The **Eyeshadow Pencils** *($7.15)* look more convenient to use than they are. The color glides on easily, but the tips are difficult to keep sharpened.

☺ **Continual Eye Color** *($9.95)* is an eyeshadow that comes in a tube; it goes on creamy and dries to a powder. There are seven colors, most rather neutral and attractive. I find this style of eyeshadow more clever than useful when it comes to blending on areas other than the lid, but it is an option. **Complete Color** *($9.95)* comes in six fairly muted earth tones and is meant to be used on the eyes, lips, and cheeks. It goes on fairly creamy and dries to a soft powder. Coordinating the whole face with one color is an intriguing concept, but blending this product on the cheeks and eyes takes some skill, and the applicator isn't best for the cheek area.

☹ <u>EYE AND BROW SHAPER:</u> **Eye Definer** *($4.95)* is a standard pencil in a small array of colors that, except for Brown and Black, are quite poor: too blue, green, or shiny. **Brow & Lash Gel** *($6.50)* is a clear mascara/hairspray sort of product. It will keep brows in place and can help get a little more distance on your lashes. **Lash & Line** *($9.50)* is a clever two-in-one product. One end of the tube is mascara, and the other is liquid liner. As convenient as it sounds, the liner is difficult to use because the handle of the brush is extremely small. It's clever, but relatively useless. **Black Eye Liner Pen** *($5.95)* comes in one shade; it isn't black, it's sort of brown-black. It goes on easily with the pen applicator tip, but dries sticky and shiny. It is relatively water-resistant, which would be OK for swimming, but it doesn't look or feel good at all.

☺ **Eye Brow Powder Pencils** *($5.95)* come in three colors, and at first glance appear to be a very clever alternative to standard pencils, because these have a slightly powdery feel. However, you still have to be careful with application; it can look very artificial, especially if the color doesn't match exactly.

☺ **Eye Brow Powder Makeup** *($7.95)* is an eyeshadow that's meant for the brows. It's a bit on the dry side but works well, and the three shades, though limited, are good.

☺ <u>**LIPSTICK AND LIP PENCIL:**</u> **Lipstain** *($6.95)* is applied with its penlike applicator tip. It stains the lips with deep color, then dries to almost a no-feel finish. If you don't have dry lips, Lipstain is an intriguing way to color the lips. The **Lipsticks** *($6.50)* are fairly creamy but a bit on the glossy side, in a nice range of colors. **Lip Treats** *($8.95)* are rather glossy but opaque lipsticks that are little more than a gloss in a stick form. They are supposed to contain AHAs, which they do, but only 1% at best. **Continual Lip Color** *($9.95)* comes in a tube and goes on rather thick, then dries to a relatively matte finish. It leaves behind a stain once the lip color wears off. The **Lip Liners** *($4.95)* are quite good standard lip pencils, with basic soft colors and a nice, smooth texture. **No Wander** *($6.50)* is a clear lip liner that is supposed to prevent lipstick from bleeding, and guess what, it really works!

☻ **Liptint** *($6.50)* is simply a shiny gloss in a tube. It does leave a bit of a stain once it wears off, but it's too greasy-looking for daytime business wear. **Tinted Lip Color** *($6.95)* is a gloss in the form of a lipstick: basic and emollient. **SPF 30 Lipstick** *($8.95)* is a glossy lipstick with a high SPF. It's not that exciting, and the sunscreen is probably more than anyone needs, but it is just fine.

☹ **Overcoat** *($7.50)* is basically just hairspray in a tube that you are supposed to apply over your lipstick to make it last longer. It tastes terrible, and although the package claims it doesn't sting, my lips tingled immediately when I put it on.

☻ <u>**MASCARA:**</u> **Every Day Mascara** *($4.95)* takes a while to build any length, and the lashes never seem to get very thick. It's not bad, but it isn't anything to get excited about.

☹ <u>**BRUSHES:**</u> There are some very good brushes in this collection, but also many poor ones in some strange sizes and textures. **Lipstick Concealer Brush** *($3.95)* doesn't work well with concealer (your finger or a sponge can blend that area just fine), and it's awfully tiny for lipstick; it would take forever to get the color on. **Finishing Brush** *($5.95)* is a thin fan-shaped brush whose purpose I am not quite sure of; I've never run into a professional makeup artist who used one, so it isn't necessary for you either. **Foundation Brush** *($6.50)* is meant to be used with

The Body Shop's Adjustable Coverage Foundation, but I don't recommend that foundation or this brush. **Blush Powder Brush** *($7.50)* is OK, but the bristles are a little too long and too loosely packed. **Brow Brush** *($3.95)* is stiff and scratchy, which means it will irritate the skin and stroke the brow color on poorly. I also don't recommend the **Lip Brush** *($3.95)* and the **Foam Applicator Stick** *($3.95)*. The Body Shop sells a **Brush Cleaning Fluid** *($5.95)*—a nice idea, but this one is almost all alcohol, which doesn't clean well and tends to dry out the bristles of the brush.

☺ **Contour Brush** *($6.50)* is soft but firm, and the bristles are shaped nicely. The **Blush Brush** *($8.50)* is soft and a perfect size. **Face Body Brush** *($9.95)* is a wonderful, huge brush that is really way too big for the face, but it would be fine for the body—I'm just not sure what you're supposed to put on the body with it. The **Eyeshadow Blender Brush** *($5.95)* and **Eyeshadow Blender** *($4.50)* are both excellent, particularly the Blender Brush. These are perfect all-over eyeshadow brushes. **Liner Softener** *($3.95)* is simply a rubber tip on the end of a long handle. It does the job fine and can be useful if you wear eye pencil.

Borghese

There really was a Princess Marcella Borghese; in her day she was quite a jet-setter, and she gained her title via marriage to Prince Paolo Borghese. According to information received from the company, the princess and her friendship with the late Charles Revson spawned her interest in skin care and cosmetics, and soon—*voila*, she was in business for herself. Over the past ten years, the line has changed hands a few times (the princess is no longer involved), but it stands out as a singularly Italian flavor amidst so many French and American lines. Borghese is also one of the more expensive product lines, but then what would you expect from a cosmetics line whose namesake is a princess? Regardless of the price tag, the products I liked, I really liked, and the ones I disliked, I really disliked. The eyeshadows look beautiful in the container but are mostly too shiny, as are the regular blushes, although they do go on smoothly. Be careful with all of the Borghese products; some of them are overly fragranced.

Borghese has huge, very attractive, and inaccessible counter displays that are organized loosely into three color groupings: Oro (yellow-based), Rosso (pink-based), and Neutrale (neutral/beige). These groupings are helpful but a bit more confusing than those of some of the other cosmetics lines, which divide their colors into the traditional four color families.

Most of Borghese's skin care products are touted as being based on the mineral content extracted from the water around the Montecantini area of Italy. This volcanic region is known for its healing waters, and Europeans flock there, as well as to other such spas around Europe and the Middle East, for a day or week of soaking up whatever restorative magic they can. Whether the spa is in France, Italy, or Israel, the boast is the same: skin care woes are eliminated. The only research I've seen concludes that some serious skin conditions (such as eczemas or psoriasis) are sometimes relieved after soaking in these high-mineral-content waters. Does that mean that if you use products that contain minerals extracted from these waters, your skin will be healed? Well, wrinkles or acne won't be healed, that's for sure. The chance that other skin disorders will be helped is also slim. There is absolutely no evidence that skin rashes can benefit from products that contain the stuff.

Mineral content is only a part of the lengthy ingredient lists covering Borghese's skin care products. There are interesting water-binding agents, antioxidants, anti-irritants, and emollients. Of course, many of these are at the end of the ingredient list, which means you're not getting as much of the good stuff as you would hope given the price tag. Still, there are some intriguing formulations to check out if price is no object.

Borghese Skin Care

☺ **$$$ Spa Comforting Cleanser** *($28.50 for 8.4 ounces)* is a mineral oil–based cleanser that also has a detergent cleansing agent. The long ingredient list includes all the latest water-binding agents, oils, and mineral salts, but they are too far down on the list to help the skin. Other than that, this could be a good cleanser for someone with dry skin. It can leave a greasy film on the skin.

☺ **$$$ Crema Saponetta Cleansing Creme** *($27.50 for 7 ounces)* is a standard detergent-based water-soluble cleanser that can potentially dry out the skin. It can be good for some skin types.

☹ **Gentle Cleanser Exfoliant** *($22 for 2.6 ounces)* would be a lot more gentle if it didn't contain peppermint oil and two detergent cleansing agents known for being extremely irritating and drying (sodium lauryl sulfate and sodium C14-16 olefin sulfate). Did someone at Borghese check out this ingredient list?

☺ **$$$ Gel Delicato Gentle Makeup Remover** *($24 for 8.4 ounces)* contains mostly water, slip agent, film former, several detergent cleansers, tiny amounts of mineral salts, plant extracts, water-binding agents, and preservatives. It will definitely take off makeup, but the detergent cleansing agents can be quite drying for the eye area.

☺ **$$$ Spa-Soothing Tonic for Sensitive Skin** *($25 for 8.4 ounces)* contains mostly water, film former (PVP, commonly found in hairspray), slip agent, plant extracts, silicone oil, water-binding agents, mineral salts, anti-irritant, plant oils, and preservatives. The film-forming agent can make the skin look smoother, but this much (it's the second ingredient) can be a problem for some skin types. I'm not sure "sensitive" is the right term for this toner.

☹ **Stimulating Tonic** *($25 for 8 ounces)* is a toner that contains mostly water, alcohol, talc, slip agent, and mineral salts. This is a lot of money for alcohol and salt. It would indeed be stimulating, as well as irritating and drying, for most skin types.

☺ **$$$ Cura Forte Moisture Intensifier** *($40 for 1 ounce)* contains mostly water, silicone oil, slip agents, mineral oil, plant oil, minerals, peppermint oil, water-binding agents, thickeners, and preservatives. This is a good mineral oil– and silicone oil–based moisturizer, but the peppermint oil can be a potential skin irritant. Most of the intriguing water-binding agents are at the end of the ingredient list.

☺ **$$$ Cura Notte Night Therapy for Dry-to-Very Dry Skin** *($39.50 for 1.7 ounces)* contains mostly water, thickeners, slip agent, more thickeners, plant oils, water-binding agents, salicylic acid, silicone oil, lactic acid, more water-binding agents, minerals, anti-irritant, vitamins, plant extracts, and preservatives. This is about a 3% AHA and BHA exfoliant in a very emollient moisturizing base; although I don't recommend salicylic acid for the face, if you don't mind it, this is an option.

☺ **$$$ Cura Notte Night Therapy for Normal-to-Dry Skin** *($39.50 for 1.7 ounces)* is identical to the product above but without AHAs, and the same review applies.

☺ **$$$ Cura Notte Night Therapy for Normal-to-Oily Skin** *($39.50 for 1.7 ounces)* contains mostly water, film former, slip agent, silicone oils, silica, salicylic acid, water-binding agents, lactic acid, vitamins, thickeners, minerals, more water-binding agents, and preservatives. Several ingredients in this product could cause problems for someone with oily skin, but it could be good for combination skin. It is a very low-percentage AHA and BHA product; you would not be buying this as an exfoliant, but rather as a lightweight moisturizer.

☺ **$$$ Cura Vitale Time-Defying Moisturizer for Dry-to-Very Dry Skin, SPF 8** *($39.50 for 1.7 ounces)* is OK for limited sun exposure. Otherwise, this is a good, though rather ordinary, emollient moisturizer. It contains mostly water, slip agent, silicone oil, thickeners, petrolatum, more thickeners, plant oil, water-binding agents, vitamins, minerals, and preservatives. The vitamins don't count for much in this product.

☺ **$$$ Cura Vitale Time-Defying Moisturizer for Normal-to-Dry Skin, SPF 8** *($39.50 for 1.7 ounces)* is almost identical to the moisturizer above, and the same review applies.

☺ **$$$ Cura Vitale Time-Defying Moisturizer for Normal-to-Oily Skin, SPF 8** *($39.50 for 1.7 ounces)* is fairly similar to the moisturizer above, only in a lighter moisturizing base, and the same review applies.

☺ **$$$ Equalizing Restorative SPF 4** *($37.50 for 1.7 ounces)* contains mostly water, silicone oil, slip agent, a long list of thickeners, mineral salts, plant extracts, anti-irritant, water-binding agents, vitamin E, plant oils, and preservatives. This is a good moisturizer, but the interesting ingredients are down at the end of the ingredient list and don't account for much; also, SPF 4 isn't even close to being able to protect adequately from sun damage.

☺ **$$$ Dolce Notte ReEnergizing Night Creme** *($47.50 for 1.85 ounces)* contains mostly water; a long list of thickeners; silicone oils; petrolatum; water-binding agents; mineral salts; vitamins A, D, and E (antioxidants); plant oil; plant extracts; more water-binding agents; anti-irritants; and preservatives. This is a very good moisturizer for someone with dry skin, but the exotic ingredients are all at the end of the ingredient list, and the ordinary emollients are in the largest concentration.

☺ **$$$ Skin Energy Source** *($40 for 1.5 ounces)* contains mostly water; silicone oil; thickeners; glycerin; more thickeners; petrolatum; silicone oils; water-binding agents; mineral salts; vitamins A, C, and E; anti-irritants; more water-binding agents; plant oil; and preservatives. The first ingredients are just ordinary, and the good stuff is so far down on the ingredient list as to be almost negligible. This is a good moisturizer for normal to dry skin, but there is no energy to be found in it.

☺ **$$$ Spa Lift for Eyes** *($40 for 1 ounce)* contains mostly water, thickener, silicone oils, glycerin, more thickener, mineral salts, several water-binding agents, plant extracts, anti-irritant, vitamin E (an antioxidant), more water-binding agents, and preservatives. This is a good lightweight moisturizer for the eyes, but the price is likely to hurt your vision. Once again, the really interesting ingredients are far down on the ingredient list.

☺ **$$$ Botanico Eye Compresses** *($47.50 for 60 pads)* contains mostly water, witch hazel, slip agents, water-binding agents, anti-irritant, mineral salts, and preservatives. It's good that this product contains an anti-irritant, because witch hazel can be a skin irritant. This is an OK, extremely lightweight moisturizing liquid for the eyes.

☹ **Fango Active Mud for Face and Body** *($50 for 18 ounces)* is a large jar of mud. The brochure describes it as "Fango Therapy of Montecantini." Montecantini is supposedly some kind of special volcanic clay. The product actually contains water, tallow (that's lard), detergent cleansing agent, bentonite (a white clay found in the United States), and a much smaller amount of Montecantini clay. It also contains some mineral salts and some plant oils. It does feel good when you take it off, but that's about it. The tallow can cause breakouts, and the detergent cleansing agent can dry out the skin. There are also other irritating ingredients such as peppermint oil. As a side note, the special clay from Italy isn't even the main type of mud used; clay from the good old U.S.A. is. Regardless of whose clay it is, this is a lot of money for mud and tallow.

Borghese Makeup

<u>FOUNDATION:</u> As this book went to press, Borghese was eliminating many of its foundations in preparation for introducing four new ones in August 1996. When they are available, I will review them in my newsletter, *Cosmetics Counter Update*. Here are the products that were available during my research.

☺ **$$$ Molta Bella Liquid Powder Makeup SPF 8** *($35)* works well on somewhat flawless, normal skin. If you have any dry skin at all, you may find that this foundation, which goes on wet and dries to a powder, looks tight and flaky. It has a wonderful matte dry finish and the SPF, though low, is better than nothing. **All of the colors are excellent;** there's not a bad one in the bunch.

☹ **Hydro Minerali Natural Finish Makeup SPF 4** *($27.50)* doesn't contain much sunscreen, but it is a good, lightweight, very sheer foundation that actually has better colors for darker skin tones than for lighter ones. Although it's supposed to blot oil all day, it won't; although it contains some talc, it isn't enough to eliminate shine. In fact, Hydro Minerali actually has a slight amount of shine itself. It's not all that noticeable, but someone with oily skin who wants the oil shine absorbed won't be thrilled with the sparkle. I do not recommend this foundation.

☺ **$$$ Effetto Bellezza Targeted Treatment Makeup SPF 8** *($35)* is a very creamy, surprisingly light foundation that feels great on the skin. The claim is that it can improve the skin's condition in ten days. If you have dry skin, it can help because it contains emollients, but that's about it; there are no wonder ingredients. SPF 8 is OK but not great. **All of these colors are excellent:** Natural Beige, Buffed Beige, and Richest Beige. **Avoid these colors:** Alabaster Beige, Golden Beige, and True Beige.

☺ **$$$** <u>CONCEALER:</u> **Absolute Concealer** *($25)* has a soft, creamy texture but only two good colors. Ideal Light is too pink for most skin tones, but Ideal Medium is a good neutral (slightly peach) and Ideal Deep would be good on darker skin tones.

☺ **$$$** <u>POWDER:</u> Borghese makes a titanium dioxide– and talc-based pressed powder called **Powder Milano** *($28.50)* that goes on very soft. **All of these colors are excellent:** Neutrale 1, Neutrale 2, Oro, and Terrecotte (which is supposed to be a matte bronzer but works well as a powder). The only color to avoid is Candlelight, which is extremely shiny.

☹ **Loose Powder Milano** *($37.50)* also contains titanium dioxide and talc and would be a good, although expensive, powder except all of the shades are shiny. Doesn't that negate the reason for using a powder in the first place?

☺ **$$$** <u>BLUSH:</u> **Blush Milano** *($28)* is a very satiny regular powder blush that has lovely colors. It feels great, but it can wear poorly on oily skin types because it is such a moist powder. **Most of the colors are superior; the only ones to avoid are:** Terracotte, Raphael, and Puccini Rosegold.

☺ **$$$** <u>EYESHADOW:</u> Borghese makes an appealing assortment of eyeshadow colors, but many have either some amount of shine or too much shine, so you have to look closely. The ones with minimal shine go on matte enough to consider them anyway. Most of the eyeshadows have a great silky texture, go on soft, and blend beautifully. For the **Singles** *($14)*, **Duales** *($27)*, and **Trios** *($32)*, **all of these colors are great velvety, matte to nearly matte shades:** Marrone, Caramello, Neutrale, Cammeo, Carbone, Cioccolato, Angelico, Oceano, Alabastro, Marino Nero, Caffe, Roseto, Grappa, Tuscan Tabac/Tuscan Beige, Roma Charcoal/Roma Ivory, Amalfi Coastal Plums, Amalfi Sandstones, and Titian Taupes. **All of these colors are too shiny or are difficult combinations and should be avoided:** Vino Nero, Forestra Nero, Espresso, Palermo Plum/Palermo Plum Mist, Solare, Madame Butterfly, Primavera Blue, Il Bacio Gray, Puccinin Plum, and Sensual Sage.

☺ **$$$** <u>EYE AND BROW SHAPER:</u> The **Eye Accento Pencil** *($17.50)* and **Linea Perfetta Brow Pencil** *($17.50)* are both ordinary but good. One end of the eye pencil has a sponge tip to blend the color, and the brow pencil has a mascara wand at one end.

☺ **$$$** **Brow Milano** *($17.50)* is an excellent brow gel, with a fantastic brush (which is so important for getting this type of product on right). Unfortunately, the color selection is limited—there are only three shades (and no shades for ash or black eyebrows)—but what there is, is superior.

☺ **$$$ LIPSTICK AND LIP PENCIL:** Borghese sells four types of lipstick in a limited selection of colors. **Lip Treatment Moisturizer SPF 15** *($17)* has a clear moisturizing center around a fairly greasy gloss color. It's rather ordinary for the price, but the SPF 15 is nice. **Superiore State-of-the-Art** *($17.50)* isn't exactly state of the art, but it is a good creamy lipstick. **La Moda Concentrate** *($17)* goes on matte and wears well. The package claims that the lipstick won't feather (bleed into the lines around the mouth), but it does, although not as much as some other lipsticks. Also, its dry texture isn't the most comfortable on the lips. **Perfetta Lip Pencils** *($17)* are basic pencils, just like those in a dozen other lines. They come in a good array of colors.

☹ **$$$ Lumina Lip Color** *($17)* is a group of shiny, fairly creamy/glossy lipsticks that I do not recommend, unless you're into frost.

☹ **MASCARA: Volumina Luxuriant Mascara** *($15.50)* has a wand, unlike most others on the market. One side is smooth with grooves, and the other has small stiff bristles. It does not lengthen lashes, and it flakes and smears as the day goes by.

☺ **$$$ Maximum Mascara for Sensitive Eyes** *($17)* is an excellent mascara, but it isn't any better for sensitive eyes than any other mascara on the market. It builds beautifully and doesn't clump or smear. **Superiore State of the Art Mascara** *($14)* is also an excellent mascara that builds easily and doesn't smear.

Chanel

I want to personally apologize for ever having suggested that Chanel was somehow uncooperative or discourteous while I was doing my research. Quite the contrary. Not only was Chanel's staff exceptionally forthcoming and helpful, they went over and above what I expected. I want to give specific thanks to Dr. Jack Mausner, senior vice president of research and development. The information and research data he presented to me was credible and comprehensive. There are still many points where Chanel and I part ways on philosophy and how to interpret the existing research, but I can present a much better review and more balanced information as a result of my exchange with Chanel.

In terms of shopping for Chanel products, for the most part I found that the salespeople at Chanel counters across the country really had their acts together. I guess that when your cosmetics are this expensive, you have no other choice. The salespeople dress in Chanel uniforms and are very enthusiastic about the fact that Chanel originated in France (never mind that not one of the products seems to be manufactured there). As far as Chanel's skin care products are concerned, the very length of the ingredient lists makes this company stand out—although I've never seen any research that equates expansive content with a superior cosmetic. Nevertheless, if you want to make sure you don't miss out on any exceptional or inexplicable ingredients for the skin, including everything from amniotic fluid to seashells, Chanel may be the line for you: you'll probably find every single ingredient you've ever thought of in just one of Chanel's skin care items. However, a great number of Chanel's products are stunningly basic, with the same standard thickening agents, emollients, oils, and sunscreens that everyone else uses. The only difference for Chanel is the price tag.

Chanel's counter displays are set up in such a way that you need a salesperson to help you test the products. All of the blushes, lipsticks, and eye and lip pencils are attractively divided into very helpful color groupings called Les Violettes (pink/plum), Les Rose Bleus (red/blue), Les Naturels (soft tones of brown/peach), and Les Soleils (yellow/coral). These are then subdivided by intensity. The eyeshadows are grouped similarly, but I was confused about how some of the shades relate to the color groups. Based on its color groupings and intensity categories, Chanel claims that any woman can wear any color group (yellow tones, blue tones, pink tones, and natural tones, according to its charts) as long as she wears the correct intensity of the color. That may be a valid theory, but most women who know their colors would disagree. If you are interested in trying a different color palette, you may be curious enough to give this a try, but be very skeptical. I think it's just another angle to sell more products. By the way, some of Chanel's color line is simply beautiful. Chanel's foundations are particularly smooth and silky, although a few are supposed to have light diffusing properties; if they do, it doesn't show up on the skin. The mascaras are quite good; regrettably, most of the eyeshadows are still shiny, as are most of the blushes.

Chanel Skin Care

☺ **$$$ Foaming Gel Cleanser** *($32.50 for 6.8 ounces)* is a standard detergent-based water-soluble cleanser that can be drying for some skin types. It also contains a tiny amount of animal protein, a water-binding agent, far down on the ingredient list, along with some plant oils, which are listed after the preservatives. Those are interesting ingredients, but the amounts are too tiny to matter.

☺ **$$$ Gentle Cleansing Bar** *($25 for 4.4 ounces)* is a detergent-based bar cleanser that contains tallow and a small amount of water-binding agents. It can be quite drying for some skin types, and the tallow may cause breakouts.

☺ **$$$ Gentle Purifying Bar** *($22.50 for 4.4 ounces)* is a detergent-based cleansing bar with some vitamins, water-binding agents, and an anti-irritant. That's nice, but this is still very expensive for a standard bar cleanser, and the vitamins and water-binding agents aren't useful in a cleanser because they are washed away.

☺ **$$$ Oil Relief Purifying Bar** *($22.50 for 4.4 ounces)* is identical to the soap above except that it also contains witch hazel, which won't relieve or purify anything.

☺ **$$$ Total Cleansing Milk** *($32.50 for 6.8 ounces)* is a standard mineral oil–based cleanser that contains some water-binding agents and vitamins, but again, they are far down on the ingredient list, and even if they did have an effect on the skin, they would be wiped away before that could happen. This product can leave a greasy film on the skin.

☺ **$$$ Gentle Exfoliating Cleanser** *($32.50 for 2.5 ounces)* is a mineral oil–based cleanser that uses shells for the scrub particles. This rather overpriced, but indeed gentle, scrub also contains some water-binding agents and vitamins far down on the ingredient list, which means they're barely there. Anyway, in a cleanser, their effectiveness is washed away. This product can leave a greasy film on the skin.

☺ **$$$ Dual Phase Eye Makeup Remover** *($23.50 for 3.4 ounces)* contains mostly water, silicone oil, slip agents, film former, and preservatives. This will take off eye makeup, but the ingredient list is fairly ordinary for the money.

☺ **$$$ Gentle Eye Makeup Remover** *($23.50 for 3.4 ounces)* is just silicone oil and mineral oil with some preservatives and a tiny amount of anti-irritant. Pure mineral oil can give you the same effect for much less.

☺ **$$$ Firming Freshener** *($32.50 for 6.8 ounces)* contains mostly water, slip agents, lanolin oil, plant extract, more slip agents, water-binding agents, soothing agent, fragrance, and preservatives. This won't firm anything, but it is a good emollient toner for someone with dry skin. The lanolin oil can be a problem for some skin types.

☹ **Refining Toner** *($32.50 for 6.8 ounces)* is alcohol-based and won't refine anything, but it will irritate and dry the skin.

☺ **$$$ Creme No. 1, Skin Recovery Cream** *($95 for 1 ounce)* contains, as the second ingredient listed, amniotic fluid. It doesn't say where the stuff came from. I have seen no evidence that amniotic fluid provides any benefit for the skin, but the implication is that it will make skin look younger—back to the womb, as it were. For $95 an ounce, it should do something, but I'm afraid all the long list of ingredients can do is to provide good standard moisturizing for dry skin. The cream does contain some good emollients and water-binding agents (including a minute amount of lactic acid, which works as a water-binding agent in this quantity and not an exfoliant), but it offers nothing you can't get elsewhere, and for less.

☺ **$$$ Emulsion No. 1, Skin Recovery Emulsion** *($58.50 for 1 ounce)* is almost identical to the cream above, and the same review applies.

☺ **$$$ Daily Protective Complex** *($52 for 1.35 ounces)* contains mostly water, slip agents, several thickeners, water-binding agents, more thickeners, anti-irritant, silicone oil, plant extracts, more water-binding agents, vitamins, and preservatives. This is a very good moisturizer for someone with dry skin, but some of the more exotic ingredients are at the end of the ingredient list, which means they're barely present.

☻ **$$$ Hydra Serum Multi-Vitamin Moisture Supplement** *($50 for 1 ounce)* contains mostly water, alcohol, silicone oil, water binding agents, film former, vitamins, fragrance, and preservatives. Alcohol can be an irritant, but in this product it is probably more an emulsifying agent than anything else. This is a good lightweight moisturizer for someone with normal to slightly dry skin, but there aren't enough vitamins in it to even mention.

☺ **$$$ Hydra-Systeme Maximum Moisture Cream** *($52.50 for 1.7 ounces)* contains mostly water, thickeners, water-binding agents, more thickeners, more water-binding agents, fragrance, more water-binding agents, and preservatives. This is a very good moisturizer for someone with dry skin; we won't get into the price tag this time.

☺ **$$$ Hydra-Systeme Maximum Moisture Lotion** *($50 for 1.7 ounces)* contains mostly water, slip agent, a long list of thickeners, silicone oil, water-binding agents, and preservatives. This is a rather ordinary but good moisturizer for someone with normal to dry skin. The really interesting water-binding agents are at the end of the ingredient list, though.

☺ **$$$ Protection Totale Total Defense Moisture Lotion SPF 15** *($48.50 for 1.7 ounces)* contains mostly water; thickeners; plant oil; silicone oil; vitamins A, C, and E; melanin; several water-binding agents; plant extracts; more thickeners; mineral oil; and preservatives. This is a good emollient sunscreen for someone with dry skin (and money to waste). The antioxidants are high on the ingredient list, which may be of interest to some, but they aren't unique to Chanel products.

☺ **$$$ Protection Totale Total Defense Oil Control Moisture Lotion SPF 15** *($48.50 for 1.7 ounces)* contains mostly water; several thickeners; vitamins A, C, and E; melanin; several water-binding agents; plant extracts; more thickeners;

silicone oil; mineral oil; and preservatives. Nothing in this product can control oil, and there are enough thickening agents and mineral oil to make it a problem for someone with oily skin. However, it would be fine for someone with normal to dry skin. The antioxidants are high on the ingredient list, which may be of interest to some, but they aren't unique to Chanel.

☺ **$$$ Creme No. 1, Skin Recovery Eye Cream** *($70 for 0.5 ounce)* contains mostly water, thickeners, mineral oil, water-binding agent, more thickeners, lanolin, plant oil, anti-irritant, silicone oil, several more water-binding agents, a tiny amount of lactic acid, and preservatives. This is a good, emollient moisturizer for dry skin, but surprisingly basic. It's the price tag that's anything but basic.

☹ **$$$ Day Lift Plus Multi-Hydroxy Refining Cream SPF 8** *($48.50 for 1 ounce)* is OK for limited sun exposure, but I prefer a higher SPF. Other than that, this is a good moisturizer for dry skin with about 4% AHA and BHA, an enormous amount of water-binding agents, and several antioxidants. If there is any ingredient you want to put on your face, it's probably in here.

☹ **$$$ Day Lift Plus Multi-Hydroxy Refining Lotion SPF 8** *($48.50 for 1 ounce)* is similar to the cream above, and the same review applies.

☹ **$$$ Day Lift Plus Oil-Free Multi-Hydroxy Refining Lotion SPF 8** *($48.50 for 1 ounce)* contains more AHAs than the two products above and is definitely a less emollient formula. However, it contains thickeners that could be a problem for someone with oily skin. This product is best for someone with normal to combination skin.

☹ **$$$ Night Lift Plus, Multi-Hydroxy Overnight Refining Treatment** *($68.50 for 1.7 ounces)* is about a 4% AHA and BHA moisturizer. It contains several thickening agents, plant oil, more thickeners, silicone oil, vitamins, water-binding agents, more plant oil, more water-binding agents, and preservatives. This has the most amazing list of water-binding agents you may ever see anywhere. Of course, the product contains only a token amount of almost all of them, but if you're afraid of missing out on some special ingredient, it's probably in here. This is a good emollient AHA/BHA product for someone with dry skin, although the 4% concentration doesn't assure the best exfoliation, and I don't recommend BHAs as exfoliating agents for the face.

☹ **Pure Response Firming Control Gel** *($50 for 1.7 ounces)* contains, as the second ingredient, aluminum starch—yes, the same ingredient you find in deodorants. It doesn't firm the skin, but it can irritate and cause breakouts.

☺ **$$$ Lift Serum Extreme, Advanced Corrective Complex** (*$70 for 1 ounce*) contains mostly water, water-binding agents, thickeners, more water-binding agents, more thickeners, vitamin E, silicone oils, plant extracts, anti-irritant, and preservatives. This is a good moisturizing lotion for someone with dry skin, and it does contain a host of interesting water-binding agents, but it won't lift your skin anywhere.

☹ **$$$ Eye Lift Corrective Eye Complex** (*$60 for 0.6 ounce*) contains mostly water, rose water, witch hazel, slip agents, water-binding agents, several plant extracts, film former, thickeners, anti-irritant, vitamins, more water-binding agents, and preservatives. I'm not fond of witch hazel on the face or near the eyes. Other than that this is an OK lightweight moisturizer for normal to slightly dry skin.

☺ **$$$ Firming Eye Cream** (*$50 for 0.5 ounce*) contains mostly water, rose water, plant oils, water-binding agent, thickeners, slip agents, plant extract, anti-irritant, more water-binding agents, and preservatives. This would be a good moisturizer for someone with dry skin, but it won't firm anything.

☹ **$$$ Gentle Cleansing Mask** (*$42 for 2.5 ounces*) is a basic clay mask that contains mostly clay, witch hazel, slip agents, thickeners, and preservatives. It can be drying for some skin types.

☹ **$$$ Environmental Purifying Mask** (*$42 for 2.5 ounces*) contains mostly water, alcohol, film former, slip agents, thickeners, vitamin E, and plant extracts. It won't purify the skin, but when you take it off, the skin will feel smooth. The alcohol and film-forming agent can be irritating for some skin types.

☺ **$$$ Maximum Moisture Mask** (*$42 for 2.5 ounces*) contains mostly water, mineral oil, a long list of thickeners, slip agents, water-binding agents, silicone oil, fragrance, more water-binding agents, vitamins, and preservatives. Many of the impressive water-binding agents come after the fragrance on the ingredient list, which means they are barely present. This is still a good emollient mask for someone with dry skin.

☺ **$$$ Natural Exfoliating Mask** (*$42 for 2.5 ounces*) contains mostly water, petrolatum, lanolin, thickeners, and preservatives. This is a very ordinary, but very emollient, mask for someone with dry skin. This is a lot of money for Vaseline and some lanolin, though.

☺ **$$$ Maximum Moisture Lip Treatment** (*$25 for 0.13 ounce*) is little more than an emollient lip balm with wax thickeners, lanolin, and petrolatum. It's about as standard as they come; only the price is above par.

Chanel Makeup

☺ **$$$ FOUNDATION:** **Teint Pur Matte SPF 8** *($47.50)* **has an incredible color selection**; it would be hard to make a mistake. The foundation does contain aluminum starch, which can be an irritant for some skin types and cause breakouts. It also comes in a pump bottle, which is not my favorite type of container, and the pump doesn't reach the bottom of the bottle. It does have a good lightweight texture and a matte, sheer finish, however.

☺ **$$$** **Teint Naturel SPF 8** *($50)* has a sheer, moist finish and would be excellent for someone with normal to dry skin. **These colors are excellent:** Fawn, Alabaster, Porcelain, Soft Bisque, Warm Beige, Tawny Beige, and Golden Beige. **These colors are too peach or rose:** Porcelain Ivory and Natural Beige.

☺ **$$$** **Teint Facettes Lumiere Perfecting Compact Makeup** *($40)* is a cream-to-powder foundation that has a very silky feel and goes on very sheer although somewhat greasy for someone with combination to oily skin. It does dry to a soft powder finish. This is a wonderful product, and **the color selection is excellent.**

☺ **$$$** **Teint Extreme Lumiere with Non-Chemical SPF 8** *($47.50)* contains mostly water, talc, and silicone, and has a nice texture for someone with normal to slightly dry or slightly combination skin. **All of the colors are excellent.** It comes in an attractive, innovative pump container that pushes the color up from the bottom and prevents waste—which is nice, because at this price, wasting even a drop is expensive.

☺ **$$$** **Teint Lumiere Creme with Non-Chemical SPF 8** *($55)* is mostly water and mineral oil. It has a creamy texture that would be appropriate only for someone with dry skin. The titanium dioxide SPF 8 provides protection for limited sun exposure. **These are the best colors:** Alabaster, Fawn, Porcelain Ivory, Soft Bisque, Beige Naturel, Beige Intense, and Golden Beige. **These colors are too peach, orange, or ash:** Porcelain and Tawny Beige.

☹ **$$$** **Perfect Colour Matte**, **Perfect Colour Creme**, and **Perfect Colour Pearle** *($52 each)* are semi-opaque tints that lay a sheer white or colored layer over the face, supposedly to make the skin look fair and flawless. In my opinion, these undercoats make the skin look chalky or give it a strange color that you then cover up with foundation. **Perfect Colour Bronze** and **Perfect Colour Blush** *($52 each)* are two of the sheerest face tints on the market—best for fair to medium skin tones only. All these products have an SPF of 8, which is nice, but layering sunscreen is not the best for the skin. Optimum protection comes from a single SPF 15 product.

☹ **CONCEALER:** Chanel's under-eye **Estompe Corrective Concealer** *($26)* has a slightly greasy texture, and **the colors are not as good as they could be:** Professional is too blue/green and combines poorly with the foundation; Light is slightly pink, but may be acceptable for some skin tones; Medium can turn slightly rosy. Also, this concealer can crease. **Extreme Estompe Cover Up** *($30)* has a beautiful creamy texture and the colors, Light, Medium, and Deep, are quite good. What a shame it creases so easily into the lines around the eyes and continues to all day long.

☺ **$$$ POWDER:** Perfecting Pressed Powder *($38)* tends to go on very dry in spite of its lovely silky texture. It is just a standard talc- and mineral oil-based powder for an unusually high price tag. **All of the colors are excellent. Perfecting Loose Powder** *($38)* comes in three shades that are supposed to have "light-reflecting properties," but they are just shiny powders; the shine sort of negates the purpose of using a finishing powder, doesn't it? The first ingredient for the loose powder is aluminum starch, which can be a skin irritant and cause breakouts. **Luxury Powder Compact** *($95)* is a stunning gold compact; it would be worth the money if it were a necklace, but it's not. The compact is refillable. **Perfecting Bronzing Powder** *($38)* comes in two shades; Golden Bronze is very shiny and Deep Bronze is nicely matte.

☺ **$$$ BLUSH:** Powder Blush *($35)* goes on fairly smooth and the color selection is rather attractive, but only four of the shades are matte: Pink Dusk, Coral Fire, Cedar Rose, and Satin Rose. The rest are too shiny to recommend. **Contour Colour Blush** *($35)* is somehow supposed to be different from the Powder Blush, but it is essentially the same texture and the colors are pastel and attractive. There is nothing contouring about these shades. The only difference is that these colors are applied with a thin fan-like brush. They have only a slight amount of shine and there are some great colors. **The only colors to avoid are:** Peach Gold and Nude. **Cheek Rouge** *($35)* is a liquid-to-powder blush that dries to a soft powder finish. It blends on beautifully and would be a great option except that almost all the colors are shiny.

☹ **EYESHADOW:** Chanel has a thing for shiny eyeshadows. Haven't they noticed how well other lines are doing with matte shadows? The only matte **Eyeshadow** *($40/$50)* is Les Mats Naturels 4 and Soft Taupe. The rest are too shiny to recommend. **Eye Blush** *($25)* is a creamy, almost liquid eyeshadow that squeezes out of a small tube and goes on intensely shiny. It dries to a soft powdery finish, but that shine, now that's intense! **Eye Essentials** *($52)* are three products in one: an eyeliner, eyeshadow, and cake mascara all in the same color. It isn't in the least essential; in fact, it is impractical and overpriced for what you get. The eyeshadow section is too tiny to get a brush through, the eyeliner is very standard, and the cake mascara, well, who wants to bother with that?

☺ **$$$ EYE AND BROW SHAPER:** **Precision Eye Definers** *($25)* are simply very expensive standard pencils and one end has a smudge tip. **Professional Eyeliner** *($43.50)* isn't all that professional. It is just a powder that can go on dry or wet. It comes in three choices of two colors each. The color combinations are a bit strange; you would be better off buying one deep-colored (not shiny) eyeshadow and lining your eyes with it. **Instant Eyeliner** *($25)* is a black liquid in a pot; it goes on very severe and will remind you of Twiggy lashes (if you're old enough). **Precision Brow Definer** *($28)* goes on rather hard, which means it doesn't look so greasy, but it still tends to make hard lines. One end of the pencil is a mascara wand, which can help soften the line you draw on.

☺ **$$$** **Brow Shaper** *($28)* is a brow gel with a small color selection: Soft Brown, Taupe, Black, and Clear. There are no shades for brunettes, blondes, or redheads, but brows definitely stay in place and the gel goes on easily, without smearing, which is very important for this type of product.

☹ **$$$ LIPSTICK AND LIP PENCIL:** Chanel makes one of the few lip products that actually prevents lipstick from bleeding into the lines around the mouth; it is called **Protective Colour Control** *($26)*. Unfortunately, it tends to cake as you apply more lipstick over it, and it's expensive. The price may be worth it for those who suffer from feathering, but I have found cheaper drugstore products that work just as well. **Creme Lipstick** *($20)* isn't as creamy as it is glossy and tends to bleed easily into the lines around the mouth. **Sheer Lipstick** *($20)* is, as the name implies, more gloss than lipstick. It's nice but standard, and doesn't last. **Matte Finish Lipstick** *($20)* is not all that matte, except in comparison to Chanel's other lip products. All of Chanel's lip colors have a slight stain so they tend to stay around slightly longer on the lips.

☹ **Professional Lip Basics** *($37)* is a lip color that goes on in two layers: a wet powder that you let dry over the lips and a gloss that you then apply over that. Interesting option, but it didn't last any longer than most other lipsticks I've tested, it was too much trouble to apply, and it ended up looking gooey and glossy. **Lip Intensities** *($45)* is a compact of lip color divided into four sections, all in the same shade but with different textures. One-quarter of the compact has a creamy consistency; the others are matte, glossy, and sheer. It's hardly convenient. Most women prefer to open a lipstick tube and quickly sweep color across the lips instead of having to use a brush. Although it sounds nice to have the texture of your choice, most women prefer one over the others. If you have a problem with lipstick feathering, the gloss and the sheer will slide into the lines around your mouth. If your lips have a tendency to be dry, the matte isn't great. The creamy lipstick may be fine, but then the other three are a waste. **Precision Lip Definer** *($25)* resembles a dozen other lip pencils. This one happens to have a lip brush on one end, which is convenient, but it doesn't warrant the steep price tag.

☺ **$$$ MASCARA:** **Instant Lash Mascara** *($20)* takes a bit of effort to build long thick lashes, but long thick lashes is what you'll get without clumping, smudging, or smearing. **Fragile Lash Mascara** *($20)* is essentially the same mascara with a different brush. They work the same, which is great.

☹ **$$$ BRUSHES:** Chanel has an attractive, satiny, fairly useful group of brushes. **Powder Brush** *($40)* and **Blush Brush** *($37.50)* are full and soft but perhaps a bit too loosely packed for optimum control, and at these prices they should be perfect. **Eye Liner Brush** *($20)*, **Contour Eyeshadow Brush** *($21)*, **Touch Up Brush** *($26)*, and **Eyeshadow Brush** *($21)* are all very good but not outstanding.

Chantal Ethocyn (Skin Care Only)

I'm sure many of you have watched the Chantal Ethocyn infomercial or seen the magazine and newspaper advertisements with the astounding before-and-after pictures of one woman's face. The side of the woman's face treated with ethocyn is smooth and practically line-free, while the other side, without ethocyn, is a mass of wrinkles. The reason for that improvement, according to the company, is that ethocyn can produce elastin.

Dr. John Bailey, director of the FDA's Office of Cosmetics and Colors, says, "The intense marketing campaign for this product reminds me of what happened with thigh creams two years ago." The Cosmetic, Toiletry, and Fragrance Association (CTFA) lists ethocyn as nothing more than a "skin-conditioning agent." Nonetheless, the product line is being endorsed by a Richard Strick, M.D., from the UCLA School of Medicine. On the surface, that endorsement is extremely impressive. However, I interviewed several dermatologists and medical researchers, including two doctors who had worked with Dr. Strick at UCLA, and not one was familiar with his work on ethocyn (work that he has been involved with since at least 1986), nor were any of them willing to say that he had discovered anything significant or worthwhile. In fact, Dr. Richard Reisner, past head of dermatology at UCLA, who has done research on ethocyn with Chantal Burnison (the creator and owner of ethocyn), said he had no information about what this ingredient does, and he doubted that it could do much of anything.

Several dermatologists told me that because data on ethocyn has never been published in any medical journal or been subject to peer review, it isn't anything they would be interested in. Only one doctor I spoke to was interested in checking out the information I had received on the product, and she was unconvinced but would not go on record with her comments. However, I was told repeatedly that building elastin might be helpful for the skin, but without at the same time building collagen, which is the major support structure of the skin, it may look interesting in the laboratory under a microscope, but it won't help remove a wrinkle. (According to the ethocyn patent, Dr. Strick claims that his product builds elastin but *decreases* collagen, because collagen gets hard with age, so you don't want it around.)

My intense skepticism was boosted by a personal letter from Dr. Strick that accompanied the package of information I received from the Chantal Pharmaceutical Corporation (formerly called Chantal Cosmetics, but that doesn't sound quite so scientific, does it?). The letter states that "[ethocyn] has been around for about 15 years or so from the time it was first discovered . . . [but] this is the company's first product to actually be sold to the general public." That simply isn't true. Chantal Ethocyn, under the name Elasyn, was retailed to the public at Saks and Bloomingdale's back in 1986, while the patent was still pending. It was also advertised in *Vogue, Harpers Bazaar,* and *Elle* magazines. It failed and was removed from the market.

It turns out that ethocyn is not exactly a natural molecule, at least not the kind of "natural" the consumer is hoping for. According to the *International Cosmetic Ingredient Dictionary,* it is a by-product of ether and alcohol that functions as a skin-conditioning agent. Ethocyn, in essence, is little more than an emollient, and a rather average one at that.

☹ **Gel Cleanser** *($23 for 6.7 ounces)* contains mostly water, alcohol, slip agents, plant oils, thickeners, and preservatives. The alcohol is a possible skin irritant and not something you should use near your eyes; other than that, this is a fairly ordinary skin cleanser.

☺ **$$$ Ethocyn Eye Cream** *($30 for 0.5 ounce)* contains mostly water, witch hazel, thickeners, plant oil, ethocyn, thickeners, and preservatives. The witch hazel is a possible skin irritant that can plump lines and cause dryness.

☺ **$$$ Ethocyn Hydrating Complex Moisturizer** *($40 for 2 ounces)* contains mostly water, silicone oils, several thickeners, slip agents, algae extract, ethocyn, several water-binding agents, and preservatives. This would be a good moisturizer for someone with normal to dry skin. The algae is a nice gimmick, but it has little to no value for the skin.

☺ **$$$ Ethocyn Essence Vials** *($50 for 0.23 ounce)* contain mostly water, several standard slip agents, thickeners, ethocyn, plant oil, and preservatives. This would be a good lightweight moisturizer for someone with dry skin, but it's incredibly expensive and not all that different from any of the other products in this line that contain ethocyn.

☹ **$$$ Revitalizing Mask** *($25 for 2 ounces)* is a standard clay mask with a tiny amount of plant oils. Clay is a potential irritant for some skin types.

Charles of the Ritz

Charles of the Ritz is overlooked by many women, perhaps because it is usually found at lower-end department stores. But take notice: this low- to medium- to high-priced line has an impressive range of products. They even offer great colors in all of their products for women of color. One minor irritation: many of the product names are silly and childish (pressed powders called Toast of the Town and Baby Bare; foundations called The Naked Truth and Tisket-a-Bisquit). It's hard for adults to relate to cosmetics that sound like a lame joke.

The display unit is a bit confusing, but the basic concept is a good one. The board is divided into two color groups: Cameo and Rose. Cameo is composed of yellow and earth-tone colors, and Rose contains pastel and vibrant blue-tone colors. The palette is further divided into smaller groups of blush, eyeshadow, lipstick, lip liner, and nail polish that are all color-coordinated. This is helpful but almost too specific, allowing the consumer little visual room to play with her own color combinations. Still, it can be helpful for those who need help coordinating all the color elements of a makeup look.

Charles of the Ritz Skin Care

☹ **$$$ Biocharge Cleanser** *($19 for 6.5 ounces)* contains nothing that's charged. It needs to be wiped off, and several ingredients high on the ingredient list can cause breakouts.

☹ **$$$ Revenescence Feather Touch Cleanser** *($20 for 12 ounces)* couldn't be further from a "feather touch" if it were a ton of bricks. It contains mostly mineral oil, water, lanolin, petrolatum, heavy thickeners, slip agent, and preservatives. This is a very emollient wipe-off cold cream. Does anybody really use this kind of stuff anymore?

☺ **$$$ Revenescence Moisture Cream Cleanser** *($18.50 for 4 ounces)* is actually more lightweight than the cleanser above, but it is still a standard mineral oil–based wipe-off cleanser that can leave a greasy film on the skin.

☺ **Moisture Balancing Day Care Skin Soother** *($18.50 for 2 ounces)* contains mostly water, mineral oil, slip agent, plant oil, thickeners, soothing agent, petrolatum, more thickeners, lanolin, and preservatives. It's a very emollient moisturizer for someone with extremely dry skin.

☺ **$$$ Revenescence Cream** *($40 for 4.4 ounces)* contains mostly water, glycerin, mineral oil, lanolin, heavy thickeners, and preservatives. This is a very heavy, ordinary moisturizer for someone with extremely dry skin, but the price tag is inane. It is almost identical to Revenescence Feather Touch Cleanser; you could use that product as your moisturizer and pocket the change.

☹ **Revenescence Liquid** *($32 for 4 ounces)* contains mostly water, glycerin, thickener, detergent cleansing agent, and preservatives. The detergent cleansing agent, sodium lauryl sulfate, is a skin irritant and can dry the skin. This is a pretty strange concept for a moisturizer: why would anyone want to rub a detergent into her skin?

☺ **$$$ Revenescence Moist Environment Night Treatment** *($40 for 2.2 ounces)* contains mostly water, thickeners, petrolatum, more thickeners, a tiny amount of water-binding agent, and preservatives. This is an overly expensive, very ordinary emollient moisturizer for someone with extremely dry skin. The second ingredient is isopropyl myristate, which can cause breakouts.

☺ **$$$ Revenescence Softening Lotion, 100% Alcohol Free for Dry or Sensitive Skin** *($17.50 for 8 ounces)* contains mostly water, water-binding agents, slip agent, soothing agent, plant extracts, plant oil, and preservatives. It is a very good lightweight moisturizer for someone with dry skin.

☹ **Revenescence Softening Lotion for Combination to Oily Skin** *($17.50 for 8.7 ounces)* contains alcohol and menthol, which aren't great for any skin type.

☹ **Revenescence Firmescence 770 Wrinkle Lotion** *($30 for 2 ounces)* contains mostly water, glycerin, alcohol, slip agents, lemon oil, and preservatives. If the term "wrinkle lotion" means this product can *cause* wrinkles, then it's close to accurate. Alcohol and lemon oil can irritate and dry skin. Nothing in this lotion is appropriate for wrinkles.

☺ **$$$ Special Formula Emollient** *($27 for 4 ounces)* is almost identical to Revenescence Cream above, and the same review applies.

☹ **Timeless Difference Day Recovery Lotion, SPF 6** *($28.50 for 2 ounces)* is not recommended. SPF 6 doesn't provide the best protection from the sun.

☺ **$$$ Timeless Essence Night Recovery Cream** *($35 for 1.7 ounces)* contains mostly water, water-binding agent, slip agent, mineral oil, a long list of thickeners, vitamin E, plant oils, and preservatives. This won't help skin recover from anything, but it is a good moisturizer for someone with dry skin.

☺ **$$$ Age-Zone Controller** *($30 for 0.8 ounce)* contains mostly water, slip agent, several thickeners, water-binding agents, silicone oil, soothing agent, and preservatives. Nothing in this product will control age in any way, but it is a good moisturizer for someone with normal to dry skin.

☺ **$$$ Biocharge Replacement Therapy Serum for Changing Skin** *($30 for 1.9 ounces)* contains mostly water, slip agent, thickeners, silicone oil, film former, soothing agent, vitamins, a long list of water-binding agents, plant extracts, more water-binding agents, and preservatives. This is a very good moisturizer with antioxidants for dry skin, but it won't stop aging.

☺ **$$$ Line Refine for Eyes** *($15 for 0.5 ounce)* contains mostly water, silicone oils, glycerin, a long list of thickeners, and preservatives. This won't refine anything, but it is a good moisturizer for someone with dry skin.

☺ **$$$ Timeless Difference Eye Recovery Cream** *($23 for 0.5 ounce)* contains mostly water, water-binding agent, thickeners, plant oil, slip agent, vitamin E, anti-irritants, silicone oil, more thickeners, and preservatives. This would be a very good moisturizer for dry skin, particularly around the eyes.

☹ **Disaster Cream** *($15 for 0.5 ounce)* is, to my way of thinking, a disastrous product. It contains mostly water, zinc oxide, cornstarch, clay, and preservatives. Not one of these ingredients is the least bit helpful for getting rid of blemishes. Also, cornstarch can be an irritant and may cause breakouts. How's that for a disaster?

☹ **$$$ T-Zone Controller, Skin & Color Corrector** *($17 for 2 ounces)* contains mostly water, alcohol, slip agent, thickeners, salicylic acid, and preservatives. Alcohol and salicylic acid show up in acne product after acne product. They don't control oil, and they don't stop breakouts. What a waste!

☺ **$$$ Moisture Intensive Facial** *($20 for 4 ounces)* contains mostly water, thickeners, slip agent, plant oil, several more thickeners, several water-binding agents, anti-irritants, plant oils, and preservatives. This is a good emollient facial mask for someone with dry skin.

☺ **$$$ Self Protection for Eyes** *($30 for 0.5 ounce)* contains mostly water, silicone oil, glycerin, thickeners, more silicone oil, slip agent, more thickeners, water-binding agents, plant extracts, anti-irritant, vitamin E, more water-binding agents, vitamin A, plant oils, antioxidant, thickeners, and preservatives. This is a very long ingredient list that adds up to a good moisturizer for dry skin. The specialty ingredients are too far down in the ingredient list to add much benefit for the skin.

☺ **$$$ Any Age Self Protection for Face, SPF 15** *($45 for 1.8 ounces)* contains mostly water, silicone oil, several thickeners, water-binding agents, plant extracts, vitamin A, plant oils, vitamin E, more water-binding agents, thickeners, and preservatives. This is a very good moisturizing sunscreen for someone with dry skin, but the price is completely excessive for an otherwise basic SPF 15.

Charles of the Ritz Makeup

☺ **FOUNDATION: Superior Moisture Foundation for Normal to Dry Skin** *($18.50)* provides medium coverage and has a smooth, moist finish. **These colors are very good:** Natural Ivory, Soft Beige, New Beige, and Bronzed Beige. **These colors should be avoided:** Beige Sand, Deep Beige, Beige Blush, and Tender Beige.

☺ **Superior Foundation for Normal to Oily Skin** *($18.50)* goes on light and feels great. **These colors are good choices:** Alabaster, Sunlit Beige, Simply Beige, Toffee Beige, and Toasted Beige. **These colors should be avoided:** Warmed Beige, Honey Buff, Mocha Bisque, and Beige Blush.

☹ **Perfect Finish Makeup SPF 6** *($12.50)* comes in a pump bottle (which isn't my favorite, because you tend to pump out more than you need and you can't get it back in the bottle). It blends on easily and dries to a soft, truly matte finish. Unfortunately, it contains a small amount of alcohol (and smells somewhat medicinal), so it would be appropriate only for someone with very oily skin, and even then I would test it carefully to make sure the alcohol doesn't dry out the skin. The SPF 6 isn't enough to protect from the sun. **All the colors but one are excellent. The only color to avoid:** Tisket-A-Bisquit—not because the name is obnoxious, but because the color is too rose.

☺ **Perfect Finish Solid Powder Foundation** *($17.50)* is more like a pressed powder than a foundation; it would work as a light matte finish only for someone with normal skin. (When this kind of product is used by itself as a foundation, it can look dull and powdery if your skin is dry.) **The color selection is excellent** (except for First Blush, which is too pink for most skin tones).

☹ **Complete Cover Makeup** *($20)* tends to go on rather thick, but it does blend out relatively sheer. It has a light feel on the skin, but sticks almost like a stain, and is extremely difficult to get off regardless of the cleanser used. If you want long-lasting makeup, this is one of the few that will hold up under almost any condition. **These colors are good:** Light Cameo and Soft Cameo. **These colors are too pink or peach:** Natural Cameo, Light Rose, Soft Rose, and Natural Rose.

☹ **CONCEALER: Complete Cover Concealer** *($14)* goes on rather thick and dry, and tends to crease. **The four colors are OK but not great:** Pale and Light may be too pink for some skin tones; Medium can be too peach; White can work when used minimally over or under foundation, but should never be used by itself.

☺ **POWDER: Translucent Pressed Powder** *($16.50)* is a standard talc-based powder that is quite silky and sheer and comes in three good shades: Light, Medium, and Dark. **Blemish Control Powder** *($14)* contains talc and clay. It won't control blemishes, but it is definitely on the dry side and comes in three good shades: Light, Medium, and Dark.

☺ **BLUSH: Moistureful Cheeks** *($12.50)* comes in eight beautiful colors. All have a silky, sheer texture, go on very soft, and blend on smooth and even. They may be too sheer for some skin tones.

☺ **EYESHADOW: Moistureful Eye Color** *($17.50)* comes only in sets of two shadows. The color combinations are quite impressive, with very compatible and surprisingly neutral shades. Most are slightly shiny, but they don't appear shiny on the eye. My only hesitation is that the colors blend on almost too soft and sheer. None of these shades would be appropriate if you want a dramatic look or have a darker skin tone. **The only color set to avoid:** Stormy Night/Rainy Day.

☺ **EYE AND BROW SHAPER: Classic Liners for Eyes** *($11)* are fairly standard pencils that have a slightly greasy texture. There aren't many colors, but most are just fine.

☺ **LIPSTICK AND LIP PENCIL: LipSTICK** *($14.00)* is Charles of the Ritz's version of Revlon's ColorStay, which isn't surprising, since Revlon owns Charles of the Ritz. It is an excellent, very matte lipstick that doesn't bleed, and I think it wears smoother than ColorStay. There are only a handful of colors, though, so it doesn't even begin to compete with its kissing cousin in that regard. **Classic Liners for Lips** *($11)* are fairly standard pencils that have a smooth texture, but only four colors.

☹ **Perfect Lip Color** *($10)* is not perfect, but it is very shiny and glossy. **Revenescence Moist Lip Color** *($15)* has a creamy consistency that is a bit on the greasy side, and several of the colors are shiny. The "maximum wear" claim on these lipsticks is a fair one; they have a stain that helps keep them around longer.

☺ **MASCARA: Perfect Finish Lash** *($11)* is an excellent mascara with great lengthening ability, but it does have a slight tendency to smudge by the end of the day.

☹ **Every Last Lash Mascara** *($13.50)* takes forever to build what length it can, which isn't much, and it tends to smear.

Christian Dior

Dior is a great name when it comes to fashion, but it seems to have lost its footing in the world of makeup. There is nothing particularly outstanding in this line. For the most part, the eyeshadows are all extremely shiny and the color combinations highly contrasting and hard to use, at least for daytime. Dior is one of the few lines with a five-color eyeshadow set, but the colors are almost all too shiny to recommend other than for evening wear. The foundations come in a very limited selection of colors, and although I like some of the textures and coverage very much, this line charges a fairly hefty sum for makeup that is not particularly special or unique; also, many of the colors are too pink, peach, or orange. The lipsticks are fairly creamy and have a good texture, which is nice but still not much to get excited about. The counter displays are nice enough and easily accessible, but the colors aren't organized by color families, which can make finding your color range difficult.

Christian Dior Skin Care

☺ **$$$ Hydra-Dior Cleansing Milk for Dry and Sensitive Skin** *($34 for 8.4 ounces)* is a standard mineral oil–based cleanser that is very difficult to rinse off without the use of a washcloth, which is not great for someone with sensitive skin.

☺ **$$$ Hydra-Dior Cleanser for Oily Skin** *($34 for 8.4 ounces)* contains several types of oils—not great for someone with oily skin. It doesn't rinse off easily, and it leaves a greasy film on the skin.

☹ **Equite Gentle Cleansing Bar** *($24.50 for 3.5 ounces)* is a detergent cleansing bar that uses sodium lauryl sulfate, which can be very irritating, as the cleansing agent. It also contains tallow, which can cause breakouts and clog pores.

☺ **$$$ Equite Gentle Gel Face Wash** *($24.50 for 4.2 ounces)* is a mineral oil–based cleanser that can leave a greasy residue on the skin. It may indeed be gentle, but it is also a remarkably ordinary wipe-off cleanser.

☹ **Equite Wash Off Cleansing Gel** *($24.50 for 6.8 ounces)* is a standard detergent-based, water-soluble cleanser that uses sodium C14-16 olefin sulfate as the cleansing agent, which is exceptionally drying and irritating for the skin.

☺ **$$$ Equite Face and Eye Makeup Remover** *($24.50 for 6.8 ounces)* contains mostly water, mineral oil, thickeners, plant extract, glycerin, more thickeners, preservatives, and fragrance. This is a lot of money for mineral oil; it will wipe off makeup but may leave a greasy film on the skin.

☺ **$$$ Equite Clear Eye Makeup Remover** *($19.50 for 3.4 ounces)* is an average makeup remover that contains slip agents and a few emulsifiers, standard cosmetic ingredients that can cut through oil and makeup. Most eye makeup removers contain the same ingredients, but in this product they cost four times as much for half the amount.

☺ **$$$ Equite Very Gentle Makeup Remover for the Face, for Dry Skin** *($24.50 for 5 ounces)* contains mostly water, mineral oil, and thickeners. It is gentle, but it's also boring and overpriced.

☺ **$$$ Equite Waterproof Eye Makeup Remover Lotion** *($19.50 for 3.4 ounces)* contains mostly water, slip agent, thickeners, and preservatives. This product will wipe off makeup, but why pay this price?

☺ **$$$ Equite Exfoliating Gel** *($25 for 3.6 ounces)* contains mostly water, glycerin, thickeners, mineral oil, fragrance, and preservatives. This is a gentle exfoliator, but it's not worth the money; it uses the same standard synthetic exfoliating agent (polyethylene) as most scrubs of this nature (most of which are considerably cheaper). The mineral oil can leave skin feeling greasy.

☺ **$$$ Equite Alcohol-Free Soothing Lotion for Dry Skin** *($24.50 for 6.8 ounces)* contains mostly water, thickeners, glycerin, fragrance, film former, preservatives, alcohol (so it's obviously not alcohol-free), water-binding agent, and more preservatives. It contains some emollients, but nothing of special interest. It also contains a minute amount of anti-irritant, but hardly enough to affect the skin at all. There isn't enough alcohol in this product to be an irritant for most skin types, but why add it at all?

☺ **$$$ Equite Alcohol-Free Softening Lotion for Dry Skin** *($24.50 for 6.8 ounces)* is almost identical to the lotion above, and the same review applies.

☹ **Equite Stimulating Toner for Normal & Combination Skin** *($24.50 for 6.8 ounces)* is an alcohol-based toner that you could call stimulating, but "irritating" and "drying" would be more accurate.

☹ **Equite Vitalizing Toner** *($21 for 6.8 ounces)* is a standard alcohol-based toner that contains mostly water, alcohol, water-binding agents, fragrance, and preservatives. It is too irritating for most skin types.

☺ **$$$ Hydra-Star Dry Skin Moisture Creme** *($42 for 1.7 ounces)* contains mostly water, film former, a long list of thickening agents, silicone oil, more thickeners, vitamin E, plant extract, a long list of water-binding agents, fragrance, film former, and preservatives. This would be a very good moisturizer for someone with dry skin, but a lot of the interesting ingredients are at the end of a very long list. Unfortunately, the film former is rather high up; although it can help make skin look smooth, it is also a potential skin irritant.

☺ **$$$ Hydra-Star Dry Skin Moisture Creme Emulsion** *($42 for 1.7 ounces)* is identical to the product above except for texture differences, and the same review applies.

☺ **$$$ Hydra-Star Dry Skin Moisture Emulsion** *($42 for 1.7 ounces)* is similar to Hydra-Star Dry Skin Moisture Creme except for texture differences, and the same review applies.

☺ **$$$ Hydra-Star Dry Skin Night Treatment Creme** *($52 for 1.7 ounces)* is similar to Hydra-Star Dry Skin Moisture Creme except for texture differences, and the same review applies.

☺ **$$$ Hydra-Star Normal and Combination Skin Night Treatment Creme** *($52 for 1.7 ounces)* is similar to Hydra-Star Dry Skin Moisture Creme except for texture differences, and the same review applies.

☺ **$$$ Hydra-Star Normal and Combination Skin Moisture Creme** *($42 for 1.7 ounces)* is similar to Hydra-Star Dry Skin Moisture Creme except for texture differences, and the same review applies.

☺ **$$$ Hydra-Star Normal and Combination Skin Moisture Emulsion** *($42 for 1.7 ounces)* is similar to Hydra-Star Dry Skin Moisture Creme except for texture differences, and the same review applies. I would not recommend this product for someone with combination skin; it contains ingredients that are not good for that skin type.

☺ **$$$ Hydra-Star Normal and Combination Skin Moisture Fluide** (*$42 for 1.7 ounces*) is a very lightweight moisturizer that contains water, thickeners, vitamin E, water-binding agents, silicone oil, film former, and preservatives. It would be a good moisturizer with antioxidant for normal to slightly dry or combination skin.

☺ **$$$ Capture Lift, Firming Night Treatment for the Face** (*$58 for 1 ounce*) contains mostly water, water-binding agents, thickener, and preservatives. Minuscule amounts of vitamins and other water-binding agents also appear on the ingredient list way after the preservative, which means they don't count for much. There is also a tiny amount of film former, which can temporarily make the skin look smooth. This is a good, but extremely average, moisturizer for normal to dry skin, but to call this "firming" or a "treatment" is almost funny.

☺ **$$$ Capture for Face** (*$74 for 1.7 ounces*) contains mostly water, glycerin, plant extract, slip agent, water-binding agents, preservatives, film former, and fragrance. This may be a good moisturizer for someone with dry skin, but the price is not justified by the ingredients, which are extremely ordinary. It also contains soybean extract, which can be an irritant for some skin types.

☺ **$$$ Capture for Eyes** (*$40 for 0.5 ounce*) contains mostly water, glycerin, thickeners, plant extract, film former, preservatives, fragrance, water-binding agents, and more preservatives. Many of the more interesting ingredients are listed after the preservatives and fragrance, meaning they are present only in minute amounts. This is a good, but rather average, moisturizer for the eye area, although the film-forming ingredients can be skin irritants. It also contains soybean extract, which can be an irritant for some skin types.

☹ **$$$ Capture Rides Multi-Action Wrinkle Creme, SPF 8** (*$68 for 1.7 ounces*) is OK for limited sun exposure. It contains mostly water, thickener, film former, a long list of more thickeners, several water-binding agents, preservatives, and fragrance. The film formers can help the skin look smoother but may also be a skin irritant. Otherwise, this is a good moisturizer for someone with normal to dry skin, but it isn't exceptional or unique in any way.

☺ **$$$ Resultante Moisturizing Day Cream for Wrinkles** (*$66 for 1 ounce*) contains mostly water, thickeners, mineral oil, more thickeners, slip agent, plant oil, water-binding agent, silicone oil, fragrance, and preservatives. This is a good moisturizer for someone with dry skin, but it's not worth this amount of money.

☺ **$$$ Resultante Revitalizing Wrinkle Cream** *($80 for 1 ounce)* contains mostly water, mineral oil, thickeners, plant oil, more thickeners, lanolin, anti-irritant, water-binding agents, and preservatives. This is a good moisturizer, but it's not any more impressive than the less expensive moisturizers in Dior's lineup. Besides, $80 for a mineral oil–based moisturizer is absurd.

☹ **$$$ Resultante Firming Wrinkle Cream** *($80 for 1 ounce)* might help your dry skin, but it could also cause breakouts. The second ingredient is isopropyl myristate, which can clog pores. Other than that, this mineral oil–based moisturizer contains a long list of thickening agents, some water-binding agents, and that's it. The interesting ingredients are at the end of the list and hardly amount to a dusting.

☹ **Resultante Eye Care Cream** *($70 for 0.5 ounce)* leaves me speechless. For a whopping $2,240 a pound you get mostly water, isopropyl myristate (which can cause blackheads), thickeners, glycerin, more thickeners, water-binding agents, fragrance, and preservatives. And it isn't even a very good moisturizer!

☺ **$$$ Resultante Throat Cream** *($76 for 1 ounce)* contains mostly water, thickeners, lanolin oil, slip agent, more thickeners, water-binding agents, fragrance, and preservatives. There isn't anything in this cream that is better for the neck than for your face or elbows. It is a good emollient moisturizer for dry skin, but the throat distinction is purely a marketing tactic.

☺ **$$$ Icone Principe Regulateur for All Types of Dryness** *($44 for 1 ounce)* contains mostly water, plant oil, thickener, glycerin, more thickeners, water-binding agents, more thickeners, silicone oil, more water-binding agents, preservative, and fragrance. Several more ingredients are listed after the fragrance, some of them quite good for dry skin, but there's not enough to count for much. This is a good moisturizer for someone with dry skin, but it won't regulate a thing.

☹ **$$$ Icone Hypersensitive Skin, Emulsion for the Face** *($54 for 1 ounce)* contains mostly water, thickeners, glycerin, silicone oil, slip agent, water-binding agents, more thickeners, anti-irritants, film former, preservative, and fragrance. Additional interesting water-binding agents are listed after the preservative, but there's not enough to count for anything. This would be a good moisturizer for someone with normal to dry skin, but nothing about it makes it more suitable for sensitive skin.

☹ **$$$ Icone Sebum Control Treatment, Oil-Free Fluid** *($40 for 1 ounce)* contains mostly water, glycerin, water-binding agents, oil absorber, and preservatives. It would be OK as an extremely lightweight moisturizer, but I wouldn't recommend using it to control oil because the product is not all that absorbent.

☺ **$$$ Equite Instant Radiance Relaxing Mask** *($32.50 for 2.5 ounces)* comes in two parts: a creamy "moisturizing emulsion," which contains mostly water, plant oil, thickeners, lanolin, silicone oil, anti-irritant, fragrance, and preservatives; and a "radiance gel," which contains mostly water, glycerin, slip agent, thickeners, preservatives, water-binding agent, and more preservatives. This would be a good mask for someone with dry skin.

☺ **$$$ Equite Instant Radiance Purifying Mask** *($32.50 for 2.5 ounces)* comes in two parts: a "purifying gel," which contains water, glycerin, slip agent, thickeners, plant extract, and preservatives; and a "radiance gel," which contains almost the same ingredients. For the money, this is an incredibly boring list of ingredients. This mask won't purify anything, but it would be OK for someone with normal to slightly dry skin.

☹ **Svelte Cellulite Control Complex** *($49 for 6.8 ounces)* isn't for the face, but I couldn't stop myself—I had to review it for you anyway. It contains mostly alcohol, water, thickeners, plant extracts, anti-irritant, and preservatives. If you want to believe that rubbing alcohol and plant extracts on your thighs can do anything but swell and irritate the skin (the same as any astringent), it's up to you. However, you would be better off rubbing the $49 you spent on this product on your thighs, because at least it won't dry out your skin.

Christian Dior Makeup

☺ **$$$ FOUNDATION: Teint Eclat Demi-Mat** *($38)* has a great soft texture and provides light coverage. It blends on evenly, giving the face a smooth, slightly matte appearance. It isn't matte enough to please someone with oily skin, but other skin types might like the finish. What a shame the color selection is so poor. **All of these colors are great:** Soft Beige, Medium Beige, and Beige. **These colors are too pink, peach, or orange for almost all skin tones:** Soft Golden, Light Golden, Medium Golden, Dore Golden, Soft Rose, and Light Rose.

☹ **Teint Ideal Mat** *($38)* is hardly ideal; in fact, it is a problem. It is alcohol-based, which means it can irritate and dry the skin; also, most of the colors are terrible.

☺ **$$$ Teint Dior Eclat Satin** *($38)* is a light, soft foundation designed for normal to dry skin. **All of these colors are excellent:** Light Golden Beige, Barely Beige, Medium Beige, and Soft Beige. **Avoid these colors:** Tres Claire Beige, Natural Golden Beige, Beige, and Soft Rose.

☺ **$$$ Teint Actuel** *($39.50)* supposedly softens lines. Don't count on it, but this thicker, moist, creamy foundation would work nicely for someone with extremely dry skin. It blends better than you would think from the look of it. **All of these colors are beautiful:** Soft Golden Beige, Soft Beige, Medium Beige, and Beige. **These colors are too peach or pink for most skin tones:** Tender Rose Beige, Delicate Rose Beige, Rose Beige, Golden Beige, and True Golden Beige.

☺ **$$$ Teint Poudre** *($39.50)* is a talc-based pressed powder that is more powder than foundation. It is slightly heavier than some pressed powders and is meant to be used either as an all-over foundation or as a powder. **All nine colors are excellent.**

☹ **Basic Teint** *($38)* is a sheer tint with sunscreen. The SPF 15 is good, but the colors are strange. One is white; the others are pink, peach, and shiny bronze.

☹ **CONCEALER: Stick Corrector** *($16)* has a dry texture that tends to crease into the lines around the eyes and comes in only two colors.

☺ **$$$ POWDER:** There are eight **Pressed Powders** *($30)* and **Loose Powders** *($37)* that come in identical shades, though the color selection leaves much to be desired. **These colors are too white, pink, peach, or rose:** Pale Mauve, White Porcelain, Florentine Blonde, Scandinavian Rose, Sahara Beige, and Invisible Plus. Summer Sun is **the only great color** in the loose powder lineup. The three pressed powders that come in natural skin shades are good, have a soft consistency, and go on sheer: Invisible Plus (has a slight pink tint), Sahara Beige, and Summer Sun (great color for tan skin tones). **Sun Powders** *($38.00)* are bronzers and, refreshingly, two kinds are beautifully matte; if that's what you're looking for, they're perfect. There are also two shiny ones, but you can just ignore those.

☺ **$$$ BLUSH: Blush Final** *($30)* has a wonderfully silky consistency and texture, although it is slightly shiny. The colors are mostly beautiful.

☺ **$$$ Powder Blush Trio** *($30)* is an interesting option, but not one to get too excited about. Of the three colors in the set, one is shiny (for highlighting), one is a brown tone (for contouring), and one is for blushing.

☹ **EYESHADOW:** All of Dior's eyeshadow **Duo** sets *($28.50)* contain one color that is too intensely shiny. The **Five Colour Eyeshadow Compact** *($47.50)* is very pretty to look at but not great to use. All the colors are shiny, and the combinations are too contrasting.

☺ **$$$ Powder Eyeshadow and Eyeliner Palette** *($47.50)* are four different sets of matte (well, fairly matte) colors with five shades each, and one dark powder eyeliner color. This product is actually quite good, with a wonderful silky texture, but the color combinations are a bit strange. Six colors might seem like a deal, but the amounts you are get almost negligible. **The best grouping:** Brown and Blue (the blue is the eyeliner color, which is really almost black).

☺ **$$$ EYE AND BROW SHAPER:** The **Eye Pencil** *($18)* is standard fare; like dozens of other cosmetics pencils. One end has a foam tip to soften the liner. **Brow Pencils** *($17)* come in only three shades; each has a rather dry texture and a brush at one end. Even though I don't care to use a pencil on the brow, this one isn't bad, although any pencil with a similar texture and a separate brow brush could function as well.

☺ **$$$ LIPSTICK AND LIP PENCIL:** **Rouge a Levres (Cream)** *($18)* feels very moist and creamy, almost luscious, and there are some great colors, but watch out for the frosted ones. **Rouge Accent (Matte)** *($18)* is a small collection of lipsticks that aren't all that matte, but they do go on thick and come in more vivid colors.

☺ **$$$ Rouge Brilliant (Sheers)** *($18)* is a fairly standard lip gloss that comes in a tube. The **Lip Pencil** *($18)* is fairly standard but comes in a nice array of colors. It's overpriced for what you get.

☺ **$$$ MASCARA:** **Lengthening Mascara with Cashmere** *($18)* is about 1% something called cashmere hydrolysate, goat hair broken down with water. Soft wool in a mascara might sound great, but it's useless, particularly this tiny amount. Nevertheless, this mascara builds quickly, lengthens, and stays all day. It also comes in colors appropriate for redheads. **Mascara Parfait** *($15)* goes on great, building beautiful thick lashes without clumping; unfortunately, it can smear by the end of the day.

Circle of Beauty

Probably the first thing you think of when you hear the name Sears is washing machines, power tools, lawn mowers, or even vacuum cleaners. Call me a snob, but even though Sears sells some impressive cosmetics lines (including Iman and Color Me Beautiful), I wouldn't exactly encourage anyone to go there for fashion inspiration. When I heard that Sears was introducing a new line of skin care and makeup products, and that Sears had also created and developed the line, I was eager to take a look, but also very skeptical. (Actually, I'm always skeptical, no matter who makes the products or where they're sold.)

Circle of Beauty is a huge line, with more than 600 items, retailed in a very inviting, very user-friendly display. (Appropriately, the counters form a complete circle with the products on the outside.) You can play to your heart's content, with easy access to every single product, but you'll never get to all of them.

The good news is that Colorworks, Circle of Beauty's makeup line, offers some remarkable, reasonably priced products. A significant strong point is that color choices are available for a wide range of skin tones, from the very light to the very dark. Of four foundation types, two are superior—one for a matte finish and the other for a more sheer, moist application. When it comes to blushes, both the powder and the cream-to-powder are excellent. The line also has good eye pencils, a superior cream/matte lipstick in 49 shades, and a superior concealer.

The bad news is that the line falls abysmally on its face with the cream-to-powder foundation, a sticky, dry mess that stains the skin and comes in a limited selection of very dark orange colors, and the simply awful eyeshadows, which flake, smear, and streak for no apparent reason. Didn't anyone test the eyeshadows before retailing them? Even the two salespeople I talked to said they were embarrassed about the way the eyeshadows went on.

Skinplicity, Circle of Beauty's skin care group, has five "circles" of products for five different skin types: oily, combination/oily, combination/dry, dry, and dehydrated. That's 25 products, plus an array of specialty products. For a new cosmetics line, that's a lot of items to start with. Sometimes there isn't much of a difference between related products in the different groupings. This can be confusing for both the consumer and the salespeople. Despite this, some products are very impressive; of course, there are some products you should absolutely ignore.

One particularly striking aspect of the skin care line is that almost every product contains three anti-irritants known for their skin-soothing properties: bisabolol, kola nut extract, and green tea extract. Circle of Beauty refers to this as its exclusive "Trisoothal Irritation Shield." These anti-irritants are often rather high on the ingredient list. Unfortunately, many of the products also contain a batch of "essential" oils that can be skin irritants. Ylang ylang oil, lemon oil, lavender oil, geranium oil, and bergamot oil are all well-known skin sensitizers. These ingredients are really more of a nuisance than a help, although the consumer usually thinks that the "naturalness" of these oils means they are good for the skin.

Depending on what you are looking for, there are definite finds at Sears' Circle of Beauty, and when you're done you can check out the appliance department or buy a set of screwdrivers.

Circle of Beauty Skin Care

☹ **Come Clean Cleanser Oily Type 1** *($8.50 for 6 ounces)* is a standard detergent-based water-soluble cleanser that uses TEA-lauryl sulfate, which is fairly drying and can be too irritating for most skin types, as the cleansing agent. Several anti-irritants in the product will help the irritation, but not the dryness. This cleanser also contains several plant oils that can be sensitizing, particularly around the eyes.

☹ **Come Clean Cleanser Combination Oily Type 2** *($8.50 for 6 ounces)* is almost identical to the Type 1 cleanser, and the same review applies. However, the Type 2 cleanser also contains sodium hydroxide (lye), which can be more drying and irritating for the skin, high on the ingredient list.

☹ **Come Clean Cleanser Combination Dry Type 3** *($8.50 for 6 ounces)* is almost identical to the Type 1 cleanser, and the same review applies.

☹ **Come Clean Cleanser Dry Type 4** *($8.50 for 6 ounces)* is more a wipe-off cleanser than a water-soluble one. It contains several thickeners, plant oil, anti-irritants, more plant oils, and preservatives. It could be good for someone with dry skin, although the plant oils can be skin sensitizers and could cause problems in the eye area.

☹ **Come Clean Cleanser Dehydrated Type 5** *($8.50 for 6 ounces)* is similar to the Type 4 cleanser, and the same review applies.

☹ **Skin Refiner Oily Type 1** *($8.50 for 8 ounces)* is an alcohol-based toner that is too irritating and drying for all skin types. Alcohol can cause problems for the skin.

☹ **Skin Refiner Type 2** *($8.50 for 8 ounces)* is almost identical to the Type 1 refiner, and the same review applies.

☹ **Skin Refiner Combination Dry Type 3** *($8.50 for 8 ounces)* is very similar to the Type 1 refiner, and the same review applies.

☺ **Skin Refiner Dry Type 4** *($8.50 for 8 ounces)* is a good alcohol-free, moisturizing toner that contains mostly water, slip agent, anti-irritants, water-binding agent, vitamin E, several plant oils, and preservatives. Some of the plant oils can be skin sensitizers for some skin types.

☺ **Skin Refiner Dehydrated Type 5** *($8.50 for 8 ounces)* is similar to the Type 4 refiner, and the same review applies.

☺ **Action + Moisture Lotion SPF 8 Oily Type 1** *($16.50 for 4 ounces)* contains mostly water, silicone oil, water-binding agent, anti-irritants, thickeners, vitamin E (antioxidant), plant oils, more water-binding agents, and preservatives. The anti-irritants are great, but the plant oils can be sensitizers and should be avoided by someone with oily skin. SPF 8 is OK for limited sun exposure, but I recommend SPF 15 because you never know how much sun you're really going to get.

☺ **Action + Moisture Lotion SPF 8 Combination Oily Type 2** *($16.50 for 4 ounces)* is similar to the Type 1 SPF 8 lotion, and the same review applies.

☺ **Action + Moisture Lotion SPF 8 Combination Dry Type 3** *($16.50 for 4 ounces)* contains mostly water, mineral oil, silicone oil, thickener, water-binding agents, anti-irritants, vitamin C (antioxidant), more thickeners, plant oils, and preservatives. Someone with combination skin wouldn't be thrilled with the mineral oil, but if your skin is more dry than oily, this could be a good moisturizer. The plant oils can be skin sensitizers. SPF 8 is OK for limited sun exposure, but I recommend SPF 15 because you never know how much sun you're really going to get.

☺ **Action + Moisture Lotion SPF 8 Dry Type 4** *($16.50 for 4 ounces)* contains mostly water, mineral oil, thickeners, silicone oil, anti-irritants, water-binding agents, vitamin E (antioxidant), more thickeners, plant oil, and preservatives. This is a very good emollient moisturizer for someone with dry skin. Some of the plant oils can be sensitizers for some skin types.

☺ **Action + Moisture Lotion SPF 8 Dehydrated Type 5** *($16.50 for 4 ounces)* is similar to the Type 4 SPF 8 lotion, and the same review applies.

☺ **Action + Moisture Cream SPF 8 Oily Type 1** *($16 for 4 ounces)* is one of two types of moisturizers Skinplicity offers for each skin type. The lotions (above) and the creams both have an SPF of 8 and differ only in texture. The brochure tells you to choose which texture you prefer and then wear that product for both day and night. That recommendation is foolhardy and completely ill-advised. Wearing a sunscreen at night is as senseless as wearing sunglasses in the dark. Not only are sunscreen ingredients unnecessary at night, there is also a risk that wearing sunscreen both day and night may cause skin sensitivity and irritation.

☺ **Action + Moisture Cream SPF 8 Combination Oily Type 2** *($16.50 for 4 ounces)* is similar to the Type 1 cream, and the same review applies.

☺ **Action + Moisture Cream Combination Dry Type 3** *($16.50 for 4 ounces)* is similar to the Type 1 cream, and the same review applies.

☺ **Action + Moisture Cream SPF 8 Dry Type 4** *($16.50 for 4 ounces)* is similar to the Type 1 cream, and the same review applies.

☺ **Action + Moisture Cream SPF 8 Dehydrated Type 5** *($16.50 for 4 ounces)* is similar to the Type 1 cream, and the same review applies.

☺ **All Even AHA Serum Oily Type 1, 2, 3, 4, 5** *($15 for 1 ounce)* contains mostly water, lactic acid (about 8%), silicone oil, antioxidants, anti-irritants, water-binding agents, plant oils, and preservatives. This would be a very good AHA product for someone with normal to somewhat dry skin. The anti-irritants are particularly helpful in this kind of product. However, plant oils could cause problems for someone with oily skin, although there may not be enough to affect normal to slightly oily skin.

☹ **Moisture Wrap Peel Off Mask** *($8.50 for 5.5 ounces)* contains mostly plastic, alcohol, anti-irritants, plant oils, and preservatives. Alcohol and plastic won't moisturize anyone's skin.

☺ **Pore Purge Clay Mask** *($10.50 for 8 ounces)* is a standard clay mask with the same anti-irritants and plant oils as the rest of the Skinplicity line. It would be good for someone with normal to oily skin, but it can't empty pores any better than any other clay mask, which is to say, it will do practically nothing.

☺ **De Puff Eye Gel** *($8.50 for 0.6 ounce)* contains mostly water, water-binding agents, thickeners, anti-irritants, plant extracts, vitamin E, and preservatives. The anti-irritants make this product worth a try. The vitamin E is present in too tiny an amount to be significant.

☺ **Overnight Eye Treatment** *($15 for 0.6 ounce)* contains mostly water, thickener, mineral oil, more thickeners, anti-irritants, more thickeners, and preservatives. This isn't much of a treatment, but it is emollient, and the anti-irritants could be good for the eye area.

Circle of Beauty Makeup

☺ **FOUNDATION:** I was very impressed with two of the four foundations. **Skin Image Soft Matte Makeup SPF 8** *($11.50)* has an excellent shine-free finish and provides medium coverage, while **Skin Image Dewy Moist Makeup SPF 8** *($11.50)* has a sheer, moist texture. A higher SPF would be better, but SPF 8 is better than nothing. Both foundations come in 20 superior colors, **almost every one a wonderful, neutral shade**, in a wide scope of true skin tones. **Colors to avoid for the Matte Makeup are:** Fair Buff, which can be slightly ash, and Rich Walnut, Rich Caramel, and Rich Bronze, which can be too orange. **Colors to avoid for the Dewy Moist Makeup are:** Fair Buff and Rich Cocoa, which can be too ash, and Rich Bronze, which can be too orange.

☺ **Skin Image Wet or Dry Makeup** *($12.50)* is a standard talc-based powder that you can apply wet or dry. It is a decent alternative for a light layer of makeup, but appropriate only for someone with normal to slightly oily skin. **The eight colors are very attractive**, although Fair Porcelain and Medium Cameo can be too pink, and there are no colors for darker skin tones, which is strange given the wide range of darker shades in the other foundations.

☹ **Skin Image Cream to Powder Makeup** *($12.50)* feels thick and sticky, it blends poorly and stains the skin, and the color choices are poor to awful. Most of the colors are too orange, too peach, or too yellow. **Skin Image Primer** *($10)* is a color corrector that comes only in green. I don't recommend color correctors under makeup anyway, so don't worry about it. **Skin Image Highlighter** *($10)* is a shiny pink liquid. I wouldn't recommend using it even if I could explain how to wear it.

☺ **CONCEALER: Out of Sight Sponge-on Concealer** *($7)* comes in six shades that are mostly just fine, but none is appropriate for lighter skin tones. The texture is very dry and matte, which is great for more coverage but terrible if you have any lines under the eye, because this product will make them look more prominent. **There are only two colors to avoid:** Truly Fair, which is too pink, and Deep Beige, which can be too ash.

☺ **No Flaw Maximum Cover Concealer** *($7)* is outstanding. **The color selection is great**, the texture is soft, it doesn't crease, and, best of all, it covers well without being heavy or thick. **The only color to avoid out of the six is** Medium Beige, which can be too rosy for most skin tones.

☺ **POWDER: Natural Finish Press Powder** *($9)* is a standard talc-based powder with a good color selection and a sheer, soft texture. The only problem is that it tends to be on the dry side. It would be appropriate only for someone with normal to oily skin. **Natural Finish Loose Powder** *($9)* has a soft, light texture with good colors, though it too is slightly on the dry side.

☺ **BLUSH: Blush Lightly** *($10)* has a soft texture and a nice array of colors for a wide range of skin tones, but some of the colors can grab the skin, meaning they go on stronger than they appear in the container, or they tend to go on choppy, so test them before buying. **Skin Pretender Powder** *($10)* is a bronzing powder; two shades are shiny, but one is surprisingly matte and an option if you are into this sort of thing. Of course, no one thinks a colored powder dusted over the face looks like a real tan, right?

☺ **Blush Creamy Cream to Powder** *($10)* has a soft, silky-sheer texture and application. The color selection is small but beautiful.

☹ **EYESHADOW:** Both the **Soft Sweep Eyeshadow Singles** *($8)* and **Duos** *($8)* are just dreadful. They blend on choppy and flake off. What a shame, because there are some great matte colors. To add insult to injury, the Duo color combinations leave much to be desired.

☹ **EYE AND BROW SHAPER:** **Stroke Up Brow Pencil** *($7)* is a twist-up pencil that comes in four colors and has a soft, easy-to-use texture. "Twist-up" means no sharpening required, which I appreciate, but I don't recommend pencils for filling in brows. **Eye Defining Pencil** *($7)* is also a twist-up, but the texture is so greasy and smeary I don't recommend it. **Color Up Brow Cake** *($8)* is a powder for the brow; it has the same problem as the eyeshadows in this collection, and I don't recommend it. **Groom Up Brow Gel** *($7)* is simply hairspray ingredients in a clear gel. It will softly keep your brows in place.

☺ **LIPSTICK AND LIP PENCIL:** I love to find a good lipstick that doesn't bleed, since most lipsticks run into the lines around my mouth. **Satin Matte Lipstick** *($8.50)* is wonderful, and with 49 colors to choose from, you are likely to find one you like.

☹ **Rich Lasting Cream Lipstick** *($8.50)* is more greasy than creamy; I don't recommend it for regular daytime use if you're over 20, working, and want your lipstick to last. It does have a stain that makes the color last longer than usual, but once the gloss is gone the stain doesn't make the lips look great. **Sheer Treat Lipstick** *($8.50)* is just a sheer translucent hint of color, with a sunscreen—not bad if you want lip protection and a natural look. **Crystal Cream** *($6)* is a pot of gloss that comes in four colors; they are all extremely iridescent, with sparkle that doesn't quit. **Lip Comfort** *($8.50)* is a very emollient, nonirritating lip gloss that can help keep lips moist and prevent chapped lips. **Smooth-Off Lip Buffer** *($8.50)* is just a gloss with some walnut shells in it; it doesn't do much for the lips and is a waste of time and effort.

☹ **MASCARA:** Your lashes won't be able to tell the difference between the **Long and Silky Mascara** *($8)* and the **Velvety Lashes Mascara** *($8)*. Neither comes close to living up to most of the claims in the package insert. They don't build well, they don't make lashes long or thick, and though the lashes feel soft enough and don't clump, which is nice, that isn't enough to make either worth recommending.

Clarins

Clarins offers an imposing procession of skin care products. Besides their standout red-and-white packaging and French breeding (Americans think Europeans know more about skin care; meanwhile, in Europe, the sales pitch emphasizes how much the

Americans know), Clarins is also capitalizing heavily on the "botanical" craze of the '90s. The ingredient lists, full of usual and unusual herbs, flowers, and vegetables, are a veritable jungle, and the labels make the far-out promises that usually accompany these ingredients. Like Aveda, Origins, The Body Shop, and dozens of other lines, Clarins wants you to believe that a little herb concentrate can do wonders for your skin. However, according to *Rodale's Illustrated Encyclopedia of Herbs*, many of the extracts used in Clarins' products (as well as other botanical-type lines) are potentially irritating. For example, according to the encyclopedia, coltsfoot is potentially carcinogenic, and sage and horsetail extracts can cause skin irritation. Always keep in mind that "natural" and "good" are not the same thing; many natural things in the environment are bad for the skin.

One of Clarins' brochures says, "Clarins promises no miracles, only effective results [from] time-proven natural extracts." Yet claim after claim sounds like a miracle. This line even has "bust-firming" products. Other claims that sound fairly miraculous to me include "maintains firm facial features, takes advantage of the beneficial toning action of facial expressions while helping to reduce apparent slackening," and "refines skin texture, firms skin tone." "Proven" is obviously a relative term.

Clarins' foundation shades have improved, but there are still some strange colors. Almost all the eyeshadows are ultra-shiny, but the pressed powders have improved and have great skin tones. Even the mascara is now excellent. The counter display is divided into four small but nice color groups—Corals, Rose, Corals Dores, and Les Roses Lumieres—but it doesn't help the quality of the products.

Clarins Skin Care

☺ **$$$ Cleansing Milk with Alpine Herbs Dry or Normal Skin** *($25 for 8.6 ounces)* is recommended for people with dry to normal skin, according to its label, but the alpine herbs can cause skin irritation and drying, which makes it a poor product for this skin type—although the herbs come after the fragrance in the ingredient list, so there probably isn't much of them in the product anyway. Other than that, this is a standard cleanser that doesn't rinse off very well and can leave a film on the skin.

☺ **$$$ Cleansing Milk with Gentian Oily/Combination Skin** *($25 for 8.6 ounces)* is identical to the cleanser above except that the herbs are different, and they have no effect on oily skin.

☺ **$$$ Gentle Foaming Cleanser** *($18.50 for 4.4 ounces)* is an OK water-soluble cleanser for someone with oily skin. However, it can be drying for some skin types and may irritate the eyes. Potassium hydroxide, which is rather high up on the ingredient list, and one of the detergent cleansing agents can both be irritants for some skin types.

☺ **$$$ Extra-Comfort Cleansing Cream with Bio-Ecolia, Very Dry or Sensitized Skin** *($29 for 7 ounces)* contains mostly water, plant oil, several thickeners, silicone oil, and preservatives. This rather ordinary cleanser needs to be wiped off and can leave a greasy film. I am always skeptical when a product with fragrance claims to be good for sensitive skin.

☺ **$$$ Oil-Control Cleansing Gel Oily Skin with Breakout Tendencies** *($18.50 for 4.4 ounces)* is a standard detergent-based water-soluble cleanser that can be drying for some skin types. It won't control oil, but it will clean the skin.

☺ **$$$ Gentle Eye Make-Up Remover Cream-Gel** *($16 for 2.7 ounces)* isn't exactly gentle. It will take off eye makeup, but the third ingredient is fairly alkaline and can be a skin irritant.

☺ **$$$ Gentle Eye Make-Up Remover Lotion** *($15 for 3.4 ounces)* is mostly rose water (glycerin and water), plant extract, slip agents, and preservatives. It's gentle enough, but pretty ordinary and unnecessary.

☺ **$$$ Extra-Comfort Toning Lotion Very Dry or Sensitized Skin** *($24 for 8.8 ounces)* contains mostly water, aloe, silicone oil, slip agent, plant extracts, film formers, more slip agents, fragrance, and preservatives. Plenty of ingredients in this product can be problematic for sensitive skin, but it could be a good irritant-free toner for dry skin.

☺ **$$$ Toning Lotion for Combination or Oily Skin** *($21 for 8.4 ounces)* is an alcohol-free toner that contains water, aloe, plant extracts, slip agents, witch hazel, and preservatives. The plant extracts and witch hazel are possible irritants and provide no benefit for oily skin, but there isn't much of either, so this could be an OK toner.

☺ **$$$ Toning Lotion for Dry to Normal Skin** *($21 for 8.4 ounces)* contains mostly water, slip agents, plant extract, fragrance, and preservatives. This is a fairly good irritant-free toner.

☺ **$$$ Gentle Exfoliating Refiner** *($21 for 1.7 ounces)* contains mostly water, several thickeners, plant extract, and preservatives. The exfoliation comes from plant skin, which among these ordinary ingredients would indeed be gentle.

☺ **$$$ Gentle Facial Peeling** *($25 for 1.4 ounces)* will exfoliate the skin, something that happens any time you rub wax or clay over the skin, which is what you would be doing with this product. That isn't bad, but rubbing can be hard on the skin. There are easier ways to exfoliate.

☺ **$$$ Face Treatment Cream for Dry or Reddened Skin** *($23.50 for 1.7 ounces)* is a good, emollient moisturizer that contains mostly water, mineral oil, vegetable oils, thickeners, rice bran oil, a small amount of sunscreen (not enough to protect the skin), lanolin oil, water-binding agents, preservatives, and herb extracts. At this price, the least they could do is put in more herb extracts than preservatives; there are almost no herbs in this product to speak of.

☺ **$$$ Face Treatment Plant Cream for Dehydrated Skin** *($28 for 1.7 ounces)* is a good standard mineral oil–based moisturizer for dry skin. It contains mostly water, mineral oil, plant oil, thickeners, silicone oil, lanolin oil, plant extracts, fragrance, and preservatives. The tiny amounts of vitamins at the end of the ingredient list are wasted, and the plant extracts are also barely present.

☺ **$$$ Face Treatment Plant Cream for Dry or Extra Dry Skin** *($28 for 1.7 ounces)* is almost identical to the cream above, and the same review applies.

☹ **Face Treatment Plant Cream for Combination Skin Prone to Oiliness** *($28 for 1.7 ounces)* is virtually identical to the cream above. Someone with oily skin does not need more oil on her skin. What was Clarins thinking?

☻ **$$$ Gentle Day Cream for Sensitive Skin** *($37.50 for 1.7 ounces)* contains mostly water, mineral oil, several thickeners, silicone oil, more thickeners, anti-irritants, and preservatives. This is a very good, but rather ordinary, mineral oil–based moisturizer for dry skin. Because it contains no sunscreen, it isn't best for daytime wear, unless your foundation contains one.

☺ **$$$ Gentle Night Cream for Sensitive Skin** *($47.50 for 1.7 ounces)* is almost identical to the cream above, and the same review applies. Vitamins are present in this cream, but only in negligible quantities. Why this product is more expensive than the one above is a complete mystery.

☺ **$$$ Hydration-Plus Moisture Lotion, All Skin Types** *($27 for 1.7 ounces)* contains mostly water, slip agent, thickener, silicone oil, film former, more thickeners, water-binding agents, plant extracts, more slip agents, vitamin E, and preservatives. This is a good lightweight moisturizer for someone with normal to somewhat dry skin.

☺ **$$$ Hydration-Plus Moisture Lotion SPF 15 for All Skin Types** *($27 for 1.7 ounces)* is similar to the Hydration-Plus above, only with sunscreen (part titanium dioxide). Now this is a daytime sunscreen your skin can live with.

☺ **$$$ Multi-Active Day Cream for All Skin Types** *($43 for 1.7 ounces)* is a good, though extremely ordinary, moisturizer that contains mostly water, thickeners, aloe, silicone oil, plant oils, fragrance, soothing agents, and preservatives. The soothing agents are at the end of the ingredient list, so there probably aren't enough to be all that soothing. Also, without sunscreen this isn't a good daytime moisturizer.

☺ **$$$ Multi-Active Day Cream "Speciale" for Very Dry Skin** *($43 for 1.7 ounces)* isn't all that special or all that different from the cream above, and the same review applies. It is slightly more emollient, but only slightly. It does contain a tiny amount of vitamins, but not enough to make a difference.

☺ **$$$ Multi-Active Night Lotion for All Skin Types** *($48 for 1.7 ounces)* contains mostly water, thickeners, plant oil, film former, more thickeners, plant extracts, more thickeners, more film formers, more plant oils, and preservatives. This is a good moisturizer for someone with dry skin, but other skin types will find the oil and thickening agents too emollient. It does contain a tiny amount of vitamins, but not enough to help your skin at all.

☺ **$$$ Multi-Active Night Lotion Very Dry Skin** *($48 for 1.7 ounces)* is almost identical to the lotion above, and the same review applies.

☺ **$$$ Multi-Regenerante Treatment Cream for All Skin Types** *($65 for 1.7 ounces)* is an amazingly standard mineral oil–based moisturizer that would be good for women with dry skin (not for all skin types, as the name implies) if they can get over the absurd price. It contains mostly water, mineral oil, a long list of thickeners, slip agent, water-binding agent, plant oils, anti-irritant, fragrance, and preservatives.

☺ **$$$ Multi-Regenerante Treatment Cream "Special" for Very Dry, Very Devitalized Skin** *($65 for 1.7 ounces)* is a very emollient moisturizer for someone with very dry skin, but the ingredients are absolutely nothing unique or special. It contains mostly water, mineral oil, thickener, plant oil, more thickeners, lanolin oil, water-binding agents, more thickeners, fragrance, and preservatives. A minuscule amount of plant extracts are at the very end of the ingredient list.

☹ **Oil Control Moisture Lotion** *($24.50 for 1.06 ounces)* contains little that will control oil, but some ingredients could be problematic for someone with oily skin. The main ingredients are water, silicone oil, several thickeners, orrisroot, fragrance, and preservatives. There are negligible amounts of zinc sulfate, nylon, and hawthorn extract, which won't help oily skin but may cause irritation.

☺ **$$$ Revitalizing Moisture Cream with Plant Marine "Cell Extract"** *($47.50 for 1.7 ounces)* contains boring ingredients, in contrast to its long, beguiling name. It contains mostly water, mineral oil, several thickeners, glycerin, petrolatum, more thickeners, water-binding agents, a tiny amount of plant extracts, fragrance, and preservatives. The amount of plant marine extract is so minuscule as to make the company look silly for putting it in the name of the product. This is a good, but exceedingly overpriced, moisturizer for someone with dry skin.

☺ **$$$ Revitalizing Moisture Base with Plant Marine "Cell Extract" for All Skin Types** *($28.50 for 1.1 ounces)* is identical to the cream above except that it contains a higher concentration of mineral oil and petrolatum, and the same review applies. Vaseline and mineral oil don't work well for all skin types, only dry skin; regardless they aren't worth this kind of money.

☺ **$$$ Double Serum Total Skin Supplement, Plant Based Concentrate Hydro Serum and Lipo Serum** *($70 for two 0.5-ounce bottles)* claims to control the appearance of aging, but mixing these two liquids together does little to control aging or anything else. Together they contain mostly water, rose water, silicone oils, plant oils, mineral oil, water-binding agents, film former, slip agents, plant extracts, and preservatives. Vitamins, plant extracts, and oyster extracts are also present, in amounts so tiny they are virtually nonexistent. This would be a good lightweight moisturizer for most skin types, but the claims are absurd.

☺ **$$$ Eye Contour Balm** *($27.50 for 0.7 ounces)* contains water, thickeners, water-binding agent, film former, and preservatives. This would be an OK but ordinary moisturizer for dry skin.

☺ **$$$ Eye Contour Balm "Special" for Very Dry Skin** *($28.50 for 0.7 ounce)* contains mostly water, thickeners, mineral oil, plant oil, more thickeners, water-binding agent, anti-irritant, silicone oil, plant extracts, and preservatives. This isn't special—it's actually quite typical—but it would be a good moisturizer for someone with dry skin.

☹ **Eye Contour Gel** *($28.50 for 0.7 ounce)* is mostly water, plant extracts, witch hazel, thickeners, and preservatives. Because of the witch hazel, this product can irritate the skin around the eyes. The company claims it is soothing, but I doubt it.

☹ **Face Treatment Oil for Dry or Reddened Skin** *($32 for 1.4 ounces)* contains hazelnut, sandalwood, cardamom, parsley seed, hayflower, and lavender oils. Sandalwood, parsley, and lavender oils can all cause skin irritation, which isn't great for someone with reddened skin.

☹ **Face Treatment Oil for Combination Skin Prone to Oiliness** (*$32 for 1.4 ounces*) contains hazelnut oil, geranium oil, fragrance, rosemary oil, lotus extract, chamomile oil, and sage oil. This product is supposed to help "balance" surface oils. What it does is place more oils on the skin, and the chamomile, rosemary, and sage oils can be irritants. Someone with oily skin could end up with oilier, more irritated skin.

☹ **Face Treatment Oil for Dehydrated Skin** (*$32 for 1.4 ounces*) contains hazelnut oil, patchouli oil (mint), rosewood oil, fragrance, and orchid extract. The patchouli oil and fragrance can be irritating to the skin.

☹ **Multi-Tenseur Skin Firming Concentrate** (*$45 for 1 ounce*) contains mostly water, aloe, plant extracts, water-binding agent, slip agents, preservatives, and fragrance— rather ordinary ingredients for this kind of money. However, if you believe condurango extract (from the bark of the condurango tree) can firm the skin, you probably stopped reading my book way before this review.

☺ **$$$ Skin Beauty Repair** (*$35 for 0.5 ounce*) is another eye-popper. At these prices— $1,120 a pound—you would think you were buying gold. You're not. What you are buying is plant oil, thickeners, more plant oils, vitamin A, and preservatives. Some of the plant oils in this product, particularly peppermint, can cause skin irritation. It's an OK moisturizer, but it won't repair skin damage.

☺ **$$$ Beauty Flash Balm** (*$29.50 for 1.7 ounces*) is an extremely average moisturizer that contains mostly water, slip agent, several thickeners, witch hazel, plant extract, water-binding agent, anti-irritant, and preservatives. Witch hazel can be a skin irritant; other than that, this could be a good lightweight moisturizer for someone with normal to slightly dry skin.

☺ **$$$ Balancing Night Gel** (*$20.50 for 1 ounce*) contains water, film former, slip agents, plant extracts, fragrance, and preservative. The plant extracts won't balance anything. A small amount of zinc sulfate, which may be a skin irritant, is also present.

☺ **$$$ Blemish Gel** (*$14 for 0.53 ounce*) contains water, slip agent, glycerin, plant extracts, zinc sulfate, preservatives, tea tree oil, and witch hazel, in a tiny bottle. Zinc sulfate and witch hazel can prove irritating and won't do much for blemishes. The amount of tea tree oil is too minuscule to do much good.

☹ **$$$ Purifying Plant Facial Mask** (*$22 for 1.7 ounces*) contains mostly water, talc, mineral oil, thickeners, clay, plant extracts, film former, fragrance, and preservatives. It won't purify anything, but it is a good mask for someone with dry skin.

☹ **$$$ Revitalizing Moisture Mask with Plant Marine "Cell Extract" for All Skin Types** (*$27 for 1.7 ounces*) is mostly water, thickeners, glycerin, plant extracts, water-binding agents, fragrance, and preservatives. This is a good mask for someone with dry skin, but "cell extract" is in quotation marks because it has no meaning.

☹ **$$$ Bio-Ecolia Perfecting Creme-Mask with Controlled Fruit Acids** *($37.50 for 1.7 ounces)* supposedly contains "controlled fruit acids." There is no such thing as controlled (or uncontrolled) alpha hydroxy acids. This mask contains a tiny amount of AHAs, probably not more than a 2% concentration. Otherwise, it is an OK mask for someone with normal to slightly dry skin. All of the ingredients are fairly standard cosmetics thickeners and water-binding agents. Some amino acids show up at the end of the ingredient list; they could be interesting water-binding agents, but the amount is too negligible to have an impact.

☺ **$$$ Absorbent Mask** *($19 for 1.7 ounces)* is a very standard clay mask that contains mostly water, clay, thickeners, more clay, more thickeners, some herb extracts, and preservatives. It will absorb oil, but no better than any other clay mask.

☺ **Sun Care Cream SPF 15** *($17.50 for 4.4 ounces)* is a partly nonchemical sunscreen that contains thickeners, silicone oil, film former, plant oil, water-binding agents, and preservatives. This is a good sunscreen for someone with dry skin.

☺ **$$$ Lip Beauty Multi-Treatment** *($16 for 0.09 ounce)* is a standard emollient lip gloss with standard thickeners, castor oil, emollients, and plant oils. It is good for dry lips, but to spend this kind of money on such an ordinary "gloss" is almost embarrassing.

☹ **"Cellulite" Control Gel** *($41.50 for 5.3 ounces)* presented too great a temptation. I wasn't going to review products like these and the "bust" products that follow, but I couldn't help myself. The quotation marks around the word cellulite are a way for Clarins to get around the truth-in-advertising laws. Quotes allow a great deal of leeway in how a word is legally defined. In this case, what the company legally means by "cellulite" is totally different from what they want you to think they mean. You think they are referring to the bumpy fat in your thighs, but what they legally mean is only the surface texture of the skin (the appearance of cellulite). Because of the quotation marks, the interpretation is vague enough that truth-in-advertising laws haven't been breached. The second ingredient in this product is alcohol, which irritates and swells the skin. This irritation may reduce the appearance of bumps on the surface of the skin for a few minutes. Of course, you could buy a bottle of rubbing alcohol and get the same results for 89 cents. Aside from all that, you cannot burn or beat up fat from the outside in, so save your money.

☹ **Plant Milk for Bust Beauty Tightening and Toning** *($35 for 1.7 ounces)* doesn't deserve an explanation, but for those of you who wonder what could possibly be in a product that claims to "tighten" and "tone" your breasts, the ingredients are water; mineral oil; thickeners; fragrance; more thickeners; hop, fennel, and lemon extracts (which can all cause skin sensitivities); and preservatives.

☺ **Bust Firming Gel** *($42 for 1.7 ounces)* contains water, fish protein (skin cells from a dead fish), algae extract (seaweed juice), plant extracts, and thickeners. If you believe this product can work, I have a bridge you may be interested in.

Clarins Makeup

☺ **FOUNDATION: Satin Finish Foundation** *($28.50)* has a lightweight texture, but it isn't particularly satiny. The squeeze tube makes it difficult to control the amount that comes out, so a lot will get wasted if you aren't careful. **Colors to consider:** Soft Beige, Natural Beige, Sun Lit Beige, Tender Bisque, and Fair Ivory. **Color to avoid:** Tawny Beige.

☺ **Le Teint Mat Multi Eclat Matte Finish Foundation** *($28.50)* is an exceptionally matte foundation that goes on light but can feel fairly dry. **Colors to consider:** Ivory Beige, Beige Sahara, Sun Lit Beige, Soft Chamois, Beige Champagne, Fair Ivory, and Caramel. **Colors to avoid:** Beige Claire, Golden Honey, Beige Sand, Rose Beige, and Natural Beige.

☺ **Compact Powder Foundation** *($22.50)* isn't all that different from the Pressed Powder below. It goes on soft and sheer, and **all six colors are lovely**.

☻ **CONCEALER: Concealer** *($13.50)* comes in three shades: Light, which is too pink for most skin tones; Medium, which is darker than medium but still a good color; and Dark, which isn't all that dark but is also OK. The consistency is good but not exceptional, and the concealer can crease into the lines around the eyes.

☺ **POWDER:** The **Pressed Powder** *($22.50)* is a soft, silky powder that comes in six attractive shades. **Duo Soleil** *($22.50)* is a matte bronzer with two beautiful shades.

☹ **Bronzing Duo** *($22.50)* is a single compact with two shades of brown, both shiny.

☺ **BLUSH: Cream-to-Powder Blush** *($20)* has a beautiful texture and great colors. **Colors to consider:** Fawn, Cinnamon, Fuchsia, Heather Pink, Rose Sand, and Rose Petal.

☹ **EYESHADOW: Duo Eyeshadow Sets** *($21)* are mostly too ultra-shiny, but there are some new matte shades worth considering: Biscuit/Sable, Toast/Mocha, Nude/Plum, and Wine/Malt.

☺ **EYE AND BROW SHAPER:** The **Eye Pencil** *($12.50)* is a standard pencil that has a soft texture and comes in a nice array of colors. One end has a sponge tip for softening the line. The **Brow Pencil** *($12.50)* has a firm texture and a small but good group of colors. One end is a brush, which is a nice touch for softening the effect of the pencil.

☺ **LIPSTICK AND LIP PENCIL:** The **Sheer Lipstick** *($15)* is more gloss than lipstick and has no staying power. The **Cream Lipstick** *($15)* has a soft texture and a slight tint, which helps it stay around for a while. The **Lip Pencil** *($12.50)* is a standard pencil that has a good, easy-to-apply texture and an attractive color selection. One end is a lipstick brush, which is convenient.

☺ **$$$ MASCARA:** Clarins **Mascara** *($18)* goes on easily, beautifully lengthens lashes, and doesn't smear.

Clinique

Clinique has assembled a huge line of products over the years. Several types of foundations, blushes, eyeshadows, and lipsticks make its counters almost over-whelmingly alive with choices. Strangely, despite the growth in product selection, this is still a strictly Caucasian line, with few to no choices for women of color. The foundation colors do not include deep brown to ebony skin tones, and the eyeshadows and blushes go on too softly to work on darker skin.

Clinique's products, particularly those for skin care, are aimed at oily or combination skin types, which is probably why Clinique attracts a young clientele. And the makeup line includes products and colors geared toward younger tastes, such as color rubs and tints for the cheek (best for flawless, unlined faces), very sheer blushes and eyeshadows, and a variety of clever eye pencils. Unfortunately, many of the pencils, eyeshadows, and color rubs are extremely shiny and not the best for daytime or on over-30 skin. Clinique does seem to be expanding its potential market somewhat with a new selection of matte shades, exquisite blush colors, impressive foundations, and matte lipsticks that are less greasy than the other lipsticks in the line.

Many women, regardless of age, are faithful Clinique customers, probably because they believe the products are hypoallergenic and better for their skin (they aren't). The salespeople, dressed in white lab coats, reinforce this belief. There are several counter displays available, but most of the products can be tested only with the help of a salesperson. The color products are arranged into four groupings: Nudes/Naturels (which are not all that nude), Tawnies/Corals, Pinks/Roses, and Violets/Berries. It's a little confusing, but can be a helpful if you know what color groups you look best in. One plus is that the products are more affordable than those of numerous other lines. You also get great service at the Clinique counters; there always seems to be four to six white-jacketed women dashing around behind those counters.

Clinique Skin Care

☺ **Wash-Away Gel Cleanser** *($14.50 for 6 ounces)* is a very good water-soluble cleanser that cleans all the makeup off without irritation or any sensation of dryness. This one is worth checking out if you have normal to oily skin.

☹ **Water-Dissolve Cream Cleanser** *($14.50 for 5 ounces)* leaves a greasy film on the skin and doesn't take off all the makeup without the help of a washcloth.

☹ **Crystal Clear Cleansing Oil** *($11 for 6 ounces)* is a wipe-off cleanser that contains mostly mineral oil and a small amount of vitamins E and A. The salesperson said it wouldn't leave an oily residue on my face, but it did.

☹ **Extremely Gentle Cleansing Cream** *($9.50 for 3.5 ounces; $17.50 for 10 ounces)* is a traditional cold cream product (that is, it requires wiping off) that contains mostly mineral oil, water, beeswax, petrolatum, thickeners, and preservatives. Wiping off makeup is not good for the skin.

☹ **Quick Dissolve Makeup Solvent** *($14.50 for 8 ounces)* contains mostly water, mineral oil, slip agents, thickener, plant and nut oils, more thickeners, and preservatives. You are supposed to use this water-soluble cleanser to take off your makeup before you use soap. Two products to clean the face is one too many.

☺ **Rinse-Off Foaming Cleanser** *($14.50 for 5 ounces)* is a standard detergent-based water-soluble cleanser that can be fairly drying for most skin types.

☹ **Facial Soap Extra Mild** *($8.50 for 6 ounces)* is standard-issue bar soap, meaning it is mostly lard and lye. This is a lot of money for your average, everyday bar of soap.

☹ **Facial Soap Mild** *($8.50 for 6 ounces)* is similar to the soap above, and the same review applies.

☹ **Facial Soap Extra-Strength** *($8.50 for 6 ounces)* is similar to Facial Soap Extra Mild, and the same review applies.

☺ **Rinse-Off Eye Makeup Solvent** *($10 for 4 ounces)* contains mostly water, detergent cleanser, and slip agents. It can be irritating to the eyes; also, Clinique makes other, gentler cleansers that can remove eye makeup all by themselves, without an extra product.

☺ **Extremely Gentle Eye Makeup Remover** *($8.50 for 2 ounces)* contains mostly mineral oil, thickeners, petrolatum, plant oil, and preservatives. It is gentle, but it is also just good old-fashioned cold cream like Pond's, only you pay more for less.

☺ **Clean-Up Stick** *($9.50 for 0.06 ounce)* is an interesting way to clean up leftover makeup or makeup mistakes, but a cotton swab and a moisturizer or cleanser will do the same thing—for a lot less money.

☺ **7 Day Scrub Cream** *($9.50 for 2 ounces; $14.50 for 3.5 ounces)* contains mostly mineral oil, water, beeswax, sodium borate (antiseptic), and thickeners. This very thick, heavy product can cause the same problems it's trying to eliminate, because beeswax and ozokerite (one of the thickening agents) can cause skin to break out.

☺ **Gentle Exfoliator Rinse-Off Formula** *($12.50 for 3 ounces)* contains mostly water, mineral oil, a long list of thickeners, a long list of plant extracts, soothing agent, vitamin E, more thickeners, and preservatives. This is a gentle exfoliant with very little abrasive, but I wouldn't call it rinseable. The mineral oil leaves a residue on the skin.

☺ **Exfoliating Scrub** *($12.50 for 3 ounces)* was probably added to the Clinique line because the other two scrubs make such a greasy mess. This detergent-cleanser scrub is definitely better for someone with normal to oily skin, although it does contain small amounts of menthol and salicylic acid, which can irritate the skin.

☹ **Clarifying Lotions 1, 2, 3, and 4** *($15.50 for 12 ounces)* all contain varying degrees of alcohol, salicylic acid, benzalkonium chloride, and menthol, which are all extremely irritating. Putting salicylic acid and alcohol in the same product is just asking for trouble.

☹ **Mild Clarifying Lotion** *($9.50 for 6 ounces)* is mild only in comparison to the four lotions above. It probably contains about 1% salicylic acid, which can be irritating for some skin types.

☺ **Dramatically Different Moisturizing Lotion** *($19.50 for 4 ounces)* contains mostly water, mineral oil, sesame oil, water-binding agent, thickeners, petrolatum, and preservatives. This is a good, basic moisturizer for dry skin, although it isn't "dramatically different" from other emollient moisturizers on the market.

☺ **$$$ Advanced Cream, Self Repair System** *($50 for 2 ounces)* contains mostly water, slip agent, plant oil, thickener, glycerin, mineral oil, plant oils, several thickeners, algae extract, vitamins A and E (antioxidants), silicone oil, and preservatives. This overpriced, but extremely emollient, moisturizer for someone with dry skin won't repair anything, but it will help keep dryness away.

☺ **$$$ Sub-Skin Cream** *($38.50 for 2.6 ounces)* contains mostly water; collagen; thickeners; oil; water-binding agents; slip agent; more thickeners; plant oils; soothing agents; vitamins A, C, and E; more thickeners; and preservatives. This is a very good moisturizer, but it won't tighten or firm the skin, and the amount of vitamins in it is too small to count.

☺ **Moisture Surge Treatment Formula** *($18.50 for 2 ounces)* contains mostly water, several water-binding agents, vitamins A and E, more water-binding agent, plant extracts, thickeners, and preservatives. This is a very good lightweight moisturizer with a nice amount of water-binding agents and antioxidants.

☺ **Skin Texture Lotion** *($19.50 for 1.25 ounces)* contains mostly water, water-binding agents, a long list of thickeners, more water-binding agent, vitamins A and E, soothing agent, more thickeners, and preservatives. This is a good lightweight moisturizer with antioxidants.

☺ **Skin Texture Lotion Oil-Free Formula** *($19.50 for 1.25 ounces)* contains mostly water, slip agents, thickeners, water-binding agent, vitamins A and E, more thickeners, and preservatives. This isn't oil-free; it contains silicone oil, as well as several thickening agents that can cause breakouts and would be a problem for someone with oily skin.

☹ **Turnaround Cream** *($27.50 for 2 ounces)* has a great name; it sounds as if this cream can turn your skin back to a younger time, but it can't. It contains mostly water, several thickeners, salicylic acid, silicone oil, anti-irritant, vitamin E, and preservatives. It is a fairly matte, lightweight moisturizing base that would be appropriate for someone with normal to slightly dry skin, but it won't exfoliate the way an AHA product might. Salicylic acid (a BHA) is an effective exfoliant, but unlike AHAs, it just keeps exfoliating, which can be too irritating when used on a regular basis. Also unlike AHAs, salicylic acid doesn't have the additional benefit of water-binding properties. If you are a fan of these Turn Around products, you might want to check out Almay's Clear Complexion Moisture Lotion 100% Oil-Free SPF 8 ($8.64 for 1.7 ounces). It is almost identical for almost one-third the price.

☹ **$$$ Turnaround Cream for Dry Skin** *($27.50 for 2 ounces)* contains mostly water, plant oils, several thickeners, salicylic acid, anti-irritant, water-binding agents, vitamin E, and preservatives. It is much more emollient than the cream above and would definitely be good for someone with dry skin, but the same review applies.

☺ **Turnaround Lotion Oil-Free** *($27.50 for 2 ounces)* contains mostly water, silicone oil, film former, thickeners, salicylic acid, water-binding agents, anti-irritant, vitamin E, more thickeners, and preservatives. If you have normal to slightly oily skin and are looking for a lightweight salicylic acid exfoliant, this is it, but the film former and silicone oil can cause problems for someone with really oily or combination skin.

☺ **$$$ Moisture on Call** *($30 for 1.6 ounces)* is supposed to help skin cells "remember" how to produce their own moisture barrier. The company calls this memory-booster effect "mnemonic." In fact, you can achieve the same effect with the daily use of *any* moisturizer, which is the only claim Clinique is really making. This product contains mostly water, jojoba oil, thickener, humectant, shea butter, silicone oil, water-binding agents, plant extracts, more water-binding agents, vitamin E, more thickeners, and preservatives. It is a very good emollient moisturizer for someone with dry skin, but no more special than hundreds of other moisturizers. The amount of vitamin E is negligible.

☺ **Very Emollient Cream** *($21.50 for 2 ounces)* contains mostly water, oil, water-binding agent, thickener, petrolatum, mineral oil, a long list of thickeners, vitamins E and A (antioxidants), more thickeners, and preservatives. This is a good emollient moisturizer for dry skin.

☺ **Moisture Stick** *($11.50 for 0.13 ounce)* is more like a lip gloss than anything else. It is definitely emollient and extremely greasy. Several ingredients can cause breakouts.

☺ **$$$ Daily Eye Benefits** *($25 for 0.5 ounce)* contains mostly water, slip agent, thickeners, plant oil, plant extracts, more thickeners, water-binding agents, soothing agent, aloe vera, silicone oil, vitamin A, petrolatum, and preservatives. The plant extracts are supposed to reduce puffiness around the eyes, but it's unlikely your skin would notice. This is a good emollient moisturizer with an incredibly high price tag. Slice up a cucumber and see if that can get rid of puffy eyes before investing in this product at $1,200 a pound.

☺ **$$$ Daily Eye Saver, Quick Eye-Area Fix** *($25 for 0.5 ounce)* contains mostly water, slip agent, aloe, plant oil, thickener, glycerin, plant extracts, water-binding agents, vitamin E, and preservatives. Although the price is out of this world, this is a good lightweight moisturizer. The amount of vitamin E it contains, though, is next to nothing.

☺ **Deep Cleansing Emergency Masque** *($18.50 for 3.4 ounces)* contains more salicylic acid, this time in a standard clay mask. Between this, the Turnaround Creams, and the toners, it would be a wonder if you had any skin left when you're done.

☹ **Anti Acne Spot Treatment** *($10.50 for 0.5 ounce)* is just alcohol, slip agents, and salicylic acid. Didn't we get enough alcohol and salicylic acid with the toners? This is overkill by almost anyone's standard but Clinique's.

☺ **$$$ City Block SPF 15** *($13.50 for 1.4 ounces)* many women complained when City Block went from SPF 13 to SPF 15; most thought it became too thick and heavy. It was nice of Clinique to provide better sun protection, but for some skin types, this will feel too heavy and emollient.

☹ **Oil-Free Sun Block SPF 15** *($12.50 for 4 ounces)* isn't oil-free—it contains silicone oil—and it is alcohol-based, which means it can irritate and dry the skin.

☹ **Oil-Free Sun Block SPF 15** *($12.50 for 4 ounces)* isn't exactly oil-free—it contains silicone oil—and it is alcohol-based, which is drying and irritating for most skin types.

☺ **Full-Service Sun Block SPF 20** *($12.50 for 3 ounces)* is a good sunscreen for someone with normal to dry skin.

☺ **Special Defense Sun Block SPF 25** *($13.50 for 3 ounces)* is a good nonchemical sunscreen with emollients, water-binding agents, and minimal amounts of antioxidants.

☺ **Zero-Alcohol Sun Block SPF 25** *($15 for 4 ounces)* is quite similar in texture and application to Lancome Body Protective Spray. It has a higher SPF, which may not be necessary, but it goes on extremely sheer with no noticeable after-feel.

☹ **All About Lips** *($20 for 0.5 ounce)* contains a long list of thickening agents, anti-irritants, water-binding agents, and a small amount of salicylic acid. That can help exfoliate the lips but it's not what I would recommend for daily lip care. Salicylic acid is just too strong an exfoliant for the lips.

☺ **Lip Block, SPF 15** *($6.50 for 0.15 ounce)* is a good standard, petrolatum-based lip gloss with a good sunblock. This can nicely ward off dry lips and protect from sun damage.

Clinique Makeup

☺ **FOUNDATION: Sensitive Skin Makeup SPF 15** *($18.50)* is one of the few foundations available with a nonchemical sunscreen that has a high enough SPF to truly protect the skin. It might feel a little heavy to those who want a sheer application, but you should see if it works for you. There aren't many colors, which is disappointing, **but all of them are superior. Almost Makeup SPF 15** *($16.50)* comes in **five great light colors**, which is pretty slim pickings, but it's an excellent sheer to lightweight foundation with nonchemical sunscreen.

☹ **Workout Makeup SPF 6** *($18.50)* is a puzzle. I'm not sure where you're supposed to "work out" with this minimal sun protection except indoors, but regardless, the color selection is poor and this product pales when compared to the other Clinique foundations with SPF. It's supposed to be water-resistant, but it leaves something to be desired. If you work out and don't sweat, it will stay on, but that's about it.

☺ **Stay True Oil-Free** *($14.50)* is a great oil-free foundation, and **all the color choices are great.**

☺ **Balanced Makeup Base** *($12.50)*, for normal to dry skin, is also quite good, and most of the 12 colors are excellent. **Colors to avoid because they are too peach:** Natural Glow, Creamy Peach, and Warmer.

☺ **Super Double Face Powder Foundation** *($14.50)* is a pressed powder that contains talc and mineral oil; it can be used as an all-over sheer foundation or as a finishing powder, and the colors are so sheer it's like wearing no makeup at all. **All of the colors are excellent.**

☺ **Continuous Coverage Makeup SPF 11** *($12.50)* is a very thick, heavy, opaque, oil-based foundation intended for those who want to cover scarring. It should not be used as an everyday makeup unless you need heavy coverage. **The color selection is excellent**, and it is one of the better foundations of this type. It's not a look I recommend, however.

☺ **Soft Finish Makeup** *($18.50)* is worth checking out if you have normal to dry skin. This good lightweight foundation has a smooth, even texture and blends on easily. How does it compare to Clinique's Balanced Makeup? Well, it's similar and perhaps slightly more sheer, but only slightly. **All of the colors are excellent.**

☺ **Extra Help** *($18.50)* makeup has a nice consistency and would be good for extremely dry skin. The color selection has been reformulated, and **all the colors except one are wonderful. Avoid** Fawn Beige, which is too rose for almost all skin tones.

☹ **Pore Minimizer** *($12.50)* contains mostly alcohol with talc. The alcohol is irritating, and the talc provides little to no coverage and tends to go on dry and flaky. This is a poor product. I incorrectly stated in the last edition of this book that this product had been discontinued. I am almost shocked that it is still available. **Good Day Face Correcting Tint SPF 6** *($13.50)* has a poor SPF and is too greasy for all but extremely dry skin. I dislike color correctors, and this is one more to add to my list.

☺ **CONCEALER:** **Quick Corrector** *($8.50)* comes in a tube with a wand applicator. Of the four shades, only medium is too rose; the others are excellent for light or medium skin tones. The texture is smooth without being greasy, but it can be too drying and matte for some skin types. It stays on well with only minimal creasing. **Soft Concealer Corrector** *($10.50)* has six excellent colors (although Deep can be too orange for most skin tones). It has a great consistency and goes on well with only a slight tendency to crease.

☺ **Advanced Concealer** *($10.50)* comes in a squeeze tube and goes on like a liquid but dries to a powder. It comes in two shades, Light and Medium; both are excellent. Beware: This product works only if the skin under your eyes is smooth; any dry or rough skin will look worse when this type of concealer is placed over it.

☹ **Anti-Acne Control Formula Concealer** *($10.50)* is very thick and heavy. It comes in two shades, Light and Medium, both poor. The anti-acne part of the formula is colloidal sulfur and salicylic acid, which will not get rid of a single blemish and can cause irritation. **Concealing Stick** *($10.50)* comes in just one color, which means it might work if you happen to have just the right skin tone. It can be greasy, and it creases easily.

☺ **POWDER:** **Soft Finish Pressed Powder** *($14.50)* is a talc-based powder that goes on soft and comes in only six (good) colors. **Stay Matte Sheer Pressed Powder** *($14.50)* is an oil-free talc-based powder that goes on very sheer and soft. The colors are great but they all have a slight amount of shine, which defeats the purpose of a powder. **Blended Face Powder with Brush** *($14.50)* is a loose, talc-based powder with a soft texture and a good selection of colors.

☺ **Transparent Buffer** *($14.50)* is also talc-based. It comes in only one shade, which is supposed to be transparent, but it doesn't look that way when applied over foundation. It can look chalky on some skin types.

☺ **BLUSH:** **Beyond Blusher** *($15)* has an exquisite selection of soft colors, all with a soft, light texture. **Soft Touch Creamy Blush** *($10.50)* is applied like a cream but dries to a powder, very sheer. All of these colors are beautiful: Bronzed Rose, Warm Glow, Sunny Blush, Basic Blush, Honey Wine, and Satin Mauve (which is very shiny, but may be good for evening wear). **Bronze Doubles** *($14.50)* have no shine and can be great contour colors, but be careful not to end up having your face look shades darker than your neck.

☺ **Soft Press Powder Blusher** *($14.50)* is fairly shiny but not terrible. The colors are attractive and blend on soft. **Color Rub** *($9.50)* pours out of a small bottle and spreads over the cheek or face like a very sheer liquid bronzer, but all the colors are too shiny. **Gel Rouge** *($8.50)*, a liquid that comes in a tube, is supposed to be rubbed over the cheek area to stain it with color. This is best for someone with smooth, even, almost flawless skin. **Cheek Base** *($9.50)* is a waterproof cheek color that comes in five very soft shades. It is more like a tint than a blush; it goes on like a cream and dries to a powder. It's best for someone with smooth, even skin. **Transparent Buffer** *($13.50)* isn't very transparent; both colors, Think Bronze and Sun Duster, are too shiny.

☹ **EYESHADOW: Daily Eye Treat** *($9.50)* is a liquid in a tube. All of the shades are very shiny, and the liquid dries in place, which makes blending tricky. **Lidsticks** *($12.50)* are fat pencils that come in mostly shiny colors; I don't recommend them.

☺ **Beyond Shadow** *($11.50)* is a waterproof eyeshadow. The color is squeezed out of a tube and blended over the eye area. It stays surprisingly well (it tends not to crease) and blends thin and sheer, almost as if you never put any on in the first place. Most of the colors have a little shine, but it is most evident when the shadow is first applied and then seems to blend away so that it doesn't affect the smooth look. All of these colors are soft and attractive but don't show up much on the skin: Natural, Warmth, Smoke, Brown, Bare, Plum, and Fern.

☺ **Soft Pressed Eyeshadow** *($11)* goes on very soft and silky, but most of the shades are too shiny. However, the small selection of matte shades is fine, and they do go on soft. **All of these colors are superb, neutral, and matte:** Pink Ginger, Brown Grape, Brandied Plum, Pure Cream, Pure Neutral, Brown Light, Twig, Pure Warmth, Honey Sun, Calming Ivory, Purely Porcelain, Creamy Neutral, Cooling Buff, Caring Beige, Friendly Fawn, Sunny Nature, and Tender Warmth. **All of these colors are beautiful and soft but, sadly, too shiny:** Golden Lynx, Bronze Satin, Tea Leaf, Violet Rain, Sunset Mauve, Teal Haze, Earthling, Starstruck, Twilight Mauve, Starry Rose, Fawn Satin, Star Violet, Olive Bronze, Silver Peony, Periwinkle Blue, Moon Turquoise, Nude Bronze, Rose Warmth, Grapeskin, Jet Stream, Charcoal, Seashell Pink, Extra Violet, Ivory Bisque, and Peach Silk.

☺ **Pair of Shades Eyeshadow Duo** *($13)* could have been a welcome addition to the line, but Clinique missed the boat. The color pairs are attractive and mostly neutral, with a small but soft selection of browns and grays, but, alas, they all have some amount of shine. If you're under the age of 21 the shine won't be that noticeable, but if you are at all concerned about how wrinkled your eyes look, any amount of shine is unacceptable. **Touch Base for Eyes** *($11)* is a cream-to-powder shadow that comes in 12 colors, all with some amount of shine. The major problem is that this product tends to dry out and then is almost impossible to use.

☺ **EYE AND BROW SHAPER: Eye Shading Pencils** *($9.50)* are standard pencils in a good range of colors (avoid the shiny ones) that go on soft, without feeling greasy. **Water Resistant Eyeliner** *($13.50)* is an old-fashioned cake liner that comes in three colors and can be used wet or dry. It isn't all that water-resistant, but it does create a dramatic line. **Quick Eyes** *($14.50)* have an eye pencil at one end of the stick and a powdered eyeshadow section with a sponge-tip applicator at the other. The eyeshadow is released into the sponge tip when you shake it. If the eyeshadows weren't so shiny, I would recommend this gimmicky product as a convenient tool for doing a fast eye design. **Brow Shaper** *($12)* is a powder meant to be used for the brows. It's fine, but an eyeshadow that matches your brow color would do. The brush that accompanies this compact is too hard and scratchy.

☹ Touch Liner *($13.50)* is a liquid liner in a tube. All three colors are shiny.

☺ **LIPSTICK AND LIP PENCIL:** Clinique's lipsticks come in an excellent color selection. **Semi-Lipstick** *($9.50)* is more gloss than lipstick and doesn't stay on well at all. **Sun Buffer Lipstick** *($10.50)* is similar to the Semi, but with SPF 15. **Almost Lipstick** *($12.50)* is extremely similar to the Semi and Buffer, only it's a gloss in a tube. Talk about redundancy. **Gloss Wear SPF 8** *($6.50)* is—I know this is hard to believe—another gloss, only it comes in a pot, with a brush. **Different Lipstick** *($10.50)* is slightly more creamy than the Semi, but only slightly. It does have a slight stain, which means it can last somewhat longer on the lips. **Re-Moisturizing Lipstick** *($12)* is a good basic creamy lipstick that goes on smoothly without caking or feeling thick. **Long Last Lipstick** *($12.50)* is an excellent semi-matte lipstick, even though they call it a matte. It has a beautiful consistency and doesn't bleed. This is a find! Clinique's **Lip Shaping Pencils** *($9.50)* have a soft, smooth texture and come in an excellent array of colors.

☺ **MASCARA: Naturally Glossy Mascara** *($11)* is good but not great. It goes on quickly and builds thickness, but it also tends to make lashes spiky, which isn't the best look. **Full Potential Mascara** *($11)* is also good but not great. It definitely makes the lashes look thicker and longer, but it has a slight tendency to smudge and clump. If you don't have a problem with mascara ending up on the under-eye skin, this is a good one to try; it's just not meant for everyone.

Color Me Beautiful

Carole Jackson no longer owns this line, and the Color Me Beautiful public relations department told me it would probably be best to remove her name from this introduction. Somehow that seems like sacrilege. Carole Jackson introduced the art of wearing the right colors for your skin type to an entire generation of women via her "seasons" theory, which explained what colors work best with a particular skin tone and hair color. Once a woman knew whether she was a Spring (blonde hair and pink skin tones; requires pastel colors with a yellow undertone), Summer (blonde hair and sallow skin tones; requires pastel colors with a blue undertone), Autumn (red hair and pink skin tones; requires yellow-based earth tones), or Winter (brunette or black hair and any skin color; requires vivid blue-toned pastels), she could find colors that enhanced her skin tone instead of draining the color from it. This philosophy has clearly changed the way women shop for clothing and makeup colors.

Ms. Jackson created this makeup line in response to the demand for her color expertise. Sadly, with or without her, the line doesn't deliver the color organization you may be looking for. The color trays are divided into the appropriate seasons, but many of the colors overlap and not all of the appropriate color swatches are represented. Some colors are in both the Winter drawer and the Spring drawer, which doesn't make any sense given Jackson's beliefs about color. Also, most of the eyeshadows and some of the blushes are just too shiny; there is only one type of foundation, which is incredibly limiting; and there is only one pressed powder color. Finally, the foundation colors are divided into the four seasons groupings, but because the shades overlap, there are really only two color groupings, not four. Although I agree wholeheartedly with the idea of using color to complement and enhance skin tone, all foundations should be neutral, with no pink or peach. Dividing these foundations into color groupings doesn't make sense. Just because a woman's skin has pink tones doesn't mean she needs a pink foundation. Her underlying skin color is still neutral. Adding pink to already pink skin only makes the skin look more pink and artificial. And there is never a reason to buy a peach-colored foundation. In fact, when I asked the salespeople if they sold much of the peach-colored foundations, they said no, none at all. What a surprise.

Color Me Beautiful Skin Care

☹ **Creamy Cleanser for Dry Skin** *($15.50 for 6 ounces)* is a very greasy mineral oil–based wipe-off cleanser. It is more a cold cream than anything.

☹ **Foaming Cleanser for Normal/Oily Skin** *($15.50 for 4.5 ounces)* is a standard detergent-based cleanser. Sodium lauryl sulfate is the second item on the ingredient list, making this cleanser too drying and irritating for most skin types.

☹ **Lathering Cleanser for Normal/Dry Skin** *($15.50 for 4.5 ounces)* is very similar to the cleanser above, and the same review applies.

☹ **Makeup Remover Gel for Eyes, Lips & Face** *($13 for 2 ounces)* contains mostly water, slip agents, plant extracts, and preservatives. This is a rather poor eye makeup remover, and the claim that it contains an anti-wrinkle compound is nonsense; it doesn't contain anything even vaguely moisturizing.

☺ **Balancing Tonic** *($12 for 6 ounces)* contains mostly water, plant extract, plant oils, witch hazel, slip agents, and preservatives. If you aren't allergic to the plant extracts or oils, this could be an OK toner. Witch hazel can be a skin irritant.

☺ **Refining Toner** *($13 for 6 ounces)* contains mostly water, slip agent, glycolic acid, glycerin, cleansing agent, and preservatives. There's a long list of plant extracts, vitamins, and minerals, but in such minuscule amounts they are at best insignificant. However, this could be a very good 7% AHA product in a nonirritating base.

☺ **Daily Defense Light SPF 8 for Normal/Combination Skin Moisturizer** *($17.50 for 1.6 ounces)* is a good standard moisturizer for someone with dry skin, but the SPF is good only for limited sun exposure, and the oils in this product would not be good for someone with combination skin. The company claims that this product contains antioxidants, but they come well after the preservatives on the ingredient list and are barely present.

☺ **Daily Defense Oil-Free SPF 8 for Oily Skin Moisturizer** *($17.50 for 1.6 ounces)* is similar to the moisturizer above, minus the oils, and the same review applies.

☺ **Daily Defense Rich SPF 8 for Dry Skin Moisturizer** *($17.50 for 1.6 ounces)* is similar to the two moisturizers above, only with more emollients, and the same review applies. This moisturizer could be good for someone with dry skin.

☺ **Glycolic Treatment for the Face** *($18.50 for 1 ounce)* is a good 8% glycolic acid–based AHA product. The lightweight moisturizing base would be good for someone with normal to dry skin.

☺ **$$$ Multi-Active Booster Vitasome Energizing Treatment** *($22.50 for 1 ounce)* contains mostly water; slip agent; plant extracts; water-binding agents; vitamins E, A, and D; plant oils; and preservatives. This product is supposed to "fight time with a vitamin-and-mineral-packed anti-wrinkle serum." Well, vitamins and minerals won't fight time, especially when they're present in such small amounts. And the minuscule bits of tissue, thymus, oyster shell, and sea-silt extract must be in there just to sound intriguing, because they have no benefit for the skin. This product is a lightweight moisturizer for most skin types, but that's about it.

☺ **$$$ Triple Action Eye Cream** *($18.50 for 0.5 ounce)* contains mostly water, slip agent, thickeners, plant extract, a long list of thickeners, plant oil, silicone oil, plant extract, water-binding agents, vitamins A and E, and preservatives. This is a very good moisturizer for dry skin. The vitamins are so far down on the ingredient list, they are barely present.

☺ **Visible Results for All Skin Types** *($18.50 for 1 ounce)* contains mostly water, glycolic acid, thickeners, slip agent, vitamins E and A, water-binding agents, plant extracts, and preservatives. This would be a very good 8% AHA product for normal to dry skin.

☺ **Instant Result Mask for All Skin Types** *($16.50 for 4 ounces)* contains mostly aloe, plant water, wax, synthetic scrub particles, thickeners, plant oil, cleansing agent, AHAs, a BHA, soothing agent, and preservatives. The AHAs and BHA are probably little more than 2% of the product, which means it probably won't irritate the skin; that's good, because otherwise the scrub particles could be too much when combined with the acids. This is a good moisturizing mask, but don't expect instant anything.

Color Me Beautiful Makeup

☺ **FOUNDATION:** **Liquid Foundation** *($16)* is quite good and light, but only for someone with normal to dry skin. **These colors are superior:** Ivory, Neutral Beige, Tawny, Rose Beige, Sepia Beige, Porcelain, Bisque, Sand, Tender Tan, Almond, Nutmeg, and Naturale. **These colors are too intensely peach or pink:** Beige Blush, Cool Beige, Peach Blush, Golden Beige, Warm Beige, Country Blush, Deep Topaz, and Mahogany.

☺ **Soft Focus Skin Perfecting Oil-Free Foundation SPF 8** *($19.50)* contains AHAs, but less than 1%. That means the AHAs are there as a water-binding agent, not an exfoliator. Still, this is a good matte foundation with some great colors, and it really is oil-free. **These colors are excellent:** Sand, Cool Beige, Neutral Beige, Porcelain, Ivory, Bisque, Naturale, Sepia Beige, Almond, Deep Topaz, and Mahogany. **These colors are too peach or orange:** Country Blush, Warm Beige, and Nutmeg.

☺ **Perfection Microfine Powder Foundation** *($16)* is a pressed powder–type foundation. It has a great, dry but soft texture and wonderful colors. **These colors are excellent:**

Ivory, Tabasco Beige, Creamy Beige, Whisper Beige, Sepia Beige, Toasty Beige, Fawn Beige, Cameo Beige, Cocoa Beige, Golden Glow, and Golden Sand. **These colors are too pink:** Rose Glow and Pink Sand.

☹ **Color Adjuster** *($15)* is a light mint green foundation meant to reduce pink skin tones. I dislike color correctors in general, and this one is like all the others: an extra, unnecessary step that can leave a strange hue on the face.

☹ **Eyeshadow Base** *($12)* is applied like a concealer over the eye area. It dries to a sticky powder finish, but it doesn't hold eyeshadow any better than using nothing. Plus the one color it comes in is slightly pink, and won't work for most skin tones.

☹ **CONCEALER: Cover Stick** *($8.50)* comes in four shades: Light, which is too pink, and Medium, Medium/Deep, and Deep, which are great. The texture isn't the best (it tends to be greasy), but it blends easily. Unfortunately, the color slips into the lines around the eye.

☺ **POWDER: Translucent Pressed Powder** *($10.50)* and **Translucent Loose Powder** *($12.50)* both have a smooth, wonderful silky finish. They come in three shades, and all are great.

😐 **BLUSH: Powder Blush** *($10.50)* comes in a nice array of colors, but most are either very shiny or slightly shiny, which I don't recommend. **These colors are good and go on soft:** Soft Plum, Soft Rose, Clear Pink, Whisper Pink, Azalea, Cranberry, and Desert Coral (good contour color). **These colors are too shiny:** Chestnut, Rosette, Clear Rose, Soft Rose, Cedar Rose, Flirtatious Fuchsia, Simply Red, Plum Wine, Warm Pink, Sunset Red, Clear Salmon, Pink Quartz, Carmelon, Ruby, Peach Crystal, Rose Gold Bronzer, Simply Red, Apricot, Tawny, Peach, and Copper Sun Bronzer.

😐 **EYESHADOW:** Most of the **Eye Shadow** *($8.50)* colors go on rather heavy, and some are *very* heavy, which makes them tricky to blend. Be careful: most of the colors aren't as soft as they look. Most are fairly shiny, too, so the selection is limited, but there are some great matte colors. **These colors are very good:** Espresso, Graphite, Cocoa, Claret, Putty, Buff (great neutral), Warm Pink, Honey, Taupe, Smoky Topaz, Tiger's Eye, and Peach. **These colors are too shiny and/or too blue or green:** Gray, Evergreen, Smoke, Champagne, Spruce, Violet, Silvered Mauve, Dove Gray, Periwinkle, Steel Blue, Sapphire, Teal Blue, Aegean Blue, Cool Pink, Smoky Turquoise, Wild Orchid, Teal Bright, Cornflower, Soft Aqua, Copper, Coffee, Bronze, Golden Green, Golden Brown, Sage, Mink, Sterling, Emerald, Jardite, and Olive.

☺ <u>**EYE AND BROW SHAPER:**</u> **Brow Color** *($12)* is a dry eyeshadow for the brows. It is a great way to apply brow color, although an eyeshadow that matches your brows would work just as well. The eye pencils, called **SmudgeLiner** *($9.50)*, go on well and are just like every other line's, although one end does have a sponge tip for softening or smudging the line. **Brow Fixative** *($9)* is a clear gel meant to keep eyebrows in place. It works well, but no better than hairspray on a toothbrush brushed through the brow.

☺ <u>**LIPSTICK AND LIP PENCIL:**</u> **Classic Lipstick** *($9)*, which comes in a wide range of colors, is very creamy, and even the soft colors have decent staying power. **More Than Matte Lipstick** *($9)* is a superior matte lipstick that has great staying power and doesn't bleed. This isn't ultra-matte (it does have some creamy movement), but it is indeed matte without being the least bit drying. **Lip Conditioner SPF 15** *($9.50)* is a good emollient gloss that could be great for dry chapped lips, and the SPF 15 is a welcome addition. There is a standard small **Lip Pencil** *($8)* collection; they go on easily without being greasy or dry.

☺ <u>**MASCARA:**</u> **Lush Lash** *($9)* is an excellent mascara. It goes on easily, doesn't smudge, and builds long, relatively thick lashes.

☺ **Sensitive Eyes Mascara** *($9)* doesn't go on as well as the Lush Lash and takes a long time to build any length and thickness. It may or may not be better for sensitive eyes—there doesn't seem to be much difference in the ingredient lists—but it isn't better for defining lashes.

Coppertone (Skin Care Only)

☹ **Skin Selects Sun Protecting Lotion for Oily Skin 100% Oil Free SPF 15 Hypoallergenic** *($6.12 for 4 ounces)* is not even remotely hypoallergenic. The second ingredient is aluminum starch, which can be a skin irritant, and it also contains PVP (hairspray), another potential skin irritant. Other ingredients include both triethanolamine and imidazolidinyl urea, which can be an unsafe combination. It is oil-free but not recommended unless you have very sturdy skin.

☺ **Skin Selects Sun Protecting Lotion for Sensitive Skin SPF 15 Nonirritating** *($6.12 for 4 ounces)* is definitely less irritating than the lotion for oily skin. It does contain PVP, but not very much. Other than that, this would be a good sunscreen for someone with normal to dry skin.

☺ **Skin Selects Sun Protecting Lotion for Dry Skin SPF 15 Rehydrating** *($6.12 for 4 ounces)* is a good emollient lightweight sunscreen for someone with normal to dry skin. It is similar to the lotion for sensitive skin, and the same comments apply.

Coty

Hiding in a corner of most drugstores is the perennial but sparse cosmetic line called Coty. Although this line doesn't have much I'd recommend, you shouldn't overlook it completely. Yes, the foundations lack testers (one of them is even packaged so you can't see the color in the container). And yes, most of the pressed- and loose-powder colors are hidden by the powder puff, so you can't begin to guess which color is best for you. But where Coty excels is in its varied collection of lip products. This line has some of the most innovative lipsticks around. If your lipsticks tend to bleed into the lines around your lips, Coty can save you. Also, the small selection of eye and lip pencils, though fairly standard, are every bit as good as a hundred other pencils on the scene, only cheaper. Coty has a handful of skin care products that are not widely distributed, which isn't necessarily bad news, because they aren't much to get excited about.

Coty Skin Care

☹ **Gentle Eye Makeup Remover** *($3.71 for 4 ounces)* will take off eye makeup, but may be somewhat irritating to the eye area.

☹ **Peel Away Apricot Facial Mask** *($3.19 for 3.25 ounces)* will definitely peel away a layer of skin, but the second item on the ingredient list is alcohol, which can irritate the skin.

☺ **Vitamin A-D Complex Cream** *($5.21 for 4 ounces)* contains mostly water, mineral oil, lanolin oil, glycerin, thickeners, fragrance, vitamin E, lanolin, preservatives, and tiny amounts of vitamins A and D. This very emollient moisturizer would be good for someone with extremely dry skin.

☺ **Vitamin Moisture Balancer Emollient Daytime Lotion** *($5.21 for 4 ounces)* contains mostly mineral oil, lanolin, witch hazel, water, beeswax, lecithin, thickeners, fragrance, vitamins A and D, and preservatives. This is an extremely emollient, almost greasy moisturizer for someone with extremely dry skin, but the vitamins are barely present. Witch hazel may be irritating for some skin types.

☹ **Sweet Earth Mud Mineral China Clay Facial Mask** *($3.19 for 3.5 ounces)* is a standard clay mask that also contains alcohol, which can be irritating.

☹ **Sweet Earth Mud Corrective Formula China Clay Facial Mask** *($3.19 for 3.5 ounces)* is almost identical to the mask above, and the same review applies.

Coty Makeup

☺ <u>FOUNDATION:</u> The **Line Minimizing Makeup** *($6.77)* is a soft talc-based powder; it doesn't minimize lines, but it does go on rather soft and silky and comes in some excellent shades. Like most powder/foundations, this one is more powder than foundation, but it does go on smoothly and provides light sheer coverage. Warning: It is also highly fragranced and not for everyone's nose.

☹ **Chronology Hydrating Creme Makeup** *($6.02)* has no testers at the counter, and there is no way to see even a hint of the color given its black tube. **Airspun Powderessence Liquid Matte Makeup** *($6.02)* has a terrible selection of very pink and peach shades.

☹ <u>POWDER:</u> **Correctives Pressed Powder with Natural Astringents** *($4.81)* is one of those products that make me angry enough to yell. This is supposed to be for someone with oily skin, and the label carries on about "oil-free" and "oil-absorbing" and "translucent," but what they don't tell you is that the powder is *iridescent.* That's right, it has shine. What a joke! In trying to get rid of shine, you add more. Coty, wake up and smell the coffee.

☺ <u>LIPSTICK AND LIP PENCIL:</u> **Lip Doctor Color Therapy Stick with AHA** *($3.95)* is a very emollient lip gloss in a tube that can be good for chapped lips. It does contain a small amount of menthol, which doesn't doctor the lips and can be an irritant for some skin types. It also contains about 1% AHAs, which makes it a good water-binding agent in terms of moisturizing, but it won't exfoliate or help reduce lines. **Sheer to Stay 6 Hour Lip Color** *($3.20)* is a rich emollient gloss that goes on smoothly, but to suggest it lasts six hours is stretching the truth by a few hours. It contains a small amount of tint, so it tends to stay a little better than an ordinary gloss, but not that much better. **Self-Sealing Lip Makeup** *($3.73)* is applied with a wand and goes on like a gloss, but it dries to a soft, matte, powdery texture. It is actually quite nice, and an interesting twist on the ultra-matte look. The color selection is extremely limited, but what is available is worth checking out. **'24' Hour Creme Lipstick** *($4.63)* is a matte lipstick with just enough "slip" to feel somewhat pleasant when you rub your lips together during the day. This lipstick doesn't bleed and stays on incredibly well during the day. Like all truly matte lipsticks, it tends to cake, but this one doesn't dry out the lips. **Stop It Anti-Feathering Stick for Lips** *($3.57)* and **Hold It Wear Extending Base for Lips** *($4.16)* are two of the absolute best on the market. No lipstick, not even reds, can bleed past these two clear lipstick bases. And they don't dry out the lips, cake, or peel. What a find! **Lip Writer Stayput Lipstick** *($4.50)* is another amazing lip product. It is an ultra-matte lipstick in a stick form, like a thick eye pencil. It goes on incredibly smooth, but it absolutely doesn't budge. In fact, this one is hard to get off. Worth checking out!

Silkstick Lipstick *($2.08)* is a fairly greasy cream lipstick that feels almost too slick. It's more gloss than silk, that's for sure.

Cover Girl

If names evoke an attitude, then Cover Girl establishes its attitude firmly: this line is for those who still think of themselves as "girls," or for those who really *are* girls. Although the concept of being a cover girl was appealing in the '60s and '70s, today very few women over the age of, say, 25 or 30 feel flattered when someone calls them a girl. As a result, Cover Girl's focus is on a younger market, and the company excels, in some ways, in catering to this group. (Drugstore shelves groan under the huge array of skin care and makeup products.) In the past, the dense, cloying fragrance that wafted from the products kept me from recommending almost all of them wholeheartedly, but that has changed, at least somewhat. I would hardly call the current fragrance annoying, although in some products, particularly the blush, it is still overly sweet. Cover Girl has also upgraded many other aspects of its products since I last reviewed them, and most of the colors are quite pretty.

As is true with many cosmetics lines, Cover Girl's eyeshadows are more shiny than matte. Still, the line does offer a number of matte shades, and those are OK, although they tend to go on choppy, so be careful when you're blending. Cover Girl offers several types of powder blushes in assorted packages, but I found no discernible differences in how these various products went on or how long they lasted; most of the colors went on soft but were somewhat shiny, which is not a look I recommend. If you don't mind shine though, and it isn't as bad as some, these are an excellent option. The lipsticks are good, and several of the mascaras are very good. Cover Girl divides almost all of its colors into one of three color families: Warm, Cool, and Neutral. There is a color-family chart on the back of some products, and some drugstores have a small computer-type device that helps you select your category. After you enter your hair color and skin color, it tells you which color family to select. This is a helpful, easy system to use, and the Cool and Warm categories are usually correct. However, Cover Girl says that its Neutral colors work with all skin tones, and I disagree.

Cover Girl Skin Care

☺ **Clearly Different Deep Cleansing Face Wash** *($4.50 for 3.5 ounces)* is a standard detergent-based cleanser that can be drying for some skin types.

☺ **Moisture-Rich Gentle Cleansing Beauty Wash** *($4.50 for 3.7 ounces)* isn't all that rich in moisture, but it is an OK cleanser for dry skin. It can leave a film on the skin and doesn't take off makeup very well.

☹ **Noxzema Original Skin Cream** *($2.89 for 10 ounces)* contains mostly water, thickener, plant oil, fragrance, lye, camphor, menthol, phenol, clove oil, and eucalyptus oil. This is one of the most irritating skin care products I've ever seen. It has more highly irritating ingredients in it than almost any other product I've ever reviewed. Phenol is one of the all-time worst skin care ingredients.

☹ **Noxzema Plus Cleansing Cream** *($2.89 for 10 ounces)* contains mostly water, thickener, plant oil, glycerin, thickener, lye, and preservatives. It isn't as caustic as the cream above, but it's still fairly irritating.

☺ **Noxzema Plus Cleansing Lotion** *($3.25 for 10.5 ounces)* does not contain most of the irritating ingredients in the two creams above, which makes it a fairly gentle cleanser, but it isn't great at taking off makeup.

☺ **Noxzema Sensitive Cleansing Cream** *($2.89 for 10 ounces)* is similar to the lotion above, and the same review applies.

☺ **Noxzema Sensitive Cleansing Lotion** *($3.25 for 10.5 ounces)* is similar to Noxzema Plus Cleansing Lotion above, and the same review applies.

☺ **Clean Eyes Conditioning Make-Up Remover** *($2.78 for 2 ounces)* is a mineral oil–based wipe-off makeup remover that can leave a greasy film on the skin. The second item on the ingredient list, isopropyl palmitate, can cause breakouts.

☹ **Extra-Fresh Purifying Astringent** *($4.05 for 8 ounces)* is mostly alcohol and glycerin, which is mostly very irritating and drying.

☹ **Extremely Gentle Refining Toner** *($4.05 for 8 ounces)* is alcohol-based, which is hardly gentle. It does contain some water-binding agents, but they can't put back what the alcohol takes away.

☹ **Noxzema Sensitive Toner** *($3.79 for 8 ounces)* is almost identical to the toner above, and the same review applies.

☹ **Noxzema Astringent Skin Cleanser** *($3.19 for 8 ounces)* contains alcohol and a host of irritating ingredients such as camphor, eucalyptus oil, clove oil, and mint oil.

☹ **Noxzema Normal Astringent** *($3.19 for 8 ounces)* is mostly alcohol and menthol. Need I say more?

☹ **Noxzema Oily Astringent Salicylic Acid Acne Medication** *($3.19 for 8 ounces)* is simply alcohol and 2% salicylic acid, just like dozens of other acne products that don't work either.

☹ **Clear Skin Clarifying Pads Acne Treatment** *($3.15 for 50 pads)* is similar to the product above, but it also contains eucalyptus oil, camphor, menthol, and clove oil to make sure the skin is completely irritated and red.

☹ **Noxzema 2 in 1 Pads Regular Strength** *($2.59 for 50 pads)* is very similar to the pads above, and the same review applies.

☹ **Noxzema 2 in 1 Pads Maximum Strength** *($2.88 for 50 pads)* is very similar to the Clear Skin Clarifying Pads above, and the same review applies.

☺ **Advanced Clean Moisturizing Hydrogel** *($5.62 for 2 ounces)* contains mostly water and glycerin. That isn't exactly moisturizing, but if you have oily skin it can be soothing.

☺ **Oil-Free Pure Performing Moisturizer** *($5.35 for 3.9 ounces)* isn't oil-free; it contains silicone oil, but just a bit. This product is mostly water, thickeners, silicone oil, and preservatives. Some of the thickening agents are not great for oily, acned skin.

☺ **Protective Skin Nourishing Moisturizer SPF 15** *($5.35 for 3.9 ounces)* is a decent lightweight SPF 15 moisturizer for normal to oily skin.

Cover Girl Makeup

☹ **FOUNDATION:** Unfortunately, testers for Cover Girl foundations are still not available at the counters, so I cannot include many foundations in this review. Some of the company's foundations are still highly fragranced, which would make me reluctant to recommend them even if there were testers, but they have other problems as well. For example, **Ultimate Finish Liquid Powder Makeup** *($5.49)* has a small but good color selection and decent textures, but it also contains aluminum starch (a skin irritant) as the second item on the ingredient list, as well as isopropyl myristate, which can aggravate breakouts. It may be OK for some skin types, but not many. It is too greasy for someone with normal to oily skin, and too drying for someone with normal to dry skin. **Replenishing Liquid to Powder Makeup** *($5.49)* has the most obnoxious colors you are likely to run into anywhere. Most of the other foundations in the Cover Girl collection have the same problem—they are just too glaringly pink or peach.

☺ **Balanced Complexion for Combination Skin Makeup** *($5.49)* is the one exception to this rule, and I've been wearing it regularly for some time now. It goes on incredibly light and smooth, but also surprisingly matte, and stays that way for most of the day. It also doesn't slip into lines. Wow! What a shame there aren't testers so you could try this one out. Sometimes they do sell little samples for $1, though, so you can test products before buying a full-size container. **Most of the colors are surprisingly good; the only color to avoid is** Natural Beige.

☹ **CONCEALER:** Clarifying Anti-Acne Concealer *($3.69)*, **Replenishing** *($3.05)*, **Moisture Wear SPF 8** *($3.23)*, **Moisture Wear Stick** *($3.45)*, and **Invisible Concealer** *($3.69)* all have the worst color selections I've ever seen. **Almost all of the colors are too peach or pink.**

☹ **POWDER:** The Cover Girl line offers several types of pressed powder, but you can't see the color you're buying through the packaging. How strange and inconvenient! And why package a pressed powder with a puff when it should be applied with a brush? The **Clarifying Pressed Powder** *($3.24)*, **Clarifying Loose Powder** *($3.79)*, and **Professional Translucent Powder** *($3.76)* all contain eucalyptus and camphor, which can be skin irritants, and the fragrance could knock you off your feet. They smell like Noxzema, which is supposed to smell good for the skin. By now most women know that fragrance means irritation. At any rate, I can't recommend any of these pressed powders because you can't see the color. **Clean Fragrance-Free Pressed Powder** *($3.25)* clears the air, but you still can't see the color you're considering, and the same is true for **Moisture Wear Pressed Powder** *($3.05)* and **Balanced Complexion Pressed Powder** *($3.05)*.

☺ **BLUSH:** Cover Girl has several blush types. I didn't notice much of a difference in their ingredients or in the way they went on. They are all talc-based, with varying amounts of mineral oil and kaolin (clay). Most are shiny, but not terribly, and can be an option for some skin types, particularly if you don't have lines or dry skin, and the colors were soft, went on well, and lasted. However, the fragrance was too sickeningly sweet for my taste. **Continuous Color Moisture Enriched Blush** *($3.09)*, **Instant Cheekbones** *($3.23)*, **Cheekers** *($2.85)*, **Professional Color Match Blush Duo** *($3.04)*, and **Classic Color Brush-On Blush** *($3.22)* were all good, but they would get a much better rating if most of the colors weren't iridescent.

☹ **EYESHADOW:** The eyeshadows come in lots of colors, including some good matte shades, but they also contain an abundance of shine. One cute but useless new product is **Non Stop Eye Color** *($3.79)*. It contains three eyeshadows, one of which is shiny, and an eyeshadow base that matches the color tone of the eyeshadows. Not necessary, and the shiny eyeshadow is a waste of money. **Professional Color Match** *($4.25)* and **Professional Eye Enhancers** *($4.25 for sets of eight colors, $3.25 for Trios, and $3.25 for Quads)* are hardly professional or eye-enhancing. In some, the color combinations are poor; in others, one or more of the shades are shiny.

☺ **Pro Colors Singles** *($1.81)* and **Professional Eye Enhancers Singles** *($1.81)* are both nicely labeled as matte or perle. Some of the matte shades are worth checking out, but they tend to blend on choppy or uneven.

☺ <u>**EYE AND BROW SHAPER:**</u> **Soft Radiants** *($1.39)* is a standard eye pencil that goes on smooth and even. **Liquid Pencil Soft Precision Liner** *($3.60)* is a traditional liquid liner dispensed in what looks like a soft felt-tip pen. It makes a dramatic, obvious line, but it doesn't chip or flake and can last all day and night. **Perfect Blend Eye Pencil** *($2.84)* is a fairly standard pencil that goes on somewhat more greasy than most. That means smearing is more likely. **Thick 'n Thin** *($2.88)* is a two-sided pencil. One side is slightly thinner than the other, but I couldn't tell any difference in consistency. The pencil has a smooth texture, but goes on somewhat thicker and creamier than most, which increases the chance of smearing.

☹ **Brow Enhancer** *($1.63)* is a standard pencil that goes on thicker than most, which is not great when it comes to creating a natural look.

☺ <u>**LIPSTICK AND LIP PENCIL:**</u> Cover Girl makes several very impressive lipsticks with an excellent selection of attractive bright and muted colors. **Continuous Color Self Renewing Lipstick SPF 15** and **Continuous Color Self Renewing Lipstick (No SPF)** *($3.73)* claim that all you have to do is press your lips together to refresh the color. Now, for what lipstick (besides the ultra-mattes) *isn't* that true? How silly. Nevertheless, both of these are very creamy, moist, lightweight lipsticks. I strongly suggest staying away from the frosted colors. **Remarkable Lip Color SPF 15** *($3.53)* has a great moist, creamy texture, slightly thicker than Continuous Color, and contains a good sunscreen too. **LipSlicks LipGloss SPF 15** *($2.55)* is a very slick, sheer lip gloss with a good SPF. It's quite emollient and can help keep lips nice and moist with a hint of color. **Soft Radiants** *($3.15)* is a somewhat glossy, sheer lipstick.

☺ **Luminesse Lipstick** *($3.04)* is an average, rather greasy, shiny, frosted cream lipstick. The frost makes it a poor fashion choice. With **Remarkable Lip Color Frost (No SPF)** *($3.53)*, the frost part speaks for itself, and it's just not a look I can recommend. **InCondition LipBlush SPF 15** *($2.55)* is Cover Girl's version of a "mood" lipstick. It goes on as a sheer gloss, and in a minute or two it tints your lips in a way that is supposed to enhance your own lip color. This is a very good emollient gloss with a tint that is supposed to be activated by skin temperature, but I didn't notice any color change when I put it on. **Remarkable Lip Definer Lip Pencil** *($2.53)* is a good twist-up/no-sharpen lip pencil that comes in five wonderful colors. It's only slightly more greasy than most. The package lists the Cover Girl lipstick colors that coordinate with that pencil color—nice touch.

☺ **MASCARA:** Cover Girl has some very good mascaras, with some of the best prices anywhere. **Extension Waterproof Mascara** *($3.24)* is fairly waterproof and goes on well without clumping. **Remarkable Washable Waterproof Mascara** *($3.87)* has a confusing name, but that can be forgiven because it goes on well, builds length easily, and doesn't smear. It isn't at all waterproof, although it is more difficult than some to get off. **Long 'n Lush** *($3.87)* is also very good. **Thick Lash** *($3.24)* is excellent.

☹ **Curved Brush Professional Advanced Mascara** *($3.05)* builds somewhat thicker lashes than the **Straight Brush Professional Advanced Mascara** *($3.05)*. Neither clumps, but they both tend to smear.

☺ **BRUSHES:** Cover Girl has two blush/powder brushes that are not great but not awful either. The **Large Blush Brush** *($4.79)* and the **Medium Blush Brush** *($4.50)* are both reliable and work well, but the bristles are not as soft as some and too sparse to provide the best control.

Dermablend

Dermablend is a small line of products designed to help women with major skin problems they want to cover up. For those women, Dermablend's offer is hard to ignore. The question is how well the products work and whether they are good for the skin. The **Cover Creme Foundation** *($18)*, **Leg & Body Cover** *($15)*, **Quick Fix** (cover stick) *($13)*, **Setting Loose Powder** *($20)*, and **Setting Pressed Powder** *($15)* are supposed to provide complete opaque coverage that hides any kind of scarring or birthmarks (no matter how severe) and spider veins on the legs. These are not lightweight products that magically place a camouflaging film over the face and legs. Not surprisingly, each product has an unusually thick texture that can blend out to thin but opaque coverage. Basically, this is heavy-duty stuff.

All of the colors are actually quite good and natural. If you spread an even layer of the foundation, body cover, or cover stick over your face or legs, you can be assured of a good deal of coverage that, depending on the depth of discoloration, will hide your problem from view. The deeper the discoloration, the less likely you will be able to hide it. The question is, Do you really want that much coverage? What you get in place of the discoloration is a noticeable layer of foundation. Even if you spread it on as thinly as possible, it still has a heavy texture. Plus, the thinner you blend it on, the less coverage you get. There is no way that these products can look natural, but they can cover. Also, the Leg & Body Cover can be a problem to use, because even though it is waterproof and won't come off in the rain, it will rub off, and there's nothing you can do to prevent that. The Setting Powder, a white talc powder that looks very pasty on the skin, should not be used at all. Almost any neutral pressed or loose powder will work just as well.

It's difficult for me to recommend this product line, yet I know that many women have strong feelings about their facial discolorations. I may think the heavy look of the foundation is no better than the discoloration itself, but the problem isn't on my face. Emotions are strong when it comes to this issue, so testing the products yourself is probably the only way to make a decision.

For your information, Dermablend does have a cleanser and a sunscreen.

☹ **Cleanser** *($12.50 for 6.3 ounces)* is a detergent-based cleanser. The second item on the ingredient list is TEA-lauryl sulfate, a very drying and potentially irritating cleansing agent.

☺ **Maximum Moisturizer, SPF 15, PABA-Free** *($22.50 for 2 ounces)* is a good emollient SPF 15 sunscreen for someone with normal to dry skin. It contains mostly water, petrolatum, thickeners, plant oil, mineral oil, more thickeners, and preservatives.

Dermalogica (Skin Care Only)

Image is a major factor in most women's decisions about buying products. Image can convey the value of a company's products through an appeal to emotions. A beautiful model, a charismatic actress, or a distinctive brochure and packaging can be all the impetus necessary to persuade unwary consumers to make a purchase. What other consideration is there for buying a cosmetic product—particularly a skin care product? If a cream promises to firm the skin or protect it from environmental damage, we have very little to go on other than the impression we get from the advertising and the packaging (and, of course, the salesperson).

With that in mind, I have always been most intrigued by cosmetics lines that choose to create a scientific image instead of a glamorous image. Dermalogica has honed its image to a tee. The name implies a relationship to dermatology, which sounds as if you are getting serious skin care. The subtitle on Dermalogica's products is even more commanding: "A Skin Care System Researched and Developed by the International Dermal Institute." But what is the International Dermal Institute? Are there any dermatologists there? Apparently not: the Dermal Institute is a school for facialists who want an education beyond what is required for their cosmetology license, and the classes are taught by facialists. (If you're going to get a facial, although I would not suggest you spend your hard-earned money on one, it is best to go to someone who has training from somewhere other than just a cosmetology licensing school. In that regard, the International Dermal Institute provides a good, albeit expensive, service.)

Does the professional atmosphere of the school associated with Dermalogica mean better products? The proof is in the pudding, and this pudding is just Jell-O, not chocolate mousse. The company's literature expounds at length on the ingredients the products *don't* contain, such as mineral oil (because it's greasy and sits on the skin, although the same could be said of many of the plant oils and water-binding agents that the products do contain). But some of the products contain petrolatum, from which mineral oil is derived, so even if mineral oil were a culprit in skin care products (it isn't), this line's claim that it doesn't contain any is misleading.

Dermalogica products also don't contain isopropyl myristate, lanolin, or coal tar–based dyes, because, as the brochure explains, they can cause breakouts. That is true, but Dermalogica's products do contain ceresin, beeswax, forms of acrylate, and other ingredients that can potentially clog pores and cause breakouts.

Another misleading statement is the claim that the products don't contain formaldehyde, a preservative that can cause problems for the skin. In fact, many of the products contain diazolidinyl urea, a preservative that can release formaldehyde. The products also claim to be fragrance-free, but many of the plant extracts and oils used in the products indeed provide fragrance. Fragrance, regardless of its origin, can be irritating to the skin. I could go on, but I'll let the products and their ingredient lists speak for themselves.

☹ **Essential Cleansing Solution** *($21 for 8 ounces)* contains mostly water, plant oil, thickeners, petrolatum, ceresin, beeswax, and more thickeners. It can leave skin feeling greasy and may clog pores.

☹ **Dermal Clay Cleanser** *($21 for 8 ounces)* is a standard detergent cleanser that also contains plant oil, water-binding agents, and a list of vitamins. Water-binding agents are wasted in a cleanser because they are washed away. The clay can feel thick on the skin. The product also contains menthol, which causes a burning sensation, can be drying, and should be kept away from the eyes.

☹ **Special Cleansing Gel** *($21 for 8 ounces)* is a standard detergent-based cleanser that can be OK for someone with oily or combination skin. It contains balm mint, which can be irritating for some skin types.

☺ **Soothing Eye Makeup Remover** *($15 for 2 ounces)* can take off makeup without irritating the eyes, but wiping off eye makeup with any product, regardless of its ingredients, is hardly nonirritating.

☺ **Multi-Active Toner** *($21 for 8 ounces)* contains mostly aloe vera juice (aloe mixed with water), several water-binding agents, amniotic fluid, emollients, and preservatives. This relatively nonirritating toner can be good for some skin types. It contains a couple of potentially irritating ingredients, but they are far down on the ingredient list and probably not a problem. Of course, the amniotic stuff from the cow has no proven benefit for the skin and should not be used by any line claiming to be cruelty-free.

☺ **$$$ Skin Prep Scrub** *($22 for 2.5 ounces)* is a detergent-based cleanser that uses cornmeal as the scrub. All of the natural-sounding ingredients come well after the preservatives, which means there's too little to have any effect on the skin. It would probably be better to just use cornmeal from the grocery store if you want a cornmeal scrub.

☹ **Gentle Cream Exfoliant** *($26 for 2.5 ounces)* is a scrub that contains mostly thickeners, plant oil, salicylic acid, and preservatives. Salicylic acid can be irritating, although in this product most of it would be washed off. The plant oil can leave a greasy film. Do not use a scrub if you are also using an AHA product.

☹ **Active Moist** *($26 for 1.75 ounces)* has an SPF of 4, which is not enough to protect skin from the sun. If this product had no sunscreen you could perhaps use it at night, but using it during the day would leave the skin open to sun damage.

☹ **Skin Smoothing Cream** *($28 for 1.75 ounces)* has an SPF of 6, which is not enough to protect skin from the sun. If this product had no sunscreen at all you could perhaps use it at night, but using it during the day would leave the skin open to sun damage.

☺ **$$$ Intensive Moisture Balance SPF 10** *($30 for 1.75 ounces)* is a good moisturizer for someone with normal to slightly dry skin, but its SPF is 10, which is good but not great at protecting the skin from the sun.

☺ **$$$ Intensive Moisture Concentrate** *($45 for 1 ounce)*, like many moisturizers, uses an acrylate as the main ingredient. It places an imperceptible layer of plastic over the skin that helps it temporarily look smoother. It can be irritating, but otherwise this is an OK moisturizer. The so-called nourishing ingredients—vitamins A, E, and B—can't feed the skin, although they are good antioxidants. The product also contains lavender oil, which can cause skin problems upon sun exposure.

☺ **$$$ Specific Skin Concentrate** *($45 for 1 ounce)* is similar to the moisturizer above, and the same review applies.

☺ **$$$ Gentle Soothing Booster** *($41 for 1 ounce)* contains mostly water, red raspberry juice, standard water-binding agent, and preservatives. Raspberry juice can be irritating for some skin types and may cause allergic reactions. Besides, there is no benefit in putting raspberries on the skin, especially not at $41 an ounce.

☺ **$$$ Active Firming Booster** *($41 for 1 ounce)* contains mostly plant extracts, thickener, and preservatives. This product also contains a form of castor oil that can form a plastic-like layer over the skin, which may make it temporarily look smoother, but is also a potential skin irritant. According to the brochure, the product contains 70% active plant extracts. The plant extracts are not active, they are just tea water, and the price is just ridiculous.

☺ **$$$ Special Clearing Booster** *($36 for 1 ounce)* is a fairly expensive 5% benzoyl peroxide–based product. There are much cheaper benzoyl peroxides available at the drugstore, and I would recommend starting with 3% hydrogen peroxide or 2.5% benzoyl peroxide for acne before jumping to 5% benzoyl peroxide.

☹ **Skin Renewal Booster** *($41 for 1 ounce)* is a 10% AHA product that also contains sulfur and salicylic acid. Both the sulfur and the salicylic acid can be unnecessarily irritating given the presence of the AHAs (lactic acid), and several much less expensive AHA products are available.

☺ **$$$ Super Fade** *($24 for 1.75 ounces)*, like all fade creams, contains hydroquinone, here in a 2% concentration. Hydroquinone has only a minimal effect on lightening brown sun spots.

☹ **Intensive Oil Replacement** *($30 for 0.5 ounce)* contains several plant oils, including lavender oil, which can cause problems upon sun exposure; eucalyptus oil, which can be a skin irritant; and sandalwood, which can cause an allergic reaction in sensitive skin types.

☺ **$$$ Solar Block SPF 15** *($25 for 5 ounces)* is a sunscreen your skin can live with nicely, but the price is absurd. Many excellent SPF 15 products are available for much less money.

☺ **$$$ Solar Shield SPF 15** *($9.50 for 0.75 ounce)* is just a clear lipstick with SPF 15. Similar products are available from Almay and Physicians Formula for half the price.

☺ **$$$ Skin Refining Masque** *($26 for 2.5 ounces)* is a standard clay mask that contains little else besides clay. All of the natural-sounding ingredients come well after the preservatives, which means there's too little to have any effect.

☺ **$$$ Skin Hydrating Masque** *($27.50 for 2.5 ounces)* contains mostly water, plant extracts, thickener, several water-binding agents, and preservatives. This would be a good moisturizing mask for someone with dry skin, although a good emollient moisturizer left on the skin a little thicker and a little longer than usual can have the same effect.

☺ **$$$ Intensive Moisture Masque** *($32 for 2 ounces)* contains mostly water, plant oil, thickeners, plant extracts, silicone oil, vitamins, and preservatives. This would be a good moisturizing mask for someone with dry skin, although a good emollient moisturizer left on the skin a little thicker and a little longer than usual can have the same effect.

Donna Karan New York (Skin Care Only)

Donna Karan has gone from designing clothing and accessories for the neck down to designing products for the neck up. As a rule, it is hard to know what input designers have on the products that bear their names. Yves St. Laurent and Calvin Klein have their names on more than 800 products each, most of which they've probably never even seen. But designers' names convey a certain status, and people believe that designer products are inherently better than products with names they don't recognize. Nevertheless, for skin care and cosmetics, what counts isn't who designs the products but how the products work. Donna Karan's stuff is no exception.

This line is based on the concept of simplicity—kind of like Ms. Karan's line of clothing, I imagine. Unbelievably, a mere three products comprise the line. Wouldn't it be great if skin care could really be that simple? To some extent it is, but three products cannot work for all of the skin types out there. If you have normal to slightly dry skin, you will be happy with these products, although you will probably need more than what's here. Someone with acned, dry, sensitive, sun-damaged, or oily skin isn't going to find what she needs. The prices of these three items, and the retail outlets where they are sold (Bloomingdale's, Saks, Nordstrom, and Neiman Marcus), indicate who the originators of this line expect to suck in with the designer angle.

☺ **$$$ Formula for Clean Skin** *($25 for 5 ounces)* is a fairly standard detergent cleanser with some castor oil, which might make rinsing a bit of a problem. This would be a good cleanser for someone with normal to slightly dry skin.

☺ **$$$ Formula for Facial Moisture SPF 20** *($45 for 1.5 ounces)* is a standard SPF 20 moisturizer that contains mostly water, silicone oils, thickeners, vitamins E and C, fragrance, water-binding agents, and preservatives. This would be a fine daytime moisturizer for someone with normal to dry skin. The salesperson said it could also be used as a nighttime moisturizer, but I never recommend using a sunscreen at night.

☹ **Formula for Renewed Skin Exfoliating Mask and After Mask Skin Conditioner** *($55 for two 1-ounce containers)* is a two-part facial mask system that is supposed to be used once a week. The Exfoliating Mask contains witch hazel, cornstarch, aloe vera, clay, papaya enzyme, and preservatives. Witch hazel and cornstarch can both cause skin irritation. Papaya enzyme can exfoliate the skin, but AHA products do a better job for much less money and bother. The After Mask Skin Conditioner is a witch hazel–based toner, which makes it a possible skin irritant; also, it's just too expensive for what you get.

Dove (Skin Care Only)

☹ **Beauty Bar** *($2.17 for two 4.75-ounce bars)* is a standard tallow-based bar cleanser that contains some emollients to cut the irritation and dryness caused by the detergent cleansing agents. It is still quite drying, and although it is technically not soap, the ingredients can clog pores. It is probably just fine for most skin types from the neck down, but not from the neck up.

☹ **Beauty Bar (Unscented)** *($2.49 for two 4.75-ounce bars)* is similar to the bar above, and the same review applies.

☹ **Sensitive Skin Formula Beauty Bar** *($2.49 for two 4.25-ounce bars)* is similar to the bar above, but without the tallow. That makes it better, but it still can be drying.

☹ **Beauty Wash** *($2 for 6 ounces)* is a standard detergent-based water-soluble cleanser that can be fairly drying for most skin types. This one contains a small amount of tallow, which can aggravate breakouts.

eb5 (Skin Care Only)

I usually don't like to make fun of people (which is different from critiquing what they make and sell), but does anyone else think that the guy who is supposed to have formulated eb5 Cream and Cleanser, Robert Heldfond, looks like Dr. Zorba on the old *Ben Casey* television show? Sorry, I just couldn't resist. In any case, the claims on this line's brochure are just absurd. First, you're supposed to believe that a pharmacist knows something about formulating cosmetic creams. Pharmacists are trained to deal primarily with prescription drugs; they are not chemists, and they are definitely not cosmetic chemists. Second, eb5's cream is supposed to be great for daytime, yet it doesn't contain a sunscreen. Unless it's worn with a foundation that has a high SPF, this is not a good day cream at all. Another claim is that a 4-ounce jar will last for many months. I guess "many" is relative, but a woman with dry skin who used an eb5 cream twice a day would be lucky if it lasted six weeks. Finally, the brochure states that the moisturizer helps makeup adhere better. In fact, any moisturizer has the exact same ability. There are some good things about this cream, but it isn't as unique as the brochure makes it out to be.

☺ **Cleansing Formula** *($14 for 6 ounces)*, a fairly gentle cleanser that contains a small amount of detergent cleansing agents, would be best for someone with normal to dry skin, but it doesn't do a very good job of taking off makeup.

☹ **Toning Formula** *($10 for 8 ounces)* is just alcohol with some slip agents, which means it is very drying and irritating.

☺ **$$$ Facial Cream** *($35 for 4 ounces)* contains mostly water, slip agent, vitamin E, mineral oil, thickeners, vitamin A, more vitamin E, and preservatives. This very ordinary, almost boring moisturizer would be good for someone with dry skin, but it's not worth this price.

☺ **$$$ Age Spot Formula** *($25 for 6 ounces)* is a standard 2% hydroquinone fade cream. It also contains fruit extracts, but these are not the kind of AHAs that can exfoliate the skin and help lighten brown spots.

Elizabeth Arden

Elizabeth Arden became famous by establishing the standard for day spas in the United States. During the '60s and '70s, they were the chic, if not the only, place to have every inch of yourself pampered. Of course, that has all changed now, and Arden works overtime to keep its image current and avoid seeming dated. Bringing the line beautifully into the '90s was Arden's introduction of a line of skin care products called Ceramide, which started with one product, Ceramide Time Capsules, and blossomed into an entire series of products shortly after its launch. Ceramide is a good water-binding agent, but that's about it. Still, Arden's accomplishment was to make ceramide an important skin care ingredient, much the way collagen and elastin were in the '80s. Arden offers a large number of other skin care products, including some very good ones, but the prices are pretty steep.

Arden's counter displays are very attractive and easily accessible—always a strong point. The blush and lip colors are divided into four easy-to-understand categories: Red Tray, Coral Tray, Pink Tray, and Plum Tray. There's enough variety to interest women of all skin tones. The eyeshadows are divided into two categories—Cool and Warm—that coordinate with the blushes and lipsticks in the four color trays. (The Cool eyeshadows work with the Pink and Plum trays, and the Warm eyeshadows work with the Red and Coral trays.) Unfortunately, many of the eyeshadows are too shiny and should be avoided.

The blush colors are attractive—on the shiny side, but worth a try. Arden has revamped its foundations, and they turned out beautifully. The textures are excellent, and the colors are fairly good, ranging from very light to darker skin tones.

Elizabeth Arden Skin Care

☺ **$$$ Ceramide Purifying Cleansing Cream** *($19.50 for 1.7 ounces)* won't purify anything. It is a fairly standard mineral oil–based wipe-off cleanser with ordinary thickening agents to give it a creamy appearance, and it can leave a greasy film on the skin.

☺ **$$$ Millenium Hydrating Cleanser** *($23.50 for 4.4 ounces)* is an OK water-soluble cleanser that leaves a slightly greasy film on the skin. It also may not remove all traces of makeup.

☺ **$$$ Skin Deep Milky Cleanser** *($18.50 for 6.7 ounces)* is a mineral oil–based wipe-off cleanser. This isn't milky, it's greasy, and it needs to be wiped off.

☺ **$$$ Special Benefit Cleansing Cream** *($26 for 8 ounces)* is even greasier than the cleanser above. It's mostly mineral oil, wax, Vaseline, and lanolin.

☺ **$$$ Visible Difference Deep Cleansing Lotion** *($18.50 for 6.7 ounces)* is a good water-soluble cleanser that lathers and rinses well. However, it can be drying and may burn your eyes. Also, the third item on the ingredient list is isopropyl myristate, which can cause blackheads.

☺ **$$$ Visible Difference One Great Soap** *($12.50 for 5.3 ounces)* is a surprisingly good soap with good emollients and water-binding ingredients. The detergent cleanser used is farther down the ingredient list than in most soaps, which helps make this milder than most. I recommend this only for someone with normal to oily skin who likes to use soap.

☹ **Daily Soap** *($14)* is just expensive soap, and it can be drying for most skin types. It looks nice and clear, just like Neutrogena's transparent bar soap, but a soap needs to do more than just look good.

☺ **Conditioning Waterproof Eye Makeup Remover** *($13.50 for 4 ounces)* isn't conditioning in the least; it is simply a silicone oil–based wipe-off cleanser that also contains a small amount of detergent cleansing agents. It will wipe off eye makeup, but why bother with it?

☺ **Conditioning Eye Makeup Remover** *($13 for 4 ounces)* is a standard detergent-based makeup remover. It wipes off makeup easily, but wiping is always a problem for the eyes.

☺ **Visible Difference Gentle Scrub Creme for the Face** *($17.50 for 3.5 ounces)* leaves a somewhat greasy film on the face (the second item on the ingredient list is petrolatum). It uses standard synthetic scrub particles, which are gentle enough, so this may feel good to someone with extremely dry, parched skin.

☹ **Visible Difference Refining Toner** *($15 for 6.7 ounces)* contains mostly water, witch hazel, alcohol, glycerin, and preservative. The alcohol and witch hazel make it too irritating for most skin types.

☹ **Ceramide Purifying Toner** *($18.50 for 6.7 ounces)* is a very expensive alcohol-based toner. Alcohol doesn't purify the skin, but it can cause irritation.

☹ **Millenium Revitalizing Tonic** *($22.50 for 5 ounces)* contains mostly water and alcohol. This is too irritating for most skin types.

☹ **Skin Basics Skin Lotion** *($16 for 6.7 ounces)* is a water- and alcohol-based toner that is too drying for most skin types.

☹ **Clear Solution Basic Toner** *($10.50 for 6.7 ounces)* is an alcohol-based toner. Although the price is relatively reasonable, it's a bad product at any price.

☺ **$$$ Immunage UV Defense Cream SPF 15** *($35 for 1.25 ounces)* contains mostly water, slip agents, a very long list of thickeners, plant oil, more thickeners, vitamins E and A, and preservatives. This is a good lightweight moisturizer/sunscreen with a tiny amount of antioxidants, but it's very overpriced for what you get: a basic SPF 15 sunscreen.

☺ **$$$ Immunage UV Defense Lotion SPF 15** *($35 for 1.25 ounces)* is similar to the cream above, but more lightweight.

☺ **Daily Moisture Drink Lotion SPF 15** *($10.50 for 1.7 ounces)* is reasonably priced, but not very interesting. It contains mostly water, several thickeners, and a tiny amount of water-binding agents.

☺ **$$$ Millenium Day Renewal Emulsion** *($52.50 for 2.6 ounces)* contains mostly water, plant oil, slip agent, silicone oil, thickeners (one is isopropyl myristate, which can cause blackheads), lanolin oil, more thickeners, and preservatives. This very rich, emollient moisturizer should be used only for dry skin. However, if you tend to break out, stay away from it; also, without sunscreen, it's a poor choice for daytime.

☺ **$$$ Millenium Night Renewal Creme** *($55 for 1 ounce)* is similar to the product above, and the same review applies, except that since it's a night cream, it's good that it doesn't contain a sunscreen.

☹ **Sunmist Oil-Free Sunscreen SPF 15** *($15.50 for 3.5 ounces)* would be a good lightweight sunscreen except that it's alcohol-based, and can be drying for the skin.

☺ **$$$ Sunwear Daily Face Protector SPF 15** *($18.50 for 1 ounce)* is a titanium dioxide–based sunscreen that contains mostly water, slip agent, thickeners, silicone oil, a tiny amount of anti-irritant, plant extracts, and preservatives. It's a good basic nonchemical sunscreen.

☺ **$$$ Alpha-Ceramide** *(from $55 for 1 ounce of 7.5% concentration of AHA to $100 for the starter kit, which includes three bottles with varying strengths of AHA and one bottle of the 7% concentration, depending on what you buy)* promotes a four-step process that is supposed to gradually increase your skin's tolerance to different AHA strengths. These petite green bottles, numbered 1 through 4, contain different concentrations of AHAs, in this case lactic acid. Step 1, which is supposed to be used for two weeks, contains 3% AHAs; Step 2 contains 4.5% AHAs and is to be used for two weeks; Step 3 contains 6% AHAs and is also to be used for two weeks; and Step 4 *($55 for 1 ounce)*, the largest bottle, contains 7.5% AHAs and is the bottle you are supposed to continue using for as long as you want. All the bottles contain lactic acid mixed with fairly ordinary slip agents, water-binding agents, and anti-irritants. Although they are vastly overpriced, the basic concept is rather intriguing: your skin starts the exfoliating process slowly, so you don't necessarily go through a period of being suddenly flaky. I also prefer this kind of liquid/serum with a feather-light texture.

☹ **$$$ Ceramide Night Intensive Repair Creme** *($45 for 1 ounce)* contains mostly water, glycerin, several thickeners, pH balancer, more thickeners, water-binding agents, vitamins C and E, more thickeners, fragrance, and preservatives. The ingredient list is surprisingly ordinary; the only interesting item is almost at the end of the list and barely amounts to anything. The second ingredient is a neutralized form of salicylic acid, which means the product won't exfoliate the skin. This is just an OK moisturizer.

☹ **$$$ Visible Difference Refining Moisturizer Creme Complex** *($47.50 for 2.5 ounces)* contains mostly water, thickener, glycerin, more thickeners (including isopropyl myristate, which can cause blackheads), plant oil, beeswax, and preservatives. This is a somewhat heavy, though ordinary, moisturizer for someone with very dry skin.

☹ **Visible Difference Refining Moisture Lotion SPF 4** *($28.50 for 1.35 ounces)* would be a good emollient moisturizer/sunscreen except for two things: the sunscreen ingredient is padimate-o, a derivative of PABA, which can be a skin irritant; and SPF 4 can't protect adequately from sun damage.

☺ **$$$ Visible Difference Eyecare Concentrate** *($30 for 0.5 ounce)* is an ordinary but good moisturizer for dry skin; it contains mostly water, mineral oil, silicone oil, thickeners, plant oil, more thickeners, and preservatives.

☹ **$$$ Ceramide Time Complex Cream** *($45 for 1.7 ounces)* is Arden's attempt at an AHA product. It falls short, containing only a small amount of an ingredient that sounds like an AHA but isn't. It is still a good lightweight emollient moisturizer for someone with normal to dry skin. It contains mostly water, silicone oil, several thickeners, slip agents, more silicone oil, water-binding agents, antioxidants, more water-binding agents, vitamins E and C, plant oil, and preservatives. The amount of antioxidants is negligible.

☺ **$$$ Ceramide Time Complex Capsules** *($55 for 0.97 ounce in 60 capsules)* are the most popular product Arden sells, yet these tiny gelatin capsules contain some fairly ordinary stuff: silicone oils, plant oil, water-binding agent, and vitamins A and E. This is a good lightweight, soothing moisturizer for the face, but that's about it.

☺ **$$$ Ceramide Eyes Time Complex Capsules** *($37.50 for 0.35 ounce in 60 capsules)* contain mostly silicone oil, thickener, witch hazel (can be a skin irritant, particularly around the eyes), plant extract, plant oil, water-binding agents, vitamins E and K, more plant oil, and more silicone oil. This would be a good lightweight oil to put around the eyes if your skin doesn't have a problem with the witch hazel—and if you can get over the $1,700-per-pound price tag.

☺ **$$$ Micro 2000 Stressed-Skin Concentrate** *($42.50 for 0.85 ounce)* contains mostly silicone oil, thickener, water, plant oil, more thickeners (one is isopropyl myristate, which can cause blackheads), plant oil, more thickeners, minerals, water-binding agents, and preservatives. This won't help stressed skin any more than any other moisturizer. The ingredients are just average—nothing special—but the product would be good for dry skin.

☺ **$$$ Millenium Eye Renewal Cream** *($37.50 for 0.5 ounce)* is a very rich, thick, ordinary moisturizer that contains mostly water, mineral oil, lanolin, thickeners, and preservatives. It will indeed take care of dry skin.

☺ **$$$ Skin Basics Beauty Sleep** *($32.50 for 2.5 ounces)* is a basic, but extremely emollient, moisturizer that contains mostly water, mineral oil, lanolin oil, thickeners (one is isopropyl myristate, which can cause blackheads), lanolin, more thickeners, and preservatives. Only for very, very dry skin.

☺ **$$$ Skin Basics Velva Moisture Film** *($38.50 for 6.7 ounces)* contains mostly water, isopropyl myristate (can cause blackheads), lanolin oil, thickeners, and preservatives.

This is a very emollient, rich moisturizer for very dry skin, but it can cause blackheads for some skin types.

☺ **$$$ Special Benefit Orange Skin Cream** *($31 for 8 ounces)* is a very heavy, extremely greasy moisturizer for parched, dry skin. It contains petrolatum, lanolin, vegetable oil, thickener, and preservatives.

☺ **$$$ Eight Hour Cream** *($19.50 for 4 ounces)*, one of the original products in the Arden skin care arsenal, contains mostly water, petrolatum, lanolin, mineral oil, fragrance, salicylic acid, preservatives, plant oils, vitamin E, and preservatives. The tiny amount of salicylic acid is probably not a problem and can work as a gentle exfoliant. This is basically just a very greasy, emollient moisturizer for someone with extremely dry skin.

☹ **Skin Basics Velva Cream Mask** *($20 for 3.5 ounces)* contains mostly water, thickener, zinc oxide, phenol, and preservative. This mostly zinc oxide mask won't do anything for the skin. Phenol is one of the first preservatives on the ingredient list, and it is most definitely a skin irritant.

☺ **$$$ Millenium Hydra-Exfoliating Mask** *($27.50 for 2.65 ounces)* is a clay mask that also contains some oil, wax, and a silicate (like sand). Because of the oil, it isn't as drying as most clay masks, but it is still just another clay mask.

☺ **$$$ Special Benefit, Eight Hour Cream Lip Protectant Stick, SPF 15** *($12 for 0.13 ounce)* is a very emollient, though standard, petrolatum-based lip gloss with sunscreen. It would work well to protect from dryness and the sun.

Elizabeth Arden Makeup

☺ **$$$ FOUNDATION: Flawless Finish Hydro Light Foundation** *($30)* is a soft-textured foundation that smoothes on evenly, providing medium coverage. Most of the colors are superior, and the effect is excellent for someone with dry skin. **These colors are the best:** Mocha, Buff, Ivory, Vanilla, Fawn, Honey, Sable, and Chestnut. **These colors can be too peach or orange for most skin tones:** Bronze, Bisque, Cameo, and Cream.

☺ **$$$ Flawless Finish Every Day Makeup SPF 10** *($25)* is a lightweight foundation that goes on even and sheer, leaving a soft feel on the skin, and SPF 10 is not bad. **These colors are great:** Vanilla, Bisque, Buff, Honey, Fawn, Mocha, Sable, and Chestnut. **These colors should be avoided:** Ivory, Cream, Cameo, and Bronze.

☺ **$$$ Flawless Finish Complete Control Matte Makeup SPF 10** *($25)* won't control oil, but it does go smooth and matte, with an even, soft finish, and SPF 10 is a decent number. It provides medium coverage, blends on easily, and has good staying power. **These colors are the most natural and best:** Buff, Honey, Fawn, Mocha (may turn ash), Chestnut (may turn ash), and Vanilla. **These colors should be avoided:** Bisque, Sable, Bronze, Ivory, Cream, and Cameo.

☺ **$$$ Flawless Finish Dual Perfection Makeup** *($25)* can be used wet or dry. It is a standard talc-based powder with a bit of silicone oil to make it feel silky over the face. This type of foundation works best for someone with normal to dry skin, especially when used wet. **Most of the colors are excellent.** The only one that may be a problem is Cream.

☹ **Flawless Finish Sponge-On Cream Makeup** *($25)* is fairly thick and somewhat greasy. The colors are good, but it is too heavy and greasy to recommend for most skin types.

☺ **$$$ Flawless Finish Mousse Makeup** *($17.50)* comes out like a foam and covers the face with a light, somewhat dry finish. The color selection is good, but it can take a while to master the application technique. I tend to prefer traditional foundation consistencies; this one is a bit too gimmicky. **These colors are the best:** Mocha, Champagne, Bisque, Buff, and Honey. **These colors are too orange, rose, yellow, peach, or pink for most skin tones:** Summer, Bronze, Sable, Vanilla, Natural, Melba, and Ginger.

☺ **$$$ Flawless Finish Control Matte Powder Makeup** *($25)* is a talc-based pressed powder that Arden recommends for use by itself as a foundation. It comes in a good range of colors, but the texture is rather on the dry side for use all over the face. It can be used as a regular pressed powder.

☹ **CONCEALER: Cream-On Concealer** *($14)* comes in a traditional tube and has a good consistency, but the colors are all too pink or peach. The **Concealing Cream** *($14)* also comes in poor colors, is greasy, and tends to slip into the lines around the eyes. **Perfect Covering Concealer** *($13)* comes in five excellent colors; unfortunately it creases easily and goes on somewhat thick and heavy.

☺ **$$$ POWDER: Flawless Finish Pressed Powder** *($22.50)* isn't all that flawless. It is just a standard, soft pressed powder that comes in three shades: Translucent Light, Translucent Medium (fairly peach), and Translucent Dark. All contain talc and cornstarch and are on the dry side, but they do have a sheer texture. The same can be said for the **Flawless Finish Loose Powder** *($22.50)*. **Bronzing Powder** *($18.50)* comes in two shades: Golden Bronze, which is too shiny, and Pale Copper, which is too orange for anyone's skin tone.

☹ **$$$ <u>BLUSH:</u>** **Luxury Cheek Color** *($20)* has some beautiful colors, but many of them are shiny, so look closely before you add sparkle to your face.

☹ **$$$ <u>EYESHADOW:</u>** Arden is not known for great matte eyeshadows. In fact, the line offers absurdly few. The shadows are packaged as **Singles** *($13.50)*, and **Duos** *($20)*. **These colors are excellent:** Sand/Smoke, Peach/Mesa, Bare/Fawn, Teak, Coralite, and Rain. The rest are shiny or too blue or green.

☺ **$$$ <u>EYE AND BROW SHAPER:</u>** Arden has a large array of both eye and lip pencil colors. **Slender Liners Eye Pencils** *($12.50)* are standard pencils that go on smooth and soft, with very little slip or greasy feel. **Dual Perfection Brow Shaper and Eye Liner** *($14)* is a standard pencil with a slightly drier texture than most ; it comes in five very good colors. **Smoky Eyes Powder Pencil** *($14.50)* is not all that powdery, in fact, it goes on much like any standard pencil. One end of the pencil has a smudge tip that can help soften the line. **Great Color Brow Makeup** *($13.50)* comes in five colors. Using powder instead of pencil is the way to go, and these are similar to many other brow powders.

☺ **$$$ <u>LIPSTICK AND LIP PENCIL:</u>** Both types of lipstick are easily accessible for testing and are divided into extremely helpful color groupings of Plum, Pink, Coral, and Red. **Luxury Moisturizing Lipstick** *($14.50)* goes on sheer and fairly glossy and bleeds easily. **Lip Spa** *($14.50)* is not all that different from the Luxury Moisturizing Lipsticks. It is very greasy, without much staying power, although for a glossy lipstick it's fine. **Slender Liners Lip Liner** *($12.50)* comes in a very attractive array of colors. It is just an ordinary pencil, but it goes on soft without being greasy or dry. **Lip Fix Creme** *($17.50)* is supposed to prevent lipstick from feathering. It works well for most but not all lipsticks, but I don't care for the squeeze-tube applicator. It goes on like a moisturizer and must dry before you put on your lipstick. It is less than convenient for touch-ups during the day. I prefer anti-feathering products that come in lipstick form with no waiting between applications. The ones by Coty are some of the best and least expensive.

☺ **$$$ <u>MASCARA:</u>** When it comes to mascara, Arden has its act together: these mascaras are very good. **Twice as Thick Two Brush Mascara** *($15)*, **Two Brush Mascara Regular** *($15)*, **Really Great Mascara** *($13)*, and **Defining Mascara** *($15)* are all excellent mascaras, and the Really Great Mascara *is indeed* really great. The only problem with the Two Brush Mascara is the two brushes. The idea sounds good—one brush for applying the mascara, the other for lengthening and separating— but I didn't notice a real difference between the two. I did notice, however, that this mascara dried up faster, and it's no wonder: two brushes pumping air into the tube would make any mascara dry faster than usual.

Erno Laszlo

Erno Laszlo's following is beyond me. I made a bet years ago, when the products first came out at upper-end department stores, that this line wouldn't last. I believed women would never pay $14 (now $23) for a bar of soap or use a foundation that looks powdery and flaky. I was wrong. It is still around, and it still has a following.

According to the company's brochure, "Erno Laszlo has been the authority in advanced skincare for over 50 years. No one blended the art of cosmetology with the science of dermatology before Dr. Laszlo's time." Great copy, except that Erno Laszlo was never licensed to practice medicine in this country, and some say he was never a medical doctor in Eastern Europe, where he was from, although the brochure makes it sound as if he was a dermatologist. In his time, Dr. Laszlo's claim to fame was prescribing skin care regimes for wealthy women who could afford to visit his clinic and spa. What he was truly best known for was his belief in using old-fashioned bar soap (he had women with dry skin cover their face in oil before using soap), then splashing the face 30 times with a basin full of the soapy rinse water, then splashing the face 30 times with scalding hot water. When that was done, his patients would finish by soaking their skin with apple cider vinegar. Dr. Laszlo claimed that nothing cleaned better than hot water and soap, but because soap's alkaline content destroyed the skin's pH level, apple cider vinegar was needed to restore it.

(I should mention that I totally disagree with this skin care regime, although I have to admit I admire its originality and concept. Hot water is too damaging to the skin, irritating it and causing capillaries to surface as small spider veins. I also feel that bar soap is too drying and irritating for the skin. We just aren't that dirty; this intense twice-a-day cleansing can cause more problems than it helps. The notion of restoring the skin's pH level after soap has stripped it off is a good idea, but if you clean the face gently, without destroying the pH balance in the first place, you won't need to restore it.)

After Erno Laszlo's death in the late '70s, Colgate-Palmolive bought the rights to use the doctor's name and develop the line in any way they chose. Are the current products in alignment with Laszlo's original skin care theories? For the most part, the skin care routines still include the bar soap and splashing first with soapy hot water and then with clean hot water. The rest of the routine is only loosely based on the good doctor's concepts. The toners are all alcohol-based, just like many other toners on the market. The line includes a few token makeup products, mostly foundations; they are overpriced and nothing special. You won't find any eyeshadows, lipsticks, pencils, or mascara worth checking out.

Erno Laszlo Skin Care

☹ **Sea Mud Soap for Normal, Slightly Oily, and Oily Skin** *($23 for 6 ounces)* contains standard soap ingredients of tallow and sodium cocoate, with a little sea mud thrown in. It's still soap, and the mud makes it more drying and leaves a slight film on the skin. Also, tallow can cause breakouts.

☹ **Special Skin Soap for Oily and Extremely Oily Skin** *($22 for 6 ounces)* contains standard soap ingredients of tallow and sodium cocoate, along with the detergent cleanser sodium lauryl sulfate, which is very drying and irritating. This is a fairly drying, average bar soap, and the tallow can cause breakouts.

☹ **Active pHelityl Soap for Dry and Slightly Dry Skin** *($23 for 6 ounces)* is a standard tallow-based bar of soap, with the same ingredients found in all soaps. This one does contain some plant oil, but that won't help the dryness caused by the other ingredients. This is a lot of money for a very ordinary bar of soap.

☺ **$$$ HydrapHel Cleansing Bar for Extremely Dry Skin** *($24 for 6 ounces)* doesn't contain any tallow, but it has all the other detergent cleansing agents that can cause dry skin. This is a standard bar cleanser with a tiny amount of emollients, and it's not the best for dry skin.

☺ **$$$ HydrapHel Cleansing Treatment Liquid Cleanser for Extremely Dry Skin** *($25 for 4.3 ounces)* is mostly Vaseline and thickening agents. This is little more than an expensive cold cream.

☺ **$$$ Active pHelityl Oil, Pre-Cleansing Oil for Dry to Slightly Oily Skin** *($32 for 8 ounces)* is supposed to be used before you use the soaps above, but why buy two products when all you need is one cleanser that doesn't dry out your skin? All this product contains is mineral oil, plant oil, fragrance, and preservatives. This is some of the most expensive mineral oil you're likely to find anywhere.

☺ **$$$ pHelitone Gentle Eye Makeup Remover** *($18 for 3 ounces)* does remove eye makeup, but it contains just a standard detergent cleansing agent and some slip agents.

☹ **Conditioning Preparation** *($29 for 8 ounces)* contains alcohol, water, fragrance, and preservative. This is almost pure alcohol, and very irritating to the skin.

☹ **Heavy Controlling Lotion** *($27 for 8 ounces)* contains mostly alcohol, water, talc, glycerin, thickener, and coloring agents. This won't control anything, and the alcohol makes it too drying and irritating for most skin types.

☺ **$$$ HydrapHel Skin Supplement Freshener for Extremely Dry and Dry Skin** *($29 for 8 ounces)* contains mostly water, slip agents, water-binding agent, soothing agent, film former, fragrance, and preservatives. At least this one doesn't contain any alcohol; it's about time. This would be a good nonirritating toner for most skin types.

☹ **Light Controlling Lotion Toner for Slightly Dry to Oily Skin** *($28 for 8 ounces)* contains mostly water, alcohol, slip agents, and fragrance. The alcohol is too irritating for most skin types.

☹ **Regular Controlling Lotion PM Oil Control for Slightly Dry and Normal Skin** *($30 for 8 ounces)* is an alcohol-based toner that also contains some talc and baking soda. The alcohol is too irritating and drying for most skin types.

☺ **$$$ Active pHelityl Cream PM Moisturizer for Sensitive/Slightly Dry Skin** *($30 for 2 ounces)* contains mostly petrolatum, safflower oil, thickeners, fragrance, more thickeners, and preservatives. This is a standard, emollient petrolatum-based moisturizer. You're paying a lot of money for Vaseline.

☺ **$$$ Daily Moisture Protection Lotion SPF 15 AM Moisturizer for All Skin Types** *($45 for 2.5 ounces)* is a good emollient moisturizer/sunscreen that contains mostly water; thickener; slip agent; silicone oil; more thickeners; mineral oil; more silicone oil; water-binding agents; more thickeners; plant oil; plant extracts; vitamins A, E, and C; more thickeners; and preservatives. Nothing about this sunscreen makes it worth the price tag. The vitamins don't contribute anything because they are so far down on the ingredient list.

☺ **$$$ Antioxidant Moisture Complex Cream for Extra Dry to Normal Skin** *($65 for 2 ounces)* contains mostly water; thickener; plant oil; glycerin; slip agent; silicone oils; more thickeners; vitamins A, C, and E; water-binding agents; more thickeners; and preservatives. This is a good emollient moisturizer for someone with dry skin, but the interesting stuff, including the antioxidants, is at the end of the ingredient list and barely amounts to a dusting.

☺ **$$$ Antioxidant Moisture Complex SPF 15 Oil-Free Moisturizer for All Skin Types** *($55 for 2 ounces)* is similar to the cream above, only it's more of a lotion and has less silicone oil. It would be a good sunscreen, and there are more antioxidants in this one.

☺ **$$$ HydrapHel Emulsion** *($44 for 2 ounces)* contains mostly water, a tiny amount of sunscreen (not enough to protect adequately from the sun), thickeners, plant oil, glycerin, more thickeners, water-binding agents, plant oil, soothing agents, vitamins C and E (antioxidants), more thickeners, silicone oil, mineral oil, preservatives, and fragrance. The antioxidants are too far down on the ingredient list to be significant. Other than that, this is a good emollient moisturizer with a small amount of sunscreen.

☺ **$$$ HydrapHel Complex PM Moisturizer for Extremely Dry and Dry Skin** *($54 for 2 ounces)* contains mostly water; mineral oil; waxes; plant oils; vitamins A, C, and E; and preservatives. This is a good standard emollient moisturizer, and the vitamins can be considered antioxidants.

☺ **$$$ pHelityl Cream** *($54 for 2 ounces)* contains mostly water, thickeners, silicone oil, more thickeners, mineral oil, more thickeners, petrolatum, and preservatives. This is a fairly standard emollient moisturizer for normal to dry skin. Can you believe they're charging that much for mineral oil and petrolatum?

☺ **$$$ pHelityl Lotion AM Moisturizer for Slightly Dry to Slightly Oily Skin** *($44 for 3 ounces)* contains mostly water, thickeners, mineral oil, vegetable oil, more thickeners, and preservatives. It's good, lightweight, and emollient for someone with dry skin, but overpriced for a very ordinary mineral oil–based moisturizer. Plus, no one with even slightly oily skin is going to be happy with this much oil in a product of any kind.

☺ **$$$ Total Skin Revitalizer** *($52 for 1 ounce)* is a lightweight emollient moisturizer that contains water, slip agent, silicone oil, plant oil, glycerin, water-binding ingredients, soothing agent, thickeners, fragrance, and preservatives. It won't revitalize the skin, but it will keep it moist, just like any other moisturizer.

☹ **$$$ AHA Revitalizing Complex** *($95 for 1.5 ounces)* contains mostly water, silicone oil, thickeners, slip agent, AHAs, BHAs, water-binding agents, and preservatives. The salespeople insist that information about the percentage of AHAs in a product is irrelevant and that other companies provide it only as a marketing ploy. That isn't true. All of the existing research suggests a significant relationship between the percentage of AHAs in a product and the product's effectiveness as an exfoliant. Because the sales force has to justify the insane cost, though, they say some pretty inane things to convince you it's worth the money. Several insisted that the Revitalizing Complex is unique because it contains all four of the essential AHA ingredients: lactic acid, salicylic acid, sodium hyaluronate, and retinyl palmitate. Out of those four, only lactic acid is an AHA, and salicylic acid is a BHA. This product contains about 3% to 4% AHAs and BHAs combined. It isn't a bad AHA/BHA product, and would be OK for those who want an AHA product in a lightweight emollient base.

☹ **Beta Complex Acne Treatment** *($65 for 2 ounces)* is another eye-popper. Why would anyone pay this much money for a 1% salicylic acid product that's just like the salicylic acid products you can buy at the drugstore for $5? This one contains water, silicone oils (which will no doubt thrill someone with acne), film former, anti-irritant (that's nice), thickeners, and preservatives.

☺ **$$$ Hydra-Therapy Skin Vitality Treatment** *($64 for six applications)* is a two-part system that is so amazingly overpriced it is almost embarrassing. You mix an ordinary liquid with a simple powder that is mostly salt, apply it to your face, let it set, and then rinse. The liquid contains water, film former, soothing agent, slip agent, and preservatives. The powder is made of magnesium carbonate (powder), sea salt, silica (sand), mineral salt, and calcium (powder). Ordinary ingredients, but an absurdly expensive product.

☺ **$$$ pHelitone Firming Eye Gel** *($30 for 0.5 ounce)* contains mostly water, thickener, soothing agent, a long list of plant extracts, pH balancer, more thickeners, and preservatives. This won't firm anything, but it will feel light and emollient around the eyes if you aren't allergic to the plants.

☺ **$$$ pHelitone Firming Eye Gel Mask for All Skin Types** *($30 for 0.5 ounce)* is almost identical to the gel above, and the same review applies.

☺ **$$$ pHelitone Replenishing Eye Cream for All Skin Types** *($42 for 0.5 ounce)* contains mostly water, thickener, slip agent, petrolatum, plant oils, more thickeners, vitamin E, soothing agents, more thickener, mineral oil, more thickeners, and preservatives. Pricey for a jar of petrolatum-based moisturizer, don't you think?

☺ **$$$ Total Skin Revitalizer for Eyes** *($42 for 0.5 ounce)* contains mostly water; a long list of thickeners; water-binding agent; plant oil; plant extracts; witch hazel; glycerin; vitamins A, E, and C; more thickeners; and preservatives. This is a good emollient moisturizer for the eyes (there isn't enough witch hazel to be much of an irritant), but there aren't enough vitamins to count for much.

☺ **$$$ Total Skin Revitalizer for Night** *($60 for 1 ounce)* contains water, water-binding agents, vitamins A and E, herb extracts, thickener, more water-binding agent, plant oil, a long list of thickeners, and preservatives. This is a good lightweight emollient moisturizer with antioxidants for the face, but the price tag may be painful.

☺ **$$$ Sea Mud Mask** *($30 for 4 ounces)* is basically a standard clay mask (kaolin is second on the ingredient list) with a smaller amount of clay from the sea as well as other standard thickeners and slip agents. Is sea mud good for the skin? Not any better than ordinary mud, which itself is of questionable benefit.

Erno Laszlo Makeup

☹ **FOUNDATION: Regular Normalizer Shake-It** *($30)* is mostly water, fluid oil, and talc. This is a drying foundation that goes on choppy and thin. **These colors are very good:** Honey, Neutral, Light Beige, and Suntan. **These colors are too peach or pink:** Beige, Porcelain, and Soft Beige.

☹ **Heavy Normalizer Shake-It** *($29)* contains mostly water, alcohol, talc, more alcohol, glycerin, and coloring agents. The alcohol makes this product too irritating for most skin types.

☺ **$$$ pHelitone Fluid** *($35)* is a light, creamy liquid foundation that has a good color selection. **These colors are very good:** Soft Beige (may turn peach), Beige, Light Beige, Suntan, and Golden Beige. **These colors are too peach or pink:** Honey Beige and Porcelain.

☺ **$$$ Oil-Free Normalizing Base** *($30)* won't normalize anything, although it is an OK lightweight matte foundation. **These colors are very good:** Golden Beige, Light Beige, Suntan, and Neutral (may turn peach). **These colors are too peach or pink:** Soft Beige, Beige, Honey Beige, and Porcelain.

☺ **$$$ POWDER: pHelitone Concentrating Pressed Powder** *($22)* is a fairly standard talc-based powder with a soft smooth texture.

☹ **BLUSH:** This line has a small array of **Blushing Powders** *($19)*, all too shiny. **pHelitone Emollient Duo Phase Concealer** *($28)* is half blush and half concealer. The concealer comes in only one color, and it is just OK. The blush half has three color options and is also OK, but the color selection is so small and the concealer so poor that this is one of the stranger products on the market.

Estee Lauder

What sets the venerable Estee Lauder company apart from its competition is that it owns most of the cosmetics lines it competes with. Lauder's formidable reach is exemplified by the impressive status of Clinique, Origins, and Prescriptives, all part of the Lauder family, and by its distribution arrangements with smaller but growing prestige lines such as M.A.C. and Bobbi Brown. Of course, Estee Lauder is still the grande dame of makeup lines, with a loyal following and impressive public relations. Ask any of the salespeople who work for this seasoned cosmetics company, and they will tell you the products sell themselves. A few years ago, Night Repair and Eyezone were jumping off the shelves; then Lauder's AHA product, Fruition, caught fire; and now the hot seller is Day Wear, the line's antioxidant. This is a company with dedication to selling and to training its sales staff. The counter displays are not accessible without the help of a salesperson, so the sales pressure is fairly intense. Even more intense is the almost overwhelming number of age-control, anti-wrinkle, micro-targeted, night-repair, quick-life, nourishing, and free radical–fighting products. It seems as if every wrinkle on your face has a product dedicated to it. Now, here's the question: If just one or two of their products could live up to their claims to get rid of wrinkles, why would you need an additional 50 products that claim to do the same thing? The Lauder lineup boasts some wonderful moisturizers, but also absurd prices for pretty standard products that can't live up to their more glorious claims.

Estee Lauder offers an immense array of Compact Disc eyeshadows in supposedly matte shades, but if you look closely, several are slightly shiny. (Several salespeople argued with me when I asked if Lauder was going to come out with more matte shades. They insisted the eyeshadows were not shiny; it was just a way to enhance the color. Shine by any other name is still shine, and tends to make skin look wrinkly.) The foundations are excellent, with a wonderful selection of shades for women of color. I particularly like Demi-Matte, Fresh Air, and Lucidity, but be careful when choosing colors; many of the foundations in this collection are pink and orange. Most of the blushes are lovely, and they too include a good selection for women with darker skin tones. All of the colors are divided into Warm and Cool, which is very helpful.

Estee Lauder Skin Care

☺ **$$$ Verite LightLotion Cleanser** *($22.50 for 6.7 ounces)* contains mostly water, thickener, water-binding agents, plant oils, silicone oil, more water-binding agents, plant extracts, more water-binding agent, and preservatives. This is an OK wipe-off cleanser that can leave a slightly greasy film.

☺ **$$$ Verite SoftFoam Cleanser** *($22.50 for 4.2 ounces)* contains mostly glycerin, petrolatum (Vaseline), detergent cleansing agents (including sodium C14-16 olefin sulfonate, which is considered quite drying), water, plant extracts, water-binding agents, a water softener, and preservatives. This is the only product in the entire line with a fairly irritating ingredient that is totally inappropriate for someone with sensitive skin. Also, the petrolatum can leave a greasy film on the skin. The water softener is a nice idea, but the problem ingredients don't give it a chance.

☹ **Splash Away** *($17.50 for 3.4 ounces)* is a fairly drying detergent-based cleanser. Keep it away from your eyes, because it can sting if you get even a little inside.

☺ **$$$ Instant Action Rinse-Off Cleanser** *($16.50 for 6 ounces)* is a plant oil–based cleanser and does not rinse off easily without the use of a washcloth. Its cleansing agent is quite mild, so this can be good for dry skin.

☹ **Facewash Self-Foaming System** *($16.50 for 6 ounces)* is a fairly drying water-soluble cleanser. TEA-lauryl sulfate, the second item on the ingredient list, can be a skin irritant.

☺ **$$$ Rich Results Hydrating Cleanser** *($18.50 for 4 ounces)* contains a small amount of a gentle cleansing agent, but it also contains wax and other thickeners that make it hard to rinse off without the aid of a washcloth. It can be good for very dry skin.

☹ **Re-nutriv Extremely Delicate Skin Cleanser** *($32.50 for 7 ounces)* contains mostly mineral oil, water, beeswax, petrolatum, plant oil, thickeners, lanolin, and preservatives. Why use this very greasy product when Pond's Cold Cream is essentially the same thing for a fraction of the price?

☺ **$$$ Re-nutriv Moisture Rich Creme Cleanser** *($27.50 for 3.4 ounces)* is a mineral oil–based wipe-off cleanser that can leave a greasy film on the skin.

☺ **$$$ Tender Creme Cleanser** *($25 for 8 ounces)* is a cleanser that needs to be wiped off with a tissue or a washcloth. It tends to leave a slightly greasy film and does not take off makeup all that well. It does have a decent amount of vitamins A and E, which can be good antioxidants, but in a cleanser they are just wiped away and therefore are useless.

☹ **Micro-Moisture Cleansing Bar** *($17.50 for 5 ounces)* is a standard bar cleanser made of tallow and sodium cocoate. It does contain some plant oils, which can help counteract some of the drying effect of this product, but why dry out the skin in the first place? Also, tallow can cause breakouts.

☹ **Micro-Refining Bar Cleanser** *($17.50 for 5 ounces)* is practically identical to the bar above, but with a different color and a few different oils, and the same review applies.

☹ **Solid Milk Cleansing Grains** *($18.50 for 3.5 ounces)* contains mostly corn flour, film former (PVP, a possible irritant), thickeners, chalk, nonfat dry milk, fragrance, detergent cleanser, soothing agent, and preservatives. This thick scrub uses sodium lauryl sulfate as the cleansing agent, and that is very drying for the skin; also, PVP in this amount is a skin irritant. One more warning: corn flour and milk can cause breakouts.

☺ **$$$ Gentle Eye Makeup Remover** *($12 for 3.3 ounces)* is a standard gentle eye-makeup remover. Any gentle water-soluble cleanser should do the same thing without making you wipe and pull at your eyes with an extra product.

☺ **$$$ Gentle Action Skin Polisher** *($18.50 for 4 ounces)* is supposed to be a water-soluble scrub, but it doesn't rinse off well. It contains mostly water, mineral oil, thickeners, detergent cleanser, and preservatives. Although the scrubbing effect is fairly mild, the other ingredients are emollient and rather standard thickeners that can clog pores. This could be good for someone with dry skin.

☺ **$$$ Clear Finish Purifying Toner N/D** *($15 for 6.75 ounces)* contains mostly water, slip agents, plant extracts, water-binding agents, and preservatives. This would be a good nonirritating toner for most skin types. It does contain a little bit of menthol, which can be a skin irritant for some skin types.

☺ **$$$ Clean Finish Purifying Toner N/O** *($15 for 6.75 ounces)* contains mostly water, slip agents, plant extracts, and preservatives. The plant extracts have no impact on oily skin, but this is still a good toner for normal to oily skin. It contains a little bit of menthol, which can be a skin irritant for some skin types.

☹ **Deep Sweep Skin Refiner** *($18.50 for 3.4 ounces)* costs a lot of money for what is basically alcohol and slip agents. It can dry and irritate the skin.

☺ **$$$ Verite Soothing Spray Toner** *($22.50 for 6.7 ounces)* contains mostly water, water-binding agents, plant extracts (including green tea, an anti-irritant), and preservatives. This is a very good nonirritating toner for all skin types.

☺ **$$$ Re-Nutriv Gentle Skin Toner** *($27.50 for 6.5 ounces)* is an alcohol-free toner whose second ingredient is cetrimonium chloride, a cleansing agent and disinfectant. It isn't bad for the skin; it just isn't all that gentle. There probably isn't much in this product, though, which means there is even less of everything else that follows it on the ingredient list.

☺ **$$$ Estoderme Creme** *($25 for 4 ounces)* contains mostly mineral oil, water, lanolin, thickeners, slip agent, water-binding agents, more thickeners, plant oil, more thickeners, and preservatives. This is a very emollient, rich, almost greasy moisturizer for someone with very dry skin.

☺ **$$$ Estoderme Emulsion** *($25 for 4 ounces)* is similar to the moisturizer above, and the same review applies.

☺ **$$$ Verite Moisture Relief Creme** *($50 for 1.75 ounces)* contains mostly water, silicone oil, water-binding agents, thickeners, more water-binding agents, plant extracts (including oat extract, which is considered an anti-irritant), and preservatives. This is an excellent moisturizer for someone with dry skin.

☺ **$$$ Verite Calming Fluid** *($60 for 1.7 ounces)* contains mostly water, silicone oils, glycerin, water-binding agents, plant extracts, more water-binding agents, vitamin

E, thickeners, and preservatives. It probably won't calm anything, but it is a very good moisturizer for someone with normal to dry skin. There isn't enough vitamin E in it to do any good.

☺ **$$$ Fruition Triple Reactivating Complex** *($42.50 for 1 ounce)* is Lauder's AHA product, but it contains less than 2% AHAs. It's an OK lightweight moisturizer, but not a great AHA product. The company recommends wearing it under a regular moisturizer, which is fine, but there are better AHA products on the market that don't require an extra moisturizer.

☺ **$$$ Advanced Night Repair** *($70 for 1.75 ounces)* is a good moisturizer that contains mostly water, water-binding agents, thickeners, anti-irritants, silicone oil, plant oil, more water-binding agents, vitamin A, and preservatives. It also contains a small amount of sunscreen, which doesn't make sense in a product that's meant to be used at night. This product won't repair anything, but it is a good lightweight moisturizer for dry skin.

☺ **$$$ Advanced Suncare No Chemical Sunscreen SPF 15** *($18.50 for 4 ounces)* is one of the better nonchemical sunscreens on the market, although, like all titanium dioxide–based sunscreens, it can feel thick and slightly sticky. It is best for someone with dry skin.

☺ **$$$ Advanced Suncare SunBlock Lotion Spray No Chemical Sunscreen SPF 15** *($19.50 for 4.25 ounces)* is a very good titanium dioxide–based sunscreen in a silicone oil base. This will leave a fairly nongreasy finish, but it can appear somewhat white on the skin.

☺ **$$$ Day Wear Super Anti-Oxidant Complex SPF 15** *($37.50 for 1.7 ounces)* contains mostly water, silicone oils, a very long list of thickeners, vitamins B and E, plant extracts, water-binding agents, more thickeners, and preservatives. The antioxidants are not exactly at the top of the ingredient list, so this product isn't all that super. What is good about this day cream is that it contains an SPF 15 sunscreen that is part nonchemical and part standard sunscreen agents. The combination of titanium dioxide (nonchemical) and a standard sunscreen agent such as benzophenone or methoxycinnamate is one of the better ways to protect against sun damage. In that regard, this product is right on.

☹ **$$$ Creme de la Mer** *($155 for 2 ounces)* is a very costly little cream accompanied by quite a story! Max Huber, a NASA aerospace physicist, created this product, supposedly to take care of burns he received in an accident. He sold and marketed it himself. After his death, his daughter continued selling the cream until recently, when Estee Lauder purchased the rights to manufacture and distribute it. As enticing as this dramatic story is, the reality is that this very basic cream doesn't contain anything particularly extraordinary or unique, unless you want to believe that seaweed extract (sort of like seaweed tea) can in some way heal burns and scars. Even if it could, burns and scars don't have much to do with wrinkling, and that's what this product is now being sold as: a wrinkle cream. According to Susan Brawley, professor of plant biology at the University of Maine, "Seaweed extract isn't a rare, exotic, or expensive ingredient. Seaweed extract is readily available and used in everything from cosmetics to food products and medical applications."

Creme de la Mer contains mostly seaweed extract, mineral oil, petrolatum, glycerin, waxlike thickening agents, plant oils, plant seeds, minerals, vitamins, more thickeners, and preservatives. This rather standard moisturizer contains some good antioxidants, which can help heal skin by keeping air off it, but these ingredients are also found in many other moisturizers that cost a *lot* less. According to the cosmetic chemists I've interviewed, it costs pennies, not hundreds of dollars, to stick some seaweed and vitamins in a cosmetic.

☺ **$$$ Skin Defender Sensitive Skin Protector** (*$45 for 0.9 ounce*) contains mostly water, water-binding agents, silicone oil, slip agents, thickeners, vitamin A, more water-binding agents, soothing agent, more thickeners, and preservatives. This is a very good moisturizer for someone with very dry skin. However, there is no SPF rating on the label and the sunscreen agent is not listed as active on the ingredient list, so there is no way to know how much protection it provides. Do not count on this one for use during the day.

☺ **$$$ Swiss Performing Extract Moisturizer** (*$23.50 for 1.7 ounces*) contains mostly water, plant oils, water-binding agents, slip agents, lanolin, mineral oil, thickeners, more water-binding agents, plant oil, silicone oil, and preservatives. This is a very emollient, very good moisturizer for someone with dry skin.

☺ **$$$ European Performing Cream** (*$37.50 for 3.25 ounces*) contains mostly water, thickeners, lanolin oil, plant oil, more thickeners, water-binding agents, vitamin E, more thickeners, fragrance, and preservatives. Although this is a very good emollient moisturizer for dry skin, the moisturizer above is far superior, with a more interesting arrangement of ingredients.

☺ **$$$ Age Controlling Creme** (*$35 for 1 ounce*) contains mostly water, lanolin, slip agents, plant oils, mineral oil, several thickeners, petrolatum, more thickeners, water-binding agents, soothing agent, vitamins A and E, silicone oil, and preservatives. It's very similar to the European and Swiss moisturizers above, and is also a very good moisturizer for someone with very dry skin, but why this product is for "age control" and the others aren't is anyone's guess. None of these products can affect aging–just dry skin. But dry skin does not cause wrinkles; the sun does. Dryness just makes skin look more wrinkled.

☺ **$$$ Enriched Under-Makeup Creme** *($25 for 4 ounces)* is definitely rich. It contains mostly water, mineral oil, lanolin, several thickeners, slip agent, water-binding agents, silicone oil, vitamin E, and preservatives. This is a very emollient moisturizer for someone with very dry skin.

☹ **Equalizer Oil-Free HydroGel** *($27.50 for 1.7 ounces)* isn't oil-free: it contains silicone oil. It also contains alcohol, which can dry out the skin. It does contain some water-binding agents, but what's the point of including ingredients that are supposed to keep water in the skin when the alcohol is going to dry the water up?

☺ **$$$ Future Perfect Micro-Targeted Skin Gel** *($30 for 1 ounce)* contains mostly water, film former, slip agent, silicone oil, water-binding agents, vitamins A and E, plant extracts, more thickeners, fragrance, and preservatives. This is a good lightweight emollient moisturizer with antioxidants, but the name is better than what's inside. It sounds as if you can place it over a wrinkle, zero in, and, poof, get rid of it. Not possible.

☺ **$$$ Skin Perfecting Lotion Lightweight Moisturizer** *($27.50 for 1.7 ounces)* contains mostly water, silicone oil, several thickeners, vitamins E and A, soothing agents, plant extracts, water-binding agents, and preservatives. It is lightweight but boring. There is no SPF rating on the label and the sunscreen agent is not listed as active on the ingredient list, so there is no way to know how much protection this product provides. Do not count on it for use during the day.

☺ **$$$ Skin Perfecting Creme Firming Nourisher** *($35 for 1.75 ounces)* is a lightweight moisturizer with one of the longest ingredient lists I've ever seen. If you are looking for every state-of-the-art moisturizing ingredient, look here: collagen, vitamins, marine extracts, plant oils, proteins, antioxidants, anti-irritant, and amino acids, all fairly high on the ingredient list. This would take care of dry skin as well as any concerns that you might be missing out on the latest skin care ingredients (except for AHAs).

☺ **$$$ Resilience Elastin Refirming Creme** *($42.50 for 1 ounce)* contains mostly water, plant oil, slip agent, thickeners, glycerin, water-binding agents, vitamin E, plant extracts, silicone oil, fragrance, and preservatives. This is a good, but extremely ordinary, moisturizer for someone with normal to dry skin. It is not one of Lauder's better moisturizers.

☺ **$$$ Resilience Elastin Refirming Lotion** *($42.50 for 1 ounce)* is similar to the product above, only in lotion form, and the same review applies.

☺ **$$$ Re-nutriv Creme** *($45 for 1 ounce)* contains mostly water, lanolin, mineral oil, a long list of thickeners, vitamins A and E, silicone oil, water-binding agents, more mineral oil, more thickeners, and preservatives. This is a very emollient, though ordinary, moisturizer for extremely dry skin. The amount of vitamins in this product isn't enough to even mention.

☺ **$$$ Re-nutriv Creme Lightweight** *($45 for 1 ounce)* is almost identical to the creme above, but more lightweight. The company suggests using this for normal to oily skin, but ingredients like plant oils, lanolin oil, and thick waxes make that recommendation absurd.

☺ **$$$ Re-nutriv Firming Eye Creme** *($42.50 for 1 ounce)* contains mostly water, water-binding agents, slip agent, several thickeners, lanolin oil, plant extract, more water-binding agents, vitamins A and E, mineral oil, more thickeners, and preservatives. This won't firm the eye area, and the fancy water-binding agents (amino acids and collagen) cannot get rid of wrinkles, but this is a very good emollient moisturizer for dry skin.

☺ **$$$ Resilience Eye Creme** *($42.50 for 0.5 ounce)* contains thickeners, silicone oil, film former, water-binding agents, plant extracts, vitamin E, more water-binding agents, more thickeners, and preservatives. This is a good emollient moisturizer, although the acrylate can cause skin sensitivities.

☺ **$$$ Time Zone Eyes Ultra-Hydrating Complex** *($40 for 0.5 ounce)* contains mostly water, aloe, glycerin, slip agent, seaweed, water-binding agents, film former, plant extracts, vitamins A and E, thickeners, and preservatives. This is a lightweight moisturizer for normal to dry skin. Seaweed won't hydrate the skin, but the water-binding agents are nice. There aren't enough vitamins to make a difference.

☺ **$$$ Eyezone Repair Gel** *($35 for 0.5 ounce)* contains mostly water, film former, plant extract, water-binding agents, thickeners, and preservatives. I was told it would last six months because you use so little, but you would have to use none for a half-ounce to last that long. The film former can be a skin irritant, but it can also make the skin look smooth. It won't repair the skin, but it is an OK lightweight moisturizer.

☺ **$$$ Maximum Care Eye Creme, Extra Forte** *($20 for 0.5 ounce)* contains mostly water, water-binding agent, thickeners, plant oil, more water-binding agents, soothing agent, silicone oil, more thickeners, and preservatives. This is a good emollient moisturizer for dry skin. The second item on the ingredient list is collagen, but we all know that collagen in a moisturizer can't add to or shore up the collagen in skin, right?

☺ **$$$ Re-nutriv Intensive Firming Plus** *($95 for 1.7 ounces)* contains mostly water, silicone oils, thickener, slip agent, anti-irritant, film former, fruit extracts, water-binding agent, thickeners, and preservatives. Although AHAs are derived from fruit, there are many fruit extracts that have nothing to do with AHAs, and many acids that sound like AHAs but are not. It's all too vague, making it impossible to determine what you are really buying. This product is a good moisturizer, but it won't firm anything and isn't a very good AHA product.

☺ **$$$ Re-nutriv Liquid** *($55 for 1.75 ounces)* contains mostly water, mineral oil, lanolin, plant oil, thickeners, silicone oil, vitamin A, more thickeners, water-binding agents, more thickeners, and preservatives. This is an extremely emollient, though standard, moisturizer for someone with extremely dry skin.

☺ **$$$ Re-nutriv Replenishing Creme** *($60 for 1 ounce, $78 for 1.7 ounces)* is similar to the moisturizer above, only not as greasy, and the same review applies.

☹ **Equalizer Oil-Free Gel** *($27.50 for 1.75 ounces)* is supposed to "monitor" and "disperse" excess oil concentration, but it simply can't do that. The ingredients are mostly water, alcohol, slip agent, water-binding agents, almond meal, vitamin A, and preservatives. The alcohol can irritate the skin, making it oilier.

☺ **$$$ Non-Oily Skin Supplement** *($37.50 for 3.25 ounces)* isn't exactly oil-free, but maybe that's not what the company means by "non-oily." It contains mostly water, slip agents, water-binding agents, plant oil, aloe, plant extracts, vitamin E, a long list of thickeners, and preservatives. It would be a good lightweight moisturizer for someone with normal to dry skin. It contains many ingredients that would be a problem for someone with oily skin, though.

☹ **Counter-Blemish Lotion** *($12 for 0.45 ounce)* contains alcohol, thickener, and salicylic acid. Another alcohol and salicylic acid product for acne: how trite. This won't stop a blemish or cure one, and it can be irritating to most skin types.

☹ **Almond Clay Mask** *($18.50 for 4 ounces)* contains mostly water, thickeners, clay, more thickeners, almond meal, more clay, a small amount of salicylic acid, and preservatives. This is a fairly standard clay mask with the addition of a gritty substance (almonds) and a peeling agent (salicylic acid). It's not bad, just potentially irritating for some skin types.

☺ **$$$ Quick Lift 4-Minute Mask N/D** *($18.50 for 3.4 ounces)* is a standard clay mask that also contains tiny amounts of water-binding agents and anti-irritants. It won't lift your skin anywhere, but it is a decent, though basic, clay mask.

☺ **$$$ Quick Lift 4-Minute Mask N/O** *($18.50 for 3.4 ounces)* is similar to the mask above, and the same review applies, although this mask has a few ingredients that make it better for oily skin than dry skin.

☺ **$$$ Stress Relief Eye Mask** *($27.50 for ten 0.4-ounce packets)* contains mostly water, glycerin, slip agents, water-binding agents, plant extracts, and preservatives. This is a good lightweight moisturizing mask. It won't change the amount of stress in your life, but if you lie down a while (with or without this mask), chances are you will feel less stressed.

☺ **$$$ Triple Creme Hydrating Mask** *($27.50 for 2.5 ounces)* contains mostly water, thickeners, plant oil, slip agent, more thickeners, standard water-binding agent, more thickeners, plant oil, more water-binding agents, more thickeners, and preservatives. These are good moisturizing ingredients, so they would feel good if left on the face for a while.

☺ **Soothing Creme Facial** *($18.50 for 3.4 ounces)* is supposed to be a deep-cleansing mask. It isn't all that deep-cleansing, but it is a fairly emollient clay mask that can be good for someone with normal to dry skin. It contains mostly water, slip agent, thickeners, water-binding agents, clay, plant oil, more thickeners, anti-irritant, cleansing agents, and preservatives.

Estee Lauder Makeup

☺ **$$$ FOUNDATION: Impeccable SPF 20** *($27.50)* has a great name; what a pity this foundation can't live up to it. This greasy foundation in a compact form blends evenly, with medium to heavy coverage. Unfortunately, it can slip into lines on the face, and the third ingredient is aluminum starch, which can cause breakouts. The color selection is wonderful, and the SPF 20 rating is impressive. This foundation would only be appropriate for someone with dry skin. **These colors are wonderful:** Ecru, Seashell, Linen, Vanilla, True Beige, Golden Honey, Sun Kiss, and Rich Cocoa. **These colors are either too peach, orange, or ash:** Nude Beige, Almond, and Fresh Ginger.

☺ **Maximum Coverage with Non-Chemical SPF 10** *($25)* goes on creamy and smooth and then seems to stick to the skin, which can feel uncomfortable. It doesn't provide as much coverage as the name implies—this isn't Dermablend, although it does cover well. There is a limited assortment of colors to choose from, but the available colors are great.

☺ **Demi-Matte** *($20)* is a superior oil-free foundation. **These colors are very good:** Fresh Beige (may turn slightly rose on some skin tones), Champagne Beige, Wheat Beige (may be too yellow), Rose Beige (may turn slightly rose), Natural Ivory, Golden Beige (may be too yellow), Ivory Beige, and Sun Bronze. **The only color to avoid is** Rose Ivory; the name speaks for itself.

☺ **Country Mist** *($18.50)* is recommended for normal to dry skin, according to the company. It would be an excellent medium-coverage foundation for dry skin, though I don't recommend it for normal skin types. **These colors are wonderful:** Suntan Beige, Golden Beige, Clear Beige, Warm Beige, Misty Tan (may turn slightly rose), Tender Beige, Beige Light, and Vanilla Beige.

☹ **Polished Performance** *($25)* gives sheer, natural coverage and is an excellent liquid foundation for normal and dry skin types, although the colors all have a rose tint, which would be a problem for most skin tones. **The only two colors to consider:** Butternut Bronze and Tawny Almond.

☺ **Lucidity Light Diffusing Makeup** *($27.50)* can't diffuse light, although it is a good liquid foundation for someone with normal to dry skin. **These colors are very good:** Gold Alabaster (excellent pale shade), Ivory Beige (slightly peach), Rich Ginger (may turn peach), Sun Bronze (may turn rose), Gold Caramel, Gold Sand, Bronze Mocha, Medium Beige (slightly rose), Sun Beige, Coffee, and Sable. **These colors are too peach or pink for most skin tones:** Neutral Beige, Gold Ivory, Cool Beige, Outdoor Beige, and Vanilla Beige.

☺ **Just Perfect Light Diffusing Makeup** *($35)* is also supposed to be light-diffusing, but it doesn't change the face or erase wrinkles. It does provide good coverage and is quite creamy for someone with normal to dry skin. **These colors are very good:** Golden Alabaster (may be too yellow for some skin tones), Golden Ivory (may be too peach), Natural Beige, Rich Ginger, Sun Bronze, Hazelnut, Cappuccino, Bronze Mocha, and Golden Caramel. **These colors are too peach or pink for most skin tones:** Sienna, Pale Ivory, Cool Beige, and Vanilla Beige.

☺ **More Than Powder** *($21)* is a pressed powder that the company recommends for use as a foundation. It has a nice consistency but works best on normal skin. **These** colors are excellent: Ivory, Barely Beige, Warm Honey, Tawny Beige, Tan Bisque, Cinnamon Sun, Toasted Walnut, and Honey Toast. **These colors are too peach or pink for most skin tones:** Sand Beige, Dawn Beige, Radiant Beige, and Blush Beige.

☺ **Enlighten Skin-Enhancing Makeup with SPF 10** *($27.50)* is a superior foundation with a nonchemical sunscreen. What a shame it's rated only SPF 10; that isn't bad, but I prefer SPF 15. It is supposed to be oil-free, but the second and fourth items on the ingredient list are silicone oils, making the claim completely erroneous. However, the application is smooth and delicate, leaving a beautiful soft matte finish. It is best for someone with normal to combination skin. **These colors are excellent:** Day Break, Natural Linen, Sun Swept, and Soft Chestnut. **These colors are too peach, pink, or copper for most skin tones:** Vanilla Beige, Neutral Beige, Outdoor Beige, and Rich Ginger.

☺ **Compact Finish Double Performance Makeup** *($25)* is a standard powder foundation with a superior soft, silky finish; it works well alone or with foundation. There are a number of impressive shades to choose from, and all are just beautiful. The only colors to consider carefully are Ivory Beige (may be too pink) and Ivory (can be too peach).

☺ **Re-nutriv Souffle Makeup** *($32.50)* is a very emollient, extremely creamy foundation that provides medium to heavy coverage. It is only appropriate for someone with very dry skin, and even then could be somewhat greasy. Still, all five colors, though limited, are very good.

☹ **Color Primer** *($15)* comes in three shades that are supposed to do the same thing everyone else's color primer or corrector does: change the skin tone. It doesn't work well at all, and adds an unnecessary layer to the makeup.

☹ **Shadow Stay Eyelid Foundation** *($12.50)* absolutely didn't work: my eyeshadows creased within a few hours.

☺ **CONCEALER: Smoothing Creme Concealer with SPF 8** *($16)* provides good coverage and has a great soft texture and some terrific colors, but—and this is always the clincher when it comes to concealers—it tends to crease into the lines around the eyes, which accentuates them and looks sloppy. **These colors are very impressive:** Smooth Light, Smooth Cocoa, Smooth Deep, and Caramel. **These are the colors to avoid:** Smooth Medium and Smooth Ivory. **Automatic Concealer** *($12.50)* comes in six very impressive shades: Light, Medium, Medium Dark, Warm Medium, Warm Dark, and Dark. The Light is fairly pink, but the other shades are great. The consistency is on the dry side, but it stays on well. Chances are it won't crease, but test it first.

☺ **POWDER:** **Demi-Matte Oil-Free Loose Powder** *($17.50)* and **Demi-Matte Oil-Free Pressed Powder** *($16.50)*, for oily skin, are both standard talc-based powders. **Lucidity Translucent Loose Powder** *($23)* and **Lucidity Translucent Pressed Powder** *($23)*, for all skin types, are also standard talc-based powders. All of these have great color selections. Demi-Matte has a great texture, but most of the colors go on a bit too chalky. Lucidity is supposed to change the way light focuses on your face. It feels good, but it doesn't look any different than dozens of other powders I've tested. **Moisture Balanced Translucent Face Powder Pressed** *($18.50)* and **Moisture Balanced Translucent Face Powder Loose** *($16.50)* are just standard talc-based powders, but they do have a good color selection.

☺ **BLUSH:** **Blushing Natural Cheek Color** *($20)* is a standard cream blush in a small array of rather pretty colors that are somewhat shiny. I dislike cream blush because it can be tricky to blend and only works for flawless skin. Shiny and creamy are not something I can recommend.

☺ **Just Blush! Eye and Cheek Powder** *($25)* has a wonderful selection of soft colors that are meant to work on both the cheek and the eye. It comes with a retractable brush that's a nice size.

☺ **EYESHADOW:** **Compact Disc Eyeshadows** *($10)* come in 80 single colors that are almost all matte but only almost; most have some amount of shine, so look carefully. This amount of shine isn't the worst for an eyeshadow but it isn't the best either. The shadows are numbered 1 through 8 and grouped in the following categories: Neutrals, Blues, Teals, Greens, Naturals, Oranges, Browns, Corals, Pinks, and Violets. Concentrate your attention on the Neutrals, Naturals, Browns, Corals, and Pinks. **These are the only true matte shades:** Brown 1, Brown 2, Brown 5, Taupe 3, Coral 3, Natural 7, Natural 8, Neutral 1.1, and Neutral 2.2.

☹ **Eye-Coloring Liquid-to-Powder Eyeshadow** *($15)* comes in 12 extremely shiny shades. These are supposed to be waterproof, but you don't want this much shine around your eyes, dry or wet.

☺ **Singles** *($15)* and **Duos** *($20)* are not from the Compact Disc collection. **These colors are lovely:** Arizona, Sand, Cactus, Colorado, Foliage, Sierra, Clouds, Twilight, Casa Rosa, Granite, Moors, Island, and Aurora. **These colors are too shiny, come in strange combinations, or are a difficult shape to use:** Gala, Trapeze, Rivers, Rainflowers, Oceanic, Bronzewood, and Peach Cream.

☺ **$$$ EYE AND BROW SHAPER:** **Automatic Pencil Liner for Eyes** *($22.50; $8 for a refill)* is a standard twist-up pencil in a very nonstandard, elegant container. It is among the most expensive pencils on the market, but the refills are a bargain and then you have the sexy container, if you're into that kind of thing. Some of the colors are too shiny and fairly greasy, so be careful. **Eye Defining Pencil** *($13)* is a standard pencil in a nice array of colors. **Liquid Liner** *($13.50)* is a fairly standard liner that draws a wet, serious line across the lid. **Two-in-One Eyeliner/Brow Color** *($25)* goes on wet or dry. It comes in one compact with two colors: Brown and Black. That's rather limited, especially when you consider that any matte eyeshadow could do the same thing. **Automatic Pencil for Brows** *($22.50; $8 for a refill)* is identical to the Automatic Pencil Liner for Eyes. It comes in a pretty container, but penciling is not the best option for a natural-looking brow. **Brow Gel** *($12)* is a clear, hairspray-like product that holds the brow in place. It works fairly well, but no better than hairspray on a toothbrush.

☺ <u>LIPSTICK AND LIP PENCIL:</u> **Perfect Lipstick** *($15)*, **All Day Lipstick** *($12.50)*, and **Polish Performance** are wonderful: very creamy and rich. **True Lipstick** *($16)* is supposed to have great staying power without bleeding. Well, it doesn't stay any better, nor is it more "true," than a hundred other lipsticks at the drugstore and cosmetics counters. This one bleeds right into the lines around the mouth—rather quickly, too, I might add. **Double Color Lipstick** *($15)* is rather greasy and has poor staying power. **Double Matte Lipstick** *($15)* isn't all that matte, but it is quite creamy, which is good, unless you want a truly matte lip color. Both of these lipsticks tend to feather. **Lip Defining Pencil** *($13)* is a standard lip pencil that comes in a great assembly of colors. **Automatic Pencil Liner for Lips** *($22.50; $8 for refills)* is a very standard twist-up pencil in a very elegant container; the refills are great and inexpensive, so in the long run it probably balances out.

☺ <u>MASCARA:</u> **More Than Mascara** *($15)* isn't more than mascara, it's just mascara. Nevertheless, it goes on easily while building nice thick lashes without clumping. **Luscious Creme Mascara** *($12.50)* is an excellent mascara that goes on easily and builds long beautiful lashes without clumping or smearing.

☹ **Lash Primer** *($12.50)* is supposed to help make lashes even longer if you apply it before the mascara. It is unnecessary; Lauder's mascara goes on just fine without help.

☺ <u>BRUSHES:</u> Lauder has a small but nice array of brushes. They are not the best I've ever seen, given those at the M.A.C., Trish McEvoy, and Bobbi Brown counters, or at The Body Shop, or the Joan Simmons brushes at Sears and J.C. Penney, but they are worth checking out. **Blush** *($18.50)* is a nice soft brush that would work well for blush. **Square Shading for Eye** *($15)* is a good all-over eyeshadow brush. **Angled**

Eyeshadow and Brow *($12.50)* is a standard soft angled brush that can work for some eyeshadow blending and filling in a brow. **Eyeshadow Shading and Contouring** *($12.50)* is a good basic eyeshadow brush. Lauder also offers an outrageously priced set of four **Professional Brushes** *($75)*. These are good brushes, but there are better ones on the market for a lot less money.

☺ Face *($18.50)* is recommended for blending foundation, but that is better done with a sponge. It has a flat top, which makes it difficult to create a soft edge. **Eye Liner** *($12.50)* is a stiff square brush that is too firm for eyeshadow and too large to control a line along the lashes. **Concealing** *($12.50)* works fine, but your finger works much better. **Tapered Blending For Eye** *($15)* is too long and floppy to provide much control for placement of eyeshadows.

Eucerin (Skin Care Only)

☺ **Cleansing Bar** *($4 for 3 ounces)* is a detergent-based bar cleanser. It is milder than most, and can be good for some skin types, but it is best used from the neck down and not on the face.

☺ **Original Moisturizing Creme** *($4.19 for 2 ounces)* is an extremely rich, rather heavy moisturizer that contains mostly water, petrolatum, mineral oil, thickeners, and preservatives. It would be best for someone with extremely dry, parched skin.

☺ **Original Moisturizing Lotion** *($10 for 8 ounces)* contains mostly water, mineral oil, isopropyl myristate (which can cause blackheads), several thickeners, and preservatives. This product is basically just thickeners and mineral oil, which makes it a mediocre but OK moisturizer for very dry skin.

☺ **Daily Facial Lotion SPF 20** *($8 for 4 ounces)* is a good emollient daytime moisturizer/sunscreen that contains mostly water, thickeners, glycerin, petrolatum, more thickeners, water-binding agents, silicone oil, and preservatives.

☺ **Plus Alpha Hydroxy Moisturizing Lotion** *($7.49 for 6 ounces)* is a mineral oil–based moisturizer with several thickeners, anti-irritant, and preservatives. It contains about 5% AHAs. This AHA moisturizer is OK for someone with dry, sensitive skin.

☺ **Plus Alpha Hydroxy Moisturizing Creme** *($7.49 for 6 ounces)* is similar to the lotion above, but with 2.5% AHAs. That makes it a poor exfoliant but a good moisturizer.

Expressions Brushes (Available Only in Canada)

Most Canadian drugstores carry these reasonably priced, professional-size brushes *($2.50 to $5)*. All of the brushes are very good and are a great way to affordably invest in the basics necessary for a good makeup application. **The best brushes are:** the Retractable Lip Brush, the Eye Lining Brush, the Fluff Brush, the Blusher Brush, and the Super Powder. **The only brushes to avoid are:** the **Lip Liner/Eye Liner Brush**, which is really too thin to line lips and too thick to line eyes; the **Fantail Brush**, which is pretty but not very practical; and the **Eye Shading Brush**, which is a little too flimsy to be very useful or long-lasting.

Fashion Fair

There are three major cosmetics lines dedicated just to women of color: Fashion Fair, Flori Roberts, and Iman. Of the three, Iman leads the pack in color choices and product quality, while Fashion Fair comes in a not-so-distant second. (Flori Roberts just can't compete with the selection of colors and product types the other two companies offer.) With its large selection of lipsticks, foundations, blushes, and concealing creams, the Fashion Fair line, though not perfect, offers many options. I must mention one major drawback, however: almost all of Fashion Fair's eyeshadows are intensely shiny and the lipsticks fairly greasy. I don't recommend shiny eyeshadow for women of color any more than I do for women with lighter skin tones. Shiny eyeshadows make eyelids look wrinkly, and they are always inappropriate in daytime. However, Fashion Fair has a line of fragrance-free products that is worth looking at, as well as oil-free foundations, blushes, concealer creams, and lipsticks. The display units are not user-friendly: it is necessary to have a salesperson get testers for you and the products are poorly organized (there are no color groupings to help you make selections).

One area of utter disappointment is the skin care products. They are mostly greasy cold cream–like cleansers, water-soluble cleansers with strongly irritating cleansing agents, alcohol-based toners, and greasy moisturizers. Even more glaring a defect is the lack of sunscreens or AHA products. Surely by now Fashion Fair knows that darker skin tones still run the risk of sun damage and all the problems that come with unprotected skin, and AHAs can help reduce the ashy skin discoloration that darker skin tones often experience.

Fashion Fair Skin Care

☹ **Deep Cleansing Lotion Balanced for All Skin Types** (*$14.25 for 8 ounces*) is a fairly greasy cleanser that needs to be wiped off. It contains several ingredients that could cause breakouts, including lanolin and isopropyl palmitate. Calling this suitable for all skin types is absurd.

☺ **Cleansing Creme with Aloe Vera** *($13.25 for 4 ounces)* is a standard mineral oil–based wipe-off cleanser that can leave a greasy film.

☹ **Facial Shampoo Original Formula for Normal or Oily Skin** *($10 for 2.1 ounces)* is a standard detergent-based water-soluble cleanser that uses sodium lauryl sulfate as the main cleansing agent. It can be very drying and irritating for most skin types, and I do not recommend it.

☺ **Gentle Facial Shampoo Mild for Dry, Sensitive Skin** *($10 for 2.1 ounces)* is definitely gentler than the shampoo above and could be very good for someone with normal to oily skin. Its fragrance and foaming agents make it a poor choice for someone with sensitive skin, though.

☺ **Eye Makeup Remover** *($8.50 for 2 ounces)* is a silicone oil–based wipe-off cleanser that can be fairly gentle. It should never be necessary to wipe off makeup, however.

☺ **Gentle Facial Polisher for All Skin Types** *($13.25 for 2.1 ounces)* is a detergent cleanser that also contains synthetic scrub particles. It would be a fairly gentle exfoliant for most skin types. It does contain a tiny amount of menthol, but this small an amount is probably not a problem.

☹ **Skin Freshener I Normal to Oily Skin** *($11.50 for 6 ounces)* contains mostly alcohol, which is very drying, not to mention irritating.

☹ **Skin Freshener II Dry or Sensitive Skin** *($11.50 for 6 ounces)* has basically the same ingredients as Skin Freshener I and can be just as drying.

☹ **Deep Pore Astringent Regular for Normal to Oily Skin** *($13.25 for 8 ounces)* is similar to the Skin Fresheners above; the alcohol is just too irritating for almost all skin types.

☹ **Toning Lotion Mild for Dry Sensitive Skin** *($13.25 for 8 ounces)* is an alcohol-based toner; alcohol isn't good for even the hardiest skin type, much less dry, sensitive skin.

☺ **$$$ All Purpose Protein Creme** *($29.50 for 1.9 ounces)* contains mostly water, several thickeners, water-binding agent (protein), silicone oil, and preservatives. It would be a good but ordinary moisturizer for someone with dry skin. The protein is OK for dry skin, but it isn't anything that warrants the increased price.

☺ **$$$ Enriched Night Creme** *($23.50 for 1.9 ounces)* contains, as the second item on the ingredient list, isopropyl myristate, which can cause breakouts. It also contains water, slip agent, petrolatum, thickeners, lanolin oil, more thickeners, and preservatives. All the specialty ingredients in this product are at the end of the ingredient list, meaning they are barely present. This is a good emollient moisturizer, but it's ordinary and can be a problem for some skin types.

☺ **Moisturizing Creme with Aloe Vera for Dry Skin** *($18.50 for 4 ounces)* is a very emollient moisturizer that would work well on very dry skin, but not because of the aloe. It contains mostly water, thickeners, mineral oil, plant oils, slip agent, preservatives, water-binding agents, more plant oils, and insignificant amounts of vitamins A, E, and D.

☻ **Moisturizing Lotion** *($18.50 for 4 ounces)* is a basic moisturizer containing mostly water, slip agent, petrolatum, several thickeners, and preservatives. This is just an OK, average moisturizer—nothing special.

☻ **Moisture Lotion for All Day Beauty** *($14.75 for 4 ounces)* contains mostly water, mineral oil, slip agent, thickeners, silicone oil, and preservatives. It's a standard emollient moisturizer for someone with dry skin.

☺ **Dry Skin Emollient for Excessively Dry Skin** *($21 for 2 ounces)* contains mostly mineral oil, water, wax, petrolatum, more thickeners, and preservatives. The amount of vitamins at the end of the ingredient list is almost too tiny to mention. This is a good, almost greasy moisturizer for someone with very dry skin.

☺ **Special Beauty Creme with Collagen** *($19.50 for 2 ounces)* contains mostly water, mineral oil, collagen, thickeners, more collagen, lanolin, and preservatives. The vitamins are at the end of the ingredient list, so there's almost too little to mention. This is a good moisturizer for someone with very dry skin. Collagen is a good water-binding agent, but it doesn't affect the collagen in your skin one little bit.

☹ **Oil-Free Moisturizer** *($19.50 for 4 ounces)* is indeed an oil-free moisturizer that contains mostly slip agent, thickeners, and preservatives. It also contains isopropyl myristate (fourth on the ingredient list), which can cause blackheads.

☹ **Oil-Control Lotion** *($15 for 3 ounces)* contains mostly alcohol and some minerals that have some ability to absorb oil. The alcohol causes more problems than the minerals can help.

☻ **$$$ Eye Cream** *($19 for 0.5 ounce)* is a somewhat thick but very basic moisturizer that contains water, thickener, mineral oil, more thickeners, plant oils, and preservatives. It also contains collagen, elastin, vitamins, and amino acids, but they come after the preservatives, meaning the amount is negligible. Nevertheless, this is a good emollient moisturizer for dry skin, although it might be too heavy for around the eyes.

☹ **Deep Pore Cleansing Masque for Normal to Oily Skin** *($15.25 for 2 ounces)* contains mostly water, synthetic scrub particles, glycerin, aluminum chlorohydrate (also found in deodorant; it can be a skin irritant), thickeners, and preservatives. I do not recommend this mask.

☹ **Skin Enhancing Creme** *($24.90 for 1.9 ounces)* is supposed to be a blend of antioxidant vitamins and beta hydroxy acids. The amount of vitamins is minimal and I found no discernible BHA on the ingredient list. There are vastly better BHA or AHA products on the market.

☺ **Vantex Skin Bleaching Creme with Sunscreens** *($14 for 2 ounces)* doesn't contain enough sunscreen to protect skin from any amount of sun damage. The bleaching agent, hydroquinone (2%), is the same one found in almost every other fade cream. It doesn't work all that well, but if you have dry skin this cream is as good as any.

Fashion Fair Makeup

☺ **FOUNDATION: Fragrance-Free Oil-Free Souffle** *($21)* goes on thick and creamy but dries to a matte sheer finish. It can be tricky to blend, but the color selection and coverage are excellent (although it may look somewhat pasty on normal to dry skin). **These colors are superior:** Amber Glo, Honey Glo, Tawny Glo, Tender Glo, Topaz Glo, Mocha Glo, Cocoa Glo, Pure Brown Glo, Ebony Brown Glo. **These colors are too peach for most skin tones:** Copper Glo, Brown Blaze Glo, and Bronze Glo.

☺ **Fragrance-Free Oil-Free Liquid** *($17.50)* is an excellent foundation for someone with oily skin. It goes on creamy but dries very matte, and has a good color selection. **These colors are very good:** ToffeeTone, Tender Brown, Rich Topaz, Warm Caramel, Bare Bronze, and Sheer Espresso. **These colors are poor:** Honey Amber, Tawny, Copper Tan, and Copper Blaze.

☺ **Liquid Sheer Foundation** *($12.50)* works best on dry skin, and comes in a superior array of colors. **These colors are beautiful:** Vanilla, ToffeeTone, Rich Topaz, Tender Brown, Warm Caramel, Bare Bronze, Sheer Espresso, and Ebony Brown. **These colors are not recommended:** Honey Amber, Tawny, Copper Blaze, and Copper Tan.

☹ **Perfect Finish Creme Makeup** *($15)* is a fairly greasy compact foundation, but it does blend sheer. The amount of oil in this can cause the color to turn orange. Foundations for women of color, and women with darker skin tones in particular, contain more pigment, and the oil intensifies the pigment, so wear this one for a while to see how the color will end up looking all day on your skin. **These are colors to consider:** Pure Pearl, Honey Glo, Topaz Glo, Mocha Glo, Beige Glo, Tender Glo, Cocoa Glo, Pure Brown Glo, and Ebony Brown Glo. **These colors are not recommended:** Tawny Glo, Bronze Glo, Amber Glo, Copper Glo, and Brown Blaze.

☺ **CONCEALER: Cover Tone Concealing Creme Fragrance-Free** *($13)* is for use under the eyes or over blemishes and scars. It has a very dry, thick consistency and provides fairly heavy coverage with a slightly sticky finish. It you need a lot of coverage this is an option; if not, this product is not in the least bit natural looking. **All of the colors are very good.**

☹ **Fragrance-Free Coverstick** *($10)* has a drier consistency for oily skin. It can be difficult to blend and the two colors, Medium and Dark, are too peach or orange for most skin tones. The regular **Coverstick** *($10)* has fragrance and a much creamier formula. It does blend sheer, but can slip into lines around the eye. Most of the colors are either too peach or orange. The only neutral color is Very Light.

☹ **POWDER:** **Loose Powder** *($15.50)* and **TransGlo Pressed Powder** (**Fragrance and Fragrance-Free**) *($12)* both contain talc and mineral oil, while **Oil-Control Loose Powder** *($13)* and **Oil-Control Pressed Powder** *($13)* are oil-free. All four have good textures and are available in an excellent range of colors, but they all have shine. The salesperson insisted they didn't, but the sparkle was clearly evident. Perhaps these would be OK for evening wear, but they certainly won't reduce the shine of a foundation.

☺ **BLUSH:** **Blush** *($13)* comes in a wonderful variety of colors, both fragranced and fragrance-free. They go on dry but smooth and include both vivid and subtle shades, but be careful: many of the colors are also quite shiny. **All of these colors are matte:** Wild Plum, Royal Red, Plum Rose, Bronze, Earth Red, Warm Sand, and Plum Rich. **All of these colors are shiny:** Paradise Pink, Moonlit Mauve, Chocolate Chip, Fiesta Pink, Quiet Coral, Ginger Berry, Raspberry Ice, Pearly Paprika, Crystal Rose, Golden Sunset, Sunlit Rose, and Golden Lights.

☹ **EYESHADOW:** **Ultimate Eyes** *($14.50)*, **Quads** *($14.50)*, **Trios** *($12.50)*, and **Singles** *($7)*, are all extremely shiny. They are a poor option for women of any color. The two shades of brown that aren't shiny each come packaged in a set of four colors, and the other three are shiny. I do not recommend any of the Fashion Fair eyeshadows except possibly for evening wear.

☺ **EYE AND BROW SHAPER:** **Slim Line Eye Liner Pencils** *($10)* is a standard eye pencil with a smudge tip on one end. **Brow Pencil** *($7)* is similar to the eye pencil except one end has a brush.

☺ **LIPSTICK AND LIP PENCIL:** Since the range of shades appropriate for women of color is so extensive, it would be nice if Fashion Fair's **Lipsticks** (**Fragrance and Fragrance-Free**) *($10.50)* were more creamy and less greasy. Even the **Forever Matte Lipstick** *($12.50)* is relatively greasy, and almost all the colors are shiny.

☺ **Slim Line Lip Liner Pencils** *($8.50)* come in a small but attractive array of colors and go on smoothly.

☹ **MASCARA: Mascara** *($11)* never builds any length or thickness, and it smears faster than any other mascara I've tested.

Flori Roberts

Flori Roberts is by far the weakest of the three major cosmetics lines designed specifically for women of color, with an abundance of shiny eyeshadows, poor foundation textures and shades, and dry, grainy blushes. Women of color require stronger colors (which tend to cause grainy texture), but that doesn't mean the blushes can't be silky smooth and have stronger pigment at the same time. (Many other lines have accomplished this feat.) And darker skin tones do not require shiny eyeshadows. If the blushes can be matte, surely the eyeshadows can too. It's time to give women of color the products they need. If Prescriptives, Maybelline, Revlon, and M.A.C. can do it, so can Flori Roberts.

Flori Roberts also offers some interesting skin care products. This line has definitely discovered AHAs, which can alleviate ashiness in darker skin tones. However, it also has its share of greasy moisturizers and drying toners, which can create problems that weren't there before.

Flori Roberts Skin Care

☺ **My Everything Treatment Foaming Gel Cleanser, Alpha-Melanix** *($10 for 6 ounces)* is a gentle detergent-based water-soluble cleanser that contains a small percentage of lactic acid (an AHA). In a cleanser, this small amount of AHA isn't a problem; the lactic acid is more a moisturizing agent than an exfoliant.

☺ **Optima Gel Cleanser Gold Oil-Free** *($15 for 6 ounces)* is a fairly good water-soluble cleanser that should work well for someone with oily skin. It can be drying for some skin types.

☹ **Double O Soap Gold** *($12.50 for 4 ounces)* is a standard bar soap with many ingredients, such as peppermint oil, eucalyptus oil, and camphor, that are very irritating and drying.

☺ **My Everything Treatment Exfoliating Facial Scrub and Primer** *($12.50 for 4 ounces)* contains mostly thickener, peanut meal, water, slip agent, synthetic scrub agent, more thickeners, and preservatives. This would be an OK and gentle exfoliant, but it can be tricky to rinse off.

☹ **Double O Complex Gold for Oily, Oily Skin** *($15 for 8 ounces)* contains alcohol and a host of irritating ingredients, such as peppermint oil, eucalyptus oil, clove oil, and camphor. This toner does nothing for the skin other than irritate and dry it.

☹ **My Everything Treatment Skin Balancing Astringent/Toner** *($15 for 6 ounces)* contains mostly water, witch hazel, slip agent, lactic acid, soothing agent, and preservatives. This is about a 5% AHA product. The witch hazel makes it more irritating than necessary and is not suitable for most skin types.

☺ **Optima Refining Lotion Gold Oil-Free** *($14.50 for 6 ounces)* contains mostly water, slip agent, witch hazel, cleansing agent, and preservatives. Water and witch hazel provide no real benefit for the skin. The lotion does contain a tiny amount of protein, but it is nothing more than a water-binding agent, and there's not enough of it to help the skin.

☺ **Hydrophilic Moisture Complex** *($20 for 2 ounces)* contains mostly water, glycerin, mineral oil, thickeners, collagen, preservatives, a tiny amount of AHAs, and more preservatives. This is an OK lightweight moisturizer for normal to dry skin, but as an exfoliant it doesn't even rate.

☺ **My Everything Creme** *($25 for 3.25 ounces)* contains mostly water, thickeners, glycerin, isopropyl myristate (can cause blackheads), plant oils, thickeners, vitamin A, soothing agents, and preservatives. This would be a good emollient moisturizer for someone with dry skin who isn't prone to breakouts.

☹ **My Everything Treatment Advanced Formula Creme, Alpha-Melanix with Sunscreen** *($28.50 for 3.25 ounces)* doesn't contain enough sunscreen to protect skin from sun damage. It contains mostly water, thickeners, silicone oil, plant oil, more thickeners, more silicone oil, glycolic acid, vitamins E and A, and preservatives. This is a very good lightweight moisturizer for someone with dry skin, but it doesn't contain even 1% or 2% AHAs. If you buy this as an AHA product or a sunscreen, you will be disappointed.

☹ **My Everything Treatment Revitalized Protection Moisturizer, Alpha-Melanix with Sunscreen** *($16.50 for 4 ounces)* is similar to the moisturizer above, and the same review applies.

☺ **Chromatone Fade Creme Plus Gold** *($15 for 4 ounces)* is a standard 2% hydroquinone fade cream in an emollient base. Hydroquinone has minimal ability to lighten the skin, but if you are curious to see how it works for you, this is a good fade cream for very dry skin.

☺ **My Everything Treatment Advanced Chromatone Plus with Alpha-Melanix Fade Cream with Sunscreen** *($14 for 1.7 ounces)* is a standard 2% hydroquinone fade cream in an emollient base. Hydroquinone has minimal ability to lighten the skin. This product contains a tiny amount of lactic acid, not enough to exfoliate the skin or help the hydroquinone perform more effectively.

☹ **T-Zone Oil Block** *($13 for 2.3 ounces)* contains mostly water and alcohol, which may make skin more oily, and definitely won't reduce oil.

Flori Roberts Makeup

☹ **FOUNDATION: Touche Satin Finish** *($15)* is a cream-to-powder makeup that stays more creamy than powdery on the skin. It provides good, even coverage, but the color choice leaves much to be desired. These just aren't realistic skin tones for women of color.

☹ **Touche Cream to Powder Matte Finish** *($15)* is a thick, heavy, sticky foundation that is difficult to blend and has a poor color selection.

☺ **Maximum Matte Souffle Oil-Free Makeup** *($20)* has a gorgeous smooth texture and blends on easily and evenly. The finish is truly matte and light, and all the colors are beautiful. This foundation is absolutely worth checking out if you have normal to oily skin.

☺ **Hydrophillic Oil-Free Foundation** *($20)* isn't oil-free—it contains silicone oil— but does have a somewhat matte finish. There are only six colors, and most are not best for darker skin tones. **These colors are good:** Chroma A and Chroma B. **These colors are too orange or copper:** Chroma C, Chorma D, Chroma E, and Chroma F.

☺ **POWDER: Melanin Face Powder Loose** *($14)* has a rather soft but moist texture. The colors may be too red for most skin tones. **Chromatic Loose Powder** *($14)* has a soft, dry finish. It comes in three shades, but Light and Medium are too peach for most skin tones. The only possible shade is Deep.

☺ **Compact Face Powder with Oil-Control** *($14)* has a dry texture, but blends on evenly. All four colors are very good. **Pressed Powder** *($14)* has a dry sheer finish. **These colors are good:** 5 and 7. 3 can be too red for most skin tones.

☺ **BLUSH: Radiance Blush** *($12.50)* has some great colors for darker skin tones, but they tend to have a grainy dry texture that can look heavy and thick. For the most part these colors would be good only for women with darker skin tones. **More Than Blush** *($12.50)* is intensely shiny and comes in only one shade.

☹ **EYESHADOW:** Signature Eyeshadow Trios *($14.50)* are all very shiny and the color selection is poor.

☺ **EYE AND BROW SHAPER:** Eye Contour Pencils *($8)* are fairly standard, but a bit drier than most on the market. This makes them a little harder to apply, but they also don't smear as fast. **Matte Brows** *(10.50)* is a powder shadow meant for use on the brows. It comes in two colors, Brown and Black, and is a great option.

☺ **LIPSTICK AND LIP PENCIL:** Flori Roberts excels in this arena. **Lipstick** *($9.50)* has a wide selection of colors and a good creamy texture almost bordering on greasy. **Matte Lipstick** *($10)* isn't really all that matte; it's actually creamy and slightly on the greasy side. **Gold Hydrophillic Lipstick** *($12.50)* has a light, creamy texture, but it also contains a stain, so the color tends to hang around longer than with the other lipsticks. There is also a small but nice selection of standard tube glosses called **Liquid Lip Gloss** *($10)* that are OK if you want a more opaque gloss, but slightly sticky. **Lip Contour Pencil** *($8)* is a standard pencil that has a slightly drier texture than most.

☹ **MASCARA:** **Lash Set Mascara** *($10.50)* goes on well and builds thick long lashes, but it does tend to clump.

Forever Spring (Skin Care Only)

Actress Connie Stevens promotes this line as the reason she looks so wonderful. Well, Connie, you do look wonderful (at least in the pictures), but I'm fairly certain it has nothing to do with these products. These are just skin care products with ingredients similar to a hundred others on the market. I also have a rough time with the name of the company. Any cosmetics-company name that implies that you won't get wrinkles if you use its products (such as Sudden Youth, Instant Youth, Instant Lift, and so on) is, well, insulting. Having let off steam, I can now be more objective and tell you that some of these products are quite good. (Only the cleanser and the exfoliator are problems.) But the **Time Machine** *($120)* is definitely one of the bigger wastes of money in the world of cosmetics. It is supposed to exercise facial muscles through topical stimulation. Facial muscles, just like body muscles, cannot be built up through artificial exercise; if they could, why would a bodybuilder ever bother to lift weights? Even if this machine did work, the muscles would simply bulge, not lift skin (you'd look like many an older bodybuilder, with muscles *and* sagging skin). In addition, this machine can create damage by breaking delicate surface capillaries. It is supposed to increase circulation, but there are better ways to increase circulation than with voltage. Running up and down your stairs for 20 minutes will not only increase your circulation but also help your heart and build energy.

☺ **Collagen Facial Cleanser** *($14.25 for 4 ounces)* is a fairly standard, greasy wipe-off cleanser that is not water-soluble. It contains mineral oil, thickeners, lanolin oil, collagen, and safflower oil. The directions say to wipe up, never down, but regardless of whether you pull the skin up or down, you're still causing it to stretch, and that causes sagging.

☺ **Glycerin Soap** *($4.75 for 3 ounces)* is a standard detergent-based bar soap that contains tallow, which can cause breakouts. This soap would be OK from the neck down, but not from the neck up.

☹ **Honey Almond Apricot Scuffer** *($13.25 for 4 ounces)* is a detergent-based cleanser that uses sodium lauryl sulfate as the cleansing agent. It would be very drying and irritating for most skin types.

☺ **Ambrosia Skin Refresher** *($9.25 for 8 ounces)* is a very good irritant-free toner that contains good water-binding agents and soothing ingredients.

☺ **Collagen Skin Quencher** *($22.75 for 4 ounces)* contains mostly water, slip agent, water-binding agents (collagen and elastin), aloe, glycerin, and preservatives. This is a good moisturizer for someone with dry skin, but the collagen and elastin can't do anything for the collagen in your skin. This moisturizer is supposed to be used with the Time Machine; you know what I know think of that.

☺ **Ginseng Facial Feed** *($21.25 for 4 ounces)* is a very good emollient moisturizer for dry skin, but nothing more. It contains mostly water, slip agent, plant oil, mineral oil, thickeners, ginseng, more plant oil, water-binding agents, silicone oil, vitamins E and A (antioxidants), and preservatives. There aren't enough vitamins in this product to make a difference.

☺ **$$$ Lift and Taut Spring Skin Serum** *($26.95 for 1 ounce)* contains mostly arnica extract (potential skin irritant), thickeners, slip agent, water-binding agent, glycerin, more thickeners, plant extracts, vitamins A and E, more water-binding agents, soothing agent, silicone oil, fragrance, and preservatives. I suspect the arnica swells the skin and makes it look temporarily smoother. Irritation of any kind can be a problem for skin. Other than that, this would be a good moisturizer for someone with dry skin.

☺ **$$$ Mandarin Liposome Oxygen Booster** *($24.95 for 1 ounce)* contains mostly water, slip agent, thickeners, plant extracts, glycerin, plant oil, water-binding agents, and preservatives. This product lists liposomes as an ingredient, which is strange, because liposomes are a delivery system (a way of formulating a product), not an ingredient. In any case, this product can't deliver oxygen into the skin, although it would be a good moisturizer for someone with normal to dry skin. Mandarin extract and oil sound good, but provide no special benefits.

☺ **$$$ Retrieve** *($26.95 for 1 ounce)* contains mostly water, aloe, slip agent, glycerin, AHAs, plant oil, plant extracts, water-binding agents, salicylic acid, more plant oil, vitamins A and E, thickeners, preservatives, and fragrance. This is about a 4% to 5% mixed AHA and BHA exfoliant in a good emollient base for someone with dry skin. I am not fond of products that contain almost any amount of BHA (salicylic acid), but this is a good possibility if you are interested in this type of product. There aren't enough vitamins to make a difference.

☺ **$$$ Super Rich Emollience** *($24.50 for 4 ounces)* contains mostly water, slip agents, plant oils, several thickeners, water-binding agents, vitamins A and E, silicone oil, mineral oil, preservatives, and fragrance. This would be a very good emollient moisturizer for someone with very dry skin. There aren't enough vitamins in it to make a difference.

☹ **$$$ Bio Eye and Throat Intensive Lubrication** *($24.50 for 2 ounces)* contains mostly water, several thickeners, plant oil, soothing agent, water-binding agent, vitamins E and A, preservatives, and fragrance. This would be a good emollient moisturizer for someone with dry skin, but it isn't as interesting as some of the others in the Forever Spring collection. There aren't enough vitamins in it to make a difference.

☺ **$$$ Petal Soft Eye Cream** *($14 for 0.5 ounce)* contains mostly water, mineral oil, thickeners, slip agent, petrolatum, water-binding agents, and preservatives. This would be a very good emollient, but standard, moisturizer for someone with dry skin.

☹ **$$$ Fibro Eye Soother** *($14 for 0.5 ounce)* contains mostly water, silicone oil, glycerin, plant extract, water-binding agents, vitamin A, preservatives, and fragrance. This product is almost all water and silicone oil, and little else. It is soothing, but hardly exceptional or unique.

☺ **$$$ Baby Soft Facial Clay** *($15 for 4 ounces)* is a standard clay mask that contains mostly water, clays, glycerin, water-binding agent, thickener, plant extract, and preservatives. If you want a clay mask, this would be fine, and it can make the skin feel soft, but no clay mask is capable of making skin "baby soft."

Freeman Beautiful Skin (Skin Care Only)

☺ **Beautiful Skin Blueberry & Lavender Facial Gel Cleanser** *($2.49 for 6 ounces)* is a standard detergent-based cleanser that contains its share of plant extracts. The blueberry and lavender are nice, but serve no real purpose. This could be a good cleanser for someone with oily skin, however. It can be quite drying for some skin types.

☺ **Beautiful Skin Lemon & Yogurt Cleansing Milk** *($3.59 for 6 ounces)* is supposed to be water-soluble, but it doesn't rinse very well and leaves a film.

☹ **Beautiful Skin Pineapple & Papaya Foaming Enzyme Facial Wash with Alpha-Hydroxy Acids** *($3.49 for 8 ounces)* is a standard detergent-based cleanser that contains a tiny amount of fruit extracts, which aren't the same as AHAs, as well as papain (papaya enzyme) and bromelain (pineapple enzyme). The enzymes, in this situation, are little more than exfoliants, and there aren't very many of them. AHAs and exfoliants in general are a problem in cleansers because of the potential for getting them in the eyes, and most of their effectiveness is washed down the drain. This is more a marketing issue than a real problem for the skin, but I advise avoiding even the possibility of problems.

☹ **Beautiful Skin Sugar Cane and Meadowsweet Alpha-Hydroxy Facial Scrub** *($3.99 for 5.3 ounces)* is similar to the product above, with the same basic considerations, and the same review applies.

☺ **Beautiful Skin Apricot & Sea Kelp Facial Scrub** *($3.59 for 6 ounces)* is a walnut shell–based scrub that also contains plant oil, thickeners, soothing agents, and preservatives. The plant oil makes this product good only for someone with dry skin. It can leave a greasy film.

☺ **Beautiful Skin Honey and Vitamin E Night Creme** *($2.49 for 8 ounces)* contains mostly water, mineral oil, thickeners, slip agent, glycerin, vitamins E and A, soothing agent, plant extracts, water-binding agents, and preservatives. This is a very good emollient moisturizer for someone with dry skin.

☺ **Beautiful Skin Honey & Vitamin E Revitalizing Antioxidant Creme** *($3.49 for 4.6 ounces)* contains mostly water, plant oil, thickeners, petrolatum, more thickeners, vitamins E and A, soothing agents, preservatives, and fragrance. This is a very good moisturizer for someone with dry skin, but there isn't enough vitamin E for it to be an antioxidant, despite its name.

☺ **Beautiful Skin Honey Dew & Orchid Moisture Mist** *($2.49 for 8 ounces)* contains mostly water, glycerin, plant extracts, water-binding agents, vitamin E, silicone oil, slip agent, preservative, and fragrance. This is a very good moisturizer for someone with normal to dry skin.

☹ **Beautiful Skin Sunflower & Aloe Perfect Moisturizer SPF 6** *($2.49 for 4.6 ounces)* is hardly "perfect." Its SPF rating is only 6, which is not adequate to protect against sun damage.

☺ **Beautiful Skin Chamomile & Allantoin Lite Moisturizer** *($3.59 for 6 ounces)* contains mostly water, standard water-binding agent, thickeners, slip agent, chamomile extract, vitamins A and E, and preservatives. This is a good lightweight moisturizer.

☺ **Beautiful Skin Avocado & Oatmeal Facial Masque** *($3.59 for 6 ounces)* is a standard clay mask with a small amount of oil, which can prevent it from being too drying. If you want to use a clay mask, this is a good one for an exceptionally reasonable price.

☺ **Beautiful Skin Blackberry & Tangerine Mud Mask** *($2.49 for 6 ounces)* is a standard clay mask that also contains a small amount of plant oil, slip agents, plant extracts, minerals, preservatives, and fragrance. Some of the plant oils can be skin irritants, but this is an OK mud mask if you want one.

☺ **Beautiful Skin Cucumber & Ginseng Peel-Off Masque** *($3.59 for 6 ounces)* contains mostly water, film former (a plastic-like ingredient), alcohol, plant extracts, preservatives, and fragrance. This peel-off mask can make the skin feel smooth, but the polyvinyl film former can be an irritant.

☺ **Beautiful Skin Sugar Cane & Guava Alpha-Hydroxy Peel-Off Masque** *($2.49 for 6 ounces)* is identical to the mask above except it contains fruit extracts. That doesn't make this an AHA product, because there is no way to tell exactly what these fruit extracts are. This mask probably won't be a problem for the face, but it's not an effective AHA product.

Galderma (Skin Care Only)

Galderma is the company that manufactures Cetaphil. Those of you who have been familiar with my work from the beginning know that Cetaphil is a facial cleanser I have been impressed with for quite some time. In 1983, when I first discovered this obscure little cleanser, it was almost exclusively being recommended by dermatologists, because no one else knew about it. Back then there were very few good products available for women to clean their faces with. Until recently, the only options were cold cream or cold cream–like products, which had to be wiped off and left the face greasy, and bar cleansers or soaps, which left the face dried out and irritated. Cetaphil was one of the only water-soluble cleansers available that cleaned the face without drying it out or leaving it feeling greasy. Times have changed, of course, and there are now many more alternatives for cleaning the face, but Cetaphil remains a primary option for women with dry, sensitive skin who don't wear much makeup. (Unfortunately, Cetaphil is not very good for removing makeup, but it is dynamite in the morning or if you wear minimal makeup.) Galderma also makes a number of other products besides Cetaphil, and it's about time I reviewed all of them for you.

☺ **Cetaphil Cleanser** (*$8.31 for 16 ounces*) is a very good cleanser for someone with dry, sensitive skin.

☺ **Cetaphil Gentle Cleansing Bar for Dry, Sensitive Skin** (*$3.29 for 4.5 ounces*) is a standard bar cleanser that uses a detergent cleansing agent. It does contain tallow, which can cause breakouts. It is best used from the neck down.

☺ **Cetaphil Moisturizing Lotion** (*$7.49 for 16 ounces*) contains mostly water, glycerin, thickeners, plant oil, silicone oil, more thickeners, and preservatives. This is a good moisturizer for someone with sensitive normal to dry skin.

☺ **Nutraderm Original Formula** (*$7.49 for 16 ounces*) contains mostly water, mineral oil, thickeners, and preservatives. This is a good basic moisturizer for someone with dry, sensitive skin.

☺ **Nutraderm 30** (*$7.49 for 16 ounces*) contains mostly water, glycerin, petrolatum, thickeners, silicone oil, water-binding agents, AHAs, more thickeners, preservatives, and fragrance. This is a good moisturizer for someone with normal to dry skin. It contains about 2% AHAs (the same as Lauder's Fruition), which is fine as a water-binding agent, but isn't enough to be an exfoliant.

☺ **Candermyl Cream Advanced Facial Moisturizer with Non-Ionic Liposomes for Dry, Sensitive Skin** (*$11.98 for 1 ounce*) was one of the first products to use liposomes as a delivery system. It is a good moisturizer for someone with dry skin, and the liposomes can help keep the moisturizer around longer than many similar products.

Guerlain

I've been asked repeatedly why I bother to review extravagant, expensive lines like Guerlain, La Prairie, and Orlane. Why would someone who's looking to save money and find the best buys want to know whether or not Guerlain has good products? The women who can afford Guerlain, or who hope that spending that kind of money on skin care can save their youth, probably aren't reading this book. They do not want to hear that they are wasting their money on a poor product or spending ten times more than they need to for a good one.

I like to review a diverse range of cosmetics lines for several reasons, including: (1) Even women who can afford to spend (waste) a lot of money deserve consumer information; (2) No matter what the price, it is never OK for women to be misled or be misinformed; (3) It is essential for me to stay informed about what is currently available in the world of cosmetics, because I never know where I might find the best products, which would then set the standard for my reviews; and (4) Reviewing expensive products almost always helps to reconfirm that "expensive" rarely means "better." Guerlain proves my last contention better than most.

If any cosmetics line can be considered sensual, luxurious, and elitist, Guerlain is it. Without even taking quality into consideration, it is hard to ignore the lavish gold packaging, intricate design, and awesome price tag that accompany everything from eyeliner to powder. A refillable powder compact sells for over $140 and a lipstick compact sells for $80! They are exquisite containers bedecked with gold and faux jewels. If it were chic to powder your nose and put lipstick on in public, you would be the talk of the party. But that's the problem with overkill packaging: it is essentially a waste, because no one but you and your makeup bag see it. All that counts when it comes to makeup is how it looks on your face. Beautiful containers are nice, but if the product is only a blush and the lipstick only a lipstick, there is no real reason to lust after a container.

Still, for many women the issue isn't effectiveness but a sense of being "worth it." I would like to suggest that the question isn't whether you're worth it, but whether it is worth your time and effort to be misled by unreal product claims. Bottom line: Don't worry if you can't afford this line; you won't be left out to wrinkle alone in the cold.

Guerlain's skin care products contain standard cosmetic ingredients that you've seen before; some are very good and some are very average. In terms of the color line, the strong points are the blushes and foundations, while the weaknesses are the shiny eyeshadows and pressed powder. To be fair, I should add that Guerlain is not the most expensive product line at the cosmetics counters, although it's definitely up there.

Guerlain Skin Care

☹ **$$$ Evolution Complete Cleanser** *($30 for 8.2 ounces)* is a standard mineral oil–based cleanser that doesn't rinse off well without the help of a washcloth, and it can leave a greasy film on the skin. This is a lot of money for a product that's basically cold cream.

☺ **$$$ Evolution Purifying Foaming Gel** *($32 for 5.4 ounces)* is a standard detergent-based cleanser that would be good for someone with normal to oily skin. It can be drying for some skin types.

☺ **$$$ Evolution Exfoliating Creme for the Face** *($26 for 1.7 ounces)* is a standard scrub that uses synthetic particles as the exfoliant. Other than that, it contains a long list of thickeners and detergent cleansing agents. It can be good for someone with normal to dry skin.

☹ **Evolution Clarifying Toner** *($32 for 8.5 ounces)* is a standard alcohol-based toner that is too irritating for most skin types. This won't clarify anything, but it can be quite irritating and drying.

☹ **Evolution Refreshing Tonic Vitale** *($30 for 8.5 ounces)* is a standard alcohol-based toner that is too irritating for most skin types. There is nothing refreshing about this toner, but it can be quite drying and sensitizing.

☺ **$$$ Evolution Sublicreme No. 1 Light Day and Night Care** *($50 for 1.7 ounces)* contains mostly water, a long list of thickeners, water-binding agents, fragrance, more thickeners, and preservatives. There are a lot of interesting ingredients, but they come after the fragrance and preservatives, which means they amount to nothing. This is a good lightweight, but very ordinary, moisturizer for normal to dry skin. It does contain a minuscule amount of DNA—but we all know DNA can't help repair skin cells, right? And without any measurable sunscreen, this product is not appropriate for day wear, contrary to its name.

☺ **$$$ Evolution Sublicreme No. 2 Rich Day and Night Care** *($50 for 1.7 ounces)* is almost identical to the moisturizer above except that it is slightly more emollient, and the same review applies.

☺ **$$$ Evolution Sublifluide Day and Night Care** *($50 for 1.7 ounces)* contains mostly water, several thickeners, slip agents, more thickeners, water-binding agents, fragrance, a tiny amount of sunscreen, vitamins A and E, and preservatives. This is a good lightweight moisturizer for someone with normal to slightly dry skin. Most of the interesting ingredients come after the fragrance, though, which means they are barely present; and there isn't enough sunscreen to even begin to protect from sun damage.

☺ **$$$ Evolution Divinaura Beauty Enhancer** *($59 for 1 ounce)* contains incredibly standard ingredients—water, slip agents, thickeners, preservatives, fragrances, and—are you ready for this?—gold. How much gold? Six milligrams, which is about 0.000353 ounce. What is this microscopic amount of gold supposed to be for? Stimulating and energizing the skin, according to the label. Skin can't absorb gold, though, so I imagine that rubbing a gold necklace over my face should do the same thing, and save me a lot of money in the bargain.

☺ **$$$ Evolution Sublilift A.R.T. Recontouring Serum for the Face** *($55 for 1 ounce)* contains mostly water, a long list of thickeners, vitamin E, fragrance, and preservatives. As in many Guerlain products, most of the interesting water-binding agents are found after the preservative on the ingredient list, and in amounts so small they are barely worth mentioning. This is a good, but extremely ordinary, moisturizer for someone with normal to dry skin; it won't recontour anything.

☺ **$$$ Evolution Specific Eye Contour Care** *($35 for 0.5 ounce)* contains mostly water, thickeners, silicone oil, lanolin, standard water-binding agents, more thickeners, more water-binding agents, vitamin E, and preservatives. This is a good emollient moisturizer, but the amino acids won't change a wrinkle.

☺ **$$$ Evolution Fresh Complexion Mask** *($35 for 1.7 ounces)* contains mostly water, slip agents, glycerin, thickeners, and preservatives. It's a very ordinary lightweight mask for someone with normal to slightly dry skin.

☺ **$$$ Evolution Treatment Mask with Revitenol** *($37 for 1.8 ounces)* is an extremely standard clay mask that also contains thickening agents, film former, more thickeners, vitamin E, fragrance, and preservatives. It does contain a minuscule amount of DNA, but that has no effect on the skin.

☺ **$$$ Issima Creme Cleanser** *($42 for 6.8 ounces)* is a standard mineral oil–based cleanser with ordinary thickeners and slip agents. It doesn't rinse off well without .the aid of a washcloth, and it can leave a film.

☺ **$$$ Issima Moisturizing Lotion** *($42 for 6.8 ounces)* contains mostly water, slip agent, thickener, fragrance, and preservatives. This product is almost embarrassingly ordinary. It is an irritant-free toner, but it contains nothing to comment about one way or the other.

☺ **$$$ Issima Aquaserum Long Term Rehydrating Formula** *($125 for 1.7 ounces)* contains mostly water, thickener, mineral oil, more thickeners, vitamin E, water-binding agent, a tiny amount of sunscreen, plant oil, more thickeners, AHAs, fragrance, and preservatives. This is a good mineral oil–based moisturizer for someone with normal to dry skin, but the price is so absurd and the product so ordinary that buying it would be like spending $125 on a box of Duncan Hines chocolate cake mix. The amount of AHAs in this product is about 1%; that makes it an OK water-binding agent, but that's about it.

☺ **$$$ Issima Intensive Protective Emulsion** *($89 for 1.7 ounces)* contains mostly water, thickeners, plant oil, a very long list of other thickeners, silicone oil, vitamin

E, AHAs, fragrance, and preservatives. This is a good moisturizer for someone with dry skin, but the price could make you feel worse than any amount of flaky skin ever could.

☺ **$$$ Issima Intensive Revitalizing Creme** *($120 for 1.7 ounces)* is similar to the product above, and the same review applies.

☺ **$$$ Issima Super Aquaserum Optimum Hydrating Revitalizer** *($125 for 1.7 ounces)* contains mostly water, plant oil, glycerin, slip agent, a long list of thickening agents, AHAs, water-binding agents, vitamin E, more thickeners, fragrance, and preservatives. This is about a 2% to 3% AHA product, which means it doesn't contain enough AHAs to exfoliate much, but the AHAs are good water-binding agents. I can't even comment about the prices anymore—they are too preposterous to believe.

☺ **$$$ Issima Midnight Secret Late Night Special Treatment** *($89 for 1 ounce)* contains mostly water, thickeners, mineral oil, silicone oil, vitamin E, fragrance, a tiny amount of AHAs, and preservatives. This is a good, extremely ordinary moisturizer for normal to dry skin, but nothing more. The secret is that there's nothing interesting inside the bottle.

☺ **$$$ Issima Anti-Wrinkle Eye Contour Fluid** *($63 for 0.5 ounce)* contains water, slip agent, plant extract, thickeners, a small amount of sunscreen, vitamin E, water-binding agents, more thickeners, more plant extracts, vitamin A, and preservatives. This is a good lightweight emollient, but the price tag is way out of line for these average ingredients.

☹ **$$$ Issima Serenissime Restructuring Treatment with Active Genesium** *($175 for 1 ounce)* is one of the most expensive skin care products on the market. What are you buying for $2,800 a pound? Extremely standard ingredients and something called "genesium," which supposedly can tackle all the things that cause the skin to age. Not on your life! Serenissime does not contain a sunscreen. Without a sunscreen it can't handle the number-one cause of aged-looking skin, and that's sun damage. It does have some good water-binding ingredients and some antioxidants, but they are overwhelmed by the waxy thickening agents and mineral oil, which you can find in a hundred other products. Even the interesting ingredients come after the fragrance and preservatives, meaning they are barely present. What an expensive waste! But being expensive is what makes this line so seductive. Not everyone can have it. Will you be $175 more beautiful or younger-looking than someone else? Of course not.

☺ **$$$ Issima Intenserum Beauty Treatment** *($165 for ten 0.08-ounce ampoules)* is, to say the least, overpriced. For $3,300 per pound, you get mostly water, slip agents, thickeners, silicone oil, vitamin E, fragrance, water-binding agents, and preservatives. It isn't worth it. To be fair, it is a good lightweight moisturizer for someone with normal to dry skin, but these ingredients do not warrant a price tag that's even one-tenth of that amount.

☺ **$$$ Issima Aquamasque** *($65 for 2.5 ounces)* contains mostly water, thickeners, plant oil, silicone oil, slip agent, vitamin E, water-binding agents, and preservatives. It is a good mask for someone with dry skin.

☹ **Odelys Gentle Foaming Cleanser** *($20 for 5 ounces)* is a standard detergent cleanser that also contains tallow and lanolin. Both tallow and lanolin can cause breakouts and allergic reactions. The Odelys product line is supposed to be for sensitive skin, but I don't think Guerlain noticed the ingredients.

☺ **$$$ Odelys Instant Relaxing Cleanser** *($27 for 7 ounces)* is a standard mineral oil–based wipe-off cleanser that can leave a greasy film on the skin. This is more like a cold cream than anything else.

☺ **$$$ Odelys Delicate Eye Makeup Remover** *($19 for 2.5 ounces)* contains mostly water, slip agent, detergent cleanser, and preservatives. It will take off eye makeup.

☺ **$$$ Odelys Soothing Toner** *($25 for 6.8 ounces)* is an OK irritant-free toner that contains mostly water, slip agents, vitamin E, and preservatives. There are some good soothing agents and water-binding agents, but they are listed after the preservatives, which means there isn't enough to benefit the skin in the least.

☺ **$$$ Odelys Perfect Care #1 Day and Night (Light)** *($49 for 1.7 ounces)* contains mostly water, thickeners, slip agents, more thickeners, plant oil, vitamin E, more thickeners, and preservatives. This product has a huge list of ingredients, most of which come after the preservatives, which means they amount to little more than window dressing. This is a good, but extremely ordinary, moisturizer for someone with normal to dry skin.

☺ **$$$ Odelys Perfect Care #2 Day and Night (Rich)** *($49 for 1.7 ounces)* is similar to the moisturizer above, only more emollient, and the same review applies.

☺ **$$$ Odelys Perfect Eye Contour Care** *($30 for 0.7 ounces)* contains mostly water, thickeners, film former, slip agents, more thickeners, and preservatives. This is a good moisturizer for someone with dry skin. The film former can be a skin irritant.

☺ **$$$ Odelys Moisturizing Creme Mask** *($30 for 2.6 ounces)* contains mostly water, thickeners, plant oil, slip agents, more thickeners, clay, mineral oil, vitamin E, more slip agents, fragrance, and preservatives. This is a good emollient clay mask for someone with normal to dry skin.

☺ **$$$ Alphabella Gentle Action with AHA for Dry or Weakened Skin** *($58 for 1 ounce)* is not even an average AHA product. This highly fragranced lightweight moisturizer contains about 2% AHAs. That makes it a poor exfoliant but a good water-binding agent; still, at these prices, it should do what you expect an AHA product to do.

☹ **$$$ Alphabella Intense Action with AHA for Combination or Oily Skin** *($58 for 1 ounce)* is similar to the moisturizer above, but with 3.5% AHAs. That's not even a competitor in the AHA arena, which for someone with oily skin would be exceedingly disappointing, not to mention financially draining.

Guerlain Makeup

☹ <u>FOUNDATION:</u> **Elysemat Liquid Make-up** *($39)* has a lovely texture, but the colors are all too peach, pink, or rose.

☺ **$$$ Issima Foundation** *($49)* has a creamy moist texture and the colors, though extremely limited, are all excellent. Didn't they notice when formulating these colors that they look natural and the Elysemat above looks like paint?

☺ **$$$ Treatment Powder Foundation** *($45)* is a standard pressed powder, not a treatment. The color choice is for the mostly great, but watch out for 3 and 9.

☹ **$$$ Teint Hydro-Lifting Firming Foundation** *($40)* won't lift your face, but it does blend on soft and sheer with a moist finish. This is another disappointment. **These are the only colors to consider:** Creme 3 and Vanille 2. **All of the other colors are too peach or pink.**

☹ <u>CONCEALER:</u> **Corrective Concealer** *($25)* comes in only two shades. It blends on very smooth and creamy but dries to a matte finish and creases into lines during the day.

☹ **$$$ POWDER: Pressed Powder** *($38)* is pretty standard, with a soft, dry texture. The color choice is limited but OK. **These colors are very good:** Transparent, Perlee, and Ambree. **This color is too pink for most skin tones:** Azalee. **Loose Powder** *($38)* comes in three great colors that have a soft, smooth, but dry finish.

☺ **$$$ BLUSH: Powder Blush** *($30)* doesn't have many shades, but the ones they do have are beautiful and silky. **Meteorites** *($39)* are small multicolored beads that mix together to make one pastel shade that is supposed to react only to your skin. The Body Shop makes a similar product for one-fourth the price.

☹ **Bronzing Powder** *($30)* comes in three shades that are all shiny to ultra-shiny.

☹ **EYESHADOW:** Almost all of the **Mono** and **Duo** *($26/$32)* eyeshadows are either too shiny, too blue, too green, or the combinations are too strange. Even the texture is poor. **Contouring Eyeshadow Powder-Creme** *($25)* comes in a tube, blends on like a thick liquid, and dries to a powder finish. **Most of the colors are shiny, except for one:** Brun Tabac.

☺ **$$$ EYE AND BROW SHAPER:** The small, attractive containers contain a tiny vial of ordinary but good liquid **Eye-Liner** *($22)*. One drawback is the container that is too small for easy application. Avoid the shiny silver (Ligne d'Argent) and shiny gold (Ligne d'Or) liners. **Eye and Brow Pencils** *($17)* are, well, eye and brow pencils. They go on thicker and drier than most, but are still standard and over-priced.

☺ **$$$ LIPSTICK AND LIP PENCIL:** **Kiss Kiss with SPF 8** *($21)* are beautiful creamy lipsticks. **Treatment Lipsticks** *($19)* won't treat anything, but they are good standard glossy, almost greasy lipsticks. **Multicolor Lip Gloss** *($18)* is an attractive-looking gloss that looks like a rainbow of colors in the tube. Of course, it goes on as one color just like any other gloss. **Lip Liner Pencil** *($17)* goes on thicker and greasier than most but comes in a nice array of colors.

☺ **$$$ MASCARA:** **Beauty Treatment Mascara** *($20)* takes forever to build any length, and even then it never makes much difference. The container is handsome, but that won't help your lashes look any better.

H$_2$O Plus (Skin Care Only)

Water, water everywhere, but not a drop to drink? Well, the name sounds like a fountain for skin, which is what this company absolutely wants you to believe. Once you see the H$_2$O Plus displays, the company's marketing angle becomes crystal clear. The gurgling tubes of colored water are very attractive, and they solidly establish the company's theme: "Hydration is everything and fun is important too, which is why you'll find exciting textures, colors, and fragrances that look and smell as good as they feel." As women mature, they fear that losing moisture in their skin will cause it to age, which makes this line extremely attractive to baby boomers.

This is the first cosmetics company I've heard declare that *fun* should be part of a woman's skin care routine. As much as I would like to think of cosmetics as fun, I am skeptical about whether adding coloring agents (standard FD&C and D&C colors) and fragrances to products makes them more fun. Coloring agents can cause problems in skin care products that might get into the eyes, such as H$_2$O Plus's Firming Eye Gel,

Natural Cucumber Cleansing Lotion, and Face Oasis. And fragrances are always potential skin sensitizers. I recommend using skin care products that have no coloring agents or fragrance, but they aren't always easy to come by because the manufacturers and marketers know that plain white fragrance-free products are less interesting to the consumer. Whether or not it's good for them, women like their cosmetics to smell good and look pretty.

Like most cosmetics companies in the '90s, H$_2$O Plus uses plant extracts and oils to give consumers the natural slant they've come to expect. Regardless of what the brochure says, are these products botanically based? Mostly they aren't, but there are plants in them. Are the products good? Some are. Are they reasonably priced? For a department-store line, yes, they are. The major question to be answered is, Will these products provide skin with more moisturizing (water-retaining) benefits than other products on the market? The answer is no, but given the fear many women have of losing the moisture in their skin, the alluring name brings eager buyers flocking to the H$_2$O Plus counters and storefronts.

☺ **Cleansing Gel** *($15 for 4 ounces)* is a standard detergent-based cleanser that can effectively clean the skin without leaving skin feeling dry or oily. It's best for oily and combination skin types; it can be drying for some skin types.

☺ **Natural Cucumber Cleansing Lotion** *($15 for 8 ounces)* is a standard wipe-off cleanser containing mostly shea butter and plant oils and a small amount of detergent cleansing agent. This can be a good cleanser for someone with very dry skin, but it can leave a greasy film.

☺ **Eye Cleanser/Makeup Remover** *($12.50 for 4 ounces)* contains water, detergent cleansing agent, soothing agents, more detergent agents, slip agents, thickeners, and preservatives. This standard detergent-based cleanser will indeed remove eye makeup, but an extra cleanser is unnecessary if the face cleanser is gentle, and this one can possibly irritate the eye area.

☹ **Facial Scrub** *($14 for 4.2 ounces)* is a detergent-based cleanser with standard synthetic scrub particles. It contains TEA-lauryl sulfate, a detergent cleansing agent that can be very drying and irritating.

☺ **Alcohol-Free Toner** *($10 for 8 ounces)* contains mostly water, slip agent, plant extract, soothing agent, film former, and preservatives. This is an OK alcohol-free toner, but the film-forming agent can be a skin irritant.

☹ **Toner Plus** *($12.50 for 8 ounces)* is an alcohol-based toner with some plant extracts, witch hazel (which is about 70% ethanol alcohol), and preservatives. It can be irritating, and I do not recommend it.

☺ **Day Lotion** *($18.50 for 4 ounces)* contains mostly water, mineral oil, slip agent, plant oil, thickeners, petrolatum, lanolin, vitamin E, and preservatives. This would be a very good moisturizer for someone with dry to extremely dry skin.

☹ **Oil-Controlling Day Gel** *($20 for 2 ounces)* contains mostly water, film former, slip agent, silicone oil, thickener, witch hazel, water-binding agents, thickeners, plant extracts, fragrance, and preservatives. This won't control oil, and the witch hazel and film former can be irritants, but it may be OK as a lightweight moisturizer for some skin types.

☺ **Botanical Nite Gel** *($20 for 2 ounces)* contains water, glycerin, water-binding agents, silicone oil, several plant extracts, thickeners, and preservatives. Some of the plant extracts may be a problem for allergy-prone individuals, but this would be a good lightweight moisturizer for someone with slightly dry or combination skin.

☺ **Pro-Vitamin Nite Treatment** *($22 for 2 ounces)* contains mostly chamomile water, plant oil, glycerin, thickeners, water-binding agents, silicone oil, vitamins A and C, and preservatives. The plant oil in this product is soybean oil, which can be irritating and may cause breakouts. It doesn't contain enough vitamins to count for much, but it is an OK moisturizer for someone with dry skin.

☹ **Face Oasis Moisture Replenishing Treatment** *($25 for 2 ounces)* contains mostly water, film former, slip agent, water-binding agents, silicone oil, plant extract, thickeners, and preservatives. This would be a good lightweight moisturizer for someone with slightly dry or combination skin, but the film former can be a skin irritant.

☹ **Firming Eye Gel** *($17.50 for 0.5 ounce)* contains mostly water, witch hazel, soothing agents, plant extracts, thickeners, and preservatives. Witch hazel can be a skin irritant, and might create the appearance of firmer skin by partially swelling it.

☺ **Hydrating Eye Cream** *($22 for 0.5 ounce)* contains mostly water, glycerin, thickener, plant extract, water-binding agents, silicone oil, vitamins A and E, more thickeners, and preservatives. This would be a very good lightweight moisturizer for someone with dry to combination skin. The vitamins could be considered antioxidants.

☹ **Hydraspa Moisture Mist** *($8.75 for 4 ounces)* contains mostly water, water-binding agents, slip agents, soothing agents, vitamin E, plant extracts, and preservatives. Because this is a mist, most of the ingredients could evaporate before being absorbed into the skin. But it could feel temporarily soothing on the skin and provide some moisture.

☺ **$$$ Dual Delivery Fruit Acid Complex** *($28 for 1 ounce)* is about an 8% AHA product that contains mixed fruit acids. Most of the research on AHAs has been done on glycolic and lactic acids. Those are the types I recommend because of the information available. Although this might be a good AHA product, there is not enough data available to evaluate its AHAs. It is a lightweight AHA product in a good moisturizing base for someone with normal to combination skin.

☹ **Protective Sun Care SPF 15** *($8 for 4.2 ounces)* has a great SPF, but the third item on the ingredient list is a film former (PVP), a substance found in hairspray; it can be a skin irritant and cause breakouts.

☹ **Facial Mud** *($25 for 4.2 ounces)* is a standard clay mask with a handful of plant extracts and minerals thrown in for appearances. It contains witch hazel, which can be a skin irritant.

☹ **Natural Honey Almond Mask** *($22 for 4.2 ounces)* contains mostly honey and almond meal. It would be a good exfoliant for someone with normal to oily skin, but it could be irritating for some skin types.

Hydron (Skin Care Only)

Hydron is sold on QVC, and it is simply captivating to watch the host of the show swear by it while enthusiastic callers echo the sentiment. The presentation is *very* convincing, but before you pick up your phone and order, you need more information than just what the company wants you to know.

The Best Defense Collection by Hydron supposedly can restore your skin's natural moisture balance by creating a water-insoluble film over the surface of your skin. According to the company, "Hydron is a polymer, which is an extremely high-molecular-weight compound." That means it is too large to penetrate the skin, so it sits on top and covers the surface. This water-insoluble film also has water-binding properties, which are nice and can benefit dry skin, but the film is hardly miraculous or rare or the only way to keep water in the skin. Hydron itself is mostly a film former, a standard cosmetic ingredient found in hundreds of products; it has more in common with hairspray than anything else. In this way, Hydron can stay on the surface of the skin and not be affected by perspiration (just the way hairspray is not affected by humidity). Film-forming agents like the one in Hydron help keep water in the skin and can also give the appearance of smooth skin.

A new wrinkle in Hydron's advertising is its comparison of skin to rawhide. Skin cannot be compared to rawhide (nor to a dead leaf, contrary to a Pond's demonstration years ago on a dried-up oak leaf). The causes of wrinkling have nothing to do with dry skin. *Dry skin and wrinkles are not associated.* The Hydron ad demonstrates that oil does not provide water (moisture) to the skin; although that is true, it is not exactly shocking news. However, it does take oil or other water-binding agents to *keep* water in the skin. For dry skin, the issue is getting water to the skin and keeping it there. That process can be as simple as spraying the face with water before you use a moisturizer. (You don't need to spray expensive toners on your face; water will do, and the moisturizer will trap the water underneath.)

Although Hydron claims to be a unique water-delivery system, it is by no means the only one. It uses liposomes, which were developed by Lancome/L'Oreal more than 15 years ago. One more point: All of the ingredients listed on Hydron's products are completely standard. That doesn't make them bad, but they're not the skin sensation they claim to be.

☺ **Best Defense Gentle Cleansing Creme** *($16.50 for 6 ounces)* is supposedly a rinseable cleanser that contains mostly thickeners and a detergent cleansing agent. It can be a good cleanser for someone with normal to dry skin, but it can leave a film.

☺ **Best Defense Micro-Exfoliating Creme** *($16.75 for 3.6 ounces)* contains mostly water, thickeners, synthetic scrub agent, more thickeners, slip agent, detergent cleansing agent, and preservatives. It can be a good standard scrub for someone with dry skin.

☺ **Best Defense Botanical Toner** *($14.50 for 6.5 ounces)* contains mostly plant water, slip agents, water-binding agents, film former, detergent cleansing agent, and preservatives. There are plenty of plant extracts in it for people who believe that's important. If you are not allergic to plants, this would be a good nonirritating toner for most skin types.

☹ **Best Defense Tri-Activating Skin Clarifier** *($37.75 for 1 ounce)* is Hydron's version of an AHA product, but the ingredient list just says it contains sugarcane extracts, and doesn't tell you *what* has been extracted from the sugarcane. It sounds natural, but if you want to be certain you're getting an effective AHA product, look for glycolic or lactic acid on the ingredient list, not fruit or sugarcane extract.

☺ **$$$ Best Defense Facial Moisturizer Oil-Free with SPF 15** *($29 for 2 ounces)* contains mostly water, slip agent, aloe, film former, thickeners, water-binding agents, antioxidant, vitamins A and E, lanolin, and preservatives. It is indeed oil-free, but there are plenty of thickening agents (including lanolin) that can be a problem for someone with oily skin. Also, most of the interesting ingredients come at the end of the ingredient list. Still, this is a good moisturizing sunscreen for someone with normal to dry skin.

☺ **$$$ Best Defense Moisture Balance Restorative Overnight Liposome Complex** *($36 for 2 ounces)* contains mostly water, slip agent, aloe, plant oils, thickener, water-binding agents, more thickeners, more water-binding agents, film former, vitamins A and E, and preservatives. This would be a good emollient moisturizer for someone with dry skin.

☹ **Best Defense All Over Moisturizer Oil-Free** *($15.50 for 2.25 ounces)* contains mostly water, slip agents, alcohol, thickeners, film former, lanolin, and preservatives. This may indeed be oil-free, but it contains lanolin and isopropyl palmitate, which can be a problem for someone with oily skin. This would be appropriate only for someone with normal to dry skin.

☺ **$$$ Best Defense Fragile Eye Moisturizer** *($26 for 0.5 ounce)* contains mostly water, slip agent, aloe, thickener, water-binding agents, more thickeners, plant oil, more water-binding agents, film former, vitamins A and E, more thickeners, and preservatives. This is a good emollient moisturizer that can be used all over the face, not just around the eyes. What a shame you get so little for so much money.

☹ **$$$ Best Defense Five-Minute Revitalizing Masque** *($24 for 2.65 ounces)* is a standard clay mask that also contains plant extracts, glycerin, thickeners, silicone oil, and preservatives. The plant extracts include eucalyptus, balm mint, pine needle, sage, and thyme, all potential skin irritants. The mask also contains some water-binding agents and a detergent cleansing agent. The water-binding agents are nice, but the detergent cleansing agent is sodium lauryl sulfate, which can be a skin irritant.

Il Makiage (Makeup Only)

A lot of you have been watching QVC lately, haven't you? How can I tell? I've received an number of queries about the makeup-only line Il Makiage, which is sold primarily through TV. Il Makiage attempts to market itself as the makeup artists' makeup line, but it isn't my kind of cosmetics line, nor is it that of many of the other professional makeup artists I've worked with. It does offer a large range of matte blushes in a wonderful range of colors, as well as matte eyeshadows in a nice selection of neutral shades that have a great texture and blend easily. Unfortunately, the foundations are poor, the mascara doesn't build any length or thickness no matter how much you put on, the brushes are mostly just OK, and the concealers are heavy and greasy and tend to crease.

A special feature of the Il Makiage color line is an assortment of makeup kits that are quite attractive and convenient, but should nevertheless be avoided for the same reason

I advise against buying sets of eyeshadow: not all of the items and colors will be appropriate for you. Apart from my feelings about the quality of the products, it is incredibly risky to buy color cosmetics from a brochure or a television show. At the very least you need to see, and preferably try on, foundations and lipsticks, and often blushes and eyeshadows too. If you are in an area where Il Makiage is sold through a hair salon or spa, you may want to consider checking it out. To find a location near you, call (800) 722-1011.

☺ FOUNDATION: **Liquid Foundation** *($15)*, **Creme Foundation** *($30)*, and **Dual Finish Foundation** *($25)* are products I can't recommend because of the risk involved when you can't try them on. You are taking a shot in the dark. Getting the foundation wrong is a grievous error in makeup application. If I were you, I wouldn't risk it.

☹ **Even Tones** *($10.50)* are standard color correctors that are supposed to be worn under foundation to even out skin tone. Almost without exception, foundation does a fine job of evening out skin tone (especially when the foundation matches your skin exactly). This adds an unnecessary layer of makeup, and the effect isn't very convincing anyway.

☹ CONCEALER: **TV Touch Concealer** *($12)* and **TV Touch Compact Combination** *($24 for two colors)* are too heavy and greasy for everyday use. The colors are interesting, but I suspect the pink, yellow, violet, and rose shades are for corrective use, a technique that really isn't used anymore (at least not in any of the TV makeup rooms I've been in over the past several years).

☺ POWDER: **Translucent Face Powder** *($14)* is a standard talc-based powder that has a soft texture and goes on fairly translucent. There are some strange colors, such as a vivid pink and a deep lavender, but also some good neutral ones. Again, because you can't see or try it before you buy it, you could end up having to send it back.

☺ BLUSH: **Color Rouge** *($12)* comes in a large assortment of attractive matte colors that go on soft but can still build good depth for darker skin tones.

☺ EYESHADOW: **Color Shadow** *($12)* is available in some great neutral matte colors, but there are also glaring shades of blue, green, and orange, and some iridescent choices. The matte neutral shades are all worth checking out; they go on very soft and blend easily.

☹ EYE AND BROW SHAPER: **Cake Eye Liner** *($12)* is just what it says: a cake eyeliner that creates the perfect Marilyn Monroe look (shades of the early '60s!). The line looks quite dramatic and is surprisingly easy to apply. **Brow Set** *($12)* is little more than bottled hairspray with a brush, but it will keep brows in place. **Jumbo Pencils** *($9.50)* are hard to sharpen, and the color selection for these are poor.

☺ **Slim Pencils** *($9.50)*, for lips, eyes, and brows, are standard pencils that go on easily without being too greasy. Color selection is limited, but all of the shades (except for the vivid blue) are quite good.

☺ **LIPSTICK AND LIP PENCIL: Lipstick** *($12)* comes in four types: creams, iridescents, sheers, and mattes. The creams have a nice texture but can be slightly greasy; the iridescents are just that and are also on the greasy side; the sheers are more like gloss; and the mattes, though quite matte, come in only five shades, all of which are rather dark. These are all just OK and not particularly exciting. **Lip Gloss** *($9)* is very glossy and comes in a nice range of colors.

☺ **MASCARA: Mascara** *($12)* doesn't smear, but it also doesn't build any length or thickness.

☺ **SPECIALTY PRODUCTS: Summer, Fall, Winter,** and **Spring Face Kits** *($55)* offer very nice blush and eyeshadow colors, but the lipstick is in an open spot in the middle and the concealer is in an open spot on the side. Every time you put a brush into the blush or eyeshadow, it gets all over the lipstick and concealer. Also, the likelihood that you will use all the products is slim.

☺ **Model Kit** *($80)* comes in three different color groupings: Neutral Light, Neutral Dark, and Mauve. You will probably be disappointed with what you get for this price: a tiny concealer, small brushes, a lip pencil, an eye pencil, mascara, a fairly glossy lipstick (in a tiny pot, so it is inconvenient), four matte eyeshadows, two shiny eyeshadows, two blushes, and a black cake eyeliner. The matte eyeshadows are nice, but the blushes are just OK, I never recommend shiny eyeshadows, the mascara is not the best, and the brushes are only passable.

☺ **Lip Kit** *($50)* offers a good selection of little pots of color. They are all on the greasy side, but if you like playing with a lot of different colors and don't have a problem with lipstick bleeding, this just may be an option.

Iman

Only a handful of women are known by their first name alone: they include Madonna, Cher, Ann-Margret, and, of course, the exquisite, regal Iman. Considered a classic Ethiopian beauty, Iman broke the color line, along with model Beverly Johnson, gracing the covers of fashion magazines that had previously deemed black women unacceptable as cover models. She also became known for her social life as part of Europe's and New York's jet set (with David Bowie as her escort). Although on the surface she appears imperious and removed, in recent years she has been active in food and aid relief for her war-torn, impoverished homeland, and has fought for the rights of Ethiopian women regarding the horror of female circumcision. Iman is no ordinary woman.

Venturing into the world of makeup seems a natural for this elegant, savvy aristocrat. And in some areas Iman has achieved breakthroughs that other cosmetics lines could learn from. Regrettably, her line loses considerable ground with its skin care products, called Liquid Assets. Whoever put these products together for her doesn't seem to have had a plan, or to have realized that different skin types exist. The cleansers are disappointing, the toners are mediocre, the AHA product is limited, and the oil-free products contain ingredients that can cause breakouts. Additionally, not one of the daytime moisturizers contains sunscreen, even though women of color are also subject to sun damage. In fact, sun damage is often responsible for darker skin tones becoming ashen, and lighter-skinned women of color run a risk of skin cancer. Like most of the skin care lines glutting the cosmetics market right now, these products have the requisite plant extracts. But don't get too excited if you're a consumer who thinks plant extracts are what good skin care is all about; most of the green stuff comes after the preservatives, which means there isn't much.

Iman's line excels when it comes to her color collection. Most of the blush, eyeshadow, and lip colors are stunning, with a majority of matte neutral shades in a wide variety of tones that don't include blues, greens, or purples. These products are appropriate for a wide range of skin colors, from Asian to Latin and all shades of African-American skin.

Iman Skin Care

☺ **Gentle Cleansing Lotion** (*$12.50 for 3 ounces*) is a standard detergent cleanser that would be best for someone with normal to oily skin. The primary detergent cleansing agent can be a potential skin irritant.

☹ **Cleansing Bar with Grapefruit Normal/Oily Skin Formula** (*$8.50 for 3.5 ounces*) is a standard detergent-based cleansing bar that contains tallow along with some plants and grapefruit. The grapefruit supposedly makes it good for oily skin types, although there isn't much in this bar. (If there were, it would be a skin irritant. Ever get grapefruit juice on an open cut? Ouch.) Also, tallow can cause breakouts. I don't recommend soap; however, if you have a penchant for it, there are better, gentler, tallow-free soaps on the market.

☹ **Cleansing Bar with Rose Petal** *($8.50 for 3.5 ounces)* is almost identical to the Cleansing Bar with Grapefruit (including the grapefruit), and the same review applies.

☺ **Eye Makeup Remover with Aloe Vera** *($10 for 3 ounces)* contains mostly water, slip agents, detergent cleansing agents, and preservatives. This is a good, extremely standard eye makeup remover, but wiping off makeup anywhere on the face is a problem for the skin.

☺ **Skin Refresher Lotion** *($12.50 for 3 ounces)* contains mostly water, slip agents, plant extract, plant oil, menthol, soothing agent, aloe, more plant extracts, and preservatives. It may be OK for someone with normal to oily skin, but only passably. The orange oil and menthol can irritate skin.

☺ **All Day Moisture Complex** *($12.50 for 3 ounces)* is an ordinary emollient moisturizer for someone with dry skin. It contains mostly water, slip agent, thickeners, plant oil, more thickeners, preservatives, plant extracts, and vitamins. The plants, vitamins, and interesting water-binding agents come well after the preservatives, which means only minimal amounts are present. Besides, since this is a daytime moisturizer, it would be best if it had some sunscreen, preferably SPF 15.

☺ **Oil-Free Advanced Moisture** *($15 for 3 ounces)* is indeed oil-free, but it contains isopropyl myristate (fourth on the ingredient list) and shea butter, both known to cause breakouts. Neither is great for oily to combination skin.

☺ **Nighttime Complex Oil-Free Moisturizer** *($20 for 1.8 ounces)* is almost identical to the moisturizer above, only thicker and more expensive, and the same review applies.

☺ **Undercover Agent Oil-Control Lotion** *($15 for 1 ounce)* is a liquid version of Phillips' Milk of Magnesia that uses magnesium aluminum silicate instead of magnesium carbonate to absorb oil. It will do the trick, but it also contains balm mint and camphor, which can be skin irritants. It might be worth trying if you have very oily skin, but I would go for the Milk of Magnesia first.

☺ **PM Renewal Cream** *($20 for 1.8 ounces)* is a very good emollient moisturizer for someone with very dry skin. It contains mostly water, thickeners, safflower oil, wax, slip agent, more thickeners, lanolin, castor oil, vitamin E, plant extracts, and preservatives.

☺ **Eye Firming Cream with Cucumber** *($15 for 0.5 ounce)* won't firm anything, but it is a good, ordinary emollient moisturizer for someone with normal to dry skin. It contains water, thickeners, castor oil, silicone oil, and preservatives. There are plants (including cucumber) and vitamins in it, but they come after the preservatives, meaning there isn't enough worth mentioning.

☺ **$$$ Instant Replay AHA Perfecting Lotion** *($35 for 1 ounce)* has about a 4% concentration of AHA. It isn't going to perfect anything, but it is an OK AHA product for someone with dry, sensitive skin. However, it can't hold a candle to Alpha Hydrox, which you can get for a fraction of this one's cost.

☺ **Perfection Even-Tone Fade Cream** *($20 for 2 ounces)* is a standard 2% hydroquinone product in a good emollient base. It's fairly expensive, considering that similar products (many with 8% AHA, a higher percentage that helps increase the effectiveness of the hydroquinone) sell for a lot less.

Iman Makeup

☹ **FOUNDATION: Second to None Cream to Powder Foundation** *($17.50)* doesn't feel anything like a cream or a powder; it feels more like spackle. It does blend out thin, but not easily. The colors would be worth checking out if the texture weren't so exceedingly thick and heavy. What a shame!

☺ **Second to None Oil-Free Makeup with SPF 8** *($17.50)* has a very matte, dry finish, and would work well for someone with oily to combination skin. It is by far a better option than the Cream to Powder Foundation above. **These colors are excellent:** Sand 1, Sand 2, Sand 3, Sand 4, Sand 5, Earth 1, Earth 2, Earth 3, Earth 4, Earth 5, Clay 1, Clay 3, Clay 4, and Clay 5. **These colors are too peach or red:** Clay 2 and Earth 6.

☹ **CONCEALER: Corrective Concealer Camouflage** *($12)* goes on very dry and thick. If you have any lines under the eye, this concealer will make them look worse. However, it doesn't slip into the lines, so there is no creasing. If you don't have lines this could be an option.

☺ **POWDER: Luxury Pressed Powder Oil-Controlling** *($15)* is a talc-based powder that has a great range of colors and a smooth, silky, even texture.

☺ **BLUSH: Blush** *($15)* comes in a spectacular array of colors, is a pleasure to apply, and has great staying potential. However, the texture can be too dry for someone with dry skin.

☺ **EYESHADOW: Eyeshadow** *($10)* comes in an incredible array of matte neutral eyeshadow colors. **These colors are wonderful for all skin tones:** Apple, Cedar Chip, Mahogany, Vanilla, Chili, Cocoa, Brazil Nut, Almond, Walnut, Cashew, Oak, Plum, Raspberry, Grape, Iris, Orchid, Wisteria, Onyx, Pearl. **These eyeshadow are too shiny:** Nutmeg, Twigs, Violet, and Tiger Eye.

☺ **EYE AND BROW SHAPER:** The standard **Perfect Eye Pencils** *($8.50)* come in a nice range of colors and have a good dry texture that goes on easily. **Perfect Brow Pencil** *($8.50)* comes in three colors and is virtually identical to the Eye Pencils.

☺ **LIPSTICK AND LIP PENCIL:** Most of the **Luxury Moisturizing Lip Colors** *($10)* are stunning, with a wide range of matte neutral shades and a wonderful creamy but matte finish. Avoid the frosted ones, which are exceedingly greasy. **Perfect Lip Pencil** *($8.50)* comes in a nice array of colors and has a smooth, slightly creamy texture.

☹ **MASCARA:** **Perfect Mascara** *($12)* isn't perfect. It does go on easily and builds lashes quickly, but it tends to smear during the day.

Jafra

Regardless of the in-home line of products you choose to try out, each makeup/skin care demonstration begins the same way. An array of products is set in front of you, and a presentation placard of information is placed next to the salesperson or, to use the preferred term, beauty consultant. ("Beauty" isn't often the operative word, but "sales" always is. The sales force for these lines is not composed of skin care or makeup experts, but of salespeople trained to sell you products. That's fine, but you don't want to rely on them for "expert" advice.) You are then taken through a rather fun, hands-on demonstration of product usage after your skin type has been assessed. Of course, skin typing is almost always hit-or-miss, but I'll get to that in a minute. The skin care routine generally involves a minimum of six products and, more often than not, "if you really want great skin," an average of ten products. Once your face is clean and loaded up with several moisturizers, including an exfoliator, "firming" gel, protective cream, and eye lotion, the makeup application begins.

Jafra's routine is no exception, although this just as accurately describes the techniques of Mary Kay, Shaklee, Amway, and all the others. Like its peers, Jafra offers some products that are great, some that are good, some that are bad, and some that are really bad.

Jafra has been around for almost 40 years and is now a subsidiary of Gillette. The salespeople are not involved in a pyramid or multilevel selling plan. (If a consultant sponsors at least seven other people who become consultants, he or she is given an extra commission direct from the company.) No consultant makes less on commission than any other consultant, although harder work nets more money direct from the company. In that way, the pay structure is much like that of Mary Kay.

What is unique to Jafra is the way its salespeople determine skin type. They have a cute little machine called a Skin Programmer. It supposedly measures the moisture level of the skin by assessing its electrical conductivity. You hold a metal cylinder in one hand while the salesperson holds a plastic handle with a metal tip on your face. You don't feel a thing, but a very small electrical charge is generated. How long it takes that electrical charge to complete its circuit—from your cheek or chin to your hand—rates a number. The theory is that the less water (moisture) you have in your skin, the slower the electrical charge; the more water in your skin, the faster the electrical charge. Unfortunately, it only *sounds* good. It doesn't really tell you much about the true condition of your skin. There is so much room for error, it's almost a joke. The way your skin registers an electrical current will be different depending on the time of day, what skin care products you have on, and even the weather. My skin was rated as normal to dry. I explained that I've never had dry skin in my life. I was told that my skin may look oily, but it is only compensating for the dry skin underneath.

That would be fine if oil production worked that way, but it doesn't. If it did, women with dry skin would automatically have oily skin too, since their oil glands would react to the state of dryness, but oil is not activated by the amount of dry skin you have. Oil production seems to be genetically determined, although it can be increased by irritation.

My skin hasn't seen a dry flake since I stopped using astringents, toners, and soap over 15 years ago. But I received more emollient products than you could imagine during my Jafra demonstration, and I left looking and feeling like one big grease ball. Over the next several days, I broke out. Moreover, the number of products the salespeople recommended was astounding. It still amazes me when I see how women are encouraged to pile products on their faces in hopes of firming, toning, moisturizing, and protecting the skin. You would do much better to follow the skin-type suggestions in Jafra's brochures, which are standard and pretty much right on, and ignore the output of the Skin Programmer.

Jafra's color collection has a few fairly interesting selections. It is a rather straight-forward line, with all the basics and some good options for a wide range of skin tones. The color line is divided into Warm, Cool, and Neutral, which is helpful, except that some of the Neutrals tend to be warm rather than truly neutral.

Jafra Skin Care

☺ **Cleansing Lotion for Dry to Normal Skin** *($10.50 for 8.4 ounces)* is an oil-based cleanser that needs to be wiped off and can leave skin feeling greasy. I never recommend wiping off makeup for any skin type, and assuredly not for someone with normal skin.

☹ **Cleansing Lotion for Normal to Oily Skin** *($10.50 for 8.4 ounces)* is meant to be wiped off with a washcloth, which is essential, because it won't come off with simple splashing, as any self-respecting water-soluble cleanser should, especially one for oily skin. This cleanser leaves skin feeling greasy, which is not great for someone with oily skin.

☺ **Cleansing Cream for Dry Skin** *($10.50 for 4.2 ounces)* is a thicker version of the lotion above; the same review applies, but even more so.

☺ **Gentle Exfoliating Scrub for All Skin Types** *($11 for 2.5 ounces)* is indeed gentle, but also fairly greasy. It contains standard synthetic scrub particles, plus several plant oils and other emollient thickeners that make it very hard to rinse off. It can leave a greasy film on the skin.

☺ **Eye Makeup Remover Gel** *($7.75 for 0.75 ounce)* is a mineral oil–based eye makeup remover. Using it is pretty much like using plain mineral oil, except that it's in a gel form. It's still mostly mineral oil, effective but greasy. Plain mineral oil is cheaper.

☺ **Skin Freshener for Dry to Normal Skin** *($11.50 for 8.4 ounces)* contains mostly water, water-binding agent, witch hazel, rose water, plant oils, soothing agent, and preservatives. Witch hazel and sandalwood oil (one of the plant oils) can both be skin irritants.

☹ **Skin Freshener for Normal to Oily Skin** *($11.50 for 8.4 ounces)* contains a lot of alcohol, which can dry and irritate the skin (causing it to become more oily). It also contains plant oils, the last thing somebody with oily skin would want on her face.

☹ **Day Cream Moisturizer for Dry to Normal Skin SPF 6** *($13.50 for 1.7 ounces)* is inadequate for protection from sun damage.

☹ **Day Lotion for Normal to Oily Skin SPF 6** *($13.50 for 4.2 ounces)* is inadequate for protection from sun damage.

☺ **Night Cream Moisturizer for Dry to Normal Skin** *($13.50 for 1.7 ounces)* contains mostly water, several thickeners, slip agent, silicone oils, more thickeners, several water-binding agents, soothing agents, and preservatives. Someone with normal skin will probably find this too emollient, but it is a good moisturizer for someone with dry skin.

☺ **Night Cream for Normal to Oily Skin** *($13.50 for 1.7 ounces)* contains mostly water, slip agents, film former, silicone oils, water-binding agents, soothing agent, thickeners, plant oil, vitamin E, and preservatives. Women with oily skin could find themselves with clogged pores and more oil than they started out with, but it could be a good moisturizer for normal to dry skin types.

☺ **Refreshing Moisture Mask for Dry and Dry to Normal Skin** *($11 for 2.5 ounces)* contains mostly water, plant oil, several thickeners, clay, more plant oils, slip agents, water-binding agents, minuscule amounts of plant extracts, vitamin E, and preservatives. Although I'm not one to recommend clay masks for dry skin, this one contains such a small amount of clay that it would be quite a good emollient mask.

☹ **Deep Cleansing Mask for Normal to Oily Skin** *($11 for 2.5 ounces)* is a fairly standard clay-based mask that also contains a small amount of plant oil, silicone oil, plant extracts, and lots of thickening agents. This would be an OK clay mask for someone with normal to dry skin. However, someone with oily skin would not be pleased with any amount of oil or with the emollient thickeners this mask contains.

☺ **Extra Care Cream Unscented** *($6 for 0.5 ounce)* contains mostly petrolatum, mineral oil, thickeners, plant oil, and preservatives. This is a very emollient moisturizer for someone with very dry skin.

☹ **Rediscover Alpha Hydroxy Complex** *($28 for 1 ounce)* contains several fruit extracts, but there is no way of knowing what they are. As I've mentioned throughout this book, although alpha hydroxy acids are derived from fruit, there are innumerable fruit extracts that have nothing to do with AHAs. This product also contains lavender oil, which can make the skin sensitive to sun exposure.

☺ **$$$ Skin Firming Complex** *($28 for 1 ounce)* contains mostly water, several water-binding agents, thickeners, soothing agent, silicone oil, and preservatives. This would be a very good lightweight moisturizer for someone with normal to oily skin.

☹ **Time Protector Moisture System** *($34 for 1.7 ounce)* isn't appropriate for daytime use because SPF 6 isn't enough to adequately protect skin from sun damage.

☺ **Eye Revitalizing Concentrate** *($14 for 0.75 ounce)* contains mostly water, thickeners, plant oil, more thickeners, several water-binding agents, and preservatives. This is a good emollient moisturizer for someone with normal to dry skin.

☺ **Sunblock Cream SPF 15** *($10.50 for 4.2 ounces)* is the only SPF 15 product in the entire Jafra line; all the other products with sunscreen are SPF 8 or less. This one can definitely protect from the sun, but it would work only for someone with dry skin.

☹ **$$$ Royal Jelly Milk Balm Moisture Lotion** *($60 for 1 ounce)* contains mostly water, several thickeners, royal jelly, more thickeners, water-binding agents, and preservatives. You may be wondering why this otherwise standard moisturizer sells for $60 an ounce. Jafra touts royal jelly as a miracle ingredient. The salesperson told me it could heal burns, get rid of scars, and erase wrinkles. It sure sounds like a miracle. Is it? Well, bee larvae who get fed *fresh* royal jelly turn into queen bees. But if you try to sneak *stored* royal jelly into them, they don't turn into queens. Does this tell you anything about royal jelly and its effectiveness on the skin? Absolutely not. There is no evidence that royal jelly has any benefit to the skin.

Jafra Makeup

☺ <u>FOUNDATION:</u> There are two types of foundation in the Jafra line: **Supertone Moisturizing Makeup SPF 6** *($11.25)* and **Supertone Makeup Oil Controlling SPF 6** *($11.25)*. SPF 6 is a poor choice as far as really protecting the skin from sun damage, but these two foundations are quite good at providing even, light to medium coverage, and the color selection is very good. **These are the only colors to avoid:** Ivory Beige and Rose Beige, which can be too rose for most skin types, and Peach Beige, which is too peach for all skin types.

☹ <u>CONCEALER:</u> **Cream Concealer** *($8)* comes in a stick form, with three rather mediocre colors: Fair is too pink for most skin tones, Medium is too peach, and Dark, although neutral, isn't all that dark and would be appropriate only for medium skin tones. The texture is somewhat thick and heavy, and it does tend to crease.

☺ **White Souffle** *($8)* is a liquid concealer that is indeed white, but it goes on very subtly, requiring just a tiny bit to lighten a shadow under the eye or along the corners of the mouth or nose. It is appropriate only for use over or under foundation.

☺ <u>POWDER:</u> **Pressed Powder** *($11.25)* is a standard talc-based powder with a soft but dry texture; it comes in three colors: Fair is too pink for most skin tones, Medium can be too peach for most skin tones, and Dark is an excellent color, although not all that dark. **Moisturizing Translucent Face Powder** *($11.25)* is not the least bit moisturizing. It has a very drying, granular texture, although the finish is indeed translucent.

☺ <u>BLUSH:</u> **Powder Blush** *($11)* has a great soft texture and blends on smoothly and evenly. All of the colors are great, including a basic selection for darker skin tones (a couple have a slight amount of shine that doesn't show up much on the face), and Terra-cotta, Desert, and Copper Blaze are excellent contour colors. **Water Colour Blushing Gel** *($4)* is a tube of liquid tint that tends to stain the cheek. It is tricky to blend, and once it's on, it's on, but it can give a soft even blush to the cheek if you have a knack for blending. It comes in only three colors.

☺ <u>EYESHADOW:</u> All of Jafra's eyeshadows come packaged in **Eyeshadow Trios** *($12.50)*. The line simply does not sell single eyeshadow colors, which is disappointing. Some of the combinations are best described as too weird or too shiny.

However, despite the fact that I think buying sets of three is a great way to waste money (you rarely use all of the colors), there are a handful of surprisingly neutral, workable groupings. **These are good matte color combinations:** Bazaar, Kashmir, Mirage, Camouflage, and Spice.

☺ <u>EYE AND BROW SHAPER:</u> **Eye and Brow Pencils** *($7.25)* are standard pencils just like the majority of pencils sold by most cosmetics lines. There is a nice array of colors, but some are shiny or too blue and green. **Liquid Eyeliner** *($7.50)* is a standard tube liner that goes on dramatically and tends not to chip or flake.

☺ <u>LIPSTICK:</u> I was surprised how much I liked Jafra's **Lasting Lip Color** *($7.50)*, because it really lasted and tended not to feather into the lines around the mouth, and the color choices are beautiful. **Moisturizing Lipstick SPF 6** *($7.50)* is more glossy than creamy, which means it doesn't last very long. Also, the color selection isn't as good as the Lasting Lip Color, and SPF 6 isn't much in the way of sun protection. An emollient, almost sticky **Lip Gloss** *($6)* comes in six shades, most of them shiny and recommended only for evening. Standard **Lip Pencils** *($7.25)*, identical to the eye pencils, come in a small but attractive color selection.

☹ <u>MASCARA:</u> **Creme Mascara** *($7)* doesn't smudge or clump, but it also doesn't build much length or thickness. You could apply this mascara for hours and never see any major changes in your eyelashes. If you have lashes that are already long and thick and you only want to add some color, this might be the mascara for you; otherwise, it would just be frustrating.

☹ <u>BRUSHES:</u> There is nothing professional about Jafra's **Professional Cosmetic Brush Collection** *($27)*. The eyeshadow brushes are too sparse, too soft, and too small to work on most eyes. The blush brush is OK, but too floppy and soft to hold the color well and control placement.

☺ **Deluxe Face Powder Brush** *($10.50)* is nice enough and feels soft on the skin, which is great for a powder brush.

Jane (Makeup Only)

See Dick run. See Jane run. See Jane get a cosmetics line named after her. I received many requests asking me to review the small line of makeup products simply called Jane, available in drugstores. It was clear from the brochures accompanying its display that Jane is aimed at teenagers. Bright young faces bemoaned the beauty problems of adolescence and found cute makeup and skin care solutions. For example, one pamphlet examined the reasons for wearing makeup with these probing fill-in-the-blank questions:

"Is looking cute the best way to get a guy?" or "How can I look older?" Inside were these answers: "Looking cute doesn't hurt. But if that's all it took to get and keep a boyfriend, we'd all be in deep doo-doo." And "Why do you want to look older? If you're trying to get into a real hip club, a little lipstick will definitely make you look like you've been there before."

The brochures might be directed at teenagers and the product line's name may have been chosen to appeal to them, but the simple black packaging, neutral colors, and vivid, creamy lipstick colors seem to be much more in alignment with what adults would be interested in. The prices are more than reasonable, and many of the colors are appropriate for a wide range of skin tones, but I get the feeling you won't be able to find these products much longer because adults will discover they don't quite live up to all their needs, and they aren't what most teens are looking for either.

☺ **FOUNDATION: Oil-Free Foundation** *($2.99)* isn't oil-free (it contains silicone oil, and a lot of it), so the color tends to separate as you blend it on. What a shame, because there are some great neutral colors.

☺ **True to You Sheer Finish Foundation** *($2.99)* has a rather good range of neutral colors and a nice, smooth texture that goes on quite sheer and matte. There are generally no testers, and I rarely recommend foundations you can't try on before buying. Sometimes they sell small samples, and you can take advantage of that to find a great color that matches your skin exactly.

☹ **CONCEALER: No Show Concealer** *($2.29)* comes in stick form, but has a surprisingly satiny texture. It comes in three decent colors and has a slight tendency to slip into the lines around the eyes as the day goes by, although it's not as bad as most (it isn't a problem if you don't have any lines, so it just depends on how old you are).

☺ **Clueless Two Way Concealer** *($2.29)* is surprisingly good, with soft coverage, good staying power, and little to no slippage into the lines around the eyes. The color choices are limited, but work well.

☺ **POWDER: Oil-Free Finishing Powder** *($2.29)* has a soft, silky, dry texture and goes on quite sheer and even. It comes in an attractive assortment of neutral colors.

☺ **BLUSH: Blushing Cheeks** *($2.29)* offers a good, muted, matte color selection, and all the shades go on fairly smooth and even.

☹ **EYESHADOW: Eyeshadows** *($2.29)* are all slightly iridescent and shiny, which might be good for someone under 18, but it isn't best for anyone who wants a more sophisticated look and doesn't want to accentuate wrinkles.

☺ **EYE AND BROW SHAPER:** The fairly standard **Eye and Brow Pencils** *($2.29)* go on well without being greasy, and are an option regardless of age. Of course, brow powders or eyeshadows are preferable.

☹ **LIPSTICK AND LIP PENCIL: Satin Lipstick** *($2.29)* is probably too creamy for teens and too greasy for adults; the colors are good, but the texture can be a problem. **Shimmer Lipstick** *($2.29)* is simply Satin Lipstick with frost. **Sheer Lipstick** *($2.29)* is more like a gloss than a lipstick, but it is nice sheer color for a teenager. **Matte Lipstick** *($2.29)* is nice and creamy but not the least bit matte; it doesn't feel any different from the Satin Lipstick.

☺ **One Liners Lip Liners** *($2.99)* come in a twist-up container, so they don't require sharpening, plus they have a wonderful smooth texture and a great color selection. **Shaping Sticks** *($2.29)* are standard pencils with a great texture, not too dry and not too greasy, that come in a nice assortment of colors.

☺ **MASCARA: Flashes Ultra Rich Mascara** *($2.29)* is surprisingly good; it goes on fast, building thick, even lashes with little to no smearing.

☹ **BRUSHES:** Jane's brushes aren't awful, they are just the wrong shape. The eyeshadow brushes are all too small or too thin, while the powder and blush brushes are soft enough but not the best size.

Jergens (Skin Care Only)

☹ **All-Purpose Face Cream** *($2.79 for 6 ounces)* is definitely all-purpose; it's also fairly greasy and thick. It contains mostly mineral oil, water, thickeners, and fragrance. It would be OK for someone with dry skin, but only minimally so.

☹ **Naturals Soap with Aloe & Lanolin for Normal to Dry Skin** *($1.89 for 9.5 ounces)* is a standard tallow-based bar soap that also contains some lanolin. The lanolin won't undo the drying effect of the soap or prevent the breakouts tallow can cause.

☹ **Naturals Soap with Vitamin E & Chamomile for Sensitive Skin** *($1.89 for 9.5 ounces)* is almost identical to the soap above, and the same review applies. Nothing about this soap makes it appropriate for sensitive skin.

☹ **Naturals Soap with Baking Soda** *($1.89 for 9.5 ounces)* is almost identical to the soaps above, and the same review applies.

☺ **Advanced Therapy Lotion, Aloe Enriched** *($2.75 for 10 ounces)* contains mostly water, glycerin, thickeners, aloe, lanolin, silicone oil, mineral oil, more thickeners, and preservatives. This very emollient moisturizer would be good for someone with dry to very dry skin.

☺ **Advanced Therapy Lotion Daily Care Moisturizer with Original Scent** *($2.75 for 10 ounces)* is similar to the lotion above, and the same review applies.

☺ **Advanced Therapy Lotion, Dry Skin Care with Vitamin E & Lanolin** *($2.75 for 10 ounces)* is similar to the lotions above, and the same review applies.

☺ **Advanced Therapy Lotion, Light Care** *($2.75 for 10 ounces)* is similar to the lotions above, and the same review applies.

☺ **Advanced Therapy Lotion, Ultra Healing Extra Dry Skin Treatment** *($2.75 for 10 ounces)* contains mostly water, glycerin, thickener, petrolatum, mineral oil, more thickeners, soothing agent, silicone oils, and preservatives. This is a good moisturizer for someone with very dry skin, but nothing in it makes it ultra-healing.

☺ **Advanced Therapy Dual Healing Cream** *($4.29 for 4 ounces)* is similar to the lotion above, and the same review applies.

☹ **Ever Soft Dry Skin Lotion** *($5.29 for 10 ounces)* is similar to most other Jergens products, only with aluminum starch as the third item on the ingredient list. This thickening agent can cause breakouts and allergic reactions.

☺ **Replenaderm Moisturizing Therapy Cream** *($5.60 for 4 ounces)* contains mostly water, silicone oils, glycerin, thickeners, slip agent, more thickeners, soothing agent, a tiny amount of AHAs, and preservatives. This is a good moisturizer for someone with dry skin, but a poor AHA product.

☺ **Replenaderm Moisturizing Therapy Lotion** *($6.79 for 8 ounces)* is similar to the cream above, and the same review applies.

Joan Simmons Brushes

Imagine a tailor without a sewing machine or a needle and thread, or a stockbroker without a computer and *The Wall Street Journal*. Every task requires appropriate tools in order to perform the labor properly. Applying makeup is no different. Using professional-size brushes is the only way to apply makeup successfully, period. The little sponge-tip applicators, tiny blush brushes, and scratchy eyebrow brushes that come with cosmetics are a total waste and serve no purpose for professional makeup application. Joan Simmons Brushes *($5 to $13)* are as good an option as you will find for professional-size brushes, and they are reasonably priced. I have found these brushes at major department stores all over the country. Look for them at Nordstrom, Macy's, Saks, or any upper-end department store in your area.

There are more than a dozen brushes, and most are very good, but some are positively a waste of money. **Foundation Applicator** *($7)* has a big sponge on one end of the handle. Although the idea isn't bad, a thin round hand-held sponge is easier to use and a fraction of the price. **Lash Whirly** *($5)* is a dry mascara brush meant to separate the lashes if they clump together. You could easily take an old mascara brush, wash it, and use it instead for free. **Blush Blender** *($7)* is a flat-edged, severely shaped brush that can't blend blush well at all. The best it can do is stripe on the color. All of the other brushes are superior and, depending on your makeup needs, worth a closer look. Call (212) 675-3136 to find out if these brushes are distributed in your area.

Kiehl's Since 1851 (Skin Care Only)

How did this very expensive, remote skin care line become so well known? Especially when you consider that the company doesn't advertise (although it does have a PR firm that handles its press relations). Obviously, there are ways to create attention without advertising, as several other cosmetics companies have proven.

As the company's name implies, the line has been around for quite some time; it has its origins in a family-owned pharmacy. Still, the products hardly warrant excitement or even mild enthusiasm. Most of them are surprisingly ordinary, with a dusting of natural ingredients almost always at the very end of the ingredient list, well past the preservatives. That amounts to little more than a token attempt to make the products appear more natural to consumers, who want to believe a plant or vitamin must somehow be better for the skin than something that sounds more chemical. Nevertheless, that token amount is enough to allow Kiehl's to brag about how its products nourish the skin or are more environmentally friendly, even though that may only be true for less than 1 percent of the product's content.

Of course, those who know better understand that vitamins can't nourish the skin; that using nonfat milk and plant extracts means the amount of preservative in a product must be increased to prevent deterioration; and that while plant oils may be moisturizing, they are not wonder ingredients.

The company's most interesting claim is that its products are all made by hand, just the way they were when the original Kiehl's pharmacy began selling cosmetics in 1851. Today, given the wide distribution of Kiehl's products—they are available at Bergdorf Goodman, Neiman Marcus, Barneys, Harrods, and many other stores—that claim is extremely hard to swallow. The person I talked to at Kiehl's said each product is made the way I would make a cake. But I've never baked thousands of cakes at once, or baked one cake that could serve thousands of people. I can't stir 100 pounds of flour and water; how can someone stir 100 pounds of water and waxes? Yes, it's all hand-stirred, she insisted. Even if that were true, which I strongly doubt, what extra benefit is there to hand-stirring a cosmetic anyway? It's just more personal, she said; there's better control. It may *sound* more personal, but the possibility of error or contamination is much greater.

Regardless of how the products are processed, the bottom line is, Can they do what they claim and are they worth the money? In this case, the products consist of totally ordinary ingredients, despite the fact that they are called special or natural. Many ingredients are questionable for sensitive skin types and in some instances would be irritating for any skin type.

☺ **Oil-Based Cleanser and Makeup Remover** *($10.50 for 4 ounces)* at least has an honest name. This very greasy cleanser needs to be wiped off like cold cream and can leave a film on the face. The second ingredient is isopropyl myristate, notorious for causing breakouts. The cleanser also contains lanolin oil, which is emollient but can be a problem for sensitive skin types.

☺ **Ultra Moisturizing Cleansing Cream** *($16.95 for 8 ounces)* contains mostly water, thickeners, plant oil, more thickeners, preservatives, and plant oil. This is a very ordinary, greasy wipe-off cleanser that can leave a film on the skin.

☹ **Washable Cleansing Milk, A Moisturizing Cleanser for Dry or Sensitive Skin** *($13.50 for 8 ounces)* is not what I would consider a "washable" cleanser. It contains oils that can leave a greasy film on the skin. Protein, nonfat milk, and other "natural ingredients" are at the very end of the ingredient list, well after the preservatives, but there isn't enough to make this product even vaguely milky.

☹ **Gentle Foaming Facial Cleanser for Dry to Normal Skin Types** *($13.50 for 8 ounces)* contains mostly detergent cleansing agent, preservatives, and plant oils. The detergent cleanser can dry the skin, and the plant oils can leave a greasy film.

☹ **Foaming Non-Detergent Washable Cleanser** *($13.50 for 8 ounces)* is not in the least a nondetergent cleanser: the second ingredient is sodium C14-16 olefin sulfate, a cleansing agent in shampoos that is known for stripping hair color. I would call this a standard detergent facial cleanser that can dry out the skin.

☹ **Rare-Earth Oatmeal Milk Facial Cleanser #1 (Mild)** *($17.50 for 8 ounces)* doesn't contain any earth that is remotely rare, just standard kaolin and bentonite, better known as clay. But I guess if you want to charge this kind of money for clay and standard detergent cleansers, you have to call it rare. The minuscule amounts of vitamins, nonfat milk, and oat flour are included to boost the natural appearance of a completely unnatural product.

☹ **Rare-Earth Oatmeal Milk Facial Cleanser #2 (Medium Strength)** *($17.50 for 8 ounces)* is very similar to the facial cleanser above, only much more drying.

☹ **Rare-Earth Foaming Cleanser #2 (Medium Strength)** *($17.50 for 8 ounces)* contains sodium lauryl sulfate as the main detergent cleansing agent. I don't recommend sodium lauryl sulfate in shampoos because it can be so drying and because it strips hair color. I definitely would not recommend this for the face. The standard natural ingredients are listed well after the preservatives, and they won't make this cleanser any less irritating.

☺ **Ultra Moisturizing Buffing Cream with Scrub Particles** *($10.50 for 4 ounces)* is a scrub that uses a synthetic scrub agent; it also contains thickening agents and oils. It would be suitable for someone with very dry skin.

☺ **Milk, Honey, and Almond Scrub** *($18.50 for 6 ounces)* is a standard abrasive scrub that also contains talc and flour, which can be hard to rinse off and can be irritating when rubbed into the skin. The nonfat milk, plant oils, and vitamins are at the end of the ingredient list. The oils may leave a greasy residue.

☹ **$$$ Pineapple and Papaya Facial Scrub, Made with Real Fruit** *($26.50 for 4 ounces)* does contain real pineapple and papaya, but they come at the very end of the ingredient list, after the preservatives, making them a token addition. This is a standard detergent cleanser with cornmeal as a scrub. You can use plain cornmeal if you want a scrub similar to this for a lot less money.

☹ **Rare-Earth Foaming Cleaner #1 (Mild) with Scrub Grains** *($18.50 for 8 ounces)* uses sodium lauryl sulfate, which can be extremely drying and irritating, as the main detergent cleansing agent. It also contains clays and talc, which are hardly rare. This scrub can be drying and irritating, so don't expect it to be mild.

☹ **Liquid Body Scrub and Cleanser with Natural Scrub Particles** *($18.50 for 8 ounces)* is mostly TEA-lauryl sulfate and cornmeal. Like sodium lauryl sulfate, TEA-lauryl sulfate can be drying and irritating. If you want to use cornmeal as a scrub, buy it at the grocery store and save your money.

☺ **Cucumber Herbal Alcohol-Free Toner for Dry or Sensitive Skin** *($13.95 for 8 ounces)* is alcohol-free, but not irritant-free. It contains balm mint, pine needle, camphor, and sulfonated oils, all of which can be irritating. Although there isn't much of those ingredients in the toner, they can still cause problems for someone with sensitive skin.

☺ **French Rosewater** *($10.50 for 8 ounces)*, as the name implies, is mostly rose water, which is merely fragranced glycerin.

☺ **Calendula Herbal Extract Toner (Alcohol-Free)** *($18.50 for 4 ounces)* contains plant extracts (tea) and preservatives. The plants used can be soothing in their original, fresh form (if you aren't allergic to them), but it is doubtful whether they retain any of their original properties when preserved in a cosmetic.

☺ **Herbal Toner with Mixed Berries and Extracts** *($19.95 for 8 ounces)* uses different herbs than the toner above, and the herbs and fruit used in this one can be irritating, but most come well after the preservative on the ingredient list and don't amount to much more than a meager presence.

☹ **Rosewater Facial Freshener-Toner** *($11.50 for 8 ounces)* is mostly alcohol with rose fragrance. It can be irritating and drying.

☹ **Blue Astringent Herbal Lotion** *($11.95 for 8 ounces; $22 for 16 ounces)* contains mostly water, alcohol, and aluminum chlorohydrate. Yes, that's right, aluminum chlorohydrate, used in *antiperspirants.* Not only is the alcohol drying and irritating, but the aluminum chlorohydrate can cause infection of the hair follicle. What were the chemists who made this product thinking?

☺ **Sodium PCA Oil-Free Moisturizer** *($22.50 for 4 ounces)* is not oil-free; the second ingredient is silicone oil. It also contains thickeners, water-binding agent, and preservatives. This would still be a good moisturizer for someone with normal to dry skin. It also contains vitamins, but they are well after the preservatives on the ingredient list, meaning there aren't enough to matter.

☺ **$$$ Ultra Facial Moisturizer with SPF 13** *($27 for 4 ounces)* has a decent SPF but is fairly pricey for what you get. It contains simply water, plant oil, thickeners, and preservatives. There are far less expensive sunscreens with better SPF ratings than this one.

☹ **Superb Total Dermal Protection Face Cream with SPF 8** *($22.95 for 2 ounces; $39.99 for 4 ounces)* is exaggerating when it claims to provide "total dermal protection" with an SPF of only 8. No product should be allowed to get away with that, especially for this kind of money. All the other ingredients are very standard oils and wax-like thickeners.

☺ **$$$ Ultra Protection Moisturizing Face Gel with SPF 15** *($52.95 for 2 ounces)* has a good SPF number, but the price is intolerable.

☺ **Panthenol Protein Moisturizing Face Cream** *($22.50 for 4 ounces)* contains mostly water, thickeners, glycerin, panthenol (an emollient), vitamin E, and preservatives. This is a good ordinary moisturizer for someone with dry skin. The really interesting ingredients are listed way after the preservatives and hardly worth mentioning.

☺ **$$$ Creme d'Elegance Repairateur Superb Tissue Repairateur Creme** *($25.50 for 2 ounces)* contains mostly water, plant oil, thickeners, slip agent, more thickeners, lanolin oil, more thickeners, petrolatum, lanolin, and preservatives. Regardless of what language you say it in, this cream will not repair skin. It would be a good moisturizer for someone with very dry skin, but the price can sting a bit. All of the fancy natural-sounding ingredients are at the end of the list, and you know what that means.

☹ **Light Nourishing Eye Cream** *($15.95 for 0.5 ounce)* uses a film-forming agent as a way to smooth the skin and keep water in. Other than that, it is an OK moisturizer. The so-called nourishing ingredients, vitamins A and E, can't nourish the skin, but there is enough that they could be considered antioxidants.

☹ **$$$ Ultra Protection Moisturizing Eye Gel with SPF 18 Hyaluronic Acid Vitamin A and Vitamin E** *($28.50 for 0.5 ounce)* does indeed contain hyaluronic acid, which is a good water-binding agent, but hardly rare or exceptional. The SPF 18 is good, but unnecessary in a separate eye product. It also contains a film former similar to the one in the eye cream above, as well as vitamins, and the same review applies.

☹ **Dermal Protection Eye and Throat Cream with SPF 6** *($27.95 for 2 ounces)* does not provide dermal protection with an SPF of only 6.

☹ **Original Formula Eye Cream, Ultra Nourishing** *($10.50 for 0.5 ounce)* contains mostly plant oil, thickeners, and preservatives. It isn't even vaguely nourishing, but it is an OK, ordinary moisturizer for someone with dry skin.

☺ **Imperiale Repairateur Moisturizing Eye Balm with Pure Vitamins A & E** *($14.50 for 0.5 ounce)* contains mostly plant oils, thickeners, vitamins E and A, more plant oil, lanolin oil, cocoa butter, and preservatives. This is a good moisturizer for dry skin. The vitamins can be considered antioxidants.

☺ **Ultra Moisturizing Eye Stick with SPF 18 and Vitamin E** *($15.95 for 0.5 ounce)* is identical to the eye balm above, only with sunscreen, and the same review applies.

☹ **Ultra Moisturizing Concealing Stick with SPF 26 and Vitamin E (Matte) #3** *($19.50 for 0.5 ounce)* is identical to the eye balm above, only with more sunscreen and color. This is a fairly greasy concealer that can crease into the lines around the eyes. If you are already using a sunscreen on your face, using another one in your makeup is completely unnecessary and can cause irritation.

☺ **Imperiale Repairateur Moisturizing Masque** *($35 for 2 ounces)* contains mostly water, plant oils, thickeners, and preservatives. It is indeed moisturizing and good for someone with dry skin. All of the fancy natural-sounding ingredients are at the end of the ingredient list, but even if there were more, they still couldn't repair skin.

☺ **$$$ Soothing and Cleansing Algae Masque for Balancing Skin Types** *($39.95 for 4.5 ounces)* contains nothing that can balance skin and is certainly not suitable for all skin types, particularly not for someone with oily or combination skin. It contains mostly slip agent, thickeners, algae, more thickener, plant oils, and preservatives. All of the natural-sounding ingredients are at the end of the list.

☺ **Rare-Earth Facial Cleansing Masque** *($16.50 for 5 ounces)* is mostly water and clay, and there is nothing rare about clay. It also contains cornstarch, which can be a skin irritant. It is an OK clay mask, but clay can't do much for the skin except dry it out.

☺ **Lip Balm #1** *($4.95 for 0.7 ounce)* is a very emollient lip gloss that contains mostly petrolatum, plant oils, lanolin, and preservatives.

La Prairie

Many of the makeup products in this line are called "Cellular Treatment." After a while it starts sounding silly. Even the mascara is called "Cellular Treatment Intensified Mascara." It's all rather gimmicky. And even if your skin could remarkably improve with these products, the prices might kill you. So what do the few women who can afford these prices get for their money? The prestige of knowing they can afford the imperial price tag. High-priced skin care lines attract women who think that the dollars they spend will buy them something special most other women can't afford. To some extent, they're right: they get an immense amount of hype. If you could read and understand the ingredient lists, you would find the prices as ludicrous as I do. Many of La Prairie's claims are based on the use of ingredients such as placental protein, flower and herb extracts, marine collagen, and amino acids. There is no research that indicates any of these ingredients can alter the skin, and product lines in all price ranges contain them, but that doesn't stop La Prairie from trying to convince you that its versions are worth the sky-high prices. To satisfy your curiosity, I suggest you compare ingredient lists. You will notice that most of the ingredients in La Prairie's products are found in lots of other lines. Also, you can tell that the amount of "specialty" ingredients in the products is almost negligible, because they are located near the end of a stupendously long ingredient list.

La Prairie's claim to fame is its Clinic La Prairie in Montreux, Switzerland, where the rich come for injections of sheep placenta extract. Does it make a difference? The clinic says it does, but there are no independent studies that prove its claim. The question I ask myself is, Why hasn't this supposedly superior skin care wonder come to the United States? If sheep injections work, why not do it in America? I suspect it's because the company would never get away with it under the watchful eye of the FDA.

La Prairie Skin Care

☺ **$$$ Essential Purifying Gel Cleanser** *($50 for 7.3 ounces)* contains mostly water, detergent cleanser, thickener, slip agent, more thickener, more detergent cleanser, and preservative. There are some herb extracts, but they are at the end of the ingredient list, in too minuscule an amount to matter. This cleanser does rinse off, but it leaves a slight film on the skin.

☺ **$$$ Foam Cleanser** *($50 for 4 ounces)* is a standard detergent-based cleanser that is about as ordinary as they come. It does contain some petrolatum (Vaseline) and silicone oil to cut the drying effect of the cleansing agents, as well as some anti-irritants, but those are nothing special either.

☺ **$$$ Purifying Creme Cleanser** *($50 for 6.8 ounces)* is meant to be rinsed off, but it actually requires a washcloth. This cleanser contains emollient thickening agents, as well as mineral oil and petrolatum, which means it leaves a film on the skin. This is merely a very expensive cold cream.

☺ **$$$ Cellular Eye Make-Up Remover** *($40 for 4.2 ounces)* is a silicone oil–based wipe-off cleanser that contains some plant extracts and anti-irritants. That's nice, but I wonder if the executives for these companies laugh about the women who believe they're getting something special when they spend this kind of money for an ordinary product.

☺ **$$$ Essential Exfoliator** *($50 for 7 ounces)* is a standard facial scrub that contains mostly water, mineral oil, thickener, apricot powder, more thickeners, detergent cleanser, and preservative. This is a good scrub for dry skin, but it doesn't rinse off very well and, to say the least, is overpriced for what you get.

☹ **Cellular Purifying Lotion** *($55 for 8.2 ounces)* is a standard alcohol-based toner with a small amount of placental protein thrown in, but that can't compensate for the irritation and dryness caused by the alcohol. Besides, at best, protein extracted from the placenta does what all proteins do for the skin: it acts as a good water-binding agent.

☺ **$$$ Cellular Refining Lotion** *($55 for 8.2 ounces)* is an irritant-free toner that contains mostly water, slip agents, water-binding agents, plant extracts, glycerin, soothing agent, and preservatives. This would be a good toner for most skin types, but the price tag is absurd.

☹ **Cellular Emergency Tonic** *($50 for 1.7 ounces)* contains mostly water, mineral oil, alcohol, propylene glycol, placental protein, and herb and flower extracts. It also contains salicylic acid, which along with the alcohol makes this a fairly irritating toner.

☺ **$$$ Age Management Balancer** *($65 for 8.4 ounces)* contains mostly water, several slip agents, plant extracts, water-binding agents, silicone oil, a tiny amount of AHA (less than 2%), anti-irritant, and preservatives. This is a good irritant-free toner, but hardly worth the price tag.

☺ **$$$ Cellular Day Creme** *($100 for 1 ounce)* contains mostly water, thickeners, slip agent, plant oil, petrolatum, glycerin, more thickeners, water-binding agent, plant extracts, and preservatives. This is a lot of money for a product that is mostly thickeners and Vaseline, but I think La Prairie was hoping you wouldn't notice.

☺ **$$$ Cellular Night Cream** *($105 for 1 ounce)* is a rather rich moisturizer for dry skin; it contains mostly water, petrolatum, thickeners, slip agent, more thickeners, glycerin, standard water-binding agent, silicone oil, and preservatives. This rather boring petrolatum-based moisturizer would be good for someone with dry skin, if she could survive the damage to her budget.

☹ **$$$ Age Management Intensified Emulsion with SPF 8** *($100 for 1.7 ounces)* contains mostly water, silicone oil, AHAs, glycerin, several thickeners, more silicone oil, film former, slip agent, plant extracts, pH balancer, more AHAs, plant extracts, water-binding agents, vitamins A and E, more water-binding agents, more thickeners, and preservatives. This is a good 6% AHA product in a good moisturizing base that would be best for someone with dry skin. SPF 8 is good for limited sun protection. I'm not even going to mention the price.

☹ **$$$ Age Management Cream Natural with SPF 8** *($125 for 1.7 ounces)* is one of the most expensive sunscreens on the market. The sunscreen is nonchemical, and it does contain about 2% AHAs (only enough to make the AHAs a water-binding agent, not an exfoliant). Other than that, it is just an emollient moisturizer with fairly standard ingredients. It does contain some good water-binding agents and vitamins, but they are too far down on the list to be significant.

☺ **$$$ Age Management Night Cream** *($125 for 1 ounce)* contains mostly water; AHAs; slip agent; pH balancer; film former; thickeners; plant extracts; more thickeners; petrolatum; silicone oil; more AHAs; anti-irritant; water-binding agents; more thickeners; more plant extracts; vitamins A, E, and C; and preservatives. This

8% AHA product in a moisturizing base would be good for someone with dry skin. But this endless ingredient list looks as if La Prairie just threw everything in, including the kitchen sink. There are a lot of interesting ingredients, but mostly just a dusting of each.

☺ **$$$ Time Management Moisturizer with SPF 15** *($75 for 1.7 ounces)* contains mostly water; thickeners; silicone oil; glycerin; plant oil; thickener; water-binding agents; vitamins A, E, and C; more water-binding agents; more plant oil; anti-irritant; and preservatives. This is a very good sunscreen in an emollient base for someone with dry skin. The interesting ingredients are so far down on the list they don't really matter. I won't comment on the price; you can see that madness for yourself.

☺ **$$$ Age Management Eye Repair** *($100 for 0.5 ounce)* contains mostly water; film former; glycerin; thickeners; plant extract; AHAs; more thickeners; plant oil; pH balancer; slip agents; silicone oil; water-binding agents; vitamins A, E, and C; anti-irritant; more water-binding agents; more thickeners; and preservatives. Like most eye creams, this one contains a film former that can help skin look smooth, but it isn't unique to La Prairie. This is a good moisturizer with about 3% AHAs, which can have minor exfoliating properties.

☺ **$$$ Age Management Intensified Serum** *($140 for 1 ounce)* contains about 8% AHAs, which is fine for an exfoliant, but a lot of other 8% AHA products can do the same thing for a *lot* less money. It contains mostly water, AHAs, pH balancer, slip agents, silicone oil, thickeners, plant extract, more AHAs, water-binding agent, more plant extracts, anti-irritant, and preservatives.

☺ **$$$ Age Management Serum** *($125 for 1 ounce)* is similar to the product above, and the same review applies.

☺ **$$$ Age Management Line Inhibitor** *($100 for 0.5 ounce)* is similar to the Age Management Intensified Serum above, and the same review applies.

☺ **$$$ Cellular Balancing Complex** *($65 for 1.7 ounces)* contains mostly water, silicone oil, thickener, slip agent, sunscreen, more silicone oil, glycerin, several thickeners, water-binding agents, vitamins A and E, and preservatives. This is a good lightweight emollient moisturizer for normal to dry skin. There isn't enough sunscreen to protect skin from sun damage, though.

☺ **$$$ Cellular Skin Conditioner** *($70 for 4 ounces)* contains mostly water, thickeners, glycerin, pH balancer, more thickeners, water-binding agents, plant extract, and preservatives. This is a fairly ordinary but good moisturizer for someone with dry skin.

☺ **$$$ Cellular Wrinkle Cream** *($105 for 1 ounce)* contains mostly mineral oil, water, petrolatum, thickeners, slip agent, more thickeners, placental protein, and preservatives. This standard mineral oil–based moisturizer is very emollient and would be good for someone with dry skin, but calling this product ordinary is an understatement. Please don't fall for the notion that placental protein can somehow restore youth to your skin. It can't.

☺ **$$$ Cellular Eye Contour Creme** *($80 for 0.5 ounce)* comes in at $2,560 per pound, yet it is nothing more than a petrolatum-based moisturizer. It is a good emollient moisturizer for someone with dry skin, but the ingredients you think you're buying come after the preservatives and don't amount to anything more than a dusting.

☺ **$$$ Skin Caviar** *($100 for 2 ounces)* is mostly silicone oil, some water, and slip agents, contained in small gelatin pellets that break open when you rub them on the skin. It's a cute idea, but paying $100 for a cute idea isn't all that cute.

☺ **$$$ Essence of Skin Caviar Cellular Face Complex with Caviar Extract** *($85 for 1 ounce)* contains mostly water, silicone oils, glycerin, thickeners, water-binding agents, vitamins A and E, plant extracts, soothing agent, and preservatives. This is a good lightweight moisturizer for someone with dry skin.

☺ **$$$ Essence of Skin Caviar Cellular Eye Complex with Caviar Extract** *($85 for 0.5 ounce)* contains mostly water, slip agents, thickener, water-binding agents, soothing agent, thickener, and preservatives. This is a good lightweight moisturizer for someone with dry skin. It does contain 0.04% caviar, which amounts to half an egg—now, isn't that exciting?

☹ **$$$ Cellular Balancing Mask** *($55 for six 0.24-ounce treatments)* is a two-part mask that you mix together. The liquid is mostly water, citric acid (an astringent and possible skin irritant), aloe vera, and preservatives. The powder contains mostly sodium bicarbonate (yes, baking soda), clay, thickeners, talc, placental protein, collagen, and fragrance. Minuscule amounts of aloe vera and baking soda are not going to balance anyone's skin, and the placental protein is a water-binding agent, nothing more.

☹ **$$$ Cellular Cycle Ampoules for the Face** *($250 for seven 0.1-ounce treatments)*. This one prices out to about $5,700 a pound! They can't be serious. This two-part self-mixed treatment contains the most ordinary assembly of ingredients you could imagine. The liquid contains water, slip agent, water-binding agent, plant extracts, thickeners, fragrance, and preservatives. The powder contains thickener, water, water-binding agents, and more thickener. This isn't even as interesting as a lot of other La Prairie products. Are there really women willing to buy this?

La Prairie Makeup

☺ **$$$ FOUNDATION: Cellular Perfection Flawless with SPF 8** *($55)* has a beautiful soft, smooth texture that feels wonderful on the skin, and SPF 8 is OK for limited sun exposure. If the handful of good colors happen to match your skin tone, you might want to check this out. **These colors are the best: 200, 300, 500, and 600. These are the colors to avoid: 100, 400, 700, and 800.**

☺ **$$$ Cellular Oil-Free Matte Foundation with SPF 8** *($55)* isn't oil-free (it contains silicone oil), but it does have a decent matte texture and blends on soft and even. The limited color selection is impressive, and the SPF 8 is OK for limited sun exposure. **These colors are the best: 15, 20, 30, 50, 70, and 80. These are the only colors to avoid: 40 and 60.**

☺ **$$$ Cellular Treatment Foundation Satin with SPF 8** *($55)* offers only a handful of colors, and most are terrible. It is a thick but moist foundation that provides medium coverage, but can feel heavy instead of moist on the skin. **These are the best colors: 4, 4.5, and 5.5. These colors are too peach, pink, or rose: 1, 3.2, 3.5, 5.7, and 6.7.**

☺ **$$$ Cellular Treatment Perfecting Primer** *($50)* is a sheer light moisturizer that is white and, not surprisingly, leaves a white finish on the skin. If you think giving your face a white cast will "perfect" your look, this is for you, but I think it's an inane waste.

☺ **$$$ POWDER: Protective Pressed Powder** *($36)* isn't protective but it is a good standard talc-powder with a smooth silky finish. **Foundation Finish Loose Powder** *($35)* is a standard powder with a very soft satiny finish.

☹ **BLUSH: Cellular Treatment Powder Blush** *($35)* has a small selection of soft and pretty colors. The texture is almost too soft, and it can blend on choppy. **Cellular Treatment Creme Blush** *($35)* has a soft but dry finish, which isn't bad, but all the colors are shiny.

☹ **EYESHADOW: Cellular Treatment Eye Colour Singles** *($30)* are all shiny. That way, after you've spent a fortune on La Prairie's skin care products to get rid of wrinkles, you can buy its makeup that helps the eye area look more wrinkly. **Cellular Treatment Eye Colour Coordinates** *($35)* come in colors that are indeed coordinated, but they are also all ultra-shiny and should be avoided.

☺ **$$$ EYE AND BROW SHAPER:** At least the pencils aren't called "Cellular Treatment." **Eye Pencils** *($25)* and **Brow Pencils** *($25)* are just standard pencils. There is a handful of OK colors, but it is foolish to spend this kind of money on something so ordinary.

☺ **$$$ <u>LIPSTICK AND LIP PENCIL:</u> Matte Lipstick** *($27)* isn't what you and I would call matte, but it does go on rather thick and creamy. **Sheer Lipstick** *($27)*, as the name implies, is more gloss than lipstick. **Moisturizing Tint** *($27)* is fairly sheer, more gloss than lipstick. **Lip Pencils** *($25)* are standard pencils that have a handful of OK colors, but why spend this kind of money?

☺ **$$$ <u>MASCARA:</u> Cellular Treatment Intensified Mascara** *($25)*, at this price, should be amazing. It isn't, but it is a good mascara that makes the lashes long, thick, and soft, and doesn't smudge.

Lancôme

Lancôme is very popular among baby boomers, and its color line is one of my favorites. Prices are steep but relatively reasonable (I use the term "reasonable" loosely) given Lancôme's place at the high end of the cosmetics world. This very French line maintains a more casual, but still professional, air than the other French lines sold at the department stores.

I like the Lancôme display units very much. They are accessible and easy to use, particularly if you want to experiment on your own. I do wish, however, that Lancôme would follow the trend of the other makeup lines and divide its blushes, eyeshadows, lipsticks, and lip liners into color groups. Still, their foundation colors are divided into three groups: D for golden, N for neutral, and R for Rose (which isn't all that rose—it's really more peach). There are many superb colors for a wide range of skin tones, from light to dark (including several suitable for African-American skin tones), that you can test on your own jawline. A few stores in selected cities now sport "super counters" that take up an entire island.

One word of caution: These days Lancôme is into color striping, the technique for selecting a foundation that Prescriptives made popular. The idea is to test which foundation shade will work best by striping three or four colors on the side of your face and seeing which one "disappears" into the skin. The idea sounds good, but what often happens is that the color that "disappears" on your face is the one that matches the ruddy, ashy, or sallow tones in your skin, which is not the best one to choose; you would be blending a color all over your face that enhances the skin tones you should be toning down. I recommend always choosing the most neutral-colored foundation, with a minimal amount of pink, peach, yellow, or ash. Apply it all over an area of the face near the jawline, then check it out in *daylight*. What seems to blend into the skin in the department store light can look fairly rosy, ashy, or peachy in daylight.

Lancome Skin Care

☺ **$$$ Respectee Extremely Gentle Creme Gel Cleanser (pump)** *($22.50 for 6.8 ounces)* is a detergent cleanser that also contains plant oil, which can leave a greasy film on the skin.

☺ **$$$ Ablutia Fraicheur Purifying Foam Cleanser** *($19.50 for 6.8 ounces)* is a standard detergent-based cleanser that can be drying for some skin types.

☺ **$$$ Galatee Douceur Milky Creme Cleanser** *($19.50 for 6.8 ounces)* is supposed to be a splash- or tissue-off cleanser for all skin types. It is fairly greasy for oily or combination skin, and it doesn't rinse off without the use of a washcloth. It also contains isopropyl myristate (the third ingredient), which can cause blackheads. However, it may be good for extremely dry skin.

☺ **$$$ Clarifiance Oil-Free Gel Cleanser** *($19.50 for 6.8 ounces)* is a very good water-soluble cleanser that takes off all the makeup without irritating the eyes or drying out the skin.

☹ **Pur Controle Cleanser for Oily and Normal to Oily Skin** *($17.50 for 4.1 ounces)* is a very drying detergent cleanser that contains several cleansing agents known for their harsh effect on the skin, including potassium hydroxide, rather high up on the ingredient list. This cleanser would be quite drying and irritating for most skin types, creating more problems than it would help.

☺ **$$$ Exfoliance Delicate Facial Buff** *($19.50 for 3.5 ounces)* is an OK detergent-based exfoliator that uses synthetic particles as the scrub. It's rather standard and can be drying for some skin types.

☺ **$$$ Bi-Facil Double-Action Eye Makeup Remover** *($16 for 4 ounces)* is a silicone oil–based wipe-off cleanser, nothing more. The price is very steep for what you get.

☺ **$$$ Effacile Gentle Eye Makeup Remover** *($15.50 for 4 ounces)* is a detergent-based eye-makeup remover that isn't all that gentle, but it will take off eye makeup.

☺ **$$$ Clarifiance Alcohol-Free Natural Astringent** *($16.50 for 6.8 ounces)* contains mostly water, alum (a powdered astringent), preservatives, and slip agent. It is alcohol-free, but alum isn't the best for the skin, at least not in terms of oily skin or acne.

☺ **$$$ Tonique Douceur Non-Alcoholic Freshener for Dry/Sensitive Skin** *($17.50 for 6.8 ounces)* is indeed alcohol-free; it contains mostly water, glycerin, pH balancer, soothing agents, and preservatives. It's good, but the price is steep for what you get.

☹ **Tonique Fraicheur Mild Astringent for Normal/Oily Skin** *($17.50 for 6.8 ounces)* is an alcohol-based toner and can be irritating to the skin.

☹ **Tonique Controle Toner for Oily and Normal to Oily Skin** *($17.50 for 6.8 ounces)* is basically just alcohol and a small amount of zinc. The zinc will absorb oil, but the alcohol is likely to cause more oil, so it creates a vicious cycle for your face.

☺ **$$$ Bienfait Total SPF 15** *($30 for 1.7 ounces)* is an OK sunscreen, but hardly exceptional. Lancome salespeople like pointing out its AHA content, but it isn't even 1% of the product, hardly worth mentioning. It contains mostly water, thickener, glycerin, more thickeners, shea butter, vitamin E, slip agent, fragrance, more thickeners, and preservatives. For this money you would expect at least a few interesting water-binding agents and emollients, but there are none in this product. It does contain aluminum starch, which can be a skin irritant.

☺ **$$$ Hydrative Continuous Hydrating Resource** *($38 for 1.75 ounces)* contains mostly water, shea butter, glycerin, standard water-binding agents, mineral oil, thickeners, a small amount of sunscreen, more thickeners, fragrance, vitamin E, and preservatives. This is a good emollient moisturizer for very dry skin.

☺ **$$$ Noctosome Renewal Night Treatment** *($50 for 1.75 ounces)* is a rich, emollient moisturizer for dry skin. It contains mostly water, plant oil, standard water-binding agents, tallow (a thickener that can cause blackheads), plant oil, protein, more thickener, water-binding agents, fragrance, vitamin E, more protein, and preservatives.

☺ **$$$ Nutribel Nourishing Hydrating Emulsion** *($36.50 for 2.5 ounces)* is a good, very emollient moisturizer that contains mostly water, plant oil, glycerin, mineral oil, more plant oils, thickeners, water-binding agents, fragrance, more thickeners, and preservatives.

☺ **$$$ Nutriforce Double Nutrition Fortifying Nourishing Creme** *($37 for 1.7 ounces)* contains mostly water, plant oil, silicone oil, thickeners, plant extracts, fragrance, and preservatives. This is a good basic (but ordinary) moisturizer for someone with dry skin.

☺ **$$$ Respectee Extremely Gentle Conditioning Lotion, Alcohol-Free** *($20 for 6.8 ounces)* contains mostly water, glycerin, slip agent, and preservative. This is as lightweight and ordinary a moisturizer as I've seen anywhere.

☺ **$$$ Trans-Hydrix** *($34 for 1.9 ounces)* contains mostly water, plant oil, shea butter, mineral oil, several thickeners, slip agents, fragrance, preservative, water-binding agents, and more preservatives. This is a good standard emollient moisturizer for dry skin.

☺ **$$$ Forte-Vital Serum Raffermissant Skin Firming Serum** *($45 for 0.84 ounce)* contains mostly water, glycerin, water-binding agent, thickeners, fragrance, and preservatives. This is an OK lightweight moisturizer, but that's about it. Nothing in it will help firm skin.

☺ **$$$ Niosome + Perfected Age Treatment** *($55 for 2.5 ounces)* is an OK lightweight moisturizer that contains mostly water, glycerin, silicone oil, plant oil, water-binding agents, thickener, fragrance, and preservatives. There are some antioxidants in it, but in such negligible amounts that they don't count for much. It's a good moisturizer, but "perfected age treatment"? They've got to be kidding.

☺ **$$$ Nutrix Soothing Treatment Creme** *($30 for 1.9 ounces)* contains mostly mineral oil, water, petrolatum, lanolin, thickeners, water-binding agents, fragrance, protein (way down at the end of the ingredient list, too little to even notice), and preservatives. This is a lot of money for mineral oil and Vaseline, but it would be good for someone with very dry skin.

☹ **$$$ Oligo-Major Activating Serum with Trace Elements** *($44 for 0.84 ounce)* contains mostly water, glycerin, water-binding agents, slip agents, fragrance, and preservatives. This is an OK lightweight moisturizer, but those trace elements are just that, trace.

☹ **$$$ Primordial** *($42.50 for 1 ounce)* is, according to Lancome, not a moisturizer, but should be worn under a moisturizer (preferably one of Lancome's, I imagine) to "insulate skin from premature aging factors so it's free to repair itself." Another product to get rid of wrinkles—what a surprise. It is basically an AHA and BHA product. That means it can exfoliate skin, like any of the other 200-plus AHA and BHA products on the market. It contains mostly water, silicone oils, glycerin, vitamin E, plant oil, mixed fruit acids, thickeners, film former, preservatives, and salicylic acid. A product that doesn't tell you exactly what kind of AHA it contains is leaving you a bit in the dark because not all fruit acids are created equal; some are more effective than others. The little bit of vitamin E won't insulate the skin or provide much in the way of an antioxidant.

☺ **$$$ Progres Eye Creme** *($34 for 1.5 ounces)* is a thick eye cream that contains mostly water, thickeners, petrolatum, more thickeners, glycerin, water-binding agent, and preservatives. This is a good emollient moisturizer for dry skin around the eyes or anywhere on the face, but it won't change wrinkles.

☺ **$$$ Renergie Double Performance Treatment** *($65 for 2.5 ounces)* contains mostly water, silicone oil, thickeners, petrolatum, more thickeners, water-binding agents, fragrance, vitamin E, and preservatives. This is a good emollient moisturizer for dry skin.

☺ **$$$ Hydrix Hydrating Creme** *($32.50 for 1.9 ounces)* is a traditional petrolatum-based moisturizer. It contains mostly water, petrolatum, mineral oil, lanolin, thickeners, plant oil, more lanolin, and preservative. It's a good moisturizer for very dry skin, but this is a lot of money for Vaseline and lanolin.

☹ **$$$ HydraControle** *($30 for 1 ounce)* contains mostly water, silicone oil, glycerin, several thickeners, a form of acrylate (like that in hairspray), vitamin B, more thickeners, and preservatives. It does contain a few unusual plant extracts, but they are at the end of the ingredient list and virtually nonexistent. This product won't control oil, but it is a good lightweight moisturizer (although it's not oil-free) for someone with slightly dry skin.

☹ **$$$ Vivifiance Hydrating Eye Gel** *($30 for 0.6 ounce)* contains mostly water, glycerin, aloe, and preservatives. The good water-binding agents and anti-irritants are so far down on the ingredient list that they are barely present.

☹ **$$$ Empreinte de Beaute Deep Cleansing Clay Masque** *($21 for 2.5 ounces)* is a basic clay mask that contains mostly water, clay, water-binding agents, more clay, thickeners, protein, more thickener, and preservatives.

☹ **$$$ Masque No. 10 Hydrating Masque** *($21.50 for 2.2 ounces)* contains mostly water, thickeners, and preservatives. There isn't much moisture in this mask; it is just a gel that dries on the face. Not very impressive, but your skin will feel smooth when you take it off (that's true for most masks). One of the thickeners is a potential skin irritant.

☹ **RefleXe Minceur Cellulite Refining Gel** *($40 for 6.8 ounces)*. contains mostly water, alcohol, silicone oil, caffeine, slip agents, saliclic acid, hairspray-type ingredient, plant oil, fragrance, and preservatives. Alcohol swells the skin, salicylic acid exfoliates, and hairspray and oils can smooth skin but caffeine won't change fat.

☺ **$$$ Protective Eye Creme Anti-Wrinkle with Non-Chemical SPF 15** *($20 for 0.6 ounce)* contains mostly water, thickeners, silicone oil, more thickeners, and preservatives. This is an extremely standard but good titanium dioxide–based sunscreen for someone with normal to dry skin.

☺ **$$$ Protective Face Creme SPF 15** *($22.50 for 1.7 ounces)* is similar to the creme above, only it contains traditional chemical sunscreen agents. It's a good sunscreen for someone with normal to dry skin, though it's rather ordinary for the price.

☺ **$$$ Body Protective Spray SPF 15** *($21 for 4.2 ounces)* is still one of my favorites for someone with normal to oily skin. It is incredibly lightweight, barely perceptible, and leaves a clean feel on the skin. It *can* be used on the face, so don't let the term "body" in the name influence you.

☺ **$$$ Stick Nutrix Levres, Lip Balm** *($15 for 0.13 ounce)* is a very emollient, but standard lip balm that contains mostly plant oil, lanolin oil, petrolatum, thickeners, and preservatives. It's good for dry lips, but very overpriced given its similarity to products at one-third the price.

Lancome Makeup

☺ **FOUNDATION:** Lancome has quite a large, almost overwhelming, array of foundations to choose from, all of which are excellent. There is even an impressive range of colors for darker skin tones. **MaquiVelour Hydrating Foundation** *($28.50)* is for normal to dry skin and has a soft, light texture with even coverage. **These colors are great:** Porcelain Delicate I, Clair II, Dore Clair II, Pale Clair II, Beige III, Beige Naturel III, Beige Sable III, and Beige Bisque III. **These colors are too peach, pink, or ash:** Bronze IV, Rose Clair II, and Beige Rose III.

☺ **MaquiControle** *($28.50)* has been reformulated and is no longer the heavy, thick foundation it used to be. It now provides light to medium coverage and feels great on the skin. It goes on very matte and truly dry. It is one of the better choices for someone with truly oily skin. **These colors are excellent:** Porcelain I, Porcelain d'Ivoire I, Porcelain Delicate I, Clair II, Pale Clair II, Dore Clair II, Beige III, Beige Naturel III, Beige Camee III, Beige Sable III, Bronze IV, Amande Bronze IV, and Miel Bronze IV. **These colors are too pink or peach:** Beige Rose III, Beige Bisque III, Beige Rose III, Rose Clair II, and Epice Bronze IV.

☺ **MaquiMat** *($22)* has a smooth, matte finish and feels wonderful on the skin. Unfortunately, the second ingredient is aluminum starch, which can be a problem for some skin types. **These colors are superior:** Porcelain Delicate I, Clair II, Dore Clair II, Pale Clair II, Beige III, Beige Naturel III, Beige Sable III, and Bronze IV. **These colors are too peach or pink:** Rose Clair II and Beige Bisque.

☺ **MaquiLibre SPF 15** *($30)* comes in the typical excellent assortment of Lancome color choices. It has a great light texture that goes on evenly and relatively sheer, plus an SPF of 15 with a fairly matte finish. It would be best for someone with normal to slightly oily or combination skin. **These colors are best:** Porcelaine I, Porcelaine d'Ivoire, Porcelaine Delicate I, Dore Clair II, Pale Clair II, Beige III, Amande Bronze

IV, Miel Bronze IV, Miel Fonce IV, and Cafe IV. **These are colors to avoid:** Rose Clair II, Beige Bisque, Beige Camee II, Beige Naturel III, Beige Rose III, and Beige Sable, because they can turn peach; and Clair II and Bronze IV, because they are too ash green for most skin tones.

☺ **Dual Finish Powder** *($26)* is more like a compact powder than a foundation. It comes in an excellent assortment of colors, can be used wet (although I think it tends be too powdery when used by itself), and is an option for someone with normal to slightly oily skin. It also makes a great finishing powder.

☹ **Imanance Tinted Creme SPF 8** *($25)* doesn't contain enough sunscreen to provide the best protection, but it is a very good, lightweight, sheer foundation that goes on well. It would be good for someone with normal to slightly dry skin. The color selection is quite limited, so this product definitely isn't for everyone.

☺ **MaquiDouceur** *($35 for 1 ounce)* is a great addition to an already impressive group of foundations. If you have dry skin, this foundation feels great and goes on beautifully. The fluffy formula has a light feel and provides medium coverage. There is a good color selection for all skin tones, including women of color. **These colors are good to excellent:** Beige III N, Pale Clair II D, Clair II N, Beige Neutral III N, Beige Rose III R, Bronze IV D (can turn slightly ash), Porcelain Delicat I N (can turn slightly pink), Porcelain d'Ivoire (can turn slightly pink), Beige Sable III D (may turn slightly peach), and Amande Bronzee IV R (can turn slightly peach). **These colors are too pink, orange, peach, rose, or ash for most skin types:** Rose Clair II R and Pale Clair II.

☺ **MaquiLumine** *($36)* is a cream-to-powder foundation that is more powdery than creamy and is best for someone with normal to oily skin. It is extremely reminiscent of L'Oreal's Luminair, but perhaps Lancome thought no one would notice. Nevertheless, **all of the colors are excellent; the only one to avoid** is Rose Claire II.

☹ **CONCEALER: Shadow Base** *($16)* is an eyeshadow base that is quite waterproof, which means it must be removed with an oil-based cleanser, but because of its color and consistency, it nicely tones down the intense shine of Lancome's iridescent eyeshadows and eyeshadow pencils. However, I never recommend doing two things when you can do one, so it's best to forget the Shadow Base, and instead use foundation on your lid and wear eyeshadows that are matte, not shiny. Besides, my eyeshadow lasted no longer when I wore Shadow Base than when I wore foundation. **Anti-Cernes Waterproof Protective Undereye Concealer** *($15)* comes in three shades: Light, Medium, and Dark. It goes on creamy but dries to a somewhat powdery, matte finish, and it isn't waterproof at all. The colors are too pink or peach for most skin tones, the tube applicator is hard to control, and it creases terribly into the lines around the eyes.

☺ **MaquiComplet** *($17.50)* comes in a wand and was supposedly introduced to appease Lancome customers who complained they didn't like the Anti-Cernes concealer's awkward-to-use squeeze tube. Bravo, Lancome. Maqui Complet provides wonderful coverage and doesn't crease even a little. **These colors are wonderful:** Porcelaine I, Beige III Neutral, and Bronze IV. **These colors should be avoided:** Beige III Rose, which can turn peach, and Correcteur, which is very yellow.

☺ **POWDER: Poudre Majeur Pressed Powder** *($23)* is a pressed powder without talc. It goes on smoothly, without a chalky finish. **These colors are excellent:** Translucent, Matte Beige, and Matte Bronze. **This color is too peach for most skin tones:** Matte Peche. There is also a very good loose powder with the same name as the pressed powder, **Poudre Majeur** *($26)*, which is made without talc; instead it contains clay and zinc, which can be somewhat heavier than talc. It also claims to have "micro-bubbles." Whatever that means, it's still only a powder and has the exact same effect as any other you've worn. **These colors are quite good:** Ivoire, Sand, Bisque, Rose, Honey, Bronze, and Buff.

☺ **BLUSH: Blush Majeur** *($21)* is a cream-to-powder blush with an OK consistency; all the colors have some amount of shine. The product itself tends to ball up and cake, which can make blending tricky. Most of the **Blush Subtil** *($21)* colors are indeed subtle; they are all beautiful soft shades, but they are also slightly shiny.

☺ **EYESHADOW:** Many of the **Singles** *($16.50)*, **Duos** *($16.50)*, **Trios** *($26)*, **Quartettes** *($26)*, and **Personal Eyes** *($22.50)* eyeshadow colors are shiny, but a lot are matte. Personal Eyes is a group of colors from which you can choose two and create your own duo compact. It is a good idea, but matte singles are just as convenient, and you don't have to buy two if you like only one of the colors. **These are colors to consider from all of the eyeshadow types:** Country Heather, Cream, Couleurs au Courant, Les Essentials, Couture de Lancome, Matte Brun, Matte Gris, Matte Beige, Teint Midi, Couleurs du Soleil, Couleurs du Ciel, Peche/Raisin, Abricot, Coquille, Biscotte, Praline, Rose Nuance, Cappuccino, Renard, Chocolate Brule, Terre, Le Gris, Fumee, Prune, Aubergine, Ciel du Soir, Violet Moderne, Grappe, Chameau, Parchemin, Le Pinque, Gardenia, and Khaki. **These are colors to avoid from all of the eyeshadow types:** Silversmoke/Fawn, Golden Leaf, Muscat, French Cream, Bleu Eclipse, Nose Gay (single eyeshadow), Splendeurs d'Automne, Ombres Naturelles, Couleurs Sauvages, Couleurs Impromptues, Couleurs du Moment, Pot Pourri de Lancome, Couleurs Teches, Les Neo Modernes, Ombre de Terre, Les Artistes, Metals Precieux, Effets Dores, Impressions Parisiennes, Silversmoke Fawn/Taupe Vert, Lezard, Raisin, Taupe Vert, Vert Artichoke, Vert Artiste, Sauvage Dore, Peche Cire, Golden Sun, Tiara, Tendre Lumiere, Bleu Cashmere, Bleu Gris, Bleu Fume, and Le Blanc.

☹ **L'Ombre Stylo Duo** *($22)* is an eyeshadow pen with different colors at each end, so you can pick and choose for yourself which two colors you want from a selection of eight. The idea and possible convenience, especially for touch-ups, would be worth checking out if the color choices were not so poor. **These colors are worth considering:** Matte Fumee (black), Matte Plum, and Matte Violet (which is best for darker skin tones only). Most of the rest are too shiny or too blue.

☺ **EYE AND BROW SHAPER: Le Crayon Brow Definer** *($14.50)* is a standard pencil with a comb at one end so you can brush through the line and soften it. **Avoid these colors:** Taupe, which is too shiny, and Brunette, which can be too red for many skin tones. **Le Crayon Kohl** *($12.50)* is an assortment of good (though not exceptional) eye-lining pencils; they come in a nice range of colors, but they are no better than others I've found for less money. The claim that they don't smudge once they're on is not entirely accurate; smudging is caused by several factors, not just the pencil itself.

☺ **Le Crayon Waterproof** *($13.50)* is a fairly waterproof pencil that comes in 15 colors. Unfortunately, most are shiny, though some of the darker shades, such as Brown and Black, are not. The pencil is hard to get off without using a wipe-off makeup remover, and I never suggest doing that; it is fat and hard to sharpen; and because they are not 100 percent waterproof, they come off unevenly while you are in the water (although the darker colors are more waterproof than the lighter ones).

☹ **Le Crayon Glace** *($12.50)* is a short, fat pencil that comes in—oh, no!—shiny, sparkly colors. These pencils are hard to sharpen, they tend to be greasy despite the powder finish, and the shiny colors are unforgivable.

☺ **Maquiglace Liquid Liner** *($15)* and **Automatic Eye Lining Felt Pen** *($18.50)* make very definite lines that do not blend, although the felt pen goes on softer than the liquid liner. These can be good for some eye designs. The felt pen is an interesting way to put on eyeliner. Some of these colors are fairly shiny. **Le Kohl Poudre** *($13)* is a unique pencil that goes on like a powder. It is difficult to sharpen and some of the colors are shiny, but this is quite a good option for lining the eyes softly.

☺ **Tinted Brow Groomer Modele Sourcils** *($15)* comes in only three shades: one each for redheads, brunettes, and ash blondes. That's not the best color selection, and the brush can be too large to make application reliable. It tends to go on messy and dries stiff.

☺ **Le Crayon Poudre for the Brows** *($15)* is a pencil; one end has a powder finish, while the other is a mascara wand meant to be combed through the brow to soften the look. It's a great idea, and not one of the colors is shiny. The color selection is limited, but if you find a match, give it a try.

☺ <u>**LIPSTICK AND LIP PENCIL:**</u> Lancome's lipsticks are mostly very good, the colors are beautiful, and they all have a bit of a stain, which helps the lipstick wear somewhat longer. **Hydra-Riche Hydrating Lip Colour** *($15)* is a moist, creamy lipstick with a consistency bordering on greasy. **Rouge Superb Matte Lip Colour** *($15.50)* goes on somewhat heavy and isn't really all that matte. It is fairly creamy and tends to bleed. **Rouge Sensation Superb Sheer Lip Colour** *($15.50)* is more like a gloss than a lipstick. All are worth checking out, though I didn't find their claims about long-lasting color or reduced feathering to be true. **Rouge Absolu Hydrating Long Lasting Lip Colour** *($15.50)* is supposed to be matte, but it depends on what you mean by matte. It is mostly a creamy lipstick that has a slight tint, so it will stay on longer, and it is less creamy-looking than Hydra-Riche, but compared to, say, M.A.C.'s Matte Lipstick or Revlon's ColorStay, it isn't the least bit matte. It also tends to feather. **Stylo Sport Lipstick with SPF 15** *($12.50)* is fairly greasy and shiny, more like a gloss than a lipstick, with a slight tint that helps keep the color around longer. The SPF 15 is nice, but there are much less expensive versions from Physicians Formula, Almay, and Maybelline as good or better, with more color choices. **Le Crayon** *($13)* is a standard automatic lip pencil that never needs sharpening. It's convenient to use and comes in a beautiful array of colors. **Le Lipstique Lip Colouring Stick** *($16.50)* is a surprisingly waterproof lip liner that goes on rather thick and heavy but stays on through thick and thin, leaving a stain after it has worn off. Lancome recommends wearing it all over the lips and applying lipstick over it, which is a fine option, but you can do that with any lip pencil for a longer-lasting look. However, because of the stain, the color can last somewhat longer than other lip liners.

☺ <u>**MASCARA:**</u> Lancome is known for its great, reliable mascaras that usually don't smudge. The best are the **Definils, Intencils, and Keracils** *($15.50)*. Definils builds the thickest lashes and is by far my favorite, but the others are equally excellent. Keracils is presently being reformulated. **Forticils** *($15)* is a clear mascara that is supposed to be a lash conditioner. There is no way to condition or feed lashes to make them grow or be thicker, however. This product is a waste of time and money.

☹ **Tendercils Sensitive Eyes Mascara** *($17.50)* surprised me—I had an allergic reaction to the stuff. Though I never base my reviews of a cosmetic's performance on my skin's sensitivities (because what I am allergic to may have nothing to do with what your skin is sensitive to), the very notion of having this kind of immediate reaction to a product made for sensitive eyes seemed like a bad joke. Essentially, nothing in this product makes it more appropriate for someone with sensitive eyes than any other mascara, including others from Lancome. To make matters worse, although I usually rave about Lancome's mascaras, this one isn't very good. It doesn't build very thick lashes, and it takes a long time to apply. It doesn't smear, but it still doesn't hold a candle to a lot of other mascaras on the market.

L'Oreal

It is fitting that L'Oreal follows Lancome so closely in my alphabetical listing, because both are owned by the same parent company in France. As a result, there are many products that are essentially indistinguishable present in both lines. For example, L'Oreal Luminair and Dualite are practically interchangeable with Lancome MaquiLumine and Dual Finish Powder. Likewise for L'Oreal's Sensitique Mascara and Lancome Tendercils Mascara. Skin care has its share of copycats too. L'Oreal Hydra Renewal is almost ingredient by ingredient the same as Lancome Niosome. Not every product is duplicated but enough that you would be wise to check out the drugstore line before the department store version.

L'Oreal is an overall good cosmetic line, and I feel confident about recommending many of its products, although the selections are somewhat limited. Like most eyeshadows in most lines, L'Oreal's eyeshadows are too shiny, but the line's other products are outstanding. You won't be disappointed by the foundations, blushes, lipsticks, powders, or mascaras. Both the regular blush and the cream powder blush have beautiful textures and are some of the best around. There are three types of lipsticks in this line, and the colors, wearability, textures, and consistency are all fabulous.

Please note that L'Oreal is sold at many Sear's stores around the country complete with testers and very attractive counter displays.

L'Oreal Skin Care

☺ **Plenitude Deep Cleansing Gel for Normal to Oily Skin** *($6.69 for 5 ounces)* is a standard detergent-based cleansing agent that can be drying for most skin types.

☺ **Plenitude Hydrating Cleansing Creme** *($6.69 for 6 ounces)* is supposed to be water-soluble, but it isn't. This plant oil– and mineral oil–based cleanser comes off only with the help of a washcloth and can leave a greasy film on the skin.

☺ **Plenitude Clarify-A³ Facial Gel Foaming Cleanser with Alpha-Hydroxy Complex** *($6.53 for 4 ounces)* is a standard detergent-based water-soluble cleanser that can be drying for some skin types. It contains fruit extracts, but too little to have any effect. Even if there were more, fruit extracts are not necessarily the same thing as AHAs, because there is no way to know what the "extracts" actually are.

☺ **Plenitude Refreshing Eye Makeup Remover** *($6.19 for 4.2 ounces)* contains mostly water, slip agent, detergent cleanser, and preservatives. It does take off eye makeup, but why pull at the eye, causing it to sag, if you don't have to?

☺ **Plenitude Hydrating Floral Toner** *($4.95 for 8.5 ounces)* contains mostly water, several slip agents, glycerin, pH balancer, water-binding agents, preservative, soothing agent, and more preservatives. This is a good irritant-free toner for most skin types.

☹ **Plenitude Clarify-A³ Toner** *($6.52 for 8.5 ounces)* contains mostly water, alcohol, glycerin, mixed fruit extracts, water-binding agents, and preservatives. There isn't a skin type in the world that needs to be dried out or irritated, and that is exactly what alcohol does. Also, mixed fruit extracts are not necessarily the same thing as AHAs, because there is no way to know what the "extracts" actually are.

☺ **Plenitude Action Liposomes** *($17.33 for 1.7 ounces)* is an emollient moisturizer that contains mostly water, silicone oil, plant oils, glycerin, water-binding agent, thickeners, fragrance, and preservatives. There are some interesting water-binding agents and vitamins after the preservatives, but in amounts too insignificant to even be considered.

☺ **Plenitude Active Daily Moisture Lotion Oil-Free for Normal to Oily Skin** *($7.39 for 4 ounces)* contains mostly water, silicone oil (so it obviously is not oil-free), glycerin, several thickeners, vitamin E, more thickeners, and preservatives. It also contains small amounts of balm mint and salicylic acid; both can be skin irritants, but there's probably not enough to affect the skin. This would be an OK lightweight moisturizer for someone with normal to slightly dry skin.

☺ **Plenitude Active Daily Moisture Lotion for Normal to Dry Skin** *($7.32 for 4 ounces)* contains mostly water, plant oils, glycerin, thickener, silicone oil, more thickeners, vitamin E, more thickeners, fragrance, and preservatives. It also contains small amounts of salicylic acid and balm mint; both can be skin irritants, but there's probably not enough to affect the skin. The amount of vitamin E is also insignificant. This could be a good emollient moisturizer for someone with dry skin but not for someone with sensitive skin.

☹ **Plenitude Active Daily Moisture Lotion SPF 15 and Antioxidants for All Skin Types** *($7.39 for 4 ounces)* contains mostly water, thickener, silicone oil, glycerin, plant oils, more silicone oils, slip agent, more thickeners, fragrance, and preservatives. It does contain antioxidants, but they are at the very end of a long ingredient list, which means they can't keep even a puff of air off the face. This sunscreen wouldn't be very good for someone with normal to oily skin because of the oils, or for someone with sensitive skin because it contains aluminum starch, which can be a skin irritant and cause breakouts.

☺ **Plenitude Advanced Overnight Replenisher** *($9.92 for 1.7 ounces)* contains mostly water, silicone oil, plant oil, thickeners, petrolatum, more plant oil, more water-binding agent, and preservatives. This would be a good emollient moisturizer for someone with dry skin.

☺ **Plenitude Excell-A³ Skin Revealing Cream SPF 8** *($9.89 for 1.4 ounces)* contains mostly water, silicone oil, thickeners, glycerin, water-binding agent, plant oil, fruit extracts, fragrance, and preservatives. SPF 8 is OK for limited sun protection, but this isn't an AHA product, at least not if you want the benefits of exfoliation. You can't tell what kind of fruit extracts are in it, and they probably have nothing to do with real AHAs such as glycolic or lactic acid, or they would be listed as such. Nevertheless, this is a good emollient moisturizer for someone with dry skin.

☺ **Plenitude Excell-A³ Skin Revealing Lotion SPF 8** *($6.52 for 1.4 ounces)* is similar to the lotion above, and the same review applies.

☺ **Plenitude Hydra Renewal** *($8.75 for 1.7 ounces)* is a very good emollient moisturizer for dry skin; it contains mostly water, glycerin, thickener, silicone oil, slip agent, mineral oil, plant oil, water-binding agents, a long list of other thickeners, and preservatives. There is a tiny amount of vitamin E, but too little to have much effect.

☺ **Plenitude Advanced Wrinkle Defense Cream** *($10.44 for 1.2 ounces)* contains mostly water, silicone oil, thickeners, plant oil, a small amount of sunscreen, water-binding agent, vitamin A, and preservatives. This good lightweight moisturizer won't protect skin from the sun or change wrinkles, but it can soften dry skin.

☺ **Plenitude Eye Defense Gel** *($10.44 for 0.5 ounce)* contains mostly water, plant oil, slip agent, water-binding agents, thickener, anti-irritant, and preservatives. This is a good lightweight moisturizer for someone with combination to somewhat dry skin.

☺ **Plenitude Firming Facial Serum** *($13.10 for 1 ounce)* contains mostly water, slip agent, silicone oil, glycerin, water-binding agents, and preservatives. This is a good lightweight moisturizer for someone with normal to slightly dry or combination skin.

☺ **Plenitude Revitalift Anti-Wrinkle Firming Care for Face and Neck** *($10.44 for 1.7 ounces)* contains mostly water, silicone oil, glycerin, mineral oil, thickeners, vegetable oil, water-binding agent, more thickeners, vitamin A, and preservatives. It won't change a wrinkle on your face or firm anything, but it is a good emollient moisturizer.

☹ **Plenitude Clarify-A³ Peeling Mask** *($6.52 for 4 ounces)* contains mostly water, alcohol, film former, thickener, water-binding agents, more thickeners, fruit extracts, and preservatives. A form of plastic that peels off, combined with alcohol and a little bit of silicone oil, won't help the skin. It is fun to peel a mask, and if the alcohol and plastic don't irritate your skin it can feel smoother for a while, but given the ingredients, you're taking a risk with this one.

L'Oreal Makeup

☺ <u>FOUNDATION:</u> L'Oreal is one of the few drugstore lines to sometimes make foundation tester units available, but it isn't consistent from store to store. **Hydra Perfecte Protective Hydrating Makeup SPF 10** *($7.95)* is a lightweight foundation with a wonderful texture for normal to dry skin. The SPF isn't the best, but it is definitely better than nothing. **These colors are excellent:** Pale Ivory (may be slightly pink for some skin tones), Bare Beige, Sand (may be slightly peach), Almond Beige, and Deep Beige. **This color is too peach:** Shell Pink.

☺ **Lightnesse Light Natural Makeup** *($8.75)* is almost too sheer. It would be good for someone with normal to dry skin who wants only minimal coverage. **These colors are excellent :** Ivory, Bare Beige, Ecru Beige, True Beige, Sand Beige, and Warmed Beige.

☹ **Visuelle Invisible Coverage Makeup** *($8.75)* has a great soft texture and goes on light; it is made for women with normal to dry skin. **These are the only colors to consider:** Soft Ivory and Buff. **The rest are too pink or peach.**

☺ **Dualite Powder** *($6.96)* provides fairly light to almost medium coverage, but not much more. The color selection is excellent, and it has a superior, silky, smooth texture. It is best for women with normal to somewhat dry skin. The company recommends Dualite as both a foundation and a powder. Using a powder as a foundation can be tricky: if your skin is too dry, it can look chalky; if you're trying to cover blemishes or imperfections, the coverage isn't great. If those problems don't apply to you, Dualite can work as an alternative to regular liquid foundation (most other powder foundations can as well).

☺ **Mattique Matte Oil-Free Makeup** *($8.75)* has a good, fairly matte texture, but it has a slightly sticky feel. Someone with oily skin might not like it. There are now six colors geared toward African-American women that are all quite good. **These colors are very good:** Beige Blush, Nude Beige, Buff Beige, Sand Beige, Honey Beige, and Rich Beige. **These colors should be avoided:** Soft Ivory (too pink for most skin tones) and Golden Beige (too orange for most skin tones).

☹ **Feel Perfect Foundation SPF 15** *($7.86)* has a good SPF rating, which is nice, but the amount of silicone oil in this product makes it slippery and difficult to blend evenly, and the colors are ghastly. Except for Buff, **all the colors are too peach and pink for almost all skin types.** Maybe L'Oreal should run next door and take a look at Lancome's foundation shades: nary a pink or a peach in the lot.

☺ **Luminair Cream-Powder Makeup** *($7)* has an incredibly smooth finish and goes on like a lightweight glove over the face. What a shame there are no testers; it's almost impossible to detect the right color through the window of the container. Cream-to-powder foundations are almost always best for normal to oily or combination skin types. They're just not the best for dry skin.

☺ <u>**CONCEALER:**</u> **Mattique Conceal Oil-Free Cover-Up** *($4.73)* is a very good stick concealer that goes on quite sheer and smooth, although it does have a slight tendency to crease into the lines around the eyes. **Hydra Perfecte Concealer SPF 12** *($4.73)* is a good lightweight, sheer concealer that provides even coverage. It has a slight tendency to slip into the lines around the eyes, but it's worth a try because it blends on so nicely.

☺ <u>**POWDER:**</u> **Visuelle Pressed Powder** *($6.20)* has a beautiful soft translucent finish and some great colors—not a problem shade in the bunch. It does contain wheat starch (second on the ingredient list), which can cause allergic reactions for some skin types.

☹ **Mattique Oil-Free Softly Matte Pressed Powder** *($6.24)* is supposed to be for someone with oily skin, and the product label exults that it is oil-free and oil-absorbing and controls shine, but what they don't tell you is that this powder is iridescent. It doesn't control shine, it puts more on! **Hydra Perfecte Perfecting Loose Powder** *($6.77)* is also iridescent, but it doesn't make any claims about controlling shine or oil. However, it seems contradictory to apply a powder to set makeup and reduce shine, only to end up adding sparkles.

☺ <u>**BLUSH:**</u> **Visuelle Softly Luminous Powder Blush** *($6.20)* has a wonderful soft, easy-to-blend texture and a great color selection, with some perfect contour shades as well. **Blushesse** *($5.40)* feels very similar to the Visuelle Blush and goes on just as well and evenly.

☺ EYESHADOW: **Soft Effects Singles** *($4.75)* have a handful of very good neutral shades that are mostly matte; some of the colors are labeled as perle and easy to avoid but some of the mattes also have some shine. **The best matte shades are:** Sand, Terra, Buff, and Blush. **The "matte" shades to avoid because they have some amount of shine are:** Sable, Bark, Eggplant, and Marine. Definitely avoid all of the **Trios** *($4.75)*, and **Quads** *($5.50)*; either they come in strange combinations, or one or more of the colors are shiny.

☺ EYE AND BROW SHAPER: **Le Grand Kohl Perfectly Soft Liners** *($4.13)* are extra-long pencils in fairly muted colors that go on smooth without being too greasy, and blend well without streaking. There is also a small selection of standard twist-up eye pencils. **Pencil Perfect Automatic Eye Liner** *($4.13)* isn't what I would call perfect; if anything, it tends to go on greasier than most, and that means a greater chance of smearing. **Lineur Intense** *($4.92)* is a traditional liquid liner in a tube; it goes on like the name says—intense—and stays that way all day. **Brow Elegance** *($4.13)* is a standard brow pencil, slightly greasier than most.

☺ LIPSTICK AND LIP PENCIL: Colour Supreme Long Wearing Lip Colour *($4.89)* is a very moist, thick, creamy lip color. It may be too glossy for some tastes, but the color selection is beautiful. **Colour Riche Hydrating Creme Lip Colour** *($5.22)* is very similar to the Colour Supreme. This one is fairly emollient, and slightly less thick than the Supreme, but that's only a technicality. By the way, both Colour Riche and Colour Supreme have frosted colors; they are easily identifiable, so you can avoid them. **Sheer Colour Riche SPF 15** *($4.89)* is true to its name: it goes on sheer, more like a gloss than a lipstick, but it is very moist and the SPF 15 is great. **L'Oreal Endure Stay-On Lip Colour** *($5.99)* is strikingly similar to Revlon's ColorStay, and only true aficionados of the latter will be able to tell the difference. They are both very matte, go on thickly, and stay in place. However, they both feel very dry, and regardless of Endure's claim about containing oil, there is no real emollient feel in either of these products at all. They tend to wear away by peeling, and pressing your lips together can feel strange. This product is for women who want truly matte lips. Endure has one edge over ColorStay: color choice. Where Revlon has about 12 colors, Endure has 24. Also, Revlon's colors tend to be muted and drab, while L'Oreal's are a wide assortment of pastels, vibrants, and neutrals.

☺ **Lip Precision Self-Sharpening Lip Liner** *($5.50)* is a standard twist-up lip pencil that is slightly more creamy than most. It comes in a nice array of colors.

☺ <u>MASCARA:</u> **Accentuous Precisely Defining Mascara** *($4.14)* goes on easily but tends to clump and has a slight tendency to smear. **Formula Riche** *($5.75)* has the same problems, although both separate lashes nicely without making them look spiked. **Voluminous Dramatically Thick Mascara** *($5.75)* was a disappointment; although it went on well and builds great thick lashes, it tends to smear. **Sensitique Hypoallergenic Mascara** *($3.99)* is merely a cheaper version of Lancome's Tendercils Sensitive Eyes Mascara. Did Lancome think no one would notice that their parent company, L'Oreal, had come out with an identical product? Tendercils is an OK mascara, but little about it guarantees you won't be allergic to it. The same is true for Sensitique. Sensitique goes on well, building long lashes without clumping, it doesn't smear, and it doesn't have the odor problem the Tendercils mascara has. You may or may not be allergic to the Sensitique, but it is a good mascara in general.

☺ **Lash Out Extending Mascara** *($5.75)* is excellent, but I prefer a shorter wand. It does build long, thick lashes, with only a slight tendency to smear.

Lubriderm (Skin Care Only)

☹ **Body Bar** *($2.79 for 4 ounces)* is a standard detergent-based cleansing bar that contains tallow. Tallow can cause breakouts and allergic reactions, and the detergent cleansing agent can be quite drying. The bar also contains some petrolatum and mineral oil to soften the blow, but they aren't much help. Using this from the neck down would be fine, but keep it away from the face.

☹ **Loofa Bar** *($2.79 for 4 ounces)* is similar to the bar above, only with scrub particles, and the same review applies.

☹ **One Step Facial Cleanser** *($8 for 8 ounces)* would be a great cleanser if it were really water-soluble; unfortunately, it isn't. Your skin is likely to feel greasy once you're done rinsing. This may be an option for someone with dry skin, but it would require a washcloth to get it all off.

☺ **Dry Skin Care Lotion Fragrance Free** *($6.59 for 10 ounces)* contains mostly water, mineral oil, petrolatum, thickener, lanolin, more thickeners, and preservatives. This is a very good emollient, though boring, moisturizer for someone with dry skin.

☺ **Dry Skin Care Lotion Original Fragrance** *($6.59 for 10 ounces)* is identical to the lotion above, only with fragrance, and the same review applies.

☺ **Moisture Recovery Creme** *($6.79 for 4 ounces)* is nice but nothing to get excited about. It contains 4% AHAs in an ordinary moisturizing base, and can be good for someone with normal to dry skin.

☺ **Moisture Recovery Lotion** *($10 for 8 ounces)* is similar to the cream above, but with no more than 2% AHAs, which means it is an OK moisturizer but a poor AHA product.

☺ **Moisture Recovery GelCreme** *($4.29 for 4 ounces)* contains mostly water, thickener, glycerin, mineral oil, silicone oil, thickeners, and preservatives. You won't recover from anything with this product, but it is a good emollient moisturizer for someone with dry skin.

☺ **Seriously Sensitive Lotion for Extra Sensitive Skin** *($6.59 for 10 ounces)* contains mostly water, slip agent, glycerin, mineral oil, petrolatum, thickeners, silicone oil, and preservatives. Nothing about this product makes it better for someone with sensitive skin. It is a good ordinary emollient moisturizer for someone with dry skin.

☺ **Seriously Sensitive Lotion for Extra Sensitive Dry Skin** *($6.59 for 10 ounces)* is almost identical to the lotion above, and the same review applies.

M.A.C.
(Make-up Art Cosmetics)

Once the new kid on the block, M.A.C. is now a serious contender in the prestigious world of department store cosmetics. This Toronto-based company is also a trendsetter in the truest sense of that term. What other cosmetics line would ever consider using RuPaul, probably the best-known transvestite in the fashion world, to represent its line of skin care and makeup products? There is much irony in the spectacle of a company that previously bragged about its word-of-mouth-only advertising jumping into glossy, full-color, $60,000-a-page advertising with RuPaul. I'm not sure exactly what statement M.A.C. is trying to make, or what its executives had in mind with this marketing maneuver. Notoriety? Well, that much punch it has.

M.A.C. sells its products throughout North America, exclusively in upscale department stores and freestanding boutiques. The name is a bit pretentious, but nonetheless accurate. M.A.C. claims its products are used by many professional makeup artists, and in my experience that is true. Most professional makeup artists prefer matte eyeshadows and blushes, and this line has a generous offering; the color selection for everything from blush to lipstick and foundations is exceptional too. Also, most of the makeup brushes are beautiful, full, and soft, as well as properly sized to fit the contours of the face and eyes. You will find this color line a pleasure to shop—at least for the most part.

Unfortunately, M.A.C.'s skin care line is in another category altogether. These products are supposed to be filled with vitamins, antioxidants, and oxygen boosters, and are purportedly pH-balanced. Those claims are all rather exaggerated, and the products aren't worth the steep prices, but that's to be expected—after all, this is the world of cosmetics. M.A.C. claims that these products are "based on dermatologically advanced moisturization concepts [using] noncomedogenic compounds." Although these products don't contain mineral oil, lanolin, or isopropyl myristate, they have plenty of other ingredients that could make you break out or irritate your skin. M.A.C.'s advanced moisturizing ingredients aren't so advanced anymore; in fact, lately they've become fairly standard. Also, the "latest water-binding ingredients" can't do any more for the skin than other moisturizing ingredients. No studies have proven that they affect wrinkling one way or the other. By the way, the lactic acid listed in most of the M.A.C. is there only in small concentrations, which makes it a good moisturizing ingredient but not an exfoliating ingredient.

M.A.C. Skin Care

☺ **Foaming Cleanser** *($14 for 4.4 ounces)* is an OK water-soluble cleanser for oily skin, although it may prove to be quite drying. The cleansing agent is potassium hydroxide (caustic potash), which is a strong alkaline detergent. Several of the ingredients are supposed to bind water to the skin, but they won't be all that soothing if your skin is irritated by the potassium hydroxide.

☺ **pH Balanced Cleanser** *($20 for 8.8 ounces)* is an OK water-soluble cleanser that can clean off all your makeup without burning your eyes, but it can be somewhat drying. There is a long list of water-binding ingredients that can help soothe the skin, but most will be washed away before they have a chance to do any good.

☹ **Exfoliating Cleanser** *($16 for 4.4 ounces)* will indeed take off some skin, but potassium hydroxide is an irritant, and jojoba wax (the second ingredient) can clog pores or cause allergies.

☺ **Eye Makeup Remover** *($17.50 for 4.4 ounces)* should be gentle and effective, although the detergent cleanser, listed among the first items on the ingredient list, can be too irritating for some skin types.

☹ **PA-1 Phyto-Astringent Purifying Toner** *($17.50 for 4.4 ounces)* is basically water, alcohol, cucumber extract, and witch hazel. The alcohol and witch hazel can be quite irritating, making oily skin worse. The cucumber extract is supposed to nourish the skin; it can't, but it does produce a nice cooling sensation. The seventh ingredient is whole wheat amino acids, which can help water penetrate the skin but won't prevent irritation from the other ingredients.

☹ **PA-2 Phyto-Astringent Purifying Toner** *($17.50 for 4.4 ounces)* is almost identical to PA-1, with some orange and papaya extract added. Both can cause skin irritations, and the alcohol and witch hazel are a problem for most skin types.

☺ **PA-3 Phyto-Astringent Purifying Toner** *($17.50 for 4.4 ounces)* is probably a very good irritant-free toner. Witch hazel is one of the last items on the ingredient list; since there isn't much, there is little chance it will irritate the skin. Some of the herb extracts can produce skin sensitivities, but it should be fine for most skin types.

☹ **PA-S Phyto-Astringent Purifying Toner** *($17.50 for 4.4 ounces)* would be a great toner if the second ingredient weren't witch hazel, which can irritate some skin types. These toners are overpriced for what you get, and they won't purify anything, although they contain some good water-binding agents.

☺ **$$$ EP-1 Environmental Protective Day Emulsion SPF 8** *($28 for 2.1 ounces)* contains mostly water, thickeners, pollen extract, plant oils, and preservatives. This very good, although overly expensive, emollient moisturizer for someone with dry skin has all the trendy moisturizing ingredients, plus SPF 8 sunscreen (which is OK for limited sun exposure). The fourth item on the ingredient list is pollen extract, which has a slight possibility of causing allergic reactions.

☺ **$$$ EP-2 Environmental Protective Day Emulsion** *($28 for 2.1 ounces)* is almost identical to EP-1, and the same review applies.

☺ **$$$ EP-3 Environmental Protective Day Emulsion** *($28 for 2.1 ounces)* is almost identical to EP-1 and EP-2, and the same review applies.

☺ **$$$ CR-1 Cellular Recovery Night Emulsion** *($35 for 2.1 ounces)* is almost identical to EP-1, EP-2, and EP-3 (the price is even higher), and the same review applies. The major difference, according to M.A.C., is the "live yeast extract," which supposedly supplies the skin cells with oxygen, improving cell renewal. It's unlikely that anything in the cream is alive, given the amount of preservatives present and the way cosmetics are formulated. M.A.C. doesn't have to back up its claims with scientific studies, so it can say whatever it wants to.

☺ **$$$ CR-2 Cellular Recovery Night Emulsion** *($35 for 2.1 ounces)* is almost identical to CR-1. It is a very good moisturizer, but it can't help your cells recover from anything.

☺ **$$$ EZR Eye Zone Repair** *($35 for 1 ounce)* is very similar to all the other M.A.C. moisturizers. It contains a long list of water-binding ingredients and oils, as well as cucumber, chamomile, and yeast extract. See the review of CR-1 Cellular Recovery

Night Emulsion, above, for a brief discussion of yeast; you already know not to expect much from the plant extracts.

☺ **NMF Moisture Regulated Formula** *($20 for 4.4 ounces)* contains many of the same ingredients as the other moisturizers, as well as a sunscreen of SPF 8, appropriate only for limited sun exposure.

☹ **VM-1 Vitamin and Mineral Hydrating Mask** *($16 for 2.1 ounces)* contains water, clay, glycerin, antiseptic (a potential skin irritant), detergent, more clay, alcohol, thickeners, vitamins A and E, and preservatives. This is just a standard clay mask with some extra irritating ingredients.

☺ **VM-2 Vitamin and Mineral Hydrating Mask** *($16 for 2.1 ounces)* contains water, clay, glycerin, sesame oil, standard slip agents, more clay, thickeners, vitamins A and E, and preservatives. This is a standard clay mask with some oil added to reduce the dryness caused by the clay. If you want a clay mask, this one is OK for some skin types.

M.A.C. Makeup

☺ **FOUNDATION: Matte Finish** *($17.50)* isn't all that matte. Someone with oily skin would not be pleased with this formulation. It's best for someone with normal to dry skin. **These colors are great:** N1, N3, N4, N5, N9, N10, C2, C3, C4, C5, and Brunette. **These colors are too pink, peach, or ashy:** N2, N6, C6, C7, and Summer Dusk.

☺ **Satin Finish** *($18)* has a nice emollient feel and provides medium coverage for normal to dry skin (it is surprisingly similar to the Matte Finish). **These colors are great:** N1, N2, N3, N4, N6, N7, N9, C2, C3, C4, C5, C6, and C7. **These colors are too peach for most skin tones:** Copper and N5.

☺ **Studio Fix Foundation** *($18)* is a rich powder foundation that provides medium coverage; although M.A.C. recommends it for normal to oily skin, it's really best on normal skin. **All of the shades are impressive.**

☺ **CONCEALER: TV Touch** *($10)* goes on rather heavy and thick, but it provides excellent coverage and stays on well without much slippage. M.A.C. recommends mixing it with the foundation or a little moisturizer before you apply it, probably to soften the thickness of the concealer, which can be a problem for someone who wants a more sheer application. **These colors are great:** Natural Beige, Light Beige, Medium Beige, Dark Beige, and Umber. **This color is too yellow for most skin tones:** Manila.

☺ __POWDER:__ M.A.C.'s powders are fairly standard talc-based powders. **Pressed Powder** *($18)* is an ordinary compact powder, and **Loose Powder** comes in a shake-it bottle *($14)* or a traditional tub *($19)*. Both are good, but the shake-it container is one of the most convenient ways to use loose powder. Consider this one a very good buy.

☺ __BLUSH:__ M.A.C.'s **Blushes** *($10)* are packaged just like the eyeshadows, in round see-through containers. (By the way, the see-through containers are great. You never have to fumble through your makeup bag and wonder if you've picked up the right color.) The colors are fine—they go on true, and there is a large matte assortment—but fairly standard, nothing exceptional.

☺ __EYESHADOW:__ The **Eyeshadows** *($10 and $13)* are almost all matte. There are several obnoxious shiny eyeshadows, but they are displayed separately, readily identified, and easily avoided. The primary color selection is nonshiny and surprisingly neutral: no glaring shades of pink, blue, or green here. Instead, you'll find a large group of tan shades ranging from pale cream to sable brown, taupe, gray-lavender, and every step in between. M.A.C. has one of the best neutral color palettes in the business. Warning: Some of the colors can be a bit on the heavy (greasy or grainy) side and they go on more intense than they look.

☺ __EYE AND BROW SHAPER:__ The **Eye Pencils** *($9)* like almost every other eye pencil on the market. **Creme Liner** *($9.50)* is an ultra-dramatic liner comes in a pot for a very thick matte look. Avoid the Aluminum shade.

☺ __LIPSTICK AND LIP PENCIL:__ Most of M.A.C.'s lipsticks are excellent. **Matte Lipstick** *($12)* doesn't bleed and doesn't require a sealer; which always thrills me. The only problem is that it can be very dry and make the lips peel or feel caked by the end of the day. **Satin Lipstick** *($12)* is wonderful and nicely creamy without being thick. It's supposed to be semi-matte; I don't see it, but maybe you will. **Sheer Lipstick** *($12)* is more a gloss than a lipstick; it contains a lot of vitamin E, which is a big selling point but not all that essential for the lips. **Liptone** *($12)* is a tint that goes on like a gloss, dries, and then becomes sort of a color stain on the lips. If you can get used to the texture, it's an interesting option for lip color that has some staying power. **Cream Lipstick** *($12)* is fairly standard but has a good smooth finish. The color selection for all of these lipstick groupings is fairly impressive. The **Lip Pencils** *($9)* are like almost every other lip pencil on the market.

☹ __MASCARA:__ The **Mascara** *($12)* is just OK and tends to smear slightly.

☺ **BRUSHES:** M.A.C. has one of the best selections of brushes you'll find anywhere *(38 different brushes ranging from $6 to $65)*. The big brushes are a little pricey, but they last forever if you take good care of them, so they are one of the few expensive makeup investments I recommend.

Make Up For Ever—Paris (Makeup Only)

If you've shopped the makeup counters at Nordstrom lately, you may have seen the intriguing display for this new line of color cosmetics imported from Paris. The extensive line of eyeshadows, foundations, powders, pencils, and concealers was originally created for use in the theater. Of course, the fact that a color line is used onstage does not mean it has what your face needs for daytime, or even evening wear. There is much about Make Up For Ever—Paris that makes it difficult for me to recommend. Many of the hues, shades, textures, and products are inappropriate or just too heavy for most skin types or for a soft, natural look. Even the salesperson had a rough time making this line sound tempting.

Make Up For Ever's primary and significant strength is its vast selection of colors for most skin tones, especially medium to darker skin tones, which is assuredly a welcome addition at the cosmetics counters.

☹ **FOUNDATION: Pre-Makeup Base** *($19)* is a tinted moisturizer that, like other color correctors, comes in lavender, green, orange, yellow, blue, white, and transparent. Color correctors come and go, and mostly, I believe, they should go. This unnecessary step builds up too much product and often mixes badly with the foundation.

☺ **Soft Modeling Film** *($24)* is an emollient liquid foundation that would be best for someone with normal to dry skin. It provides light to medium coverage and has an impressive selection of colors. **Most of the colors are excellent. These colors should be avoided:** 1, which is too rose; 5, 7, and 13, which are very orange; 6 and 14, which can be too ash; and 12, which can be too yellow.

☹ **Pan Stick** *($27)* contains mostly petrolatum, carnauba wax, lanolin, and castor oil. It is a greasy mess of a foundation, impossible to recommend. Just as bad, the wide range of colors displays strong tones of pink, orange, ash, rose, and peach. There are a few good colors, but why bother?

☹ **Pan Cake** *($27)* is, as the name implies, a cake of pressed powder that you can apply wet or dry. There are 16 colors, almost all too peach, orange, or ash. If the theater is your goal, these can be useful; otherwise, they are better left behind the counter.

☹ <u>CONCEALER:</u> **Eye Concealer Stick** *($16)* is a lipstick-style concealer that comes in only one shade; it is slightly pink, which is inappropriate for most, if not all, skin tones. Although it goes on rather sheer, the texture is quite greasy, and it can crease into the lines around the eye. **Pot Concealers** *($17)* are waterproof and come in an excellent array of colors for medium to darker skin tones. They provide serious coverage, but you have to put up with a dry, thick appearance. **Eye Concealer Pencil** *($17)* is a standard thin pencil that comes in two colors, one for Caucasian skin and one for darker skin tones. Each of the two pencils has a different color at each end, but the colors aren't the best, particularly the one for darker skin tones, which is strongly orange. You also have to get used to applying a concealer with a texture so dry that it feels like you're poking yourself.

☺ <u>POWDER:</u> **Poudre Libre** *($27)* is a standard talc-based loose powder with a soft texture. **Almost all of the colors are very good and neutral. These colors should be avoided:** 114 (hot pink), 2 (lavender pink), 6 (lavender), and 4 (green). **Compact Powder** *($27)* is a standard talc-based powder with a great color selection. Although nothing exceptional, it is a good powder with a nice texture.

☺ <u>EYESHADOW AND BLUSH:</u> Referred to as **Colors** *($14)*, these versatile items come in more than a hundred shades, and a good number of them are matte. The colors are strongly pigmented, so even the softest-looking pink goes on red, and the palest taupe goes on deep brown. (This is a definite drawback for those with lighter skin tones, but a strong plus for women with darker or African-American skin tones.) There are shiny colors in this mix, and several blues and greens, so pay attention. (Avoid. Avoid.) Just for the record, these colors don't hold a candle to M.A.C.'s, and M.A.C.'s cost less. Make Up For Ever also offers something called **Star Powders** *($17)*, little pots of loose iridescent powder in a fun range of colors. If you're feeling impetuous or are under 30 and want a sparkling effect, they could make an interesting splash of color somewhere, or everywhere.

☺ <u>EYE AND BROW SHAPER:</u> **Demographic Pencils** *($15)* are standard, everyday pencils for the eyes, brows, and lips. They come in an attractive collection of colors, except for the blues and greens, and they go on easily. The lip pencil colors are much more vivid than you would imagine from just looking at them, so try them on before buying.

☺ <u>LIPSTICK AND LIP PENCIL:</u> While color choice seems to be Make Up For Ever's strong point, the three lipsticks, **Matte**, **Transparent**, and **Nacre** *(all $16)*, offer a surprisingly small selection. The Matte lipsticks go on thick and matte and stay on well, with little to no bleeding. The Transparents are simply sheer, greasy lipsticks. The Nacres are standard creamy, iridescent lipsticks, something I never recommend. The Demographic Pencils, reviewed above, include lip pencils.

☺ **MASCARA:** The Mascara *($16)* goes on easily, builds long thick lashes, and stays on well without smearing.

☺ **BRUSHES:** This line features more than 15 brushes, and a few are quite usable, but the quality (the bristles are supposed to be sable and pony, but they are too soft and loose) and the price (around $25 for even the tiniest brush) may be hard to swallow. While the bristles have a wonderfully soft texture, they are too sparse to hold color well or offer good control on the cheeks or eyes.

Marcelle (Available Only in Canada)

Marcelle is one of the few lines in Canada to sport ingredient lists on most of its products. This reasonably priced drugstore line has some good products that perform well and look great. The packaging is simple, and some of the products are fragrance-free. Sad to say, this isn't an exciting line; there are almost no matte eyeshadows, and the foundations have an incredibly poor color selection. However, the blushes, one of the mascaras, and the lipsticks are worth investigating. The skin care products boast that they are hypoallergenic, but they aren't; there's no way any company can know what your skin may be allergic to. Also, many of these products contain ingredients that have a rather high potential for irritation.

Note: All prices listed for Marcelle products are in Canadian dollars.

Marcelle Skin Care

☹ **Aquarelle Aqua-Pure Cleansing Bar Oil-Free** *($5.38 for 125 g)* is a standard bar soap that can be quite drying for almost all skin types. It contains tallow, which can cause breakouts.

☹ **Hydractive Hydra-Pure Cleansing Bar for Dehydrated/Normal to Dry Skin** *($6.38 for 125 g)* is similar to the soap above, and the same review applies.

☹ **Soap Hypo-Allergenic** *($2.68 for 100 g)* is similar to the soaps above, and the same review applies.

☺ **Aquarelle Oil-Free Purifying Cleansing Gel for Oily Skin** *($10.58 for 170 ml)* is a good standard detergent cleanser for most skin types. It won't purify anything, but it can clean the skin without irritation or dryness, and it won't irritate the eyes.

☺ **Cleansing Cream Hypo-Allergenic** *($7.98 for 240 ml)* is a mineral oil–based detergent cleanser that can leave a greasy film on the skin. Calling this product hypoallergenic is stretching the facts; it absolutely contains ingredients that some skin types may react to.

☺ **Cleansing Milk for Combination Skin Hypo-Allergenic** *($9.89 for 240 ml)* is a standard detergent-based, water-soluble cleanser. It contains a tiny amount of lactic acid that probably isn't enough to be a problem for the skin or eyes. This could be a good cleanser for some skin types.

☺ **Liquid Cleanser for Combination Skin** *($10.95 for 240 ml)* is similar to the product above, and the same review applies.

☺ **Cleansing Milk for Dry/Normal Skin Hypo-Allergenic** *($9.88 for 240 ml)* is a mineral oil–based cleanser that must be wiped off. It can leave a greasy film on the skin.

☺ **Gentle Foaming Wash for Sensitive Skin Types Hypo-Allergenic** *($8.98 for 170 ml)* isn't all that gentle, but it is an OK standard detergent-based, water-soluble cleanser that can be drying for most skin types.

☺ **Hydractive Water Rinseable Cleansing Lotion for Dehydrated/Normal to Dry Skin** *($11.95 for 180 ml)* is a wipe-off cleanser that isn't all that rinseable, and isn't very good at removing makeup either. You have to use a washcloth, and that isn't a great way to remove makeup because it can be irritating and pulls at the skin. It could be OK for someone with very dry skin who doesn't wear much makeup, but it can leave a greasy film.

☺ **Liquid Cleanser for Dry/Normal Skin** *($9.88 for 240 ml)* is a standard mineral oil–based cleanser that can leave a greasy film and must be wiped off.

☺ **Quick Cleanser** *($7.98 for 120 ml)* is like a cold cream and must be wiped off. It can most definitely leave a greasy film on the skin.

☺ **Creamy Eye Make-Up Remover Hypo-Allergenic** *($6.58 for 50 ml)* is basically just mineral oil, some thickeners and slip agents, and petrolatum. It will wipe off makeup and leave a greasy film on the skin.

☺ **Eye Make-Up Remover Pads Hypo-Allergenic** *($6.98 for 60 pads)* are mineral oil–soaked pads.

☺ **Oil-Free Eye Make-Up Remover Lotion Hypo-Allergenic** *($7.48 for 120 ml)* contains detergent cleansing agents, slip agent, and preservatives. It will remove makeup, but it is hardly hypoallergenic, and could be a problem for some skin types.

☹ **Scrub Wash for All Skin Types Hypo-Allergenic** *($8.98 for 100 ml)* is a clay cleanser that also contains witch hazel, zinc oxide, alcohol, detergent cleanser, thickener, and preservatives. Not only is it *not* hypoallergenic, but the clay and zinc oxide make it hard to rinse off.

☹ **Aquarelle Oil Normalizing Toner Alcohol-Free for Oily Skin** *($9.98 for 240 ml)* contains mostly water, witch hazel, slip agents, aloe, film former, and preservatives. Technically, it is alcohol-free, but the witch hazel contains a small amount of alcohol and can be a skin irritant. This isn't a bad product, but it isn't the kind I recommend for any skin type.

☺ **Hydractive Alcohol-Free Reviving Toner for Normal to Dry Skin** *($11.25 for 180 ml)* contains mostly water, slip agent, water-binding agents, glycerin, aloe, film former, anti-irritant, and preservatives. This would be a very good nonirritating toner for most skin types.

☹ **Skin Freshener Combination Skin Hypo-Allergenic** *($8.98 for 240 ml)* is mostly just alcohol and glycerin and is not a good idea for any skin type I can think of. Calling alcohol hypoallergenic is someone's idea of a joke, right?

☹ **Skin Freshener for Dry/Normal Skin Hypo-Allergenic** *($8.98 for 240 ml)* is similar to the product above, and the same review applies. This product also contains aluminum chlorohydrate, a key ingredient in underarm deodorant, which can cause breakouts and allergic reactions.

☹ **Skin Toner Combination Skin** *($7.95 for 240 ml)* is similar to the Skin Freshener for Combination Skin above, and the same review applies.

☹ **Skin Toner for Oily Skin** *($8.98 for 240 ml)* is similar to the Skin Freshener for Combination Skin above, only it contains even more alcohol and the same review applies.

☺ **Aquarelle Aqua-Matte Hydrating Fluid** *($12.58 for 120 ml)* contains mostly water, several thickeners, fragrance, more thickeners, aloe, silicone oil, and preservatives. There are some good water-binding agents and antioxidants, but in amounts too minuscule to have value for the skin. This is an OK but ordinary moisturizer for someone with normal to slightly dry skin.

☹ **Formula 24 Cream for Oily Skin** *($7.48 for 60 ml)* contains mostly water, slip agent, thickeners, sulfur, and preservatives. Sulfur is a disinfectant that may have an effect on acne, but it doesn't make sense to put it in a cream base that contains thickeners that can cause breakouts.

☺ **Hydractive Hydra-Repair Night Treatment with Sphingolipids, Hyaluronic Acid, Echinacea Extract, Vitamins A and E** *($17.95 for 60 ml)* contains mostly water, plant extract, thickener, silicone oil, plant oil, more thickeners, more silicone oils, thickeners, water-binding agent, plant extracts, and preservatives. Of the ingredients mentioned in the name of the product, only hyaluronic acid (a good water-binding agent) comes well before the preservatives. All the others are at the end of the list, in amounts barely worth mentioning. This is a good emollient moisturizer for someone with dry skin, but more because of the standard ingredients than the fancy-sounding ones.

☺ **Moisture Cream Hypo-Allergenic** *($8.58 for 40 ml; $11.98 for 60 ml)* contains isopropyl myristate, which is known for causing breakouts, as the third ingredient: so much for hypoallergenic. Other than that, this is a good, ordinary emollient moisturizer for someone with dry skin. It does contain AHAs, but only about 2%, not enough to make it an exfoliant.

☺ **Moisture Lotion Hypo-Allergenic** *($9.88 for 90 ml; $12.58 for 120 ml)* is similar to the cream above, but without the AHAs, and the same review applies.

☺ **Multi-Defense Cream Daily Moisturizer SPF 15 Perfume-Free** *($12.95 for 60 ml)* is a good basic sunscreen for someone with dry skin. It contains mostly water, slip agent, thickeners, plant oil, more thickeners, silicone oil, water-binding agent, more plant oil, and preservatives. There are antioxidant vitamins in this cream, but not enough to have much impact.

☺ **Oil-Free Multi-Defense Lotion Daily Moisturizer SPF 15 Perfume-Free** *($13.48 for 120 ml)* contains mostly water, slip agent, thickeners, silicone oil (it's obviously not oil-free), water-binding agent, and preservatives. Someone with oily skin may not be nuts about how this lotion feels on the skin, but it is a good sunscreen for someone with normal to slightly dry skin.

☹ **Sun Block Lotion SPF 15 Perfume-Free** *($6.78 for 120 ml)* is basically sunscreen and thickeners. It's OK for someone with dry skin, but the second ingredient is isopropyl myristate, which can cause breakouts.

☺ **Sun Block Cream SPF 15 PABA-Free, Perfume-Free** *($6.78 for 90 ml)* is a good basic sunscreen for someone with dry skin.

☺ **Night Cream** *($8.58 for 40 ml)* is almost identical to the Moisture Lotion above, but it's a cream, and the same review applies.

☹ **Alpha-Radiance Cream Skin Renewal Activator with Alpha-Hydroxy Acid Hypo-Allergenic** *($14.38 for 60 ml)* doesn't contain more than 2% to 3% AHAs. It won't renew skin, although it could be an OK moisturizer for someone with dry skin.

☺ **Alpha-Radiance Lotion Skin Renewal Activator with Alpha-Hydroxy Acid Hypo-Allergenic** *($14.38 for 120 ml)* is similar to the moisturizer above, and the same review applies.

☺ **Anti-Aging Cream with Collagen and Elastin Hypo-Allergenic** *($11.95 for 40 ml)* contains mostly water, thickeners, water-binding agents, plant oil, more thickener, more water-binding agents, and preservatives. This is a very good moisturizer for someone with dry skin, but there is nothing anti-aging in this product whatsoever. Collagen and elastin are nothing more than water-binding agents; they have no effect on the collagen and elastin that are part of your skin.

☺ **Eye Care Cream Ultra-Light Hypo-Allergenic** *($7.68 for 15 ml)* contains mostly water, several thickeners, glycerin, aloe, film former, water-binding agents, vitamin E, silicone oil, and preservatives. This is a good moisturizer for someone with normal to dry skin.

☺ **Eye Cream Ultra Rich Hypo-Allergenic** *($6.78 for 15 ml)* is just mineral oil, petrolatum, wax, and preservatives. It is about as close to Vaseline as you can get, which makes it greasy and relatively hypoallergenic.

☺ **Hydractive Hydra-Replenishing Cream** *($13.78 for 40 ml)* contains mostly water, glycerin, several thickeners, film former, water-binding agent, and preservatives. It's fairly standard, but it would be a good moisturizer for someone with normal to dry skin.

☹ **Clay Mask with Kaolin Hypo-Allergenic** *($8.98 for 100 ml)* contains mostly water, witch hazel, clay, glycerin, thickener, and preservatives. This is a standard clay mask, but I wouldn't call clay or witch hazel hypoallergenic.

☹ **Moisturizing Peel-Off Mask, Dry/Normal and Combination Skin** *($9.95 for 100 ml)* contains alcohol and a plastic-forming agent, which can make the skin feel smooth, but it can also cause problems for the skin.

☹ **Peel-Off Mask, Oily Skin** *($8.98 for 100 ml)* is similar to the mask above, and the same review applies.

Marcelle Makeup

☹ **FOUNDATION: Oil-Free Makeup** *($8.25)* is half alcohol and half talc and coloring, making it hard to apply. The alcohol is too drying and irritating for most skin types. **Moisture Rich Foundation for Dry/Normal Skin** *($8.25)* would be a good foundation if the colors weren't so pink and peach. **Matte Finish Oil-Free Foundation** *($8.25)* and **All Day Protection with SPF 8** *($8.75)* both have a very poor color selection.

☹ **CONCEALER: Cover Up** *($6.25)* is a lipstick-type concealer with a terrible selection of colors, none of which I recommend. **Concealer Crayon** *($6.25)* is a fat pencil that comes in three OK shades: Light, Beige Cameo, and Dark (which isn't all that dark). The texture is workable, but it tends to crease into the lines around the eye.

☺ **POWDER: Pressed Powder** *($8.75)* is a good standard talc powder that comes in a handful of shades. **These colors are OK:** Suntan, Translucent Medium, and Translucent Dark. **These colors should be avoided:** Classic Beige, Rosy Peach, and Translucent.

☺ **BLUSH: Moisturizing Blush** *($9)* isn't all that moisturizing, but it comes in an excellent group of colors and the price is reasonable.

☺ **EYESHADOW: Eyeshadow Singles** *($6.75)* and **Duos** *($7.75)* come in some excellent matte neutral colors. **These colors and combinations are excellent:** Granite, Iris, Caramel, Blush, Chiffon, Soleil d'Or, Moss/Suede (the moss may be too green for most skin tones), Whisper/Nude, and Blue Stone/Pebble Pink (not a great combination, but the blue is grayer than most). **These colors are too shiny or blue:** Praline, Smoky Teal, Espresso/Creme Fraiche, Purple Passion/Mango (a strange combination), Algue Marine, Cote d'Azure.

☺ **EYE AND BROW SHAPER: Eye Pencil** *($6.50)* is similar to many other pencils on the market. There are two types; the waterproof one does stay on well when wet, but so does the other. Some of the colors are shiny and should be avoided.

☺ **LIPSTICK AND LIP PENCIL:** Marcelle has a good but limited selection of **Lipsticks** *($6.50)*. The fairly standard **Lip Pencils** *($5.95)* conveniently twist up so you don't have to worry about sharpening.

☹ **MASCARA: Superlash Mascara** *($8.50)* takes a long time to build definition. It would be OK if you just want a lightweight makeup look.

☺ **Ultimate Lash Mascara** *($8.50)* is an exceptional mascara that goes on beautifully and never smears or clumps. I would definitely buy this one again.

Mary Kay

Mary Kay is one of the original multilevel-marketing home-sales cosmetics companies. Since beginning her firm in 1963, Mary Kay Ash has built herself (and her sons) quite an empire. There are now more than 300,000 Mary Kay salespeople, and they sold $1.2 billion worth of cosmetics in 1992. (Of that total, $840 million was disbursed back to the sales reps.) The company also boasts a fleet of 923 pink Cadillacs—the ultimate reward for selling Mary Kay cosmetics—and 4,000 Pontiac Grand Ams. As impressive as this all sounds, and it is impressive, the average salesperson's income is more like $5,000 to $10,000 a year. Obviously, the ability to sell does not come naturally to every member of the sales force.

All the Mary Kay sales representatives I've ever met were extremely dedicated to Mary Kay and her products; their pitches sounded as if they were talking about a religion, not cosmetics. That kind of intensity is not atypical for cosmetics salespeople, particularly for in-home sales–oriented companies, but this kind of devotion to the owner of the company is unique. Regardless, their presentations were organized and systematic. At each one, I was given new demo-size brushes to use and individual samples of almost every product (including tiny eye and lip pencils).

Mary Kay's strong points are great blushes, very good foundations, and reasonably priced eye and lip pencils. The colors are conveniently divided into Cool, Warm, and Neutral. But there are lots of pitfalls to watch out for, such as a huge selection of blue eyeshadows, a cream concealer that easily creases into the lines around the eyes, lipsticks that tend toward the greasy side, and a skin care system (including foundation) that forces you to buy all of it or none of it.

Another potential problem arises from the way the products are marketed. Each salesperson buys her products and samples from the company and sells them directly to the consumer, yet because of cash flow not everyone can afford to stock all of the colors. What tends to happen is that the consumer is shown only what the salesperson has in stock.

Mary Kay's policy is not to sell a foundation to a first-time customer unless she buys the basic skin care products for her skin type, which makes this one very expensive foundation. The rationale for this unusual restriction is that the foundation is part of the skin care routine. The salespeople justify this policy by saying they want to monitor allergic reactions and perfect their assessment of your skin type. This sounds good, but all it really means is that you have to buy products that I would otherwise suggest you avoid. So I'm caught between a rock and a hard place. If I recommend these foundations, I'm also recommending a handful of other products I think aren't worth it. The list of colors I like is presented for your information, but I can't really encourage you to try them if it means you have to buy $50 worth of other products you may not need or want.

Mary Kay Skin Care

☺ **Creamy Cleanser** (*$9 for 6.5 ounces*) is indeed a creamy cleanser, but it can't be rinsed off without the aid of a washcloth. It also can leave behind traces of makeup.

☺ **Deep Cleanser** *($9 for 6.5 ounces)* is a water-soluble detergent cleanser that can be too drying for most skin types.

☺ **Gentle Cleansing Creme** *($9 for 4 ounces)* is a traditional, greasy cold cream containing mostly mineral oil, water, petrolatum, beeswax, glycerin, and other waxes. It might be gentle, but it is also quite heavy, and wiping off makeup is not good for the skin.

☺ **Extra Emollient Cleansing Creme** *($9 for 4 ounces)* is identical to the cream above, only heavier.

☹ **Purifying Bar** *($11 for 4.2 ounces)* is a standard bar soap that won't purify anything, but it may dry out the skin.

☺ **Gentle Action Freshener** *($10 for 6.5 ounces)* is a nonirritating toner that can be somewhat soothing. It does contain witch hazel, but at the very end of the ingredient list, so it shouldn't pose a problem. Some silk amino acids are also in this product; they may sound good, but even if they could do something for the skin, they come well after the preservatives, so there isn't much.

☹ **Hydrating Freshener** *($10 for 6.5 ounces)* contains mostly water, slip agent, preservative, and a small amount of arnica and peppermint, which can irritate the skin. There are a few interesting ingredients after the preservative, but the amount is so trivial as to make them completely inconsequential. This freshener is being sold as irritant-free, but the peppermint and arnica completely negate that claim.

☹ **Blemish Control Toner** *($10 for 6.5 ounces)* contains mostly water, alcohol, slip agent, more alcohol, menthol, and eucalyptus oil. It also contains salicylic acid. There is no evidence that alcohol or salicylic acid will control blemishes, and both ingredients, as well as the menthol and eucalyptus oil, are extremely irritating.

☹ **Refining Freshener** *($10 for 6.5 ounces)* contains mostly water and alcohol, which can irritate the skin.

☹ **Daily Defense Complex with SPF 4** *($25 for 1.4 ounces)* is an ordinary moisturizer with a minimal amount of sunscreen that can't defend adequately from the sun. There are a few interesting ingredients, but they come after the preservatives, so they don't count for much.

☺ **Balancing Moisturizer** *($16 for 2.4 ounces)* is a good basic moisturizer for normal to dry skin, containing mostly water, mineral oil, water-binding agents, thickeners, plant oil, and preservatives.

☺ **Enriched Moisturizer** *($16 for 1.4 ounces)* isn't all that enriched or all that different from the moisturizer above. It does contain collagen, but far down on the ingredient list, so there's not enough to really benefit the skin.

☺ **Extra Emollient Moisturizer** *($16 for 4 ounces)* is a very rich, somewhat heavy moisturizer for dry skin; it contains mostly water, wax, plant oils, water-binding agents, thickeners, collagen, and preservatives.

☺ **Extra Emollient Night Cream** *($11 for 2.5 ounces)* is a very rich, extremely heavy moisturizer for someone with severely dry skin. It contains mostly petrolatum, mineral oil, several thickeners, and preservatives.

☺ **Advanced Moisture Renewal Treatment Cream** *($19 for 2.5 ounces)* is a good rich moisturizer for dry skin, but it's nothing special; it contains mostly water, mineral oil, thickener, petrolatum, plant oil, several other thickeners, and preservatives. Some vitamin E and water-binding agents are in this product, but they come well after the preservatives, so there isn't enough to matter. .

☺ **Eye Cream Concentrate** *($12 for 0.75 ounce)* is a good emollient that contains mostly water, petrolatum, thickener, plant oil, mineral oil, more thickeners, and preservatives. Vitamin E, aloe, and collagen are at the end of the ingredient list, so there isn't enough to matter.

☹ **Triple-Action Eye Enhancer** *($15 for 0.65 ounce)* claims to have more benefits in one little product than almost any other I've ever seen. According to the company's magazine, it has much more than just triple action; I lost count after six benefits. It has free-radical scavengers, AHAs, and light-diffusing ingredients; it can be used as an eyeshadow base or as an under-eye concealer; it reduces puffiness and increases skin firmness; and, finally, it reduces the appearance of wrinkles. What's in this little miracle? Mostly silicone oil, a form of acrylate (kind of like a thin layer of plastic), a fixative (like those found in hairsprays), clay, several thickeners, more silicone oil, and preservatives. There are tiny amounts of vitamins E and A, but they are at the end of the ingredient list and therefore present in amounts so minuscule as to be completely insignificant. Then what about those benefits? Well, there aren't enough AHAs in this product to exfoliate skin, which is actually good, because you wouldn't want that on your eyelids. It doesn't have light-diffusing properties. The film-forming ingredients can form a tight layer over the skin, giving the illusion of smoother skin, but they can also cause allergic reactions. This product is a poor under-eye concealer. It would probably work well as an eyeshadow base, although for most women an eyeshadow base is unnecessary.

☹ **Skin Revival System** is a two-part product consisting of **Skin Revival Cream** *($25 for 1.5 ounces)* and **Skin Revival Serum** *($25 for 1.5 ounces)*. This is Mary Kay's answer to the AHA craze. The claims are just short of miraculous, yet it is overpriced and doesn't contain much AHA. One of the salespeople told me it contains about 5% AHAs, but I couldn't get a firm number from the company. You're supposed to apply the serum, let it dry, then apply the cream, then add an additional moisturizer if you want. That's more complicated than it needs to be. The cream is mostly a rich moisturizer with less than 1% AHAs. It also contains Nayad, a yeast that is supposed to soothe the skin. I doubt that, but it's in here if you're interested. The serum contains mostly water, alcohol, AHAs, thickener, salicylic acid (a peeling agent), and Nayad. Don't waste your time with this; there are plenty of products that contain 8% AHAs and don't include alcohol or salicylic acid, both of which can irritate the skin.

☹ **Oil-Control Lotion** *($16 for 3.4 ounces)* is a lightweight moisturizer that contains mostly water-binding agents, thickeners, and preservatives. Nothing in this product can control, change, or affect the amount of oil your skin produces. If anything, it can make the skin feel greasy.

☺ **Acne Treatment Gel** *($6 for 1.25 ounces)* contains mostly water, slip agent, and benzoyl peroxide (5%). The active ingredient is the benzoyl peroxide, and it could work as a disinfectant for acne.

☻ **Clarifying Mask** *($11 for 4 ounces)* is a standard clay mask that can definitely dry the skin, but for a clay mask it's OK.

☺ **Moisture Rich Mask** *($11 for 1.4 ounces)* is a very emollient cream that contains mostly water, thickeners, plant oil, more thickeners, standard water-binding agent, plant oils, petrolatum, more thickeners, and preservatives. It also contains an insignificant amount of vitamin A. This should feel very good on dry skin.

☹ **Revitalizing Mask** *($11 for 2.4 ounces)* is a standard clay mask that also contains a lightweight abrasive. It is thicker than most because it also contains candelilla and carnauba (as in car) wax, so it can also clog pores and be difficult to rinse off.

Mary Kay Makeup

☻ **FOUNDATION: Day Radiance Formula I Foundation for Dry Skin** *($10)* can go on a little heavy and provide too much coverage for a natural sheer look. It might be good for someone with very dry skin. **These colors are excellent:** Pure Ivory, Soft Ivory, Antique Ivory, Buffed Ivory, Dusty Beige, Almond Beige, True Beige, Toasted

Beige, Cocoa Beige, Walnut Bronze, and Mahogany Bronze. **These colors are too peach, pink, ash, yellow, or copper for most skin tones:** Rose Petal Ivory, Blush Ivory, Delicate Beige, Fawn Beige, Mocha Bronze, Bittersweet Bronze, and Rich Bronze.

☺ **Day Radiance Formula II for Normal to Dry Skin** *($10)* has a beautiful texture with a smooth, light finish and is great for someone with normal to dry skin. Day Radiance Formulas I and II both contain a titanium dioxide–based sunscreen, but their SPF is only 8, which is good for limited sun exposure. However, because these foundations are titanium dioxide–based, there is no problem or conflict wearing an SPF 15 sunscreen underneath. The foundations should either provide adequate protection or just leave it out altogether. **These colors are excellent:** Pure Ivory, Antique Ivory, Buffed Ivory, True Beige, Delicate Beige, Fawn Beige, Almond Beige, Toasted Beige, and Cocoa Beige. **These colors are too peach, pink, ash, yellow, or copper for most skin tones:** Rose Petal Ivory, Soft Ivory, Blush Ivory, Dusty Beige, Mocha Bronze, Rich Bronze, Walnut Bronze, and Mahogany Bronze.

☺ **Day Radiance Formula III Oil-Free for Oily and Combination Skin** *($10)* is a lightweight foundation that works great for oily skin types. **These colors are excellent:** Fawn Beige, Toasted Beige, True Beige, Almond Beige, Antique Ivory, Buffed Ivory, Pure Ivory, Soft Ivory, Cocoa Beige, and Mahogany Bronze. **These colors are too peach, pink, ash, yellow, or copper for most skin tones:** Delicate Beige, Dusty Beige, Blush Ivory, Rose Petal Ivory, Mocha Bronze, Bittersweet Bronze, Walnut Bronze, and Rich Bronze.

☺ <u>**CONCEALER:**</u> **Perfecting Concealer** *($7.50)* isn't perfect, but it comes close. It does not crease into lines, and the colors are wonderfully neutral. That alone is impressive.

☹ **Cream Concealer** *($7.50)* comes in only one shade: yellow. This product is greasy, it slips into the lines around the eyes, and the yellow makes you look slightly jaundiced all day long.

☺ <u>**POWDER:**</u> **Powder Perfect Loose Powder** *($12.50)* and **Powder Perfect Pressed Powder** *($7.50)* are talc-based powders with a soft consistency. They go on sheer and all three colors are quite good.

☺ <u>**BLUSH:**</u> **Powder Perfect Cheek Color** *($7 each)* is sold in separate tins that can be placed in a refillable compact. You buy the compact *($6)* separately and fill it with the colors of your choice. It's very convenient, you don't have to keep paying for a compact, and most of the colors are great. **Creamy Cheek Color** *($6)* is a standard cream blush that comes in two shades. It's not the best choice if you want a reliable, long-lasting blush color, but it's fine if you are into this kind of product.

☺ **EYESHADOW: Powder Perfect Eye Color** *($16 for two shades and compact; $6 per shade, refill only)* is sold in separate tins that can be placed in a refillable compact. You buy the compact separately and fill it with the colors of your choice. The only negative is that the eyeshadows, although matte, are not offered in the best assortment of neutral shades. **These colors are nicely matte and go on softly, perhaps too softly for some skin tones:** White Sand, Honey Glaze, Whisper Pink, Taupe, Gray Flannel, Lavender Mist (can look blue on some skin types), Marmalade, Hazelnut, Iris, Truffle, Heather Rose, Smoky Plum, and Blackest Black. **These colors are too blue, green, or shiny:** Crystalline, Gingerspice, Cranberry Ice, Olive, Misty Pine, Real Teal, Blue Lace, Brilliant Blue, and Midnight Blue.

☹ **EYE AND BROW SHAPER:** The **Eye Defining Pencils** *($6.50)* are standard pencils that have a fine texture and a reasonable price. The **Eyebrow Pencils** *($6.50)* have a slightly slick texture, which can make for a shiny brow.

☹ **LIPSTICK AND LIP PENCIL:** Mary Kay calls her lipstick **Lasting Color Lipstick** *($9)*, but that name is not accurate. The consistency is slightly greasy, and the color can feather quickly into the lines around the mouth. **Lip Liner Pencils** *($6.50)* feature great colors and textures.

☺ **MASCARA: Flawless Mascara** *($7.50)* is a decent mascara that goes on OK, but it doesn't build very thick or long lashes in comparison to a lot of other mascaras I've tested. **Conditioning Mascara** *($7.50)* can smudge, so if you have a problem with mascara smearing by the end of the day, this would not be a good choice.

Max Factor (Makeup Only)

Max Factor, *the* makeup artist for the rich and famous in the 1920s, is credited with developing the first mass-produced makeup products that were more than heavy powders or tints for the cheeks and lips. He made the men and women in films look exotic, sweet, masterful, wicked, or seductive in a way that was less obvious than on the stage, and he did it with unprecedented flair and creativity. Pancake Makeup and Erase, which have survived to this day, were the first foundation and coverstick. (I don't recommend pancake foundation for anyone, but it's nice to recognize the roots of makeup.)

In recent years Max Factor has attempted to bring its image into the '90s with an array of products called High Definition. The eyeshadows, blushes, concealer, and mascaras are interesting, and there are a couple of good new foundations, but this line is still drab and dreary. The dark navy packaging makes identifying the names and colors of the products difficult.

☹ <u>FOUNDATION:</u> **Pan-Cake Makeup** *($5.26)* and **Pan-Stick Makeup** *($5.26)* are both packaged in sealed plastic wrap that prevents you from viewing the colors. For that reason alone these are difficult for me to recommend, but in addition the textures of both the Pan-Cake and the Pan-Stick are too heavy, thick, and greasy. **Almost all of the colors are too peach or pink.** Satin Splendor Flawless Complexion Makeup *($7.50)* has a small but good color selection and decent textures, but it also contains aluminum starch, a skin irritant, as the second ingredient, as well as isopropyl myristate, which can aggravate breakouts. This product is too greasy for normal to oily skin and too drying for normal to dry skin.

☺ **Rain All Day Hydrating Makeup** *($6.20)* and **Balancing Act Skin Balancing Makeup** *($6.20)* both have a fairly smooth, even texture, provide light to medium coverage, last well, and offer a good range of colors, from very light to very dark. The formulas are almost identical, so the names are completely irrelevant. There is nothing hydrating about Rain, and nothing balancing about Balancing Act. Both would be appropriate for someone with normal to slightly oily or slightly dry skin who wants a matte finish. Drugstores often carry little trial samples of these two foundations; test them before you buy. **These Rain colors are worth considering:** Pale Porcelain, Light Champagne, Fair Ivory, True Beige, Cool Bronze, Toasted Almond, Golden Mocha, and Sable. **These Rain colors should be avoided:** Cream Beige (too rose), Rich Beige (too peach), and Sienna (too red). **These Balancing Act colors are worth considering:** True Beige, Light Champagne, Pale Porcelain, and Fair Ivory. **These Balancing Act colors should be avoided:** Cream Beige (too rose), Rich Beige (too peach), and Natural Honey (too pink).

☺ **High Definition Perfecting Makeup** *($6.20)* has a good color assortment and a soft matte, but dry finish that is excellent for someone with oily skin, but, alas, no testers. **Colour and Light Makeup** *($6.19)* is a lightweight foundation with colors specifically designed for darker skin tones, but again there are no testers.

☹ **Whipped Creme Makeup** *($5.21)* has the most awful array of foundation colors I have ever seen. Who is buying this stuff? **High Definition Compact Makeup** *($6.24)* also has terrible colors.

☺ <u>CONCEALER:</u> **Erase Colour Precise** *($3.75)* is a creamy liquid that provides medium coverage. This excellent concealer really hides dark circles and rarely creases into the lines around the eyes. It does go on fairly heavy and is not for a sheer, soft look.

☹ **Erase Secret Cover-Up** *($3.75)* concealer stick was the staple of my youthful days. The coverage is good, the consistency is creamy without being greasy, and the colors are excellent. It is not the best on dry skin, it can easily crease into the lines around the eyes, and the fragrance is too pungent for my taste.

☹ <u>POWDER:</u> **Colour and Light Pressed Powder** *($8.19)* would be a good option except that the colors are packaged so that you can't see them, and therefore it is impossible to choose wisely. **High Definition Perfecting Pressed Powder** *($6.24)* has an extremely poor selection of colors that are all overly peach or pink.

☺ <u>BLUSH:</u> **High Definition Blush** *($5.99)* is a soft, exceedingly smooth cream-to-powder blush in a subtle range of pastel colors. This isn't high definition, but it is soft and pretty.

☹ **Satin Blush** *($4.95)* would be a lovely powder blush except that all of the colors are shiny.

☹ <u>EYESHADOW:</u> **Eyeshadow Singles** *($2.46),* **Duos** *($2.64),* and **Quads** *($3.73)* are all either too shiny or poor combinations of colors.

☺ <u>EYE AND BROW SHAPER:</u> The **Brush & Brow Eyebrow Color** *($5.25)* is a powder shadow that colors the brow with a hard brush. The powder works beautifully, but the firm brush is a throwaway and shouldn't be used. A soft brush would be better. **These colors are excellent:** Smoky Gray, Soft Black, Natural Brown, Midnight Brown, and Ash Blond. **Brow Tamer** *($4.99)* is a clear gel that can keep brows in place. It works well, but you can get the same effect by spraying hairspray on a toothbrush and combing it through your brows. **Eyeliner Pen** *($4.13)* is a liquid eyeliner that is applied with a felt-tip pen applicator; it works well, although it tends to dry slightly sticky.

☺ **Kohliners** *($4.16)* are a good assortment of standard eye pencils that are a bit on the greasy side; one end is a sponge tip. **Eyebrow and Eyeliner** *($3.20)* is a standard pencil that's almost identical to the Kohliner.

☹ **Eye Designer Shadow Liner** *($3.53)* is a fat pencil that smears over the eyelids. It doesn't dry to a powder and can easily crease.

☺ <u>LIPSTICK AND LIP PENCIL:</u> Except for the fragrance, I love the Max Factor's lipsticks. **Moisture Rich Lipstick** *($4.75),* **New Definition** *($4.95),* and **Lasting Color Lipstick** *($4.75)* are all extremely creamy, and the color really lasts. If you can take the somewhat sweet odor, they're great. **Restorative Lip Care** *($4.50)* is a lip gloss with SPF 15, but it won't restore your lips. The **High Definition Lip Liner** *($4.15)* pencil is wonderful; one end is a lipstick brush, which can be convenient.

☹ **Stay Put Anti-Fade Lip Foundation** *($4.50)* does prevent lipstick from feathering, but it also tends to make the lipstick cake and dries out the lips.

☺   <u>MASCARA:</u> **2000 Calorie Mascara** *($4.95)* goes on easily, doesn't smear, and makes lashes thick and long. It tends to flake if you overbuild the lashes. Don't overdo, and it should last the whole day.

☹   **Super Lash Maker** *($4.95)* is a terrible mascara with a strange tiny brush that is difficult to use and builds no length or thickness. **S-T-R-E-T-C-H Mascara** *($4.95)* is a puzzle. Whoever came up with the name must not have tried it on. It doesn't build any length, regardless of how much is applied, and it tends to smear.

Maybelline

In early 1996 Maybelline was purchased by L'Oreal. As this book went to press, the purchase had not affected the displays or the products available, but it is hard to believe that things won't change, and possibly for the better, although Maybelline already has its act together in many aspects of skin care and makeup. There are some impressive products, particularly pressed powders, mascaras, concealers, pencils, liquid liners, and brushes, and the prices are wonderful. With a little caution, you can come away from the Maybelline counter with some great bargains and a beautiful look.

Beauty Note: Maybelline's **Shades of You** (reviewed below with the makeup products) is a very impressive group of color products for African-American skin tones. Most of the foundation, blush, and lipstick colors are excellent and worth investigating. All of the colors for both foundations are surprisingly good, with no overtones of orange or ash, often a major problem with darker-colored foundations (the liquid makeup is the better choice for a soft daytime look). Although the selection is small, if your color is available, it's worth a try. One overwhelming negative is that both foundations in this line are only for women with normal to oily skin. The company has yet to create a foundation for women of color who have dry skin.

Maybelline Skin Care

☺   **Revitalizing Alpha Hydroxy Moisture Lotion** *($11.89 for 4 ounces)* and **Revitalizing Alpha Hydroxy Moisture Cream** *($11.89 for 2 ounces)* both use a derivative of molasses (an AHA extract) as their source of AHAs; there is no information available about its effectiveness as an exfoliant. Moreover, without knowing the percentage (looking at the ingredient list, I would guess it's about 4%), there is no way to tell how effective these lotions are anyway. However, while I can't recommend them as exfoliants, both lotions would be good lightweight moisturizers for someone with normal to slightly dry skin who is not all that interested in the amount of AHAs they contain.

☹ Revitalizing Enhanced Moisture Lotion with SPF 2 *($8.97 for 4 ounces)* and Revitalizing Enhanced Moisture Cream with SPF 2 *($8.97 for 2 ounces)* would be good daytime moisturizers for someone with normal to dry skin, but SPF 2 is grossly insufficient to protect against the sun.

☺ Revitalizing Optimum Eye Treatment Cream *($8.97 for 0.45 ounce)* is a good lightweight moisturizer that would be fine to use all over the face. Unfortunately, like most eye creams, this one comes in a very small jar.

Maybelline Makeup

☺ **FOUNDATION:** For the most part, there are no testers for the foundations in this line, so I cannot recommend them. **Long-Wearing Liquid Makeup** *($3.29)*, **Shades of You Oil-Free Liquid Water-Based Makeup** *($4.25)*, and **Shades of You 100% Oil-Free Compact Creme Makeup** *($4.29)* all have some good colors and textures (but no testers).

☹ **Moisture Whip Liquid Makeup** *($4.50)*, **Shine-Free Oil-Control Liquid Makeup** *($3.95)*, and **Shine-Free Blemish Control Makeup** *($3.29)* all have an appalling selection of foundation tones. **Revitalizing Liquid Makeup** *($4.89)* is supposed to be both a good AHA product and a good sunscreen. That combination might be possible, but in this case the AHA ingredient isn't an effective exfoliant; also, the colors aren't very good.

☺ **Natural Defense Makeup with SPF 15 (Nonchemical Sunscreen)** *($4.24)* is new, and definitely worth checking out. The SPF is great and the nonchemical sunscreen is a nice option. Some of the colors are surprisingly good, and tiny trial bottles are often available so you can test your selection. This wonderfully lightweight foundation offers soft, subtle coverage. It is best for someone with normal to dry skin. The colors are generally neutral, but there isn't much for darker skin tones. **These colors are excellent:** Light Ivory, Ivory, Light Beige, Soft Beige, Deep Beige, and Golden Beige. **These colors are too peach or rose:** Medium Beige and Rose Beige.

☹ **CONCEALER:** Shine-Free Oil-Control Coverstick *($3.65)* won't control oil, and the colors aren't the best. This concealer goes on very dry and would be suitable only for someone with very oily skin; also, it has a slight tendency to crease. **Revitalizing Coverstick** *($4.99)* comes in three reliable shades, but it too tends to crease. **Revitalizing Concealer with Sunscreen** *($3.65)* has good coverage, but it tends to go on heavy and definitely creases into the lines around the eyes. **Coverstick** *($2.94)* is packaged so that you can't see the color, but even if you could, it has a terrible consistency and easily creases. **Shades of You 100% Oil Free Coverstick** *($2.95)* is a sticky, greasy mess that easily creases into lines around the eyes.

☺ **Undetectable Creme Concealer** *($3.65)* goes on easily and dries to a matte finish; it stays in place and really covers. I wouldn't exactly call it undetectable, but it does come in three good shades—Light, Medium, and Dark Medium (which isn't all that dark)—and doesn't crease. It would be best for someone who doesn't have dry skin.

☺ **POWDER:** **Translucent Pressed Powder** *($4)* contains talc and mineral oil, and **Satin Complexion Pressed Powder** *($4.33)* contains talc and no oil. Both have good colors to choose from but tend to go on chalky. **Shine-Free Oil-Control Loose Powder** *($3.53)* is packaged so that you can't see the color, and there is no way to select an appropriate color.

☺ **Revitalizing Translucent Powder** *($5.69)* is a standard talc-based powder and truly is translucent. It comes in three OK shades: Light, Medium, and Dark. **Shine-Free Oil-Control Translucent Pressed Powder** *($3.35)* won't control oil, but it is a wonderful soft, dry powder that goes on smooth and sheer. **Finish Matte Pressed Powder** *($3.29)* is also exceptional, with beautiful colors and a silky, even texture. **Shades of You 100% Oil-Free Pressed Powder** *($3.36)* has a lovely assortment of colors and a smooth, soft finish.

☹ **Moisture Whip Translucent Pressed Powder** *($3.36)* has a terrible assortment of peach and pink colors.

☺ **BLUSH:** **Natural Accents Blush** *($2.69)* comes in ten attractive, subtle (and I mean subtle) shades; all of them are somewhat shiny (although not terrible). Their texture is on the dry side, and they tend not to adhere very well. **Brush/Blush I** *($3.05)*, **II** *($3.23)*, and **III** *($3.39)* come in single, duo, and trio compacts. They are all somewhat shiny—not awful, just not great. They go on smoothly, and the colors are attractive.

☺ **Shades of You 100% Oil-Free Powder Blush** *($3.36)* has a slight shine that's hardly noticeable. It goes on silky and soft without being heavy or greasy, and there are some wonderful colors.

☹ **EYESHADOW:** **Expert Eyes Eyeshadows** *($1.95)* mostly have a large amount of shine or dreadful colors. **These colors are good and truly matte:** Earthy Taupe, Creme de Cocoa, Gray Suede, and The Suedes, but they tend to go on very powdery and somewhat choppy. **Shades of You Eyeshadow Collection** *($3.36)* comes in colors that are all too shiny.

☹ Natural Accents Eyeshadow *($2.62)* comes in a M.A.C.-like compact, but all the colors have some amount of shine. This isn't the best eyeshadow, but the colors are surprisingly soft and blend well. If you don't mind shine, these can be an option.

☺ **EYE AND BROW SHAPER:** Lineworks Felt-Tip Eye Liner *($3.94)* is a felt-tip liquid liner that dries to a smooth, dry finish with no shine. It doesn't budge once in place, and it doesn't have the slick shine of a lot of liquid liners. **Expert Eyes Brow and Eye Liner Pencil** *($3.09)* is an automatic pencil that can be sharpened to a finer point than most, but other than that, it is just a standard pencil with a dry texture, which means less smudging. **Lineworks Liquid Liner Washable** *($3.29)* is a standard liquid liner that dries to a smooth, flat finish and has good staying power. **Ultra-Brow Brush-On Brow Color** *($3.42)* is a great standard brow powder. It comes with the standard hard brush that needs to be tossed away and replaced with a good soft professional brush.

☹ Smoked Kohl Liner *($3.60)* is a standard, fairly greasy pencil that has a smudge tip at one end. **Great Line Waterproof Eye Liner** *($4.88)* has a smooth, soft texture, but it isn't all that waterproof. **Linework Ultra-Liner Waterproof Liquid Liner** *($3.75)* is a standard liquid liner that has good staying power under water, but it tends to peel off if rubbed. **Expert Eye Twin Brow and Eye Pencil** *($1.87)* is a very greasy pencil.

☺ **LIPSTICK AND LIP PENCIL:** Moisture Whip Lipstick *($3.29)* and **Long Wearing Lipstick** *($3.36)* both have a rich, creamy, slightly glossy texture; it's hard to tell the two apart. **Shades of You Lipstick** *($3.52)* and **Shades of You Long Wearing Lipstick** *($3.36)* both have a superior color selection with remarkably appropriate shades for women of color. They have a nice moist feel without being thick or greasy. **Great Lip Lip Color** *($4.72)* doesn't offer many colors, which is disappointing, but what is available provides ultra-matte competition for Revlon's ColorStay. It doesn't bleed, it stays on at least as well as any other matte lipstick, and the price is great. **Shades of You See Through Gloss** *($4.72)* and **Moisture Whip Gloss** *($3.76)* are virtually identical standard glosses in a small but pretty group of colors. **Precision Lip Liner** *($3.77)* and **Shades of You Lip Liner** *($2.73)* are also virtually identical and both are great, with a small but beautiful color selection.

☹ **MASCARA:** Great Lash Mascara *($4.20)* always gets mixed reviews: It goes on well, but it definitely smears. **Magic Mascara** *($3.95)* has an awkward curved brush that doesn't build much length or thickness. **Perfectly Natural Mascara** *($3.25)* is OK, but it doesn't build up much thickness. **Lash by Lash Mascara** *($3.49)* took forever to build any definition, it smeared later in the day, and the two products I purchased were practically dried up from the very first time I tested them.

☺ **Maybelline Great Lash Pro Vitamin** *($4.72)* is a good lengthening and thickening mascara that may slightly clump but doesn't smear. The "pro vitamin" (vitamin B) won't do anything for your lashes, though. **Illegal Lengths Mascara** *($4.55)* is excellent without being too thick or clumpy, and it doesn't smear or flake. **No Problem Mascara** *($4.20)* is quite good, one of the better Maybelline mascaras.

☺ **BRUSHES:** The **Eyeshadow Brush** *($3.05)* and **Blush Brush** *($3.46)* are extremely soft but firm, and work well.

M.D. Formulations (Skin Care Only)

In the area of serious AHA products, M.D. Formulations far surpasses its competition, offering some of the highest-percentage glycolic acid–based AHA products on the market. Not only do most of its products have over 12% AHAs (8% to 10% is the standard percentage in most other good AHA products, available from such lines as Alpha Hydrox, Avon, and Pond's), but M.D. Formulations has a new line of AHA products, called Forte, with up to 20% glycolic acid. If you're of the opinion that more is better, then look no further. However, let me warn you that I do not encourage or recommend over 15% AHAs for the skin on a daily or even semiregular basis. At this time, there have been no long-term studies that have established the effect of higher concentrations of AHA products on the skin. In fact, this much irritation of the skin on a daily basis can be harmful, and could actually cause the skin to wrinkle.

M.D. Formulations makes everything from moisturizers and acne products to shampoos (considered good for dandruff or psoriasis) and foot and nail treatments. If you want to exfoliate skin on any part of your body with an AHA concentration that can really make a difference, you will be impressed by some of these products. However, M.D. Formulations makes several products that I think are bad for the skin, and its AHA moisturizers are fairly ordinary except for the AHA content. Despite those reservations, and the fact that these products are incredibly overpriced, if you pick and choose carefully, you stand to find some very good AHA products.

M.D. Formulations is sold directly to physicians for retail sale. For more information about these products, or the name of a physician near you who sells these products, call (800) 347-2223. You can also have the products shipped to you directly by calling that same number. Under the company name Herald Pharmacal, M.D. Formulations has created a line of products called **Aqua Glyde** and **Aqua Glycolic**, sold in drugstores and priced from $8.50 to $16—they are reviewed earlier in this chapter.

One word of caution: Any time you use a product that contains more than 8% AHAs, some stinging can occur; also, you should not let the product come in contact with the eyes or any mucous membranes. Be aware that you may have an allergic reaction to AHAs. Slight stinging is expected, but continued stinging is not. Discontinue use if this should happen.

☹ **Facial Cleanser with 12% Glycolic Compound** *($25 for 8 ounces)* is a problem for most skin types. It is overkill to put AHAs in a cleanser that could accidentally get too near your eyes or mouth when splashing and cause serious irritation. I would not recommend washing the face or other body parts with this product. This is also a lot of money for an ordinary detergent cleanser.

☹ **Glycare Cleansing Gel for Oily Skin with 12% Glycolic Compound** *($25 for 8 ounces)* is similar to the cleanser above, and the same review applies.

☹ **Forte Glycare Cleansing Gel with 15% Glycolic Compound** *($25 for 8 ounces)* is similar to the Facial Cleanser 12% above, only with more AHAs, and the same review applies.

☹ **Forte Facial Cleanser with 15% Glycolic Compound** *($25 for 8 ounces)* is similar to the Facial Cleanser 12% above, only with more AHAs, and the same review applies.

☺ **Facial Cleanser Basic** *($12 for 8 ounces)* is a gentle water-soluble cleanser for most skin types. Actually, this product is pretty much a knockoff of Cetaphil.

☺ **$$$ Facial Lotion with 12% Glycolic Compound** *($45 for 2 ounces)* is just AHAs with a thickener and preservatives. This is a good basic AHA product for most skin types; however, if you have normal to dry skin, you will most likely need a moisturizer too.

☺ **$$$ Forte I Facial Lotion with 15% Glycolic Compound** *($45 for 2 ounces)* is similar to the lotion above, only with more AHAs, and the same review applies.

☹ **$$$ Forte II Facial Lotion with 20% Glycolic Compound** *($47 for 2 ounces)* is similar to the Facial Lotion 12% above, but with more AHAs, and the same review applies. The long-term effects of this much AHA are unknown.

☺ **$$$ Night Cream with 14% Glycolic Compound** *($60 for 2 ounces)* is a simple AHA cream of water, thickeners, and preservative. The ordinary moisturizing base probably would not be sufficient for someone with very dry skin, but it is a good strong AHA product.

☺ **$$$ Forte I Facial Cream with 15% Glycolic Compound** *($32 for 1 ounce)* is similar to the cream above, but with more AHAs, and the same review applies.

☹ **$$$ Forte II Facial Cream with 20% Glycolic Compound** *($35 for 1 ounce)* is similar to the creams above, but with even more AHAs, and the same review applies. This product is pretty intense and definitely not for everyone. The long-term effects of this much AHA are unknown.

☺ **$$$ Smoothing Complex with 10% Glycolic Compound** *($35 for 0.5 ounce)* is identical to the Night Cream above except it has less AHA and does not contain a few of the thickeners. It is a good overall AHA product.

☹ **$$$ Advanced Hydrating Complex Cream Formula** *($40 for 1 ounce)* contains mostly water, several thickeners, water-binding agent, slip agent, thickener, and preservative. A good water-binding agent and Nayad (yeast) are at the very end of the ingredient list, so the amount of each is negligible although there is no real evidence Nayad performs any real function for skin.

☺ **$$$ Forte Advanced Hydrating Complex Cream Formula** *($45 for 1.7 ounces)* is quite similar to the cream above, but somewhat more emollient, and the interesting ingredients are higher up on the ingredient list. This is definitely a better product for someone with normal to dry skin than the one above.

☹ **Advanced Hydrating Complex Gel Formula** *($40 for 1 ounce)* is a below-average, very expensive, non-AHA moisturizer for the eyes. It contains water, alcohol, thickener, water-binding agent, more thickeners, and preservatives. Although the moisturizer also contains a good water-binding agent and Nayad (yeast), they are at the very end of the ingredient list, so the amount of each is negligible. If the skin around your eyes is dry, this won't do much to change it, and the alcohol could make things worse.

☹ **Forte Advanced Hydrating Complex Gel Formula** *($45 for 1.7 ounces)* is quite similar to the moisturizer above, but the interesting ingredients are higher up on the ingredient list. This is definitely a better product than the one above, but the alcohol remains a problem.

☺ **$$$ Vit-A-Gel with Vitamin A Propionate** *($40 for 1 ounce)* contains mostly aloe vera, slip agents, vitamin A, more slip agent, thickeners, several water-binding agents, and preservatives. If you're looking for a good dose of vitamin A, here it is, but the best part of this product is the lightweight water-binding agents. It's pricey for what you get, but it is a good lightweight moisturizer for someone with normal to slightly dry or combination skin.

☹ **Glycare 5 for Extremely Oily or Acne-Prone Skin** *($35 for 4 ounces)* is an alcohol-based toner with 7% AHAs. I don't recommend using alcohol on anyone's skin, and the alcohol in combination with the AHAs can cause extreme irritation. The product also contains eucalyptus oil, another skin irritant.

☹ **Glycare 10 for Extremely Oily or Acne-Prone Skin** *($35 for 4 ounces)* is identical to the Glycare 5 except that it contains 12% AHAs. The same warnings about irritation apply.

☹ **Forte I Glycare with 15% Glycolic Compound** *($18 for 2 ounces)* is identical to the Glycare 5 and 10 except that it contains more AHAs. The same warnings about irritation apply.

Forte II Glycare with 20% Glycolic Compound *($20 for 2 ounces)* is identical to the Glycare 5, 10, and 15 except that it contains more AHAs. The same warnings about irritation apply. The long-term effects of this much AHA are unknown.

☺ **$$$ SPF 20 Sunblock** *($25 for 4 ounces)* is a standard non-AHA sunscreen that provides good protection for someone with normal to dry skin.

☺ **$$$ Benzoyl Peroxide 5% for Extremely Oily and Acne-Prone Skin** *($25 for 4 ounces)* is a good benzoyl peroxide toner, but you can buy similar solutions for a lot less at the drugstore.

☺ **$$$ Benzoyl Peroxide 10% for Extremely Oily and Acne-Prone Skin** *($25 for 4 ounces)* is identical to the toner above except for the proportion of benzoyl peroxide, and the same review applies.

☹ **$$$ Skin Bleaching Lotion** *($30 for 1.5 ounces)* is a standard 2% hydroquinone product. To make it more effective, use it in conjunction with one of the AHA creams or lotions.

☺ **$$$ Forte Skin Bleaching Gel with 2% Hydroquinone in a Base Containing 10% Glycolic Compound** *($30 for 1.5 ounces)* is what I recommended in the review above: hydroquinone with AHAs. It is worth a try, but don't expect dramatic, or even all that noticeable, changes in skin color; these products lighten skin only slightly.

☹ **$$$ Forte Glycare Perfection Gel, 1% Salicylic Acid in a Base Containing 5% Glycolic Compound** *($18 for 1.7 ounces)* is overpriced for what you get. According to the company there is some evidence that this combination of salicylic acid and AHAs can be beneficial for acne; I am not convinced, especially given that this product also contains alcohol, and that can dry and irritate the skin.

Merle Norman

The Merle Norman boutiques are in dire need of not just a face lift but serious surgery. All of the stores I've been to have had a slightly worn, almost eerie, outdated feel. Although some products, particularly the foundations, have been revamped, the displays are poorly organized and not very user-friendly; in fact, they appear almost haphazard. It would be much better if there were some color or style groupings. As it is, the colors have no relation to one another; they seem just strewn all over.

Merle Norman has scaled back the number of shiny eyeshadows it sells, but their overall quality hasn't changed: they leave much to be desired. There are more than half a dozen types of foundation, and several offer an enormous number of colors; unfortunately, many of the colors are exceedingly poor, with an overabundance of pink and peach shades. Some of the foundations have great textures, but an equal number are just a thick, greasy mess. The lipsticks are fairly greasy, and the concealers crease easily. And despite the large number of cleansers it offers, this line still lacks a good cleanser that doesn't leave the face greasy or dry.

Although this all sounds pretty dismal, with a few adjustments this line could really come to life. The matte blushes and eyeshadows are wonderful, there's an extensive selection for women of all skin tones and colors, and the face powders are quite good. A few color improvements and a good reorganization would bring Merle Norman into the next millennium.

Merle Norman Skin Care

☹ **Cleansing Cream, Original Formula** *($12.50 for 7.5 ounces; $16.50 for 16 ounces)* is a mineral oil–based wipe-off cleanser that contains thick waxes and cocoa butter. It's pretty much just overpriced cold cream.

☹ **Cleansing Lotion** *($12.50 for 5.5 ounces; $16.50 for 14 ounces)* is similar to the cream above, but with less wax. It is still fairly greasy and contains petrolatum, lanolin, and a thickener that can cause breakouts.

☹ **Gel Cleanser** *($11 for 4 ounces)* is an alcohol-based detergent cleanser that can be quite drying and irritating for some skin types.

☹ **Special Cleansing Bar, Soap Free** *($8.95 for 4 ounces)* is a wax-based bar cleanser that contains two detergent cleansing agents (sodium lauryl sulfate and sodium C14-16 olefin sulfate) that can be irritating and drying for most skin types.

☹ **Luxiva Skin Refining Cleanser** *($16.50 for 4 ounces)* won't refine anyone's skin. It has some scrubbing beads, which are OK for gentle exfoliation, but it also contains a fair amount of potassium hydroxide, which can be irritating. This product tends to leave a greasy film, which is not great for someone with normal to oily skin, despite the company's recommendations.

☹ **Luxiva Collagen Cleanser** *($15.50 for 6 ounces)* is a mineral oil–based wipe-off cleanser that can leave a greasy film on the skin. It does contain collagen, but who needs that in a cleanser?

☹ **Instant Eye Makeup Remover for Sensitive Eyes** *($8.95 for 3 ounces)* is a detergent-based cleanser that isn't what I would call good for sensitive skin. It's OK, but the detergent cleanser can be a problem for some skin types.

☹ **Very Gentle Eye Makeup Remover** *($8.95 for 2 ounces)* contains mostly mineral oil, which is gentle, but it's a lot like the wipe-off face cleansers above. Why bother with a second product if you're already wiping greasy stuff over your face to take off your makeup?

☺ **Luxiva Collagen Clarifier** *($13 for 6 ounces)* does indeed contain collagen; in fact, it is the third item on the ingredient list. Collagen is a good water-binding agent, but that's about it. This product would be fine for someone with normal to dry skin, but it's unnecessary.

☹ **Fresh 'N Fair Skin Freshener** *($10.50 for 5.5 ounces; $16.50 for 14 ounces)* is an alcohol-based cleanser that will leave the face feeling dry and irritated.

☹ **Milky Freshener, Normal/Dry** *($10.50 for 5.5 ounces; $16.50 for 14 ounces)* contains mostly water, slip agent, nonfat milk, and preservatives. If you leave this stuff on, it will attract bacteria, which can cause breakouts.

☹ **Refining Lotion** *($10.50 for 5.5 ounces; $16.50 for 14 ounces)* is almost all witch hazel and preservatives. The minuscule amounts of other ingredients in the lotion aren't worth mentioning. Witch hazel contains a good percentage of alcohol and is a potential skin irritant.

☹ **Cellular Therapy Toner with Alpha Hydroxy Acids** *($14.50 for 6 ounces)* contains lots of alcohol and a small amount of AHAs, which adds up to irritation. The AHAs may be OK for exfoliating, but the alcohol is a problem for all skin types.

☺ **Aqua Lube** *($10.50 for 2 ounces)* contains mostly mineral oil, water, wax, thickener, petrolatum, lanolin, more thickeners, and preservatives. "Lube" is a good name for this extremely rich moisturizer, which I would recommend only for someone with extremely dry skin; however, the company recommends it for oily skin. The only word for this is "insane."

☹ **Super Lube** *($11 for 2 ounces)* is basically petrolatum and wax. You could use Vaseline and be just as happy, but I wouldn't recommend either. Petrolatum by itself is not hydrating or emollient enough for most skin types; it's just greasy.

☺ **Intensive Moisturizer** *($13.50 for 1.25 ounces)* contains mostly water, mineral oil, slip agents, several thickeners, lanolin oil, more thickeners, lanolin oil, and preservatives. I would recommend this extremely rich moisturizer only for someone with extremely dry skin.

☺ **Moisture Emulsion** *($13.50 for 3 ounces)* contains mostly water, mineral oil, slip agent, several thickeners, and preservatives. This is an OK moisturizer for someone with dry skin, but it contains nothing of interest for most skin types.

☹ **Moisture Lotion** *($10.45 for 3 ounces)* is similar to the moisturizer above, but more lightweight. It's an OK, rather ordinary moisturizer for someone with dry skin.

☹ **Protective Veil** *($9.50 for 3 ounces)* contains mostly water, thickener, slip agents, more thickeners, and preservatives. The second thickening agent is isopropyl palmitate, which can cause breakouts. The company recommends this for someone with oily skin—big mistake.

☹ **Miracol Booster** *($10.50 for 1.25 ounces)* contains mostly water, alcohol, thickeners, and preservatives. Alcohol makes skin dry and irritated and can increase oil production.

☹ **Miracol Original Formula Revitalizing Lotion** *($13.50 for 5.5 ounces)* contains mostly water, thickener (which may cause allergic reactions), egg white, thickener, fragrance, and preservatives. This isn't revitalizing, but it can be irritating.

☹ **Miracol Creamy Formula Revitalizing Cream** *($13 for 6 ounces)* is almost identical to the lotion above, and the same review applies.

☺ **Luxiva Collagen Support** *($18.50 for 2 ounces)* contains mostly water, slip agent, collagen, elastin, water-binding agent, thickeners, preservatives, and more water-binding agents. This is a very good moisturizer for normal to dry skin types. The collagen and elastin won't change or improve wrinkles, but you already knew that, right?

☺ **$$$ Luxiva Night Creme with HC-12** *($35 for 2 ounces)* contains mostly water, slip agent, a long list of thickeners, silicone oil, shea butter, plant oils, preservatives, and plant extracts. This is a good emollient moisturizer for dry skin types, but HC-12 is just a clever marketing name for a combination of plant oils, water-binding agent, plant extracts, and vitamins.

☺ **$$$ Luxiva Day Creme with HC-12** *($22 for 2 ounces)* is identical to the cream above except that it contains a small amount of sunscreen—not enough to adequately protect the skin from sun damage.

☺ **$$$ Luxiva Cellular Therapy Emulsion with Alpha Hydroxy Acids** *($30 for 1 ounce)* contains thickeners, sugarcane extract, slip agent, plant oil, thickeners, more plant oils, anti-irritants, and preservatives. "Sugarcane extract" gives you no information about the type of AHAs you're getting. It sounds natural, but that doesn't mean it can work like an AHA.

☺ **$$$ Luxiva Energizing Concentrate** *($35 for 1 ounce)* contains mostly water, slip agents, silicone oil, plant extract, water-binding agents, and preservatives. Protein, yeast, and amino acids show up at the end of the ingredient list, which makes them barely present. This won't energize the skin, but it is a good moisturizer for normal to dry skin types.

☺ **Luxiva Eye Cream** *($17.50 for 0.5 ounce)* contains mostly water, almond oil, a very long list of thickeners, plant oil, more thickeners, petrolatum, more thickeners, and preservative. The interesting water-binding agents are at the end of the ingredient list, meaning they're almost nonexistent. This overpriced moisturizer could be good for someone with dry skin.

☺ **$$$ Luxiva Hydrosome Complex** *($32 for 1 ounce)* contains mostly water, thickeners, aloe, slip agent, silicone oil, shea butter, more thickeners, more water-binding agents, and preservatives. This is a good emollient, somewhat lightweight moisturizer for normal to dry skin types, but many of the interesting water-binding agents are at the end of the ingredient list, which means they're almost nonexistent.

☺ **$$$ Luxiva Protein Cream** *($37.50 for 4 ounces)* contains mostly water, petrolatum, a long list of thickeners, collagen, more thickeners, and preservatives. Collagen isn't a protein, and there isn't very much in here to boot. This is a good moisturizer for someone with dry skin, but it's extremely ordinary. Once you look at the price, it becomes embarrassing.

☹ **Luxiva Triple Action Eye Gel** *($19 for 0.5 ounce)* contains mostly water, slip agents, aloe, witch hazel, plant extract, water-binding agent, and preservatives. Most of the plant extracts, antioxidants, and water-binding agents are at the end of the ingredient list, which means they're practically nonexistent; the witch hazel can be an irritant.

Merle Norman Makeup

☺ **FOUNDATION: Luxiva Liquid Makeup SPF 16** *($13.50)* is an extremely light, but wonderfully emollient, foundation with a good sunscreen. **These colors are excellent:** Ivory, Alabaster, Soft Bisque, Quiet Rose, Palest Ivory (great for very light skin tones), Golden Beige, Sandy Beige, Cafe Beige, Sun Beige, Cafe Au Lait, Amber Glow, Mahogany, Toasted Almond, Bronze Glow, Creamy Beige, and Golden Brown. **These colors are too peach, yellow, or pink:** Porcelain, Palest Porcelain, Ecru, Toffee, Simply Beige, and Soft Honey.

☺ **Luxiva Ultra Powder Foundation** *($18)* is a standard talc-based powder that goes on smooth, but it's a bit on the dry side. It would be best for someone with normal to oily skin, or worn over makeup instead of by itself. **All of the colors are excellent.**

☺ **Aqua Base** *($12.50)* is an extremely creamy, rather thick foundation that is supposed to provide matte coverage. It is somewhat matte, but can feel too thick if you don't blend it carefully. If you want medium coverage and a silky feel and have normal to dry skin, this is a great foundation with some wonderful colors for a wide range of skin tones. **These colors are great:** Alabaster Beige, Ivory, Palest Porcelain (slightly pink), Champagne Beige, Delicate Beige, Cream Beige, Palest Ivory (great for light skin tones), Toasted Almond, Ecru, Maple Cream, Golden Beige, Amber Glow, Bronze Glow, Cafe Au Lait, Toffee, and Mahogany. **These colors are too pink, peach, rose, or yellow:** Translucent, Bamboo, Fawn Beige, Porcelain, Taffy Cream, Golden Birch, and Gentle Tan.

☺ **Luxiva Ultra Foundation with HC-12** *($22)* claims to "retexturize" skin with HC-12, which seems to be a combination of plant oils, water-binding agent, plant extracts, and vitamins. If you have very dry skin, they will help moisturize it; if that's what they mean by "retexturizing," this product will do that. **These colors are beautiful, with no unnatural undertones:** Ivory, Alabaster, Creamy Beige, Simply Beige, Soft Bisque, Quiet Rose, Ecru, Pure Beige, Sun Beige, and Cafe Au Lait. **These colors are too pink, peach, or yellow for most skin tones:** Palest Porcelain, Porcelain, Sandy Beige, Golden Beige, Tan Beige, Cafe Beige, Soft Honey, Toffee, and Bronzewood.

☹ **Total Finish Compact** *($15)* is as close to greasepaint as you will ever find, but even greasepaint isn't this greasy. The salesperson confided that everyone calls this the "Tammy Faye Baker foundation."

☺ **Oil-Control Makeup** *($15)* won't control oil in the slightest; it isn't even oil-free (it contains both silicone oil and plant oil). It has some talc, but that won't help much given these other ingredients. This is a light, sheer, soft foundation that would be best for someone with normal to combination skin. The color selection is good but ridiculously small. **These are good colors to consider:** 2, 4, 5, and 6. **These colors are too pink or peach:** 1 and 3.

☺ **Powder Base** *($12.50)* is more cream than powder, and initially has an almost sticky feel. It finally blends out quite sheer and smooth, but with almost no powder feel, so the name is confusing. It tends to stain the skin—it is that thick. If you have dry skin and want a soft, slightly matte finish, this is an intriguing foundation to test, but it definitely won't be to everyone's liking. **These are good colors to consider:** Palest Ivory, Ivory, Cream Beige, Alabaster Beige, Champagne Beige, Sandy Beige, Maple Cream, Fawn Beige, Spice Beige, Golden Birch, Dark, and Sunny Tan. **Avoid**

these colors at all costs: Palest Porcelain, Taffy Cream, Midtone, Rose Beige, Bamboo Beige, Rose Glow, Blushing Beige, Caramel Beige, Porcelain, Gentle Tan, Translucent, Newport Tan, and Latan.

☹ **Luxiva Liquid Creme Foundation** *($20)* has some of the most awful colors I've ever seen, and a greasy texture too.

☺ **Color Corrector** *($9.50)* comes in four shades: White, Yellow, Mint, and Lilac (really rose). My general recommendation is to avoid this type of product. If you must use it, this one would be OK only for someone with dry skin.

☹ **CONCEALER: Retouch Cover Creme** *($9)* has some good colors for darker skin tones, but it can crease into the lines around the eyes, and I do not recommend it. **Oil-Free Concealing Creme** *($9)* is oil-free but still has a fairly emollient texture. It goes on drier than the Retouch, but it also tends to crease into the lines around the eyes, and I do not recommend it.

☺ **POWDER: Remarkable Finish Loose Powder** *($16.50)* and **Remarkable Finish Pressed Powder** *($14.50)* are standard talc-based powders that go on soft and smooth. The seven good colors range from Translucent to Deep. **The only color to avoid:** Translucent Pink. Neither **Remarkable Finish Oil Control Loose Powder** *($16.50)* nor **Remarkable Finish Oil Control Pressed Powder** *($14.50)* will control oil, but they are oil-free, talc-based powders that go on soft and smooth. The seven good colors range from Translucent to Deep. **The only color to avoid:** Translucent Pink.

☺ **BLUSH: Blushing Powder** *($12.50)* textures vary a bit, but most are soft and blend on easily. There is a vast selection of blush colors for a wide range of skin tones; most have a slight amount of shine, but not enough to be bad.

☺ **EYESHADOW: Creamy Powder Rich Eyeshadows Singles** *($11)*, **Duos** *($14)*, and **Trios** *($15)* come in some very good matte shades that blend on smooth and soft. **These colors are matte and beautiful:** Taupe Suede, Cocoa, Rosy Brown, Cappuccino, Wheat, Sepia, Chestnut, Peach Blossom, Honey, Pumpkin Spice, Cashmere, Olive, Cashmere/Suede, Wine & Rose, Warm Naturals, Cool Naturals, Butternut/Spice, Sand/Wall St. Grey, Shell Pink/Burgundy. **These colors are too shiny, strange, or colorful:** Toast, Coffee Mist, Peach Parfait, Topaz, Rococo, Gilded Olive, Laurel Green, Teal, Turquoise, Sea Foam, Burnished Bronze, and Pink Shimmer/Blue Haze.

☺ **EYE AND BROW SHAPER: Trim Line Lip Pencils** *($11)* and **Trim Line Eye Pencils** *($11)* are standard pencils that come in a small but good color selection. They go on soft but not greasy.

☺ **LIPSTICK AND LIP PENCIL:** Color Rich Lip Creme with SPF 4 *($10.50)* is an all-purpose cream lipstick that is fine for daily wear, although SPF 4 i completely unimpressive. **Moist Lip Color** *($9)* is a very greasy gloss that comes in a tube and, like all glosses, has limited staying power. The **Lipsticks** *($10.50)* are creamy but on the greasy side, and don't have much staying power. **Semi-Transparent Lipstick** *($8.95)* is more gloss than lipstick and has little to no staying power. **Lip Pencil Plus** *($9.50)* is a fat pencil with a lip liner on one end and a lipstick on the other. The pencil requires a special sharpener and is difficult to sharpen, while the lipstick side is fairly greasy. Actually, the pencil side is greasy, too. **Lip Treatment Cream** *($8.95)* is supposed to prevent bleeding. It does an OK job, but it doesn't feel great and it tends to peel off.

☺ **LipSoother Plus** *($7.50)* and **Lip Moisture** *($7.50)* are good clear glosses; both are quite emollient and can help nicely with dry lips.

☹ **MASCARA:** Creamy Flo-Matic Mascara *($10)* is an OK mascara. It doesn't clump, but it also doesn't build very thick lashes. **Luxiva Ultra Thick Mascara** *($12)* does go on thick, but almost too thick. It stays on well, but the clumping makes lashes look unattractive.

Mon Amie

A few years ago I saw an impressive ad for **Charles of the Ritz Timeless Essence Night Recovery Cream** *($35 for 1.7 ounces)*, reviewed elsewhere in this chapter, and I wrote about it in the July 1993 issue of my newsletter, *Cosmetics Counter Update*. Here is an excerpt from the article I wrote:

"The primary emphasis of the ad consists of quotes and pictures of talk-show host, singer, and professional endorser Kathie Lee Gifford. 'It works,' she exclaims. '[This product produces] smoother, younger-looking skin that's virtually free of visible fine dry lines.' Timeless Essence contains mostly water, a water-binding agent, glycerin, mineral oil, thickeners, vegetable oil, silicone oil, a long list of thickeners, and preservatives. It's an OK moisturizer for normal to slightly dry skin and nothing more. Kathie Lee's proclamation must have been influenced (and financed) by an attractive endorsement contract, because the product isn't timeless. If you thought your skin (or Kathie Lee's) would recover from the effects of aging by using it, think again."

Well, Ms. Gifford has landed another lucrative endorsement contract. She is now appearing in nationwide infomercials for the new Mon Amie line of skin care and makeup products. Mon Amie must be doing very well, based on the number of letters I've received. A large part of the attraction has to be Kathie Lee herself. Her well-known visage is a channel-stopper for many women, and her sincerity and enthusiasm are contagious. The infomercial's other participants, a French makeup artist and a Beverly Hills dermatologist, pale in comparison. But let's take a minute to look at the products. What you get for the considerable kit price (*$119.85*) might surprise you.

Bottom line: Mon Amie is both friend and foe. The makeup products are impressive, but the colors may not be right for you, depending on how you determine your skin color. After telling the Mon Amie phone representative that I had a medium skin tone, I was sent a beautiful range of peach blushes and lipsticks and yellow-based eyeshadows; the only problem is that I'm a Winter, and peach makes me look washed out. The overpriced skin care line would be tolerable if the products were interesting, but they leave much to be desired. If you don't already have dry skin, you might after trying these products (as many women mentioned in their letters).

Please note that the prices for the skin care products are the company's suggested retail prices, which help make the kit look like a huge bargain in comparison (even though you get a limited amount of each product). To order, call (800) 622-5700.

Mon Amie Skin Care

☹ **Gentle Facial Cleanser** (*$14.95 for 6.7 ounces*) is a standard detergent cleanser; TEA-lauryl sulfate, the second ingredient and the primary cleansing agent, is very drying. This product is anything but gentle.

☹ **Moisturizing Skin Clarifier** (*$14.95 for 3.5 ounces*) contains mostly water, alcohol, slip agents, salicylic acid, and preservatives. It's beyond me why anyone would even think of calling this product moisturizing when it contains mostly alcohol and 5% salicylic acid. But wait a minute: the package says it *doesn't* contain alcohol. Didn't anyone look at the ingredient list? Alcohol is right there, in black and white. Salicylic acid does exfoliate the skin, but in an alcohol base it can be a problem for even the oiliest, least sensitive complexion.

☺ **$$$ Daytime Moisturizer Replenishment Complex SPF 15** (*$24.95 for 1.75 ounces*) contains mostly water, thickeners, vitamin E, water-binding agents, silicone oil, more thickeners, and preservatives. This is a very good sunscreen for someone with normal to somewhat dry skin.

☺ **$$$ Intensive Eye Serum** (*$39.95 for 0.5 ounce*) contains mostly water, thickeners, water-binding agents, vitamin E, and preservatives. This isn't all that intensive, but it is still a very good lightweight moisturizer for someone with normal to slightly dry skin.

☺ **$$$ Nighttime Renewal Complex** (*$36.95 for 1.75 ounces*) contains mostly water, thickeners, plant extract, more thickeners, silicone oil, sugar extracts (AHAs), more thickeners, water-binding agents, and preservatives. The amount of AHAs isn't much, maybe 4%, but given that the toner contains salicylic acid, how much exfoliation can your skin take? Only one product needs to be exfoliating; two is excessive, and using both can be irritating and drying for most skin types.

Mon Amie Makeup

☺ **FOUNDATION:** The **Foundation** is beautifully neutral and has a wonderful creamy texture that is fine if you have normal to dry skin. Someone with oily skin would not be pleased with the consistency, though. You get two separate colors that can be blended together to create the right shade for your skin tone. That isn't as convenient as having one foundation that matches your skin exactly, but it does reduce the chances of getting an entirely wrong shade, given that you can't try it on before you buy it.

☹ **CONCEALER:** **Concealer Stick** goes on easily; it also creases easily, which is not what concealers are supposed to do.

☺ **POWDER:** **Pressed/Translucent Powder** is a standard talc-based powder that has a soft texture and goes on dry.

☺ **EYESHADOW AND BLUSH:** The two **Blushes** and four **Eyeshadows** you receive in the kit have wonderful textures and are perfectly matte. The eyeshadows are mostly neutral shades with no garish colors, and the blushes are soft colors that are easy to apply. You may not be thrilled with the array of colors if they don't work with your skin tone or aren't colors you want, but if they do match, the quality and colors are superior.

☺ **EYE AND BROW SHAPER:** The kit also comes with a two-sided **Brow Pencil**, a two-sided **Eye Liner Pencil**, and a two-sided **Lip Pencil**. I don't recommend filling in brows with pencils, or even lining the eyes with pencils, but the colors are fine and the texture is firm but soft, with only a slightly greasy feel.

☺ **LIPSTICK AND LIP PENCIL:** The kit includes three **Lipsticks,** which seems quite generous. One is a sheer glossy lipstick that easily feathers into the lines around the mouth and may not be of much use, but the other two have nice, somewhat creamy, matte textures. Again, the colors may not be right, but the quality is there.

☺ **MASCARA:** This is a good **Mascara** that goes on well and has decent staying power. It isn't exciting, but it is reliable.

Monteil of Paris

As this book went to press, Monteil was a company in distress. It was losing its placement in upper-end department stores, and where it would end up was a mystery.

Don't be all that impressed by the French-sounding name of this line. (You may remember that Monteil of Paris used to be Germaine Monteil.) For a long time it was owned by Revlon, not nearly as prestigious a name. Revlon went crazy in the 1980s, buying up a large number of cosmetics lines, and ended up mired in management hell. It needed financing to improve the lines it had acquired, but the money just wasn't there. Monteil was bought by the Lancaster Group, but Lancaster also had some rough financial dealings and sold Monteil.

In many ways, Monteil is just another fancy, overpriced cosmetics line whose prices are beyond what is tolerable. Until the company regains its footing, there isn't all that much for me to recommend.

Monteil Skin Care

☺ **$$$ Cleanser Actif** *($18.50 for 8 ounces)* is a standard detergent-based, water-soluble cleanser that cleans makeup off well but gently. Unfortunately, it can sting the eyes and leave the skin feeling slightly dry.

☺ **$$$ Rich Whipped Cleanser** *($35 for 8 ounces)* is a standard mineral oil–based wipe-off cleanser. The long list of ingredients includes water-binding agents and vitamins, but they are present only in negligible amounts. Besides, those kinds of ingredients are completely wasted in a cleanser because they get washed off.

☺ **$$$ Ice Super Soft Rinse-Off Cleanser** *($25 for 4.2 ounces)* is a good cleanser for normal to dry skin. Its detergent cleansers are further down on the ingredient list than they are in most cleansers, so it is milder. It does take off makeup and rinses nicely.

☺ **$$$ Gentle Lift Pro Eye Makeup Remover** *($13.50 for 4 ounces)* is a standard detergent-based wipe-off cleanser. Pulling at the eyes is always a problem; if the other cleanser works, this one isn't necessary.

☹ **Freshener Actif** *($18.50 for 8 ounces)* contains mostly water, witch hazel, slip agent, soothing agent, water-binding agents, mineral salts, and preservatives. The witch hazel can be irritating to most skin types.

☹ **Toner Actif for Oily Skin** *($18.50 for 8 ounces)* is a standard alcohol-based toner; alcohol can irritate and dry the skin.

☹ **Firming Action Moisture Cream with SPF 2** *($40 for 0.6 ounce)* contains mostly water, thickener, slip agent, several water-binding agents, fragrance, and preservatives. It won't firm the skin or get rid of wrinkles; it's just a good emollient moisturizer for normal to dry skin. (SPF 2 is a joke, right?)

☹ **Firming Action Moisture Lotion with SPF 2** *($32.50 for 2 ounces)* contains mostly water, mineral oil, slip agent, several thickeners, silicone oil, water-binding agents, vitamin E, plant oil, soothing agent, more thickeners, and preservatives. This is a good emollient moisturizer for someone with normal to dry skin, but there isn't nearly enough sunscreen.

☺ **$$$ Firming Action Night Treatment** *($65 for 2.25 ounces)* won't firm anything, but it is a very good (though very overpriced) basic moisturizer for dry skin. It contains mostly water, mineral oil, slip agent, several thickeners, plant oil, more thickeners, water-binding agents, silicone oil, film former, soothing agent, vitamin E, fragrance, and preservatives.

☺ **$$$ Firming Action Eye Creme with Sunscreen SPF 2** *($32.50 for 0.5 ounce)* is identical to the product above except for its embarrassing SPF 2 rating.

☺ **$$$ Lift Extreme Nutri-Collagen Concentrate with Sunscreen SPF 2** *($47.50 for 0.46 ounce)* contains mostly water, slip agent, plant extract, thickeners, more plant extracts, water-binding agents, fragrance, and preservatives. Collagen is a good water-binding agent, but that's all. SPF 2 is ineffectual and makes this moisturizer practically useless. Otherwise, this is a good lightweight moisturizer for normal to dry skin.

☺ **$$$ Super Moist Beauty Emulsion with Sunscreen SPF 2** *($40 for 4 ounces)* contains mostly water; thickener; lanolin; plant oil; isopropyl myristate (which can cause blackheads); thickeners; mineral oil; glycerin; soothing agents; vitamins A, E, and D (antioxidants); water-binding agents; more thickeners; and preservatives. Every ingredient you can think of is in here, but most come after the preservatives. This is a very good emollient moisturizer for dry skin if you don't have a problem with breakouts and don't need sun protection.

☺ **$$$ Super Moist Beauty Creme Moisturizer with Sunscreen SPF 2** *($32.50 for 2.25 ounces)* is similar to the moisturizer above, and the same review applies.

☺ **$$$ Super Moist Night Creme** *($30 for 1.25 ounces)* is similar to the product above, only without the sunscreen, and the same review applies.

☺ **$$$ Super Moist Line-Stop Creme Concentrate** *($27.50 for 1 ounce)* contains nothing that will stop lines. There is too little sunscreen to protect against sun damage, which is what causes lines. This product is similar to the one above, only more greasy. It is good for dry lips, but overpriced for what you get.

☺ **$$$ Lightyears Eye Area Formula Contains Sunscreen** *($40 for 0.3 ounce)* contains mostly water, slip agents, thickener, water-binding agents, plant extracts, more water-binding agents, and preservatives. This is a good lightweight moisturizer for normal to dry skin, but it doesn't contain enough sunscreen to protect from sun damage which makes it almost useless.

☺ **$$$ Moisture Build Triple Action Emulsion Oil-Free with SPF 8** *($32 for 2 ounces)* contains mostly water, slip agent, several thickeners, water-binding agent, plant extracts, several more water-binding agents, plant oils, and preservatives. Perhaps Monteil should read its ingredient list before claiming its product is oil-free—what do they think plant oils are? Nevertheless, this would be a good moisturizer for someone with normal to dry skin.

☹ **$$$ Activance Energy Concentrate** *($48 for 1 ounce)* contains mostly water, thickener, slip agents, film former, plant oil, solubilized oxygen, thickener, plant extract, preservatives, fruit extracts, and water-binding agents. You're supposed to believe this product can deliver oxygen to your skin, but there isn't enough oxygen for one breath. This isn't a bad product, just a waste of money.

☺ **$$$ Acti-Vita Enriched Eye Creme** *($35 for 0.5 ounce)* contains mostly water, mineral oil, thickeners, plant oil, more thickeners, plant oil, soothing agent, and preservatives. This is a good but ordinary emollient moisturizer for someone with dry skin.

☺ **$$$ Acti-Vita Enriched Moisture Creme** *($47.50 for 1 ounce)* is similar to the moisturizer above, and the same review applies.

☺ **$$$ Acti-Vita Multi-Nutritive Creme** *($60 for 1 ounce)* is similar to the Eye Creme above, and the same review applies.

☺ **$$$ Ice Fundamental Emulsion** *($42.50 for 1.3 ounces)* is an ordinary lightweight moisturizer that contains mostly water, thickeners, soothing agent, fragrance, minute amounts of algae and grapefruit extract, and preservative. You're paying a lot of money for some algae extract that doesn't provide any benefit for the skin.

☺ **$$$ Ice Ultimate Cream Concentrate** *($47.50 for 1.3 ounces)* contains mostly water, vitamin E (an antioxidant), thickener, plant oil, more thickeners, plant extract, petrolatum, more thickeners, fragrance, aloe, and preservatives. This is a good emollient moisturizer for dry skin, with a good amount of vitamin E, if that's what you're interested in.

☺ **$$$ Skin Reform Fluid Energizer** *($30 for 6.7 ounces)* contains mostly water, thickener, honey, plant extract, AHAs, anti-irritant, slip agent, more plant extract, water-binding agents, silicone oils, and preservatives. This is a good, emollient 4%

AHA product that could be suitable for someone who wants to try an AHA product but has sensitive skin. Of course, it's absurdly overpriced for what you get. The honey has no benefit for the skin.

☺ **$$$ Skin Reform Fortifying Cream** (*$45 for 1.7 ounces*) contains mostly water, plant oils, plant extract, slip agent, several thickeners, silicone oils, preservatives, salicylic acid, and more preservatives. This emollient moisturizer contains a tiny amount of BHAs (salicylic acid). It will slightly exfoliate the skin, and may be one of the more gentle options for a BHA product.

☹ **$$$ Skin Reform Lip Line Defense Dual Phase Treatment Formula** (*$27.50 for 0.28 ounce of gel and 0.30 ounce of cream*) is a two-part product. The gel is applied to the lips and lip area as a mask and then rinsed off with a washcloth. It is supposed to exfoliate the skin, but the washcloth is probably doing most of the work. There are definitely better exfoliators than this one. The cream is an ordinary moisturizer that contains mostly water, mineral oil, and thickeners. Down at the end of the list is some protein, but it won't help the lines around your lips.

☹ **$$$ Skin-Stress Relief Dual Phase Balancing System for Oily Skin** (*$50 for 1.5 ounces for one each of the Treatment Gel and Face Creme*) is a fairly ordinary, two-part lightweight moisturizer that is supposed to coax the skin back to tranquillity. First you apply the gel, then the cream. The gel contains water, witch hazel, slip agent, thickeners, amino acid, more thickeners, plant extracts, and preservatives. The cream contains water, slip agent, thickeners, mineral salts, more thickeners, vitamin E, more thickeners, and preservatives. If you want to believe plant extracts, mineral salts, and standard thickeners can "calm" your face, then go for it. The witch hazel can be a skin irritant.

☹ **$$$ Skin-Stress Relief Dual Phase Comfort System for Dry Skin** (*$50 for 1.5 ounces for one each of the Treatment Gel and Face Creme*) does not have exactly the same ingredients as the version for oily skin, but the two products are more alike than different, and the same review applies.

☹ **$$$ Double-Action Skin Lightening Creme with Sunscreen** (*$25 for 2.1 ounces*) is a standard bleach cream that contains 2% hydroquinone, which has some ability to lighten skin discolorations, but not much. This cream also contains a small amount of sunscreen, but other than that, it is just a collection of thickeners and slip agents.

Monteil Makeup

☺ **$$$** <u>FOUNDATION:</u> **Habitat Natural Foundation with Chemical-Free SPF 4** *($30)* provides light to medium coverage and goes on silky smooth and matte; the SPF 4 isn't great (it should be at least 8), but it is chemical-free. **All of the colors are excellent.**

☺ **$$$** Soft Cover Liquid Makeup SPF 8 *($25)* has a very moist, soft texture that blends easily. **These colors are good:** Porcelain Beige, French Beige, Sheer Beige, and Natural Beige. **These colors are too peach or rose:** Rose and Ivory.

☺ **$$$** Soft Cover Creme Makeup SPF 8 *($25)* has a very rich, emollient finish. The color selection is exceptionally limited. **These colors are good:** Sheer Beige, Natural Beige, Beige, and Fresh Beige. **This color is too peach:** Ivory.

☹ <u>CONCEALER:</u> **Hides Anything Moisturizing Concealer** *($17.50)* won't hide everything and is not at all moisturizing—in fact, someone with dry skin might not like the texture at all—but it is a good under-eye concealer that provides medium coverage, although it tends to crease into the lines around the eyes. It comes in three colors; Light and Medium are both great, but Deep can turn peach on most skin tones.

☺ **$$$** <u>POWDER:</u> **Supreme Pressed Powder** *($18)* is talc-based and comes in a small but impressive assortment of colors. **These colors are quite good:** Sheer 1, Sheer 2, Sheer 3, Sheer Natural, and Tan (a bronzer without shine).

☹ **Loose Powder** *($25)* comes in only one shade. How limited can you get?

☺ **$$$** <u>BLUSH:</u> **Silk Powder Blush** *($18)* has a very attractive assortment of matte blushes. The texture is a bit on the dry side, but it blends on easily. While the label says that Matte Bronze is meant to be an overall bronzer, I recommend using it only as a contour color and not an overall face color. **These colors are too shiny:** Peche Naive and Shimmer Rose.

☺ **Creme Blush** *($13)* is a traditional, greasy cream blush with only four colors. It is hard to find this type of blush anymore because powder blush is easier to use and doesn't dissipate like cream blush. It's an OK product if cream blush is what you are looking for, though.

☺ **$$$** <u>EYESHADOW:</u> **Rich Powder Eyeshadow Singles** *($15)* and **Duos** *($17)* have a wonderful silky-smooth consistency and blend on beautifully. Only a handful are matte, but those are worth testing. **These colors are excellent:** Twilight Blush/ Twilight Oyster, Volcane, Bisque, Espresso, Fawn, Brun/Chamois, Light, Terra Rose/ Terra Wood, and Cafe/Creme. **These colors are too shiny or blue, or are a poor combination:** Ashe/Gazelle, Eden Roc/Gris Pale, Vert de Mer/Menthe, Simply

Brown/Mushroom, Rose/Petale, Mahogany/Roseblush, Silvert/Bleu, Laquene/ Ciel, Hibiscus, Raisin, Vanilla, Cocoa/Carob, and Shade/Stonewash.

☺ **EYE AND BROW SHAPER:** Eye Pencils *($12)* are average, standard pencils. They are fine and a bit drier in texture than most.

☺ **$$$ LIPSTICK AND LIP PENCIL:** Sheers *($12.50)* are almost like a lip gloss; **Tints** *($12.50)* are little more than Sheers but still pretty glossy; **Lipsticks** *($12.50)* are fairly glossy but much more opaque and much like dozens of other lipsticks. The **Lip Pencils** *($12)* are fairly standard. There is nothing very exciting in this grouping except for some great colors.

☹ **MASCARA:** Ideal Mascara *($13.50)* is hardly ideal: it builds poorly and can smear.

Murad (Skin Care Only)

Like M.D. Formulations and Neostrata, Murad is a line of skin care products that boasts an above-average AHA content. Most contain 8% to 15% glycolic acid, which makes them very reliable AHA creams and lotions. Murad also has its share of products that contain alcohol and other irritating ingredients. I should mention that the prices are a bit excessive, at around $40 per product, especially compared with Neostrata (which has a similar AHA content) at around $16 per product.

I've received many letters asking me about Dr. Murad's extremely successful infomercial. In my opinion, the doctor has crossed a line, and I fear this is a growing trend in the world of dermatologists-turned-cosmeticians. We all assume that a dermatologist knows everything there is to know about skin care products in regards to their formulation, use, and effectiveness. Most important, we expect them to know, and tell us, the absolute truth about skin care. We don't expect cosmetics-counter hype from these highly trained medical professionals.

In fact, I am highly skeptical that dermatologists are the best source of "cosmetic" skin care information. Dermatologists are trained in skin disease, not in the daily use of cosmetics. Almost all the dermatologists I've ever interviewed could not have cared less about cosmetics. Their standard advice has always been to use soap or Cetaphil, Basis soap, Lubriderm, or Lac Hydrin, among others—that is, until they started selling their own stuff. But even then, they never uttered the sorts of words you hear from the Murad camp about wrinkle creams and spa products.

Regardless of whether dermatologists know best about lotions and potions, no scrupulous doctor would, with a clear conscience, sell products using the ludicrous claims made for the extended line of Murad products. Any doctor who is willing to sell products such as Murasome Cellular Serum, claiming it neutralizes free-radical damage (when most researchers will tell you that is only a theory that has not yet been proven true for the skin), or Murad Purifying Clay Masque, saying it provides the ideal environment for cellular repair, has sold out completely. Every product has the same hype, the same unsubstantiated claims, the same exaggeration about the beneficial effects of ingredients that are present only in the tiniest amounts, without even a mention of the standard ingredients that make up the bulk of these products.

One word of caution: Any time you use a product that contains more than 8% AHAs, some stinging can occur; also, you should not let the product come in contact with the eyes or any mucous membranes. You may have an allergic reaction to AHAs. Slight stinging is expected, but continued stinging is not. Discontinue use if this should happen.

☺ **$$$ Advanced Combination Skin Formula** *($40 for 3.3 ounces)* is a lightweight gel that contains 8% to 15% AHAs and mostly water, alcohol, salicylic acid, water-binding agents, aloe vera, vitamins A and E, and preservatives. The alcohol and salicylic acid are both very drying and irritating. The AHAs should be enough to exfoliate the skin without the extra irritants.

☹ **Advanced Oily Prone Skin Formula** *($40 for 3.3 ounces)* is almost identical to the gel above, but it lacks some of that product's good water-binding agents. The alcohol and salicylic acid are too irritating, but if you're interested in these products, at least go for the one that has some soothing water-binding agents.

☺ **$$$ Advanced Skin Smoothing Lotion** *($40 for 5 ounces)* contains about 8% to 15% AHAs and water, standard water-binding agents, several thickeners, more water-binding agent, vitamin E, aloe vera, and preservatives. This is a good AHA product for normal to dry skin.

☺ **$$$ Advanced Skin Smoothing Cream** *($40 for 1.7 ounces)* contains about 8% to 15% AHAs and is almost identical to the lotion above. It also has an SPF of 8, which is not enough to protect adequately from the sun. It is still a good emollient AHA product for normal to dry skin.

☺ **$$$ Murasome Eye Complex 10** *($40 for 0.5 ounce)* is identical to the lotion above except that it has additional water-binding agents. It is a good AHA product, but you need only one; three is overdoing it.

☺ **$$$ Murasun Spectrum 15 Daily Defense** *($18.50 for 3.5 ounces)* is a good emollient, but extremely standard SPF 15 sunscreen for the face or body; it contains no AHAs.

☺ **$$$ Advanced Age Spot and Pigment Lightening Gel** *($40 for 1.7 ounces)* is a standard 2% hydroquinone product that also contains alcohol. Most skin bleaches contain hydroquinone, which can be quite drying, and the alcohol exacerbates the problem. To overcome the dryness from the alcohol and to make the hydroquinone more effective, use it in conjunction with one of the AHA creams or lotions over the discolorations. Don't expect a lot; it still can't lighten sun damage spots all that much.

Additionally, if you want non–glycolic acid products, you can get a set of the following three items from Murad for $39.95:

☺ **$$$ Refreshing Skin Cleanser** *(6 ounces)* is an extremely standard detergent-based cleanser for someone with normal to oily or combination skin. It can be drying for someone with dry skin.

☹ **$$$ Spa Formula Peach Toner** *(6 ounces)* contains mostly water, slip agent, witch hazel, peach extract, water-binding agents, more slip agents, and preservatives. Peach sounds nice, and it might be, but the witch hazel (which contains about 15% alcohol) can be irritating for some skin types.

☺ **$$$ Murasome Skin Perfecting Lotion** *(2 ounces)* contains mostly water, plant oil, glycerin, several thickeners, several water-binding agents, and preservatives. This is a good moisturizer for someone with dry skin.

Neostrata (Skin Care Only)

Murad, M.D. Formulations, and Neostrata all sell a complete line of products with high AHA concentrations. What are the differences between them? Although the people who sell these lines wax poetic about the quality of their particular company's AHA complex or compound, the truth is that the results of all these products are the same. AHAs provide good, consistent exfoliation that reduces the thickness of the skin's outer layer, which in turn can solve many skin problems, including dryness, blemishes, sun damage, and skin discolorations. Which product line should you choose? Good question. Neostrata is the most reasonably priced of these three, but other products, such as Avon's Anew and those in the Alpha Hydrox line, also contain a good percentage of AHAs.

When this book went to press, Neostrata products were not all that easy to obtain; they are available mostly through physicians. Call (800) 628-9904 to find a physician in your area who carries the products, or (609) 520-0715 to find out which drugstores in your area carry the products.

One word of caution: Any time you use a product that contains more than 8% AHAs, some stinging can occur; also, you should not let the product come in contact with the eyes or any mucous membranes. You may have an allergic reaction to AHAs. Slight stinging is expected, but continued stinging is not. Discontinue use if this should happen.

☺ **Sensitive Skin AHA Facial Cleanser** *($12.95 for 4 ounces)* is a standard detergent-based, water-soluble cleanser that contains 4% AHAs. Although that isn't much, AHAs are wasted in a cleanser and can be a problem if you get the product in your eyes.

☺ **Skin Smoothing Cream** *($15.50 for 1.75 ounces)* contains 8% AHAs as well as water, several thickeners, silicone oil, more thickeners, and preservatives. This is a good AHA product in an ordinary but emollient moisturizing base.

☺ **Skin Smoothing Lotion** *($16.95 for 6.8 ounces)* contains 10% AHAs and is quite similar to the cream above, but it's a lotion. This is a good AHA product in a good emollient base.

☹ **Solution for Oily and Acne Skin** *($16.50 for 4 ounces)* contains 8% AHAs as well as alcohol, slip agents, and preservatives. The alcohol is too irritating and drying for most skin types.

☺ **Gel for Age Spots and Skin Lightening** *($11 for 1.6 ounces)* is a standard 2% hydroquinone skin-lightening product that also contains 10% AHAs. This would be a good product to try on age (sun damage) spots, except the second item on the ingredient list is alcohol, which can be drying and irritating to most skin types.

☺ **Sensitive Skin AHA Face Cream** *($17.50 for 1.75 ounces)* contains mostly water, plant oil, thickener, AHAs, more thickeners, glycerin, silicone oil, and preservatives. This is a good emollient moisturizer with about 4% AHAs. It would indeed be good for someone with sensitive skin interested in trying an AHA product.

☺ **Sensitive Skin AHA Eye Cream** *($16.95 for 0.5 ounce)* is almost identical to the cream above, which means it is completely unnecessary.

☺ **AHA Lip Conditioner** *($3.95 for 0.1 ounce)* is basically a lip gloss with 8% AHAs. I'm not sure whether regular exfoliation offers the same benefits for the lips as it does for the face, but this product is a good option if you're interested in that kind of treatment.

Neutrogena (Skin Care Only)

Neutrogena has been around since 1954, when that first clear amber bar of soap was manufactured. How well I remember discovering it when I was a teenager. It didn't leave quite the same soapy film as most bar soaps, and the amber color just radiated purity and a deep clean that could get rid of blemishes. I knew that my acne would go away if I diligently washed my face with this little gem. Of course, that wasn't the case. It didn't change my acne one little bit, and it dried my skin just the way other bar soaps did. Oh well, so much for amber clarity.

Since then, Neutrogena has created a skin care line with many elements worth considering for all skin types, although the emphasis is still on women who worry about breakouts. The bar soaps are still here, but so are a couple of OK water-soluble cleansers, a rather good irritant-free toner, and lightweight daytime sunscreens. One point of contention: Several products are promoted as being noncomedogenic, but there is no way a company can know what might make a particular person break out. I have had reactions to many products that claimed they wouldn't cause blackheads or acne. That doesn't make these products bad; it just makes the claim misleading.

☹ **Transparent Facial Bar Original Formula Fragrance or Fragrance-Free** *($2.69 for 3.5 ounces)* is a standard bar soap with detergent cleansers that can be drying for most skin types. The first two ingredients are triethanolamine and triethanolamine stearate, which are strong irritants when present in this amount.

☹ **Transparent Facial Bar Dry Skin Formula Fragrance or Fragrance-Free** *($2.90 for 3.5 ounces)* is a standard bar soap with detergent cleansers that can be drying for most skin types. The first two ingredients are triethanolamine and triethanolamine stearate, which are strong irritants when present in these amounts. It also contains tallow, which can cause breakouts.

☹ **Transparent Facial Bar Acne-Prone Skin Formula** *($2.90 for 3.5 ounces)* is a standard bar soap that is identical to the soap above except it also contains a few stronger detergent cleansers. This soap would be even more drying and irritating than the one above, and that would be a problem for someone with acned skin.

☹ **Transparent Facial Bar Oily Skin Formula Fragrance or Fragrance-Free** *($2.90 for 3.5 ounces)* is a standard bar soap that is almost identical to the Transparent Facial Bar Dry Skin Formula; the same review, warnings, and problems apply.

☹ **Antiseptic Cleanser for Acne-Prone Skin Alcohol- and Fragrance-Free** *($5 for 4.5 ounces)* contains a large number of ingredients that are too irritating for almost all skin types, including camphor, peppermint oil, eucalyptus oil, and benzalkonium chloride. It's nice that it doesn't contain alcohol or fragrance, but other things can irritate the skin too. While the label directs you to avoid using the product on the eye area, as it will burn the skin there, it is likely to burn the skin anywhere on the face.

☹ **Antiseptic Cleansing Pads for Acne-Prone Skin Alcohol- and Fragrance-Free** *($4.75 for 40 pads)* is identical to the cleanser above, only it comes on pads, and the same review applies.

☺ **Cleansing Wash for Skin Irritated by Drying Medications or Facial Peels** *($9.20 for 6 ounces)* is a standard detergent-based, water-soluble cleanser that isn't as gentle as the name implies. It can be drying for some skin types.

☺ **Liquid Neutrogena Facial Cleansing Formula (Fragrance or Fragrance-Free)** *($9.85 for 8 ounces)* is a fairly drying water-soluble cleanser that can thoroughly clean the face but would be a problem for anyone with sensitive, dry, or combination skin. Even someone with oily skin may find this irritating. It's actually quite similar to the product above.

☺ **Fresh Foaming Cleanser Soap-Free Cleanser for Combination Skin** *($8 for 5.5 ounces)* is a very good detergent-based, water-soluble cleanser for most skin types.

☺ **Non-Drying Cleansing Lotion** *($8 for 5.5 ounces)* is an OK water-soluble cleanser for someone with dry skin; it takes off all the makeup, but tends to leave a slight film unless it's used with a washcloth (which can be quite irritating to the face).

☹ **Oil-Free Acne Wash Gentle Yet Effective Cleanser for Acne Treatment** *($6.75 for 6 ounces)* contains a very drying and irritating detergent cleansing agent, as well as 2% salicylic acid, which is wasted in a cleanser and a problem if you get it in your eyes. This isn't gentle in the least, and it isn't effective for acne either.

☺ **Alcohol-Free Toner** *($8 for 8 ounces)* is an irritant-free toner that would be quite soothing for most skin types.

☹ **Oil Absorbing Drying Gel for Oily Skin Control** *($3.50 for 0.75 ounce)* contains mostly alcohol, slip agents, and preservatives. Alcohol won't control oil, and it is definitely drying. In fact, all this product can really do is dry and irritate the skin.

☹ **Non-Drying Gel** *($3.37 for 2 ounces)* is similar to the gel above in that both contain alcohol. Why this one is considered nondrying, while the one above is drying, is a mystery.

☺ **Chemical-Free Sunblocker SPF 17** *($7.99 for 4 ounces)* isn't really chemical-free, but it is titanium dioxide–based, an excellent way to protect from the sun if you can tolerate the slightly white film it leaves on the face.

☺ **Healthy Skin Face Lotion** *($9.39 for 2.5 ounces)* appears to be a very good AHA product. It doesn't contain a buffering agent, so the pH may not be reliable, which might affect its performance as an exfoliant. It contains about 8% glycolic acid in a lightweight emollient base, but Alpha Hydrox's Lotion for Normal to Dry Skin 8% AHA gives you six ounces of product for the same amount of money. This product does contain its share of antioxidant vitamins, though, so if you're searching for those theoretical free-radical scavengers, this product can (if you'll excuse the saying) kill two birds with one stone.

☺ **Intensified Day Moisture SPF 15** *($13.85 for 2.25 ounces)* is an OK lightweight moisturizer with a good SPF. It contains mostly water, glycerin, thickeners, silicone oil, more thickeners, and preservatives.

☺ **Intensified Eye Moisture 12-Hour Hydration** *($10 for 0.5 ounce)* contains mostly water, glycerin, thickener, film former, more thickeners, water-binding agents, plant extracts, anti-irritants, and preservatives. This is a good moisturizer for normal to dry skin. It is astonishingly similar to many other eye moisturizers.

☺ **Light Night Cream Won't Clog Pores** *($13.85 for 2.25 ounces)* contains mostly water, glycerin, plant oil, thickeners, petrolatum, more thickeners, silicone oil, and preservatives. Many of the thickeners in this moisturizer could indeed clog pores. It is a good emollient moisturizer for someone with normal to dry skin, but I wouldn't call it light.

☺ **Moisture Non-Comedogenic Facial Moisturizer for Sensitive Skin** *($7.50 for 2 ounces)* contains mostly water, glycerin, thickener, silicone oil, petrolatum, more silicone oil, more thickeners, and preservatives. This is probably great for someone with dry, sensitive skin, but the thickeners could cause breakouts.

☺ **Moisture Non-Comedogenic Facial Moisturizer SPF 15 Untinted** *($12.50 for 4 ounces)* contains mostly water, thickener, glycerin, more thickeners, silicone oil, and preservatives. The noncomedogenic claim is extremely misleading: any one of these ingredients (except for water) could cause someone to break out, as they did me. This can be a good lightweight moisturizer/sunscreen for normal to dry skin.

☹ **Moisture Non-Comedogenic Facial Moisturizer SPF 15 Sheer Tint** *($12.50 for 4 ounces)* is similar to the moisturizer above, and the same review and warning apply. Also, this tint is not for everyone or even most skin tones.

☺ **Lip Moisturizer, SPF 15, With PABA-free Sunblock Protection** *($3.29 for 0.15 ounce)* is a basic but good emollient lip gloss that contains mostly castor oil, plant oil, thickener, petrolatum, and more thickeners. It is very good for dry lips and can protect from the sun.

Nivea Visage (Skin Care Only)

☹ **Foaming Facial Cleanser** *($7.19 for 5 ounces)* is a standard detergent-based, water-soluble cleanser that can be extremely drying and may irritate the eyes.

☹ **Gentle Facial Cleansing Lotion** *($7.59 for 6 ounces)* is a standard mineral oil–based cleanser that doesn't rinse off very well and doesn't take off all the makeup without the aid of a washcloth, which isn't very gentle on the skin at all.

☺ **Visage Hydro-Cleansing Gel** *($6.49 for 5.5 ounces)* is a standard detergent-based cleanser that can be quite good for someone with normal to oily skin. It can also remove eye makeup without irritation.

☹ **Moisturizing Creme Soap** *($2 for 3 ounces)* is a standard bar soap that contains tallow and a strong cleansing agent. It also contains some plant oil and petrolatum, but they won't undo the irritation this soap can cause or prevent the breakouts tallow can cause.

☺ **Alcohol Free Moisturizing Facial Toner** *($7.19 for 6.8 ounces)* is a soothing, lightly moisturizing, fairly irritant-free toner. It contains mostly water, slip agents, several water-binding agents, preservative, and fragrance.

☹ **Facial Nourishing Lotion SPF 4** *(7.59 for 4 ounces)* has such a low SPF that it isn't suitable for daytime wear.

☹ **Facial Nourishing Creme Essential Daily Moisturizer SPF 4** *($7.59 for 1.7 ounces)* has such a low SPF that it isn't suitable for daytime wear.

☹ **Optimale Cumulative Care Creme SPF 6** *($10.99 for 1.7 ounces)* doesn't have enough sunscreen to make it worthwhile for day wear. It contains mostly water; castor oil; thickeners; silicone oil; vitamins C, E, and B; and several water-binding agents. There are plenty of antioxidants in it, and it would be a good emollient moisturizer for someone with dry skin. What a shame the SPF number is so out of line.

☹ **Shine Control Mattifying Fluid Oil-Absorbing Moisturizer SPF 4** *($10.99 for 3 ounces)* contains starch for absorbing oil, which is OK but not great because it can be a skin irritant. It is mostly water, silicone oil, thickeners, vitamin E, water-binding agents, soothing agent, and preservatives. It would be a good daytime moisturizer for someone with normal to slightly oily skin, but the SPF is too low to make it good for day wear. The low SPF numbers on this product and the one above are very strange given that most cosmetics companies know about the need for higher SPF numbers.

☺ **12-Hour Deep Moisture Liposome Creme with Vitamin E** *($14.39 for 1.7 ounces)* contains mostly water, thickeners, slip agent, silicone oil, glycerin, vitamin E, water-binding agents, more thickeners, and preservatives. This is a good moisturizer for someone with normal to dry skin. The vitamin E could be considered an antioxidant.

☺ **UV Care Daily Facial Moisture Lotion SPF 15** *($10.29 for 3 ounces)* contains mostly water, thickener, mineral oil, more thickeners, glycerin, vitamin E, and preservatives. This is a fairly ordinary moisturizer with a little bit of vitamin E, but the sunscreen is great.

☺ **No Oil All Moisture Hydrogel** *($10.29 for 2 ounces)* contains mostly water, slip agent, thickeners, water-binding agent, and preservatives. This is definitely oil-free and lightweight, which can be good for someone with combination skin.

☺ **Inner Beauty Daytime Renewal Treatment Natural AlpHA Complex** *($14.39 for 1 ounce)* is a lightweight moisturizer with about 4% AHAs. It contains mostly water, thickener, silicone oil, slip agent, AHAs, vitamin E, AHAs, water-binding agents, more thickeners, and preservatives. This AHA product would be OK for someone with sensitive skin who wants to see how her skin will do with a low-percentage AHA product.

☺ **Inner Beauty Nighttime Renewal Creme Natural AlpHA Complex** *($14.39 for 1.7 ounces)* is similar to the moisturizer above, only more emollient, and the same review applies.

☺ **Eye Contour Gel with Liposomes** *($14.39 for 1 ounce)* contains mostly water, slip agents, thickener, glycerin, more slip agents, water-binding agents, and preservatives. It is a good lightweight moisturizer for normal to dry skin.

☹ **Anti-Wrinkle Cream with Vitamin E SPF 4** *($9.49 for 1.7 ounces)* is an ordinary moisturizer that can feel fairly thick. It contains only a tiny amount of vitamin E, and the SPF is too low. This moisturizer can't and won't fight wrinkles, or even dry skin, very well.

☺ **Advanced Vitality Creme** *($14.39 for 1.7 ounces)* contains mostly water, thickeners, glycerin, several more thickeners, vitamin E, plant oil, water-binding agents, and preservatives. All of the good ingredients are at the end of the list. This isn't a very advanced moisturizer at all, but it would be good for someone with dry skin.

Noevir (Skin Care Only)

When this Japanese in-home-sales, multilevel-marketed skin care line first came to the United States, its sales representatives seemed to be more assertive than those from, say, Nu Skin or Mary Kay. That has been toned down a great deal, but some of the company's more outlandish claims continue. I was told that Noevir is special because Dr. Suzuki (creator of the Noevir product line) was "one of the few scientists with a Ph.D. in cosmetics research." Actually, the area of cosmetics research is filled with Ph.D.s from all sorts of disciplines: medical, chemical, and cosmetics research. Suzuki hardly stands alone. Another quote from the literature: "The medical profession supports Noevir's belief that products with mineral oil and other petroleum-based products are not beneficial to the skin." Well, plenty of studies indicate that mineral oil and petrolatum are just fine and quite useful for the skin, and I have never seen any studies indicating the opposite.

Another problem is that Noevir doesn't have a sunscreen as part of its daily skin care routine. This philosophy is almost prehistoric. In addition, the brochure announces that Noevir products contain no preservatives or fragrances, even though those substances are listed in black and white.

Almost every Noevir product has an assortment of collagen, placental protein, vitamin E, spleen extract, thymus extract, umbilical extracts, DNA, plant extracts of every kind, and a host of water-binding agents. I explain in the introduction why these ingredients are a waste, but if you want to believe that a hunk of dead spleen or thymus can create healthy skin cells ("almost like a transplant," I was told), I have a bridge I'd like to sell you.

Noevir has six different product groupings and a host of specialty items, which are very difficult to tell apart because many of the product names are the same. Only two categories are organized according to skin type; the others seem to be all-purpose. The main distinctions seem to be price and implied quality, because the individual products are not that different from one another. This system of product classification reminds me strongly of Shiseido, another Japanese line; I imagine Noevir began as a way to compete with Shiseido's successful department store line.

To order products or get more information about Noevir, call (800) 437-2258 or (800) 872-8888. Don't believe anything the salespeople tell you, though, because as long as they are being trained by this company, they are not being told the truth and therefore can't give you straight information.

☺ **$$$ 003 Line (For All Skin Types) Deep Cleansing Cream** *($18 for 3.5 ounces)* is a fairly standard wipe-off cleanser that doesn't clean all that deeply, nor is it the least bit water-soluble. It can leave a film, and wiping off makeup pulls at the skin and can cause sagging.

☺ **$$$ 003 Simple Cleansing Foam** *($18 for 3.8 ounces)* is a standard detergent-based, water-soluble cleanser that can possibly leave a slight film on the skin because of the few oils that appear at the end of the ingredient list. The detergent cleansing agents are fairly strong and can dry out the skin.

☹ **003 Perfect Toning Rinse** *($18 for 4.3 ounces)* is a standard alcohol-based toner that can irritate and dry the skin. It contains its share of plant extracts, including balm mint and mistletoe; both can cause skin irritation.

☹ **003 Gentle Moisturizing Lotion** (*$18 for 4.3 ounces*) is not what I would call gentle. The second ingredient in this product is alcohol, which dries out the skin and has no place in any product that claims to moisturize.

☺ **$$$ 003 Protecting Cream** (*$25 for 1.2 ounces*) is a good moisturizer that contains mostly water, slip agent; thickener; plant oil; more thickeners; witch hazel (can be a skin irritant); plant extracts (including balm mint and mistletoe, which can be skin irritants); more plant oils; vitamins E, D, and A; and preservatives. The plant oils and vitamins are too far down on the ingredient list to be of any significance, and some of the plant extracts can cause problems.

☺ **$$$ 95 Herbal Cleansing Massage Cream** (*$30 for 3.5 ounces*) is a fairly greasy wipe-off cleanser that is almost identical to several cleansers in this line. Massaging it around the face may feel good, but you can do that with almost any oil-based moisturizer, most of which cost a lot less. Some of the plant extracts can be skin irritants.

☺ **$$$ 95 Herbal Facial Cleanser** (*$30 for 3.5 ounces*) is a standard detergent-based, water-soluble cleanser that can be somewhat drying for many skin types. Who thought of these prices?

☹ **95 Herbal Cleansing Rinse** (*$20 for 5 ounces*) is a standard alcohol-based toner that also contains some water-binding agents, but they won't counteract the drying and irritating effects of the alcohol.

☹ **95 Herbal Skin Balancing Lotion** (*$30 for 4 ounces*) is a standard alcohol-based toner that also contains some good water-binding agents, but they won't counteract the drying and irritating effects of the alcohol.

☹ **95 Herbal Enriched Moisturizer** (*$36 for 3.3 ounces*) would be a good moisturizer for normal to dry skin types except that the second ingredient is alcohol, which has no place in a moisturizer.

☺ **$$$ 95 Herbal Skin Cream** (*$40 for 1 ounce*) is a good emollient moisturizer for dry skin; it contains mostly water, slip agent, several thickeners, plant oils, several water-binding agents, placental protein (animal), plant extracts, and preservatives. One sales rep explained that using this cream would be like getting baby cells transplanted onto your skin. Nothing could be further from the truth.

☺ **$$$ Series 4 Deep Cleanser** (*$30 for 3.5 ounces*) is virtually identical to many of the other wipe-off cleansers Noevir sells. Why this one has a different name is anyone's guess. Wiping off makeup is always a problem for the skin. The price is ridiculous, but that's standard for this line.

☺ **$$$ Series 4 Light Cleansing Foam** *($30 for 3.5 ounces)* is virtually identical to many of the other detergent-based, water-soluble cleansers Noevir sells. It can be drying for most skin types, and it contains tallow, which can cause breakouts, high up on the ingredient list.

☹ **Series 4 Enriched Toner** *($30 for 4 ounces)* is virtually identical to all the other alcohol-based toners Noevir sells; they all dry and irritate the skin, and are a waste of your hard-earned money.

☺ **$$$ Series 4 Protective Moisturizer** *($40 for 1 ounce)* contains mostly water, plant oil, several thickeners, more plant oil, water-binding agents, vitamin E, plant extracts, preservatives, and fragrance. This would be a good emollient moisturizer for someone with dry skin. One of the thickeners is tallow, which is high up on the ingredient list and can cause breakouts.

☺ **$$$ 105 Herbal Cleansing Massage Cream** *($70 for 3.5 ounces)* is virtually identical to many of the other wipe-off cleansers Noevir sells. Wiping off makeup is always a problem for the skin. The price is even more ridiculous than those of the other cleansers.

☹ **105 Herbal Cleansing Rinse** *($32 for 4 ounces)* is a standard alcohol-based toner that also contains some water-binding agents, placental protein, and plant extracts, but they won't counteract the drying and irritating effects of the alcohol.

☺ **$$$ 105 Herbal Facial Cleanser** *($56 for 3.5 ounces)* is virtually identical to many of the other detergent-based, water-soluble cleansers Noevir sells. It can be drying for most skin types, and it contains tallow, which can cause breakouts. That anyone would charge (or spend) this much money for a cleanser is shocking.

☹ **105 Herbal Skin Balancing Lotion** *($62 for 4 ounces)* is virtually identical to all the other alcohol-based toners Noevir sells, with the same list of water-binding agents. Alcohol dries and irritates the skin no matter what else you put in with it. But if you are willing to waste your money on animal placenta, who am I to stop you?

☺ **$$$ 105 Herbal Enriched Moisturizer** *($70 for 2.6 ounces)* is virtually identical to the other moisturizers Noevir sells; the only real difference is that this one is even more expensive.

☺ **$$$ 105 Herbal Skin Cream** *($70 for 0.7 ounce)* is virtually identical to the other moisturizers Noevir sells; the only real difference is that this one is even more expensive. It contains tallow, which can cause breakouts, rather high up on the ingredient list.

☹ **505 Herbal Skin Balancing Lotion/Skin Lotion** *($88 for 5 ounces)* is another outrageous product. Surely there isn't anyone willing to lay out this kind of money for some alcohol and water-binding agents. Most of them sound pretty nifty, but they can't change, feed, or do much of anything else for your skin.

☹ **505 Herbal Enriched Moisturizer/Milk Lotion** *($132 for 3.3 ounces)* is insulting: it is incredibly overpriced and incredibly similar to the other moisturizers in this line, and alcohol is the third item on the ingredient list.

☺ **$$$ 505 Herbal Skin Cream** *($220 for 1 ounce)* is even more insulting than all of the other products combined. It is a good moisturizer, but so overpriced that it seems like a bad joke.

☹ **Medicated Skin Care Formula Cleansing Treatment** *($14 for 2.6 ounces)* is a fairly strong detergent cleanser that also contains salicylic acid, which should never be used near the eyes or lips because of its potential to irritate and burn mucous membranes.

☹ **Medicated Skin Care Clarifying Toner** *($14 for 2.3 ounces)* is an alcohol-based toner that also contains salicylic acid (see review above). This toner contains some soothing agents, but they won't help the irritation caused by the alcohol and the salicylic acid.

☹ **Medicated Skin Care Blemish Cream** *($16 for 0.7 ounce)* contains mostly water, clay, alcohol, more clay, sulfur, and preservatives. It won't get rid of acne or blackheads, and the clay and sulfur can be very drying and irritating.

☺ **$$$ Special Night Cream** *($35 for 0.7 ounce)* contains mostly thickeners, plant oils, more thickeners, fragrance, vitamin E, mink oil, and preservatives. This is a very thick, rich moisturizer for someone with very dry skin. If you are expecting a miracle from mink oil, you would want a product that contains more of it than this one does.

☺ **$$$ Eye Treatment Stick** *($30 for 0.19 ounce)* isn't much of a treatment, but it is a good lubricating emollient for dry skin.

☺ **$$$ Eye Treatment Gel** *($65 for 0.52 ounce)* contains mostly water, slip agent, water-binding agents, vitamin E, more water-binding agents, thickeners, fragrance, and preservatives. This is a good moisturizer for someone with normal to dry skin. But it's probably your head that needs treatment if you pay this kind of money for a moisturizer.

☺ **$$$ Eye Makeup Remover** *($16 for 3.3 ounces)* is a standard detergent-based wipe-off makeup remover. It does take off eye makeup, but wiping is never good for the skin.

☹ **Suspension** *($80 for 1 ounce)* contains mostly water, plant oil, glycerin, alcohol, slip agent, thickeners, water-binding agents, plant extracts, more thickeners, preservatives, and fragrance. Alcohol is fourth on the list. Need I say more? I think not.

☹ **Recovery Complex** *($45 for 1 ounce)* contains mostly water, silicone oil, alcohol (irritant), thickeners, slip agent, fruit extracts, more thickeners, plant oils, water-binding agents, vitamins A and E, plant extracts, and preservatives. Fruit extract is not the same thing as AHAs, because there is no way to know exactly what has been extracted.

☹ **Advanced Moisture Concentrate** *($65 for 0.83 ounce)* contains all the trendy water-binding agents and alcohol. You already know what I'm going to say, except at these prices I feel like screaming.

☹ **Moisturizing Formula Concentrate** *($35 for 1 ounce)* is similar to the product above, and the same review applies except that the price is slightly more tolerable.

☹ **Revitalizing Essence** *($60 for 0.24 ounce)* comes in four separate vials, which combined have a very interesting ingredient list, but alcohol comes before all of the fun stuff on the list, and it is drying and irritating for most skin types.

☹ **Night Recovery Complex** *($50 for 1 ounce)* contains all the trendy water-binding agents and alcohol. You already know what I'm going to say: "Save your money."

☹ **Ultimate Peel-Off Masque** *($35 for 2.4 ounces)* places a layer of plastic over your face; after it dries you peel it off. That can make the skin feel smooth, but this product also contains alcohol, which can dry and irritate the skin.

☹ **Clay Masque** *($23 for 3.5 ounces)* contains mostly water, glycerin, alcohol, clay, thickeners, water-binding agents, vitamin E, plant extracts, and preservatives. This line puts alcohol in almost everything. I'm getting tired of warning against it. Except for the alcohol, this could be a very good clay mask.

☺ **$$$ Sun Defense SPF 15** *($24 for 4.2 ounces)* is a good, partly nonchemical-based sunscreen. It doesn't contain any of the gimmicky ingredients all these other Noevir products do, but, ironically, it is the only one that can really protect the skin and stop wrinkles.

Noxzema

See Cover Girl Skin Care *for reviews of these products.*

Nu Skin (Skin Care Only)

Let me start by saying that Nu Skin is not a miracle, a cure, the total answer, or even part of the answer for every woman's skin care needs. Nevertheless, the people who sell this line want you to believe it can alter your life as well as your skin. Like all of the other lines I've reviewed, this one contains some very good products, some useless ones, and some that are simply a waste of money. Also, as usual, the claims are all highly exaggerated. What sets Nu Skin apart is its intense direct-marketing strategy. As in most multilevel businesses, you meet someone who is selling the line, and if you subsequently buy anything, you are then asked to become a salesperson. The promise of unlimited financial return sounds like the pot of gold at the end of the rainbow. However, the multilevel aspect of the sales arrangements means the people who got in at the beginning are more likely to make money than those who came in later. Selling isn't as lucrative as getting people to sell for you. The saturation point can be reached quickly, which is one of the reasons the Federal Trade Commission and the Securities and Exchange Commission have contacted the company (attorney generals in seven states are doing the same). According to the March 1992 issue of *Drug and Cosmetics Industry* magazine, Nu Skin International has responded to complaints and lawsuits in Ohio, Illinois, Michigan, Florida, and Pennsylvania by voluntarily consenting to change some of its marketing and sales policies. One of the problems was that sales reps, in order to keep their commission percentage up, would overbuy cosmetics and then be stuck with them. After signing agreements with the attorney generals' offices in these states, Nu Skin was supposed to refund up to 90 percent of the money its distributors paid for products that went unsold. The company was also supposed to monitor its distributors to be sure that 80 percent of their sales are to at least five customers not affiliated with the company. Unfortunately for Nu Skin, in spite of these efforts, Connecticut's attorney general has filed a new lawsuit claiming the company's advertising misleads distributors into believing they will make more than they can. Actual figures indicate that 98 percent of all Nu Skin distributors average about $38 a month in commissions.

Its distribution methods aren't the only thing that's questionable about Nu Skin. The literature that accompanies the products announces in no uncertain terms that these products are packaged miracles. "All of the good and none of the bad," the brochures and accompanying tapes proudly announce. Unfortunately, it depends on how you define "bad." The products contain preservatives that can be potentially irritating, and some also contain peppermint oil, spearmint oil, witch hazel extract, grapefruit extract, camphor, and sulfur, which are all fairly irritating and known skin sensitizers.

Another difficulty is that this product line includes almost every gimmick in the book. Some are good for the skin, but most are just for show, to cover all the necessary bases of "natural" skin care: royal bee jelly, human placenta extract, aloe vera, vitamins, wheat germ oil, walnut husks, collagen, jojoba oil, and herbal extracts. Although many of you already know that you cannot feed skin from the outside in and are aware that there is no evidence that any of these function better than other moisturizing ingredients, I want you to also realize that most of these specialty ingredients are located at the bottom of the list for each product. That means they are present in essentially the smallest amount possible. As you may have already guessed, the first ingredients—the primary components of the products—are fairly standard ingredients such as water, thickeners, water-binding agents, and plant oils. There are some good products in the line, but they are not the miracles the company would like you to believe they are.

☺ **Cleansing Lotion** (*$10 for 4 ounces*) contains mostly water, aloe, thickener, and oils. It needs to be wiped off and can leave a greasy feeling on the skin. Wiping off makeup pulls at the skin, which can cause sagging.

☺ **Facial Cleansing Bar** (*$10.30 for 3.5 ounces*) is a standard detergent-based bar cleanser. It can be drying for most skin types.

☹ **Clarifex pH Acne Medication Cleansing Scrub** (*$13.30 for 2.65 ounces*) contains too many irritating ingredients, including sulfur, sulfuric acid, and salicylic acid, to make it an option.

☹ **Exfoliant Scrub Extra Gentle** (*$11.95 for 2.5 ounces*) contains mostly water, aloe, glycerin, seashells (as an abrasive), thickeners, and peppermint oil. It exfoliates the skin quite nicely, but the peppermint oil does not make this product extra gentle. There are vitamins at the end of the ingredient list, after the preservatives, meaning only a minute amount is included.

☺ **Facial Scrub** (*$10.50 for 2 ounces*) contains mostly water, aloe vera, glycerin, walnut husks, thickeners, and preservatives. It also contains peppermint oil, which can be irritating. There are vitamins at the very end of the ingredient list, which means they are present only in negligible amounts. For the most part, this is a good scrub, although it can be irritating for some skin types.

☺ **$$$ Eye Makeup Remover** (*$15 for 2 ounces*) is a silicone oil– and plant oil–based wipe-off cleanser that can leave a greasy feel. It will remove makeup, but wiping off makeup is always a problem for skin.

☹ **pH Balance** (*$8.45 for 4.2 ounces*) contains mostly, water, aloe, witch hazel (a skin irritant), glycerin, slip agent, water-binding agents, camphor, and preservatives. For some skin types this could be a good toner, but the witch hazel and camphor can cause irritation.

☹ **$$$ Alpha Extra/Face Dramatic Moisturizer for Uncommonly Dry Skin** *($25.25 for 2 ounces)* contains a minute amount of AHAs. This is an OK moisturizer for dry skin, but the name is misleading. It is actually rather ordinary, containing mostly water, thickeners, plant oil, silicone oil, several more thickeners, AHAs, vitamin E, water-binding agents, fragrance, and preservatives.

☺ **$$$ Celltrex Skin Hydrating Fluid** *($25 for 0.4 ounce)* is a lightweight moisturizer that contains mostly water, aloe, slip agent, water-binding agents, thickener, more water-binding agents, vitamin E, and preservatives. This is a good lightweight moisturizer for normal to dry skin, but don't expect the trendy ingredients to add to or change the cells in your skin.

☺ **$$$ Enhancer Skin Conditioning Gel** *($9.15 for 2.5 ounces)* is a lightweight gel that contains mostly water, aloe, slip agents, glycerin, water-binding agents, soothing agent, fragrance, and preservatives. These ingredients can nicely retain moisture in the skin, but they won't heal the skin. The amounts of RNA and royal jelly are too minute to talk about.

☺ **$$$ NaPCA Moisturizer** *($19.80 for 2.5 ounces)* is a good lightweight moisturizer that actually contains very little NaPCA. The major ingredients are water, aloe, thickeners, plant oil, more thickeners, slip agent, more water-binding agents, plant oils, vitamins, and preservatives. This is a very good moisturizer for someone with dry skin; it contains all the latest water-binding agents, which make it quite interesting, but it won't work any miracles.

☺ **$$$ HPX Hydrating Gel** *($49.95 for 1.5 ounces)* contains mostly water, plant oil, slip agent, human placental protein (whose idea was this?), vitamin E, water-binding agent, and preservatives. The placenta doesn't deserve comment, and the rest just makes this a good moisturizer for normal to slightly dry or combination skin.

☺ **$$$ Intensive Eye Complex** *($40 for 0.75 ounce)* contains mostly water, aloe, thickener, plant oil, more thickeners, slip agent, water-binding agent, glycerin, more plant oils, several more water-binding agents, vitamins, soothing agent, and preservatives. This is a good emollient moisturizer with several good water-binding agents high on the ingredient list, but the only thing intensive about this product is the price.

☺ **$$$ Sunright 15 Maximum Protection Sunscreen** *($13 for 8 ounces)* is a good sunscreen for someone with dry skin. It has some minute amounts of vitamins, RNA, and other fashionable ingredients, but the only thing that counts is the SPF, and that's good.

☺ **$$$ Rejuvenating Cream** *($28.48 for 2.5 ounces)* won't rejuvenate the skin, although it can be a good lightweight moisturizer. It contains mostly water, aloe, slip agent, several thickeners, vitamin E, water-binding agent, vitamin A, more water-binding agents, vitamin D, and preservatives. You're supposed to believe that royal jelly, algae, and RNA, among other ingredients, can rejuvenate your skin; they can't, and there is so little in this cream that it's almost silly.

☺ **$$$ Face Lift with Activator Original Formula and Sensitive Skin Formula** *($32 for 2 ounces of the Face Lift Powder and Activator)* is really two separate items you mix together to get the results implied by the name. Basically, the Face Lift Powder is egg white, cornstarch (a possible irritant), and silica (sand). The Activator contains water, benzethonium chloride (a possible skin irritant), aloe vera, soothing agent, and water-binding agent. The Activator swells and irritates the skin, and the egg white and cornstarch in the Face Lift Powder temporarily dry it in place, which supposedly makes it look smoother. It doesn't, at least not for long. Irritation around the eyes can be a problem and might cause more wrinkles.

☺ **$$$ Clay Pack** *($11.50 for 2 ounces)* is a standard clay mask that contains mostly water, standard water-binding agents, clay, thickeners, and preservatives. Again, the vitamins and royal bee jelly are at the end of the ingredient list, meaning you get only a tiny amount. Besides the clay, this product contains no other irritants or drying agents, so it could be a fairly gentle clay mask.

☹ **Clarifex pH Acne Treatment Mud** *($13.30 for 5 ounces)* is basically just clay and sulfur. It can be drying and irritating for most skin types.

Oil of Olay (Skin Care Only)

"Oil Olay" must be a very convincing name, because the line's popularity remains strong. For the longest time I wondered if people really thought it was some kind of oil derived from an exotic plant. It's not a very exciting line, lacking any state-of-the-art moisturizing ingredients, but there are a few good products to consider.

☺ **Facial Cleansing Lotion** *($4 for 3 ounces)* is a lightweight cleanser that doesn't quite rinse off without the aid of a washcloth; it can leave a residue on the skin, but it could be OK for someone with dry skin.

☺ **Foaming Face Wash** *($4 for 3 ounces)* is a standard detergent-based, water-soluble cleanser that cleans the face well, but can be drying for some skin types.

☺ **Sensitive Skin Foaming Face Wash** *($3.37 for 3 ounces)* is a good water-soluble cleanser for most skin types, but it is definitely not the best for sensitive skin.

☹ **Refreshing Toner** *($4.50 for 7.75 ounces)* contains alcohol, witch hazel, water-binding agent, soothing agents, and more water-binding agents. Without the alcohol, this would be a decent toner, but alcohol and witch hazel irritate the skin and negate all the soothing benefits of the other ingredients.

☹ **Daily UV Protectant Beauty Fluid SPF 15 (Fragrance and Fragrance-Free)** *($6.58 for 3.5 ounces)* is an OK, but rather boring, sunscreen that contains silicone oils and thickeners. This sunscreen is supposedly noncomedogenic; that's hard to believe because it contains aluminum starch, which can be a skin irritant and cause breakouts.

☹ **Daily UV Protectant Cream SPF 15 (Fragrance and Fragrance Free)** *($6.99 for 1.7 ounces)* is similar to the sunscreen above, and the same review applies.

☺ **Hydro-Night Renewal Gel** *($10.99 for 1.7 ounces)* contains mostly water, soothing agent, glycerin, silicone oil, slip agent, and preservatives. This won't renew anything, but it is a good, extremely lightweight moisturizer for normal to slightly dry or combination skin.

☺ **Hydro-Gel** *($9.30 for 1.7 ounces)* is similar to the moisturizer above, and the same review applies.

☻ **Original Beauty Fluid** *($5.99 for 4 ounces)* is a very ordinary moisturizer that contains only water, mineral oil, and thickeners. There is nothing beautiful about this one, but it can be good for dry skin.

☻ **Oil-Free Beauty Fluid** *($7.69 for 6 ounces)* contains mostly water, glycerin, thickeners, silicone oil, more thickeners, and preservatives. This is an ordinary moisturizer that contains more thickeners than anything else, and it can be good for dry skin, but these moisturizers are so boring they are hard for me to recommend.

☻ **Sensitive Skin Beauty Fluid** *($7.25 for 4 ounces)* is similar to the moisturizer above, and the same review applies.

☻ **Moisture Replenishing Cream** *($6.86 for 2 ounces)* contains mostly water, glycerin, thickener, petrolatum, silicone oils, more thickeners, and preservatives. It is a good, but very ordinary, moisturizer for someone with dry skin.

☻ **Oil-Free Replenishing Cream** *($6.86 for 2 ounces)* isn't oil-free; it contains silicone, which is not necessarily a problem for someone with oily skin, but the other thickening agents in this cream may be. It contains mostly water, glycerin, thickener, silicone oil, more thickener, more silicone oil, fragrance, and preservatives. It won't replenish anything, but it is a good, albeit extremely ordinary, moisturizer for normal to dry skin.

☺ **Sensitive Skin Replenishing Cream** *($6.86 for 2 ounces)* is similar to the cream above, only somewhat more emollient, and the same review applies.

☺ **Night of Olay Night Care Cream** *($6.91 for 1.7 ounces)* contains mostly water, glycerin, thickeners, silicone oil, more thickeners, more silicone oil, and preservatives. This is a good, but extremely ordinary, moisturizer for normal to dry skin. One of the preservatives is dmdm hydantoin, a strong skin irritant.

☺ **Intensive Moisture Complex** *($7.63 for 1.7 ounces)* contains mostly water, mineral oil, standard water-binding agents, a long list of thickeners, and preservatives. This is an OK emollient moisturizer, but hardly intensive.

Origins

Estee Lauder started off the 1990s with a new cosmetics line called Origins, and what a concept it has. A quote from one of the brochures sums it up quite nicely: "Origins marries the forces of nature with the vigor of modern science to make provocative differences in the way you experience cosmetics." To put it in my own words: "Origins uses all of the current fads on the market to create one of the most gimmicky makeup and skin care collections around." The brochures, like most of the packaging, are made of recycled paper. The ad copy is loaded with exotic-sounding botanicals, herbs, and oils. References to ancient Egyptian and Roman know-how are frequent. No other department store line makes a more persuasive case for the glory of natural products (except maybe Clarins, but only maybe). Origins even sells sensory-therapy oils and gels that are "thousands of years old." Of course, the oils and gels aren't that old, but the idea is that whoever was around thousands of years ago used these concoctions, and they must still be good.

I was very impressed with the color presentation at the Origins counter. The lipsticks, eyeshadows, blushes, and lip pencils are all divided into three color groupings: Peach to Rust, Beige to Tan, and Ivory to Pink. All of the colors have minimal or no shine, and most are soft and muted and therefore extremely easy to use. The textures are wonderful, and the application is almost flawless. Although I like the eyeshadows, be aware that a few have some shine; many of the salespeople insisted that all the colors are matte, but they are not. The amount of flower extract in many of the Origins products is also cause for concern. If you have any hay fever–type allergies, these extracts will cause you problems. "Natural" ingredients are not necessarily the best for all skin types.

Origins (like Aveda and The Body Shop) offers skin care systems based on every fad in the book and then some, including botanicals, essential oils, recycled packaging (including a recycling service at its counters for the empty bottles and compacts), products that aren't tested on animals, "ancient" skin care treatments, anti-stress formulas, and aromatherapy. The recycling efforts and animal-free testing are praiseworthy examples. However, the ancient and natural stuff is the real bait that hooks women. The ingredients are so obscure that it's difficult, even for me, to see beyond the plants and herbs. Even the salespeople I interviewed didn't know "what all those herbs were about." As you might expect, juxtaposed around the "special" oils and herb extracts are standard skin care ingredients. Also, many of the "good" ingredients are at the end of the ingredient lists, meaning they are practically nonexistent.

Origins's basic skin care theory is that all skin wants to act normal, the way it did when we were young. As we grow up, our skin gets confused or behaves badly, not because it wants to, but because it lacks something. If skin is supplied with the correct plants and oils, according to Origins, "nature's memory" can "retrain" your skin to function the way all skin wants to function—normally. What an enticing concept. Of course, the ingredients that supposedly retrain your skin are derived from the "ancient science of essential oils," which assumes that people who lived long ago had great skin because of this special knowledge. It does sound convincing, but, alas, there aren't any ancient people around to prove or disprove those claims. Moreover, you can't retrain the skin; that claim sounds like something the FDA should take a closer look at. But I have to admit that this is one of the most creative skin care ploys I've ever seen, and that is saying a lot.

In order to review this line without writing an entire book about it, I have summarized most of the plant extracts (which are little more than plant tea) by listing them as just that: plant extracts or plant water. Keep in mind that once a plant has been put in a cosmetic and preserved, it has little, if any, benefit, regardless of whether it had any in the first place. Having said all that, I still think Origins offers some good products; you just have to read between the lines to find out what they are.

Origins Skin Care

☺ **Liquid Crystal** (*$12.50 for 5.9 ounces*) contains mostly thickeners and plant oils; it can leave a greasy film on the face, and you have to use a lot of cleanser to remove all your makeup without the aid of a washcloth.

☺ **Mint Wash** (*$13.50 for 5.9 ounces*) is a good water-soluble cleanser that doesn't dry out the skin and does take off all the makeup. Some of the plant oils can be skin irritants and may slightly burn the eyes.

☺ **Pure Cream Rinseable Cleanser You Can Also Tissue Off** (*$13.50 for 6 ounces*) is supposed to be water-soluble, but it leaves a greasy film unless it's used with a washcloth. Also, the peppermint, lime, and tangerine oils in it can burn the eyes and are potential skin irritants.

☺ **Cream Bar** *(9.50 for 5 ounces)* is a standard bar cleanser that also contains several oils. The oils can help reduce the dryness caused by the soap, but they can also be irritants for some skin types.

☺ **Well-Off** *($11 for 3.4 ounces)* is a fairly gentle eye-makeup remover, but if the cleansers worked better, this product wouldn't be necessary.

☺ **Swept Away Gentle Slougher for All Skins** *($15 for 3.15 ounces)* is a fairly gritty exfoliant based on oat flour and talc. It also contains jojoba wax and a small amount of peppermint oil; both can be skin irritants. This is supposed to be gentle for sensitive skin, but that doesn't seem to be the case, although it can be an OK scrub for some skin types.

☺ **Swept Clean Special Sloughing for Oily-Acting Skin** *($15 for 3.15 ounces)* is a very gritty exfoliator that is identical to the one above except for the addition of menthol (which can be a skin irritant) and charcoal, although there is hardly enough of either to make them much of a problem or a benefit.

☹ **Managing Solution** *($16.50 for 5.7 ounces)* is a toner that is supposed to normalize oil production, but its ingredients—plant water, essential oil, aloe vera, vitamin E, slip agents, and preservatives—won't change oil production. The oil content won't make someone with oily skin very happy.

☹ **Oil Manager** *($21 for 5.7 ounces)* contains nothing that can stop oil or close pores. It does contain some plant oils, which would be a problem for someone with oily skin. What was Origins thinking?

☺ **$$$ Zero Oil** *($10 for 0.64 ounce)* cannot stop oil production, but it can absorb some amount of oil. It contains mostly plant water, earth mineral (which can absorb oil, the way talc or magnesium can), camphor (which can be a skin irritant), slip agents, and preservatives. This is pretty much a modified version of Phillips' Milk of Magnesia, which can do the same sort of thing, only better. By the way, why do they have both a no-oil product for acne and an oil-based product for acne? I guess Origins can't make up its mind.

☺ **$$$ Spot Remover to Clear Up Acne Blemishes** *($10.50 for 0.3 ounce)* is a standard salicylic acid and alcohol solution, like dozens of much less expensive drugstore acne products. This product can irritate and dry the skin.

☺ **Comforting Solution If Your Skin Acts Sensitive** *($16.50 for 5.7 ounces)* is supposed to help sensitive skin defend itself against the environment. It can't protect against the environment; however, it is a soothing toner of sorts that contains aloe vera, plant oils, soothing agent, vitamin E, water-binding agent, and preservatives. This product contains far too many potentially sensitizing ingredients to be considered reliable for someone with sensitive skin.

☺ **$$$ Constant Comforter** *($21 for 1.85 ounces)* contains mostly plant water; slip agent; thickener; plant oils; several thickeners; plant extract; anti-irritant; vitamins E, A, and B$_6$; water-binding agent; more plant oils, and preservatives. There is a long list of oils at the very end of the ingredient list, meaning there is just a tiny amount of them in the cream. This is a good emollient moisturizer for normal to dry skin, but it won't calm anything; in fact, many of the plant oils are potential skin sensitizers.

☺ **$$$ Drenching Solution** *($16.50 for 5.7 ounces)* contains mostly plant water, aloe, plant oils, water-binding agent, plant extract, thickener, vitamin E, preservative, more thickeners, and preservatives. It is a good soothing toner of sorts, but it won't teach skin to retain water.

☺ **$$$ Steady Drencher** *($20 for 1.85 ounces)* contains mostly plant water, plant oils, aloe, slip agent, several thickeners, more plant oil, vitamins A and E, anti-irritants, more vitamins, plant oils, more water-binding agents, and preservatives. The ingredient list is huge, but after you get past the minuscule amounts of many ingredients, this is a very emollient moisturizer that will nicely take care of dry skin.

☹ **Tuning Solution** *($16.50 for 5.7 ounces)* is supposed to rebalance the oily and dry areas of your face. It doesn't contain anything capable of doing that, but it is an OK toner of sorts. It contains mostly plant water, aloe, plant oils (many are possible skin irritants), water-binding agent, vitamin E, and preservatives.

☹ **Fine Tuner** *($25 for 1.9 ounces)* is supposed to even out combination skin. None of its ingredients can change oily skin, although it does contain some oils that can definitely help dry skin. It also contains shea butter, which can be a problem for someone with oily skin. It contains mostly plant water, aloe, slip agents, plant oils, thickeners, vitamin E, water-binding agents, vitamin A, more thickeners, silicone oil, and preservatives.

☹ **Mending Solution** *($16.50 for 5.7 ounces)* is almost identical to the product above, only this one is supposed to energize the skin's "look-young systems." No one's skin has "look-young systems." But isn't it amazing that such similar products are supposed to do such disparate things for the skin?

☺ **$$$ Time Mender** *($21 for 1.85 ounces)* contains mostly plant water, thickener, slip agent, more thickeners, anti-irritant, more thickeners, vitamin E, silicone oil, preservatives, and a long list of plant oils. This is a very good moisturizer for dry skin. The company claims that this product can firm the skin, but all the plant oils and water-binding agents in the world can't do that.

☹ **$$$ Line Chaser Stop Sign for Lines** *($25 for 0.5 ounce)* can't stop wrinkles, but it is an OK lightweight moisturizer for normal skin. It contains mostly plant water, thickeners, slip agent, water-binding agents, and preservatives. It does contain a minuscule amount of vitamins A and E, but they come well after the preservatives.

☺ **$$$ Starting Over** *($22.50 for 1 ounce)* is supposed to improve cell renewal; it can't do that, but it is a good moisturizer that contains mostly plant water, silicone oil, thickeners, water-binding agents, sugarcane extract, plant oils, vitamin A, more water-binding agents, more thickeners, and preservatives. The sugarcane extract is supposed to make you think you are getting AHAs, but you aren't— and even if you were, there isn't enough of the extract to consider it an exfoliant, and that's what AHAs have to be in order to "improve cell renewal."

☹ **$$$ No Puffery** *($20 for 0.64 ounce)* claims it can release trapped fluids and toxins from the skin, but that is not possible. It contains mostly plant water, slip agent, water-binding agent, plant extracts, and preservatives.

☺ **$$$ Urgent Moisture** *($25 for 2 ounces)* contains mostly plant water, glycerin, thickeners, slip agent, water-binding agents, more thickeners, silicone oil, and preservatives. This is a good lightweight moisturizer for normal to dry skin. It is supposed to perform best in super-dry weather, but it doesn't contain enough emollients to protect the skin from serious dehydration.

☹ **$$$ Eye Doctor** *($25 for 0.5 ounce)* is not what the doctor ordered. It is mostly plant water, slip agents, several standard thickeners, plant oil, water-binding agents, more thickeners, more plant oils, more plant extracts, anti-irritant, vitamin E, silicone oil, and preservatives. The mint and wintergreen oils can be skin irritants. Otherwise, this is a good moisturizer for someone with normal to somewhat dry skin, but I would keep it away from the eyes.

☹ **Clear Improvement Active Charcoal Mask to Clear Pores** *($15 for 2 ounces)* is a standard clay mask that contains mostly plant water, clay, slip agent, thickeners, standard water-binding agent, charcoal, more thickeners, and preservatives. The charcoal is supposed to lift impurities out of the pores, but it can't do that; also, there is hardly any charcoal in this product. Otherwise, this is an OK clay mask.

☺ **$$$ Silent Treatment SPF 15** *($15 for 1.7 ounces)* is a nonchemical (titanium dioxide–based) sunscreen suspended in a silicone oil base. It is a great idea, but it can leave a slightly white cast on the skin. I was very concerned to see that this product contains lavender oil, which can cause photosensitivity (if you go out in the sun wearing lavender oil, you can get an allergic reaction). Given the frequency of application needed to protect the skin adequately (including the chest and the back of the hands), this is a pricey little sunscreen.

☺ **Let the Sunshine SPF 14 No Chemical Sunscreen** *($12.50 for 5 ounces)* is one of the better titanium dioxide–based sunscreens on the market. Origins also offers **Let The Sunshine SPF 7**, which isn't the best protection, and **Let the Sunshine SPF 21**; both are nonchemical sunscreens.

☹ **Lip Remedy** *($9 for 0.18 ounce)* isn't much of a remedy. This lip product contains a long list of thickeners, plant oil, more thickeners, and preservatives. It also contains menthol and camphor, which are more irritants than anything else. There are better emollient lip balms available that can help dry lips.

Origins Makeup

☺ **FOUNDATION:** Original Skin is the clever name for Origins' foundations, although it is hardly accurate. This stuff doesn't look like original skin, it looks like foundation—a nice foundation, but foundation nevertheless. The salesperson told me Original Skin would make my skin look like a baby's bottom and let it breathe the way it does without foundation. Although I thought Original Skin was pretty good, it did not make my skin look like a baby's bottom, nor was the product less opaque than other foundations. It also did not hide tiny lines (foundation almost always makes lines look more prominent, and this one is no exception). Don't expect anything unique in terms of ingredients, either; besides some plant extracts and a small amount of plant oils, this is just a good standard foundation. Please note that the names of the foundations reviewed below are perfectly accurate. Also, all of the foundations below are best for normal to oily skin (the salespeople will tell you that all skin types can use them, but they are not very emollient or moisturizing).

☺ **Some Coverage** *($13.50)* is almost watery, like a liquid, but it goes on sheer and blends more evenly than you would expect. **These shades are good to excellent:** Paperwhite, Ivory, Linen, Tawny (may turn slightly peach), Fair, Flax (may turn slightly rose), Tan, Amber (may turn slightly ash), Copper (may be too orange for some skin types), Bronze (may be too orange for some skin types), Sepia, and

Mahogany. **These shades are too pink, orange, peach, rose, or ash for most skin types:** Porcelain, Blushing, Beige, Rosy, Golden, and Sable.

☺ **More Coverage** *($13.50)* provides just that: more coverage than the Some Coverage foundation above. **These shades are good to excellent:** Ivory, Linen, Paperwhite, Blushing (can turn pink), Fair, Flax (can turn pink), Tan (can turn orange), Sable, Copper (can turn peach), Amber (can turn ash), Sepia, Bronze, Mahogany, and Tawny (can turn peach). **These shades are too pink, orange, peach, rose, or ash for most skin types:** Porcelain, Rosy, and Golden.

☺ **Most Coverage** *($13.50)* ups the coverage another notch and is fairly opaque. **These shades are good to excellent:** Ivory, Linen, Paperwhite, Blushing (can turn pink), Fair, Flax (can turn pink), Tan (can turn orange), Sable, Copper (can turn peach), Amber (can turn ash), Sepia, Bronze, Mahogany, and Tawny (can turn peach). **These shades are too pink, orange, peach, rose, or ash for most skin types:** Porcelain, Rosy, and Golden.

☺ **CONCEALER: Original Skin Concealer** *($10)* has a smooth, light texture and comes in six shades. Best of all, it doesn't crease and has wonderful staying power. **All of the colors are superior.**

☺ **POWDER: Original Skin Pressed Powder** *($17.50 for compact and powder refill)* and **Original Skin Loose Powder** *($15)* are soft and sheer talc-based powders. **All of the colors are beautifully neutral and natural.**

☺ **BLUSH: Brush on Color** *($15 includes compact and blush refill)* tends to go on a bit dry, but it is very attractive and would work well for someone with normal to oily or combination skin. **All 15 colors are superb. Pinch Your Cheeks** *($10)* is a tiny tube of liquid blush that tints the cheek. It is best for someone with smooth flawless skin that is neither oily nor dry. That limits who can use it, but it is a good cheek tint.

☺ **EYESHADOW:** Origins has a superb array of matte **Eye Accent Eyeshadows** *($10)*. Although I dislike almost all shades of bright blue and green eyeshadows, most of the colors in this line are worth a try. Even the blues are some of the nicest blues on the market. Warning: Not all of these colors are matte; a very few have a small amount of shine, but not enough to show up poorly on the skin.

☹ **Kohl Mine** *($6.50)* is a fat eye pencil that goes on creamy and dries to a powder. It is an interesting way to apply one color, but difficult to blend over the eye with other shades. I prefer powders, but this is a fun option; however, pencils are always tricky to keep sharpened.

☺ <u>**EYE AND BROW SHAPER:**</u> The **Eye Pencils** *($10)* come in great colors, although the selection is limited. The **Brow Pencil** *($10)*, like all brow pencils, has a slightly slick texture; I do not recommend it unless you are a wizard at penciling brows that don't look fake.

☺ **Just Browsing** *($10)* is a brow color that you apply like mascara. This is a great way to make brows look full and filled in. **All four shades are good.**

☹ <u>**LIPSTICK AND LIP PENCIL:**</u> **Lip Color** *($10)* is very glossy, and the color won't survive to your midmorning break. If you have a problem with lipstick bleeding into the lines around your mouth, you'll feel this lipstick traveling the second you put it on. **Lip Gloss** *($10)* is a standard tube gloss. **Matte Stick** *($12)* is a lipstick in the form of a fat pencil. It goes on creamy and smooth, then dries to a matte but creamy finish. It is a fun product that creates a rich but soft matte look, though keeping it sharpened isn't very convenient.

☺ **Lip Pencil** *($10)* is a standard but good pencil that comes in a very flattering array of colors.

☹ <u>**MASCARA:**</u> **Underwear for Lashes** *($10* is a gimmicky, completely unnecessary undercoating for the lashes that you apply before the mascara. The claim is that it helps the lashes grab more mascara. A good mascara should suffice; this is a wasted extra layer on fragile lashes.

☺ **Fringe Benefits Mascara** *($10)* is a good mascara that builds evenly and doesn't smear.

Orlane

I have to admit that reviewing Orlane products was, at first, a bit intimidating. If I went to the counter dressed casually, without makeup (which is how I often dress when I'm reviewing a cosmetics line), the salespeople acted as if I were wasting their time. It seemed apparent to them that I couldn't afford $70 for a half-ounce jar of wrinkle cream. They were wrong, though: I probably have one of the largest cosmetics-buying budgets in the country, totaling well over $10,000 annually. But if they thought I wasn't worth the effort, they were right: I would never waste my money on this kind of marketing hype and incredibly overpriced products.

Attracting a wealthy clientele and convincing them that what they're buying is the absolute best isn't an easy task. The issue isn't money. Women who buy Orlane products aren't wondering whether they can afford the $500-plus it costs to take care of their skin the Orlane way; they just want to be assured that what they're getting is the best of the best, regardless of cost. Orlane's slick, sapphire blue packaging with silver letters is stunning. Its opulent, elegant appearance communicates prestige. But there has to be more to marketing than brilliant packaging, right? How does Orlane seduce a woman into believing its cosmetic chemists know something no one else does?

Orlane's pitch is that a Nobel laureate created "anagesium," one of the ingredients in its Anagenese line of products. Now, *that* is a great angle. Of course, I haven't received any information on who the person is or was, or what the research revealed. But it definitely sounds good.

Orlane says that anagesium is a combination of proteins that are supposed to provide some outstanding benefit to the skin. However, the ingredient lists reveal the truth: there are no unique proteins, or unique anything, in any of the Orlane products. Every product contains standard ingredients just like those used by the rest of the industry. Most of Orlane's products contain proteins and amino acids, which can help keep water in the skin, but they are not the only ingredients that can do that, and Orlane is not the only cosmetics company using them.

Maybe I shouldn't say that all of Orlane's ingredients are standard. Two hard-to-miss components are brain and spleen extract. What the consumer is supposed to swallow (no pun intended) is that a hunk of dead cow brain or spleen can have some rejuvenating effect on the skin. La Prairie makes the same body-parts ingredient claims, but there is no evidence or research to support this contention.

All of Orlane's brochures feature gushing phrases such as "optimum functioning of the epidermis," "natural molecules called Oxytoners," and "creates the proper environment for the skin." It all sounds so impressive—until you take a closer look and notice that the claims just don't jive with the accurate information on the ingredient list. No facts, no actual research, no proof is given in anything I've read from the company. It is all hyperbole. Charts for Orlane's Anagenese Total Time Fighting Care proclaim that it has produced a 52 percent reduction in wrinkles. But nowhere are there details of how that study was done, how many women were in it, what age group was tested, whether the study was double-blind, and who measured the before-and-after results. A 52 percent reduction might appeal to your emotions and hopes, but without more data it's a meaningless number.

It is hard for me to imagine that a woman could sincerely believe that spending this kind of money on skin care products will prevent wrinkles or aging skin or make her skin more beautiful. Women who can afford the so-called best products still have to get face lifts and eye tucks. But believe these claims they do—Orlane's sales are not hurting.

To be fair, and I always try to be, the line does have several creams and lotions that have a wonderfully silky texture. As I mentioned, most Orlane products contain fancy water-binding ingredients in the form of proteins and amino acids, and although they aren't unusual, they are interesting. Proteins work primarily by staying on top of the skin and preventing dehydration, while amino acids are better able to penetrate the skin and protect against moisture loss a little more deeply. That's about it, though. Do I think that translates into some extraordinary benefit for the skin? No. But they do feel nice and can keep the skin moist.

By the way, Orlane is perhaps the most uncooperative cosmetics lines I've dealt with (and I've dealt with a few). They refused to give us their ingredient lists, which were almost impossible to obtain because they are not on the box but on an insert inside the tightly wrapped container. They also did not offer any interviews or substantiating documentation for their claims. You might think a company with so many "miracle" products would want to establish their credibility. Not Orlane. Perhaps there is nothing credible for them to tell me. My staff and I did the best we could to get information about as many products as possible; this is not all of Orlane's product line. However, it should be enough to give you an idea of what is there.

Orlane is principally a skin care line; its makeup line is rather ordinary and almost inconsequential.

Orlane Skin Care

☹ **Detoxinating Wash-Off Cleansing Cream** *($29 for 6.8 ounces)* is a detergent-based, water-soluble cleanser that uses the cleansing agent sodium lauryl sulfate, which can be very drying and irritating for the skin (and hair, for that matter). It also contains lanolin, which can be a problem for some skin types. Protein and amino acids are present in tiny amounts, but they are a waste of time in a face cleanser anyway, because they're washed off before they can benefit the skin.

☺ **$$$ Detoxinating Purifying Gel Cleanser** *($29 for 8.4 ounces)* is a good water-soluble cleanser for someone with normal to oily skin, but it won't purify anything and might be a bit drying for some skin types.

☺ **$$$ Hydralane Moisturizing Cleanser, Continuous Hydro-Active System** *($25 for 13.3 ounces)* has one of the longest ingredient lists I've ever seen, but except for that, it is a completely ordinary wipe-off cleanser and has all the problems associated with wiping off makeup, namely stretching the skin. It contains mostly water, several thickeners, silicone oil, slip agent, more silicone oil, plant oil, water-binding agent, more thickeners, more silicone oil, and preservatives. The number of ingredients that fall after the preservatives is astounding and strictly there for show, because there is too little to have an effect on the skin, particularly not in a cleanser that is wiped away.

☺ **$$$ Hydralane Moisturizing Toner, Continuous Hydro-Active System** *($25 for 13.3 ounces)* contains mostly water, slip agents, witch hazel, water-binding agents, more slip agents, and preservatives. The witch hazel can be a skin irritant, but the other rather standard ingredients are good for the skin and nonirritating.

☹ **Detoxinating Purifying Lotion** *($29 for 8.4 ounces)* contains mostly water, slip agent, plant extracts (including arnica, lemon, and oak root, which can be skin irritants), animal protein, soothing agent, salicylic acid, sulfur, alcohol, and preservatives. Besides the irritating plant extracts, salicylic acid, sulfur, and alcohol can all be irritating and drying. This product is a rash waiting to happen.

☺ **$$$ Detoxinating Soothing Lotion Without Alcohol** *($29 for 8.4 ounces)* contains mostly water, slip agent, witch hazel, water-binding agent, several plant extracts, cleansing agent, protein, soothing agent, and preservatives. The witch hazel can be a skin irritant, and the number of plants in the product can be a problem for allergy-prone people.

☹ **Reviving Toner for All Skins** *($29 for 8.4 ounces)* contains mostly water, alcohol, slip agent, protein, plant extracts, salicylic acid, peppermint oil, and preservatives. The combination of alcohol, salicylic acid, and peppermint oil makes for a strong potential skin irritant; suggesting that this is for all skins is preposterous.

☺ **$$$ B21 Bio-Energic Vivifying Lotion for All Skins** *($40 for 6.8 ounces)* contains mostly water, slip agent, water-binding agents, fragrance, and preservatives. This would be a good nonirritating toner for most skin types. The serum protein in this is just a fancy name for a standard water-binding agent.

☹ **Very Gentle Exfoliating Cream** *($28 for 2.5 ounces)* uses polyvinyl chloride, which can be a skin irritant, as the scrub. Otherwise, this is a standard detergent-based cleanser that also contains some plant oils, which can prevent dryness, but not irritation.

☺ **$$$ Anagenese Eye Contour Cream** *($40 for 0.5 ounce)* contains mostly water, thickener, brain extract, several thickeners, plant oil, more thickeners, milk protein, plant extract, silicone oil, more plant oils, and preservatives. This would be a good emollient cream for someone with dry skin around the eyes, but brain extract? Is that supposed to make your skin smarter or something?

☺ **$$$ Anagenese Total Time Fighting Care** *($70 for 2.5 ounces)* is similar to the cream above, and the same review applies.

☺ **$$$ B21 Absolute Skin Recovery Care Eye Contour** *($75 for 0.5 ounce)* contains mostly water, thickener, glycerin, mineral oil, more thickeners (including cornstarch, which can be an irritant), petrolatum, plant oil, silicone oil, plant extract, water-binding agents, spleen extract, preservative, more thickeners, and more preservatives. This is a very good but fairly ordinary moisturizer for dry skin. The interesting stuff, albeit useless, is at the end of the ingredient list and therefore mostly inconsequential.

☺ **$$$ B21 Bio-Energic Absolute Skin Recovery Care** *($130 for 1.7 ounces)* contains mostly water, silicone oil, several thickeners, more silicone oil, thickeners (one is cornstarch, which can be a skin irritant), water-binding agents, plant oil, plant extracts, fragrance, and preservatives. This can be a good moisturizer for someone with dry skin.

☺ **$$$ B21 Ultra-Light Cream for the Day** *($75 for 1.7 ounces)* contains mostly water, slip agent, thickeners, aloe, spleen extract, more thickeners, water-binding agents, more thickeners, silicone oils, and preservatives. This is a good average moisturizer for someone with normal to dry skin.

☺ **$$$ B21 Protective Oxytoning Cream, For All Skins** *($90 for 1 ounce)* contains mostly water, thickeners, silicone oil, slip agent, more thickeners, spleen extract, several more thickeners, fragrance, and preservatives. This is a rather ordinary moisturizer for someone with normal to dry skin. There's that spleen extract again, a minuscule amount for $90. This can't be real, can it?

☺ **$$$ Extrait Vital Eye Contour Cream** *($42 for 0.33 ounce)* contains water, slip agent, water-binding agent, thickener, calfskin, spleen extract, more thickeners, several water-binding agents (including a tiny amount of lactic acid, but not enough to make this an AHA product), more thickeners, and preservatives. This is a very good emollient moisturizer for someone with dry skin. I don't have to discuss the spleen or calfskin extract, right?

☺ **$$$ Extrait Vital, Vital Biological Cream** *($50 for 1.7 ounces)* contains mostly water, plant oil, slip agent, thickeners, plant extract, plant oils, more thickener, spleen extract, water-binding agents, and preservatives. This is a good emollient moisturizer for someone with dry skin, but the minuscule amounts of spleen extract and proteins aren't enough to make a difference on the skin, even if they were somehow useful, which they aren't.

☺ **$$$ Extrait Vital, Vital Biological Emulsion** *($45 for 1.3 ounces)* contains mostly water, slip agents, thickeners, mineral oil, thickener, water-binding agents, plant oil, more thickeners, and preservatives. This is a good emollient moisturizer for someone with dry skin.

☺ **$$$ Soin Hydratant Moisture Skin Care** *($45 for 1.7 ounces)* contains mostly water, honey, silicone oil, several thickeners, plant oil, more thickeners, water-binding agents, mineral oil, vitamins B and E, preservative, and fragrance. Several more water-binding agents are listed after the preservatives and fragrance on the ingredient list, which means they are insignificant. This is a good moisturizer for someone with dry skin, but is it worth the price tag? These ingredients aren't unique, and the product isn't any better than a lot of less expensive moisturizers on the market. The ingredient list is lengthy, but just because it's long doesn't mean it's better.

☺ **$$$ Hydratant Riche Enriched Moisture Care** *($45 for 1.7 ounces)* is almost identical to the product above, and the same review applies.

☺ **$$$ Hydralane Moisture Skin Care, Continuous Hydro-active System** *($45 for 1.7 ounces)* contains mostly water, honey extract, silicone oil, several thickeners, plant oil, slip agent, more thickeners, more silicone oil, water-binding agent, mineral oil, and preservatives. This is a good but fairly ordinary moisturizer for someone with normal to dry skin. The number of ingredients that fall after the preservatives is absurd.

☺ **$$$ Nutrilane Total Nutrition System for Dry or Delicate Skin** *($45 for 1.7 ounces)* contains mostly water, several thickeners, slip agent, water-binding agent, plant oil, several more thickeners, silicone oil, and preservatives. Nothing in here is even vaguely nutritional, and the gimmicky ingredients yeast and DNA are at the end of the list.

☹ **Multi-Active Revitalizer with Apple Alpha-Acids** *($70 for 1.7 ounces)* contains apple extract, which is not an AHA ingredient, at least not as far as exfoliation is concerned. Regardless, without buffering you are buying an OK moisturizer and little else.

Orlane Makeup

☹ <u>FOUNDATION:</u> **B21 Teint Absolu Foundation** *($50)* contains spleen extract, which is supposed to explain its price tag. It does have a good soft texture, but it also has an extremely poor selection of six colors. **These colors are OK:** Perle and Dore. **The other colors are too peach, ash, or pink for many skin tones.**

☺ **$$$ Satilane** *($35)* is a matte foundation with a great light finish and all of the colors are great, although there are only five to choose from.

☹ Special Effects Foundation *($40)* has the same poor colors as the others; **all of the colors tend to be too peach for most skin tones.**

☹ Powder to Creme Foundation *($40)* is a standard cream-to-powder foundation that goes on very sheer and comes in six colors. It would be an option if the colors were more neutral. **These colors should be avoided:** Extra Rose and Extra Dore, which can turn peach, and Extra Blanc, which is extra white and looks ghostly.

☹ CONCEALER: Conceal Creme *($18)* is an OK concealer that comes in two colors. Clair is good for light to medium skin tones, but Tres Clair is too pink for most skin types.

☹ POWDER: Velvet Pressed Powder *($32)* is not all that velvety, and all the colors have shine. What a waste to put shine in a product that is meant to eliminate shine.

☺ Translucent Powder *($35)* is a talc-based powder with a small amount of plant oil. It has a silky texture and all three of the shades available are excellent. There are two bronzer shades, Soleil Cuiver and Soleil Clair; both are shiny, and I do not recommend them.

☺ **$$$** BLUSH: Velvet Blusher *($32)* is not what I would call velvety, but it does have a soft texture. Most of the colors have some amount of shine. **These colors are OK:** Quest, Rose d'ete, Rouge d'ete, Vendanges, and Muscat.

☹ EYESHADOW: Velvet Eyeshadow *($32.50)* comes in duo, trio, and quad sets, and all are shiny.

☺ **$$$** EYE AND BROW SHAPER: The Eye and Brow Pencils *($20)* are the same standard German-made pencils found in every line from Almay to Chanel.

☺ **$$$** LIPSTICK AND LIP PENCIL: Orlane's small selection of Lipsticks *($19)* comes in two types, one that is matte and one that is creamy, bordering on greasy. The handful of Lip Pencils *($16.50)* are the same standard German-made pencils found in every line from Almay to Chanel.

☺ **$$$** MASCARA: Special Effect Mascara *($22.50)* goes on well and doesn't smear or smudge, but for $22.50 it should be a great mascara, and it isn't.

Paula's Choice (Skin Care Only)

Are you sitting down? I've done something some of you may find shocking: I've created my own line of skin care products, called Paula's Choice.

There, I've said it. I hope most of you are thinking that this isn't so shocking after all, and are wondering what took me so long. Of course, you may just be wondering why

I decided to create a line of skin care products at all. Isn't that like Ralph Nader designing and selling cars? Good question.

Believe me when I say I did not undertake this endeavor without much consideration. Basically, after 14 years of analyzing and reviewing hundreds of cosmetics lines and thousands upon thousands of skin care and makeup products, it seemed like a natural extension of my work. As you already know, I have been continually frustrated by the endless array of products making claims that are either untrue or misleading. And even when I find products that meet my criteria for performance, they often fall short in other ways.

For example, after years of searching for a truly nongreasy sunscreen for oily skin, I finally found two, but one is ridiculously expensive and the other contains two irritating ingredients that aren't great for skin. Many products I otherwise like contain fragrance (a major cause of skin irritation), coloring agents, problematic preservatives, test on animals, or are overpriced.

Paula's Choice is a line of skin care products that meet my criteria when it comes to skin care products. None of my products contain coloring agents, fragrance (including masking fragrances), or any of the irritating ingredients I've been warning about for years, and they aren't tested on animals. Better yet, they are inexpensive—every product is under $10 and comes in generous containers.

I've always said I want to stop the cosmetics industry from bamboozling and misleading women; that is why I continue to write books and newsletters on cosmetics. Offering a line of inexpensive products that do what they say they will do feels like an extension of that work, and not in the least a conflict.

For the past two years, I have worked diligently with a major manufacturer to establish my criteria for the ingredients, the formulations, and the way the products are supposed to work. After the basic requirements were established, more than half a dozen versions were created before I accepted the final prototypes. Then, back in January 1996, I sent out 110 sets of the products, along with a detailed survey, to women who subscribe to my newsletter, *Cosmetics Counter Update*. Fifty-five women received skin care products for normal to oily/combination skin, and 55 received products for normal to dry skin types. All 110 women returned their completed surveys. The results? About 80 percent of the women said they really liked the products they received and were quite pleased with the way they worked, about 10 percent had concerns about two of the products but thought the other three were great, and about 10 percent didn't like the products at all or had allergic reactions to them.

Several women who responded to the survey asked me to include additional products, such as eye cream, lip balm, facial masks, and a more emollient nighttime moisturizer. I am working on those products as this book goes to press. Although eight women commented that they would prefer products with fragrance, I strongly feel that fragrance can cause problems for the skin, so I will not be adding any.

A few women were concerned that I would be abandoning my cosmetics and hair care research, as well as my objectivity, for cosmetics sales. This is not my intent. I truly believe that offering women inexpensive, high-quality skin care products that live up to my expectations is a service that should not get in the way of my judgment. However, all of you will be the best judges of whether I indeed remain objective. I am committed to maintaining my standards. There will always be great products for me to recommend, and terrible overpriced products for me to caution you about. My products are an option: nothing more, nothing else.

Paula's Choice products are available by calling (800) 831-4088 or (206) 723-6300. You can also order through my WEB page at http://www.cosmeticscop.com.

I debated at length about how to review my products as if they weren't my products, and decided to just give it a go, trying to be as impartial as I could possibly be. Basically, this section is just a way to give you a better understanding of my products. I did decide to leave them unrated because I couldn't possibly be that impartial.

One Step Face Cleanser for Normal to Oily/Combination Skin *($8.95 for 8 ounces)* is similar to Clarins's and Nivea's cleansers. It is a standard detergent cleanser that takes off all the makeup, including eye makeup, without irritating or drying the skin.

One Step Face Cleanser for Normal to Dry Skin *($8.95 for 8 ounces)* is kind of a cross between Cetaphil Lotion and a cleanser by Yves St. Laurent. It is a standard detergent cleanser that takes off all the makeup, including eye makeup, without irritating or drying the skin.

Final Touch Toner for Normal to Oily/Combination Skin *($8.95 for 8 ounces)* is a nonirritating toner that contains mostly water-binding agents, slip agent, soothing agent, and preservatives. It should leave a clean, soothing feeling on the skin.

Final Touch Toner for Normal to Dry Skin *($8.95 for 8 ounces)* is a nonirritating toner that contains mostly water-binding agents, slip agent, soothing agent, and preservatives. It should leave a clean, soothing feeling on the skin.

8% Alpha Hydroxy Acid Solution *($9.95 for 4 ounces)* is an 8% serum-type AHA liquid with a pH of 4.5. It also contains an anti-irritant, water-binding agents, and preservatives. It can be mixed with other moisturizers or used under sunscreens.

Essential Moisturizing Sunscreen SPF 15 *($9.95 for 6 ounces)* is a partly titanium dioxide–based sunscreen that contains thickeners; plant oil; vitamins A, B, and E (antioxidants); and preservatives. This would be a good emollient moisturizer for someone with dry skin.

Essential Non-Greasy Sunscreen SPF 15 *($9.95 for 6 ounces)* is based on several alcohol-free SPF 15 products I've recommended in the past, only this one leaves a slightly drier feel on the skin. It does not contain titanium dioxide as the sunscreen agent because it can cause breakouts for someone with oily skin.

Completely Non-Greasy Moisturizing Lotion *($9.95 for 4 ounces)* contains mostly water, thickener, plant oil, more thickeners, water-binding agents, vitamin E, anti-irritant, and preservatives. This would be a good lightweight moisturizer for someone with normal to oily skin. It can be used around the eye area.

Completely Emollient Moisturizer *($9.95 for 4 ounces)* contains mostly water, plant oils, vitamin E, thickeners, water-binding agents, vitamins A and D, soothing agent, and preservatives. This would be a good emollient moisturizer for someone with normal to dry skin. It can be used around the eye area.

Physicians Formula

There are some great products in this line, but before I review the wonderful blushes, eyeshadows, lipsticks, and moisturizers I have to tell you how much I dislike the name Physicians Formula. You would logically assume that all of the Physicians Formula products are formulated by physicians. Wrong. According to David Lozano, vice president of marketing and research for the company, the chemists at Physicians Formula are neither doctors nor dermatologists. They are just chemists, like the ones working for every other cosmetics line. They study ingredients that have been researched in universities and reviewed in various investigative journals, and based upon their experience and knowledge they choose "reliable" supplies of ingredients. This same process is used by hundreds of other cosmetics companies. So why the name Physicians Formula, besides the fact that it sounds very professional?

In 1937, Dr. Frank Crandell, an allergist, created Physicians Formula's first product, called Le Velvet, for his wife, who had photosensitive skin; hence the name Physicians Formula. (An allergist *is* a physician, after all.) Does today's Le Velvet even remotely resemble the original product that Dr. Crandell invented 56 years ago? Well, Physicians Formula claims that it still emulates Dr. Crandell, striving to create hypoallergenic, noncomedogenic products. But given the new ingredients on the market, I would be shocked if the original formula is still in use.

According to David Lozano, you can be sure that Physicians Formula's products are hypoallergenic because they have been tested on animals in outside laboratories and were reported to cause zero allergic reactions. This is hard to believe, but I wasn't given the test results. Products are also supposedly tested on in-house employees, but again I was not provided with any results. Mr. Lozano told me that product quality is further ensured by a medical committee, which evaluates each and every product before it is put on the market. Naturally, you would expect a *medical* committee to be composed of doctors, particularly given the name of the company. Wrong again. This committee is headed by Dr. Stuart Martel, who became a board-certified dermatologist in 1955. Surprisingly (or maybe not), he is the only certified doctor on the committee. The rest of the "medical" committee is made up of sales, marketing, and consumer representatives.

Having said all this, I want to report that Physicians Formula does have some products that I can recommend as great buys. Also, this is one of the few cosmetics companies that publish a list of the irritating ingredients they *don't* use in their products, ingredients that often show up in other skin care and makeup products. None of the Physicians Formula products contain lanolin, aluminum sulfate, benzoic acid, bovine extracts, linoleic acid, oil of walnut, salicylic acid, serum proteins, or yeast extract, which for a lot of skin types is a bonus. However, the Physicians Formula product line still contains ingredients that can pose irritation and skin sensitivity problems, such as alcohol, sodium lauryl sulfate, camphor, and menthol among others. Write to Physicians Formula Cosmetics (230 South Ninth Avenue, City of Industry, CA 91746) if you want a copy of this list.

I liked Physicians Formula's Captyane line of products, which is its version of liposomes—in essence, time-release moisturizers. These are good moisturizers, even though the claims are as exaggerated as they get.

Physicians Formula Skin Care

☹ **Deep Cleanser for Normal to Oily Skin** *($4.95 for 4 ounces)* is a standard detergent cleanser that contains potassium hydroxide and the detergent cleansing agent sodium lauryl sulfate, both of which can be very drying and irritating. This cleanser may be able to deep-clean, but it can also deeply dry out the skin.

☺ **Enriched Cleansing Concentrate for Dry to Very Dry Skin** *($5.95 for 4 ounces)* is a standard mineral oil–based wipe-off cleanser that contains plant oil and petrolatum. It is like cold cream and has all the problems associated with wiping off makeup.

☺ **Gentle Cleansing Lotion for Normal to Dry Skin** *($5.50 for 4 ounces)* is similar to the product above, and the same review applies.

☺ **Gentle Cleansing Cream for Dry to Very Dry Skin** *($5.95 for 4 ounces)* is similar to the Enriched Cleansing Concentrate above, except with a detergent cleansing agent, but it can still leave a greasy film on the skin. The same basic review applies.

☹ **Gentle Cleansing Facial Bar for Normal to Dry Skin** *($3.75 for 3.5 ounces)* is a detergent-based cleansing bar that can be drying for most skin types. It does contain a tiny amount of plant oil and water-binding agents, but that won't take care of the dryness caused by the other ingredients.

☹ **Oil-Control Facial Bar for Normal to Oily Skin** *($3.75 for 3.5 ounces)* is similar to the product above, only without the plant oil, and the same review applies.

☹ **Oil-Control Deep Pore Cleansing Gel for Normal to Oily Skin** *($6.95 for 8 ounces)* is a standard detergent-based, water-soluble cleanser that can be drying for most skin types.

☺ **Eye Makeup Remover Lotion for Normal to Dry Skin** *($4.25 for 2 ounces)* is just mineral oil, some thickeners, and petrolatum. This is greasy stuff, and wiping off makeup is a problem for the skin.

☺ **Eye Makeup Remover Pads for All Skin Types** *($4.50 for 60 pads)* is similar to the product above, and the same review applies.

☺ **Oil Free Eye Makeup Remover Pads for Normal to Oily Skin** *($4.50 for 60 pads)* is a detergent-based makeup remover, but it also contains witch hazel, which can be a skin irritant.

☺ **Vital Lash Oil Free Eye Makeup Remover for Normal to Oily Skin** *($4.25 for 2 ounces)* is a standard detergent-based makeup remover. It is oil-free, but it is still meant to be wiped off.

☺ **Beauty Buffers Exfoliating Scrub** *($5.39 for 2 ounces)* is a standard detergent-based, water-soluble scrub that uses synthetic particles as the scrub agent. It can be good for someone with normal to combination skin.

☹ **Oil-Control Conditioning Skin Toner for Normal to Oily Skin** *($6.95 for 8 ounces)* is an alcohol-based toner that also contains camphor and menthol. This is extremely drying and irritating for all skin types.

☺ **Gentle Refreshing Toner for Dry to Very Dry Skin** *($4.95 for 4 ounces)* is a good nonirritating toner that contains mostly water, glycerin, plant extracts, water-binding agents, and preservatives.

☹ **Pore-Refining Skin Freshener for Normal to Dry Skin** *($4.95 for 4 ounces)* is an alcohol-based toner that also contains a little glycerin. It is extremely drying and irritating for all skin types.

☺ **Collagen Cream Concentrate for Dry to Very Dry Skin** *($8.95 for 2 ounces)* contains mostly water, plant oil, several thickeners, water-binding agents, silicone oil, more thickeners, more water-binding agent, and preservatives. This is a good emollient moisturizer for someone with dry skin.

☺ **Elastin Collagen Moisture Lotion** *($8.50 for 4 ounces)* contains mostly water, thickener, plant oil, more thickener, water-binding agents, more thickeners, mineral oil, more water-binding agents, more thickeners, and preservatives. This very emollient moisturizer would be good for dry skin. It contains elastin and collagen, but they are just water-binding agents, nothing more.

☺ **Deep Moisture Cream** *($8.50 for 4 ounces)* contains mostly water, thickener, mineral oil, glycerin, more thickeners, petrolatum, more thickeners, plant oil, and preservatives. This is an ordinary mineral oil– and petrolatum-based moisturizer, good for dry skin but boring.

☺ **Emollient Oil** *($5.25 for 2 ounces)* contains plant oils, petrolatum, slip agents, and fragrance. This is a good, very emollient oil, but no more so than a pure oil from your pantry.

☺ **Enriched Dry Skin Concentrate for Dry to Very Dry Skin** *($7 for 2 ounces)* contains mostly water, thickeners, plant oil, glycerin, more thickeners, vitamins A and E, plant oil, and preservatives. This is a good emollient moisturizer for dry skin. The vitamins are at the end of the ingredient list, meaning they are barely present.

☺ **Extra Rich Rehydrating Moisturizer** *($8.49 for 4 ounces)* contains mostly water, thickener, mineral oil, more thickeners, and preservatives. It isn't as rich or as interesting as many of the other moisturizers in this group, but it is a good, ordinary moisturizer for someone with dry skin. It's poorly named, considering the mediocre ingredient list.

☺ **Gentle Moisture Lotion** *($8.49 for 4 ounces)* contains mostly water, mineral oil, thickeners, petrolatum, more thickeners, and preservatives. It is almost identical to the product above, and the same review applies.

☺ **Intensive Therapy Moisture Cream for Dry, Rough Skin** *($8 for 2 ounces)* is similar to the product above, and the same review applies.

☺ **Intensive Therapy Moisture Lotion** *($7.75 for 6 ounces)* is similar to the product above, and the same review applies.

☺ **Nourishing Night Cream for Dry to Very Dry Skin** *($5.95 for 1 ounce)* contains mostly plant oil, water, more plant oil, petrolatum, thickener, mineral oil, more thickeners, and preservatives. This is an extremely emollient moisturizer for someone with very dry skin.

☹ **Oil-Control Oil-Free Moisturizer for Normal to Oily Skin** *($8.50 for 4 ounces)* contains mostly water, thickeners, glycerin, soothing agent, clay, more thickeners, and preservatives. I can't imagine why the company thinks thickening agents with clay and a little bit of magnesium are oil-controlling. The thickening agents can clog pores and make the skin feel slick.

☹ **Oil-Control Shine Away** *($6.95 for 1 ounce)* contains polyacrylamide as the second ingredient. Polyacrylamide creates a thin, plastic-like film on the skin (which can feel tight and smooth), but it is also a potential skin irritant. The package claim that this product is clinically proven to instantly help regulate oil product on and keep skin shine-free. Water is the first ingredient; it also contains several w x-like thickeners and two other plasticizing agents that have a smaller potential for ausing skin irritation. A lot of new products contain these plasticizing ingredients (which are normally found in hairspray) because they set the skin in place and let little else in or out. That may initially benefit the appearance of the skin somewhat, but I doubt there is any long-term benefit, particularly in the case of this product, since the waxes and the plasticizing agents can clog pores.

☺ **Luxury Eye Cream** *($5.95 for 0.5 ounce)* contains mostly water, thickeners, petrolatum, plant oils, more thickeners, mineral oil, more plant oil, and preservatives. This is a very good emollient moisturizer for someone with dry skin.

☺ **Oil Free Nourishing Eye Gel for Normal to Oily Skin** *($6.25 for 0.5 ounce)* contains mostly water, plant extract, caffeine, slip agent, more plant extract, water-binding agent, and preservatives. This is a good lightweight moisturizer for slightly dry skin. I have no information about how caffeine is supposed to help your face, but it shouldn't be a problem.

☹ **Captyane Purifying Cleansing Gel for Normal to Oily Skin** *($8 for 3.5 ounces)* is a standard detergent-based, water-soluble cleanser that can be somewhat drying. It also contains tallow, which can cause breakouts.

☹ **Captyane Purifying Cleansing Lotion for Normal to Dry Skin** *($8 for 3.5 ounces)* is a mineral oil–based wipe-off cleanser that can leave a greasy film on the skin.

☺ **Purifying Facial Toner for Normal to Dry Skin** *($8 for 6 ounces)* is a good nonirritating toner that contains mostly water, slip agents, soothing agent, plant extract, water-binding agent, plant oils, vitamin, a tiny amount of AHA, and preservatives. The amount of AHA makes it a water-binding agent, not an exfoliant, which is just fine. This toner would be very good for someone with normal to dry skin.

☹ **Purifying Facial Toner for Normal to Oily Skin** *($8 for 6 ounces)* is an alcohol-based toner that is drying and irritating for all skin types.

☺ **Captyane Replenishing Eye Complex for All Skin Types** *($11 for 0.5 ounce)* contains mostly water, mineral oil, thickeners, water-binding agents, plant oil, more water-binding agents, and preservatives. This is a good emollient moisturizer, but it won't prevent or erase wrinkles.

☺ **Captyane Replenishing Gel-Cream with Microparticles for Normal to Dry Skin** *($11 for 1 ounce)* contains mostly water, plant oil, silicone oil, glycerin, more plant oil, water-binding agents, thickeners, more water-binding agents, vitamin E, and preservatives. This is a very emollient moisturizer for dry skin.

☺ **Captyane Replenishing Gel-Cream with Microparticles for Normal to Oily Skin** *($11 for 1 ounce)* is essentially the same as the product above, and the same review applies. This one does contain cornstarch, which can be a skin irritant.

☺ **Captyane Replenishing Night Treatment for Normal to Dry Skin** *($11 for 1 ounce)* contains mostly water, silicone oil, plant oil, glycerin, mineral oil, vitamin E, thickeners, water-binding agents, and preservatives. This is a very good emollient moisturizer for someone with dry skin. It does have a few trendy ingredients such as DNA and an amino acid, which make the ingredient list look impressive but don't do anything special for the skin.

☺ **Captyane Replenishing Night Treatment for Normal to Oily Skin** *($11 for 1 ounce)* contains mostly water, thickener, egg yolk, more thickeners, vitamin E, and preservatives. This is a good, but ordinary emollient moisturizer for normal to slightly dry skin. The egg yolk is cute, but it doesn't benefit the skin in any way.

☺ **Self Defense Protective Moisturizing Lotion with SPF 15 for Normal to Dry Skin** *($5.29 for 2 ounces)* contains mostly water, several thickeners, water-binding agents, petrolatum, and preservatives. This would be a very good sunscreen for someone with dry skin.

☹ **Self Defense Protective Moisturizing Lotion with Sunscreen with SPF 15 for Normal to Oily Skin** *($5.29 for 2 ounces)* is similar to the product above. It doesn't include the petrolatum but it does contain clay, which can absorb oil to some extent. The long list of thickening agents can be a problem for someone with oily skin.

☺ **Vital Defense Moisture Concentrate with SPF 15 for Dry to Very Dry Skin** *($8.50 for 2 ounces)* isn't very emollient, which doesn't make it appealing for someone with very dry skin, and it isn't as interesting as the Self Defense Protective Moisturizing Lotion for Normal to Dry Skin above, but it can be good for someone with normal to dry skin.

☺ **Vital Defense Moisture Lotion with SPF 15 for Normal to Dry Skin** *($8 for 6 ounces)* is similar to the Self Defense Lotion for Normal to Dry Skin, and the same review applies.

☺ **Vital Defense Oil Free Lotion with SPF 15 for Normal to Oily Skin** *($8 for 6 ounces)* is similar to the Self Defense Lotion for Normal to Oily Skin, and the same review applies.

☹ **Deep Cleaning Face Mask** *($5.95 for 2.8 ounces)* is a standard clay mask that contains mostly water, witch hazel, clay, alcohol, and glycerin. The clay is drying, and the alcohol and witch hazel will only make things worse. This mask won't deep-clean, but it can deeply irritate the skin.

Physicians Formula Makeup

☺ **FOUNDATION: Le Velvet Film Makeup with Nonchemical SPF 15** *($7.25)* is a compact foundation that goes on surprisingly moist and creamy and can blend out fairly sheer. Also, it contains a good titanium dioxide–based sunscreen with an SPF of 15. What a shame there are no testers for this product, because it would be a definite option for someone with dry skin, but the colors are too difficult to judge through the container.

☺ **Le Velvet Powder Finish with Nonchemical SPF 15** *($7.25)* is a very good cream-to-powder foundation that has a smooth, even finish and feels like you have nothing on your face. It also has some great colors for light to medium skin tones, as well as a nonchemical SPF of 15. This is definitely worth checking out but it does take guesswork, because no testers are available; in three attempts, I still got the wrong color for my skin tone.

☺ **Sun Shield Liquid Makeup with SPF 15** *($5.25)* is a good option for someone with normal to dry skin, but there are no testers. It has a soft, smooth texture and more reliable colors than the other two liquid foundations, but it is risky to buy a foundation without trying it on first.

☹ **Oil Control Matte Makeup** *($5.25)* won't control oil but it is oil-free; despite the lack of oil, though, it does not have a completely matte finish and can feel heavy and thick. **Most of the shades are too peach or pink.**

☹ **Sheer Moisture Light Diffusing Makeup** *($5.25)* has a smooth, moist finish, but the phrase "light-diffusing" refers to the sparkle in the makeup. It make the skin reflect light, but if you think that will change the way a wrinkle looks, you're mistaken; it actually makes wrinkles look worse.

☺ **Refill Sponges** *($2.50)* for the Le Velvet foundation work well with any foundation. I prefer the round, thin shape to the thick wedge sponges you normally find at cosmetics counters and drugstores.

☹ <u>CONCEALER:</u> **Gentle Cover Concealer Stick** *($4.35)* comes in four shades: Green, Ice Blue, Light, and Medium. The texture is too heavy and tends to crease into the lines around the eyes. I never recommend green or blue concealers. **Gentle Cover Cream Concealer** *($4.35)* creases easily into the lines around the eyes, and all the colors are way too peach, pink, or yellow. **Color Corrective Primer** *($3.75)* comes in Mauve, Yellow, and Green. The texture is very greasy and thick and it can feel tacky under foundation.

☹ <u>POWDER:</u> **Translucent Loose Powder** *($5.75)* is a talc-based powder with a dry, powdery finish and a small amount of shine. The container is very inconvenient to use.

☺ <u>BLUSH:</u> **Matte Blush** *($5.75)* is a great find. I wouldn't call these blushes silky, but they do go on smooth and are totally matte. Only one word of warning: Most of these colors are very muted, bordering on dull. Check them out only if you are looking for a very natural tawny blush color.

☺ <u>EYESHADOW:</u> The **Matte Collection Singles** *($2.95)* and **Duos** *($4.25)* is a wonderful collection of matte eyeshadows. They go on beautifully and blend easily. **These colors are excellent:** Taupe, Cinnamon, Peaches 'N' Creme, French Vanilla, Smoke, Perfect Pink, Jade (may be too green for most skin types), Rosewood, Plum Smoke, Praline, Chocolate Fudge, Khaki, Dusty Mauve, Autumn Dusk, and Vanilla Marble. **These colors should be avoided:** Midnight Blue, Misty Blue, Stormy Skies, and Sky Blue/Pink (too blue); Teal (too green); and Flamingo (a difficult color combination of peach and green).

☹ <u>EYE AND BROW SHAPER:</u> **Gentlewear Eye Pencils** *($3.95)* are fat, which makes them hard to sharpen and hard to control. Also, most of them are shiny, and they are packaged so that you can't see the color.

☺ **Eye Definer Automatic Eye Pencil** *($4.75)* is a twist-up eye pencil that is greasier than most, which means it can smear or smudge easily.

☺ <u>LIPSTICK AND LIP PENCIL:</u> **Total Perfection Lipstick** *($4.50)* is almost too creamy; it isn't supposed to feather into the lines around the lips, but it does. **Beyond Moisture with SPF 8** *($4.95)* is a good glossy lipstick with an SPF of 8. **Vital Defense Lip Treatment** *($3.50)* and **Gloss Guard Protective Shine** *($3.95)* are petrolatum-based emollient lip glosses with an SPF of 15; the Lip Treatment comes in a Chapstick-like container, and the other is in a squeeze tube.

☺ **Lip Defining Automatic Pencil** *($4.50)* is a very good twist pencil that has a smooth, dry texture.

☹ **MASCARA: Length-Plus Mascara** *($4.50)* and **Full Lash Mascara** *($4.50)* don't build much length or thickness, and they tend to smear. **Plentiful Length-Plus Lengthening Mascara** *($3.72)* and **Plentiful Full Lash Thickening Mascara** *($3.72)* neither lengthen nor thicken. Furthermore, by midday they smear and smudge all over the place.

Pond's (Skin Care Only)

Pond's is spending over $36 million to advertise its line of AHA products, called Age Defying Complex, so it has likely caught your attention by now. Six-page ads in major fashion magazines and several sultry television commercials are the company's way of letting you know it has seriously joined the AHA competition. The ads carry on about tests showing that Pond's AHA products improved the skin of women who used them over a six-month period. Of course, the ads don't mention whether any other AHA products were tested or what other products the women were using beforehand. They probably figured that most women wouldn't want to be bothered with such details. The ads don't really give you any information you can use to make a decision. Having said all that, even though I consider the ads to be totally bogus, I do happen to think that Pond's has created two very good AHA moisturizers, and one of its water-soluble cleansers is terrific.

☺ **Cleansing Lotion & Moisturizer in One for Normal to Dry Skin** *($4.39 for 4 ounces)* isn't all that water-soluble, and there isn't much in it that can clean off makeup; you'll need to use a washcloth, which means wiping and pulling the skin. This isn't a bad product, but I don't recommend it.

☺ **Foaming Cleanser & Toner in One** *($4.39 for 4 ounces)* is a good water-soluble cleanser that can take off all your eye makeup without causing irritation. It may be drying for some skin types.

☹ **Self-Foaming Facial Cleanser** *($6.99 for 8 ounces)* definitely foams, and, as the box says, you've never seen anything like it. I haven't, at least not in a facial cleanser. It is reminiscent of a man's shaving foam. I have to admit I found the self-foaming part rather fun and unique, but the novelty wore off the second I asked myself the basic questions pertaining to any facial cleanser: Unfortunately, while this product cleans well, the foam was difficult to spread and it can dry out the skin. The detergent cleansing agent is extremely drying and potentially irritating.

☹ **Lemon Cold Cream Deep Cleanser** *($4.39 for 3.5 ounces)* is mostly mineral oil and wax; that's pretty much cold cream, and it's a greasy mess when you wipe it off.

☹ **Water Rinseable Cleanser** *($4.50 for 5.5 ounces)* is not at all water-soluble. The main ingredients are water, mineral oil, and beeswax. If anything, the cleanser leaves an oily film on the skin.

☹ **Moisturizing Cleansing Bar with Moisture Complex** *($1.99 for 3.25 ounces)* is a standard bar cleanser that has no ingredients that would moisturize the skin. This soap would be quite drying for most skin types.

☹ **Clarifying Astringent** *($4.39 for 7 ounces)* is a standard alcohol-based toner that also contains witch hazel, menthol, and eucalyptus, all of which can seriously irritate the skin.

☺ **Dry Skin Extra Rich Skin Cream** *($5.49 for 6.5 ounces)* is a standard mineral oil– and petrolatum-based moisturizer with thickeners and preservatives. It would be good for dry skin, but its ingredients are very ordinary and boring.

☺ **Nourishing Moisturizer Cream Oil-Free** *($6.29 for 2 ounces)* can't nourish the skin and it definitely isn't oil-free, but it is a good moisturizer for normal to dry skin. It contains mostly water, glycerin, silicone oils, thickeners, vitamins A and E (antioxidants), water-binding agents, and preservatives.

☺ **Nourishing Moisturizer Lotion Oil-Free** *($6.29 for 4 ounces)* is similar to the product above, and the same review applies.

☺ **Nourishing Moisture Lotion with SPF 15** *($5.99 for 2.5 ounces)* won't nourish anyone's skin, but it does contain several thickeners, silicone oil, vitamins A and E, water-binding agents, and preservatives. This would be a very good sunscreen with antioxidants for someone with dry skin.

☺ **Nourishing Moisturizer Lotion Oil-Free with SPF 15** *($5.99 for 2.5 ounces)* isn't oil-free (it contains silicone oil), but it is still a good, partly nonchemical sunscreen for someone with normal to dry skin. It does contain vitamins (antioxidants) and water-binding agents.

☺ **Overnight Nourishing Complex Cream Oil-Free** *($6.29 for 2 ounces)* contains mostly water, silicone oil (it obviously isn't oil-free), thickeners, slip agent, more thickeners, vitamins A and E, water-binding agents, fragrance, and preservatives. This is a good emollient moisturizer for dry skin, but the vitamins can't nourish the skin; they are just good antioxidants. One of the thickening agents high up on the ingredient list is isopropyl myristate, which can cause breakouts.

☺ **Dramatic Results Skin Smoothing Capsules with Nutrium** *($11.59 for 0.26 ounce)* contains mostly silicone oils, plant oil, thickener, vitamins A and E, and water-binding agents. The results won't be dramatic, but this is certainly a good product for someone with dry skin.

☺ **Revitalizing Eye Capsules, Delicate Eye Area** *($11.59 for 0.13 ounce)* is similar to the product above, and the same review applies.

☹ **Revitalizing Eye Gel with Vitamin E** *($5.99 for 0.5 ounce)* contains mostly water, witch hazel, slip agent, vitamin E, plant extracts, and preservatives. Witch hazel is a possible skin irritant and a problem in a product meant to be used near the delicate skin around the eyes.

☺ **Age Defying Complex** *($11.59 for 2 ounces)* and **Age Defying Complex for Delicate Skin** *($11.59 for 2 ounces)* are both very good AHA products. Although the two creams are labeled differently (one for delicate skin and the other presumably for all skin types), they are practically identical except for the amount of AHAs; the Delicate Skin formula contains 4% AHAs; the other, 8%. These are rather impressive, reasonably priced AHA products for normal to dry skin. You can start at a weaker strength and then move to a higher-percentage product when you see how your skin reacts.

☺ **Age Defying Lotion** *($11.59 for 3 ounces)* and **Age Defying Lotion for Delicate Skin** *($11.59 for 3 ounces)* are similar to the products above, only in lotion form, and the same review applies. They contain 8% and 4% AHAs, respectively.

☺ **Age Defying System with SPF 8** *($14.99 for two products, totaling 2.5 ounces)* is simply a repackaging of the Age Defying Complex AHA cream and a sunscreen. The sunscreen part is called Prevent, and its SPF is 8, which is good only for limited sun exposure. The Age Defying Complex is a good AHA product, with about an 8% concentration. Packaging an AHA product with a sunscreen is a nice concept, but this is an expensive way to do it. You can buy a good SPF 15 sunscreen for a lot less and buy the Age Defying Complex individually for less and get more of both.

Prescriptives

What comes to mind when you hear the name of Prescriptives' new line of skin care products, Prescriptives Px? A physician's prescription, maybe? Even some of the packaging has a medicinal or clinical appearance. What a great marketing concept. Of course, there is nothing medical, clinical, unique, or even particularly interesting about this new group of products, other than the marketing contrivance. There are six Prescriptives Px products, each one supposedly necessary to solve a specific skin problem. The brochure poses a question and then answers it with a product, but the one question it doesn't include is why the prices are so absurdly high.

Prescriptives prides itself on having a wide range of colors that are appropriate for almost every skin color. For this, the line wins high marks. Prescriptives has an outstanding selection of matte eyeshadows and blushes, neutral-colored foundations, and a handsome array of lip colors for every skin tone you can think of. It's also one of the few department-store cosmetics lines that is almost entirely fragrance-free.

Prescriptives is an extension of Estee Lauder, but the lines have very little in common. The major problem you may have with Prescriptives is that selecting a product is somewhat complicated. The counter personnel I interviewed had varying amounts of training, and this line requires training—you're better off talking to someone who has been with the line for a while. (Actually, that's true of almost all lines, but it's especially true of this one.)

Prescriptives' counter displays are incredibly well organized, and most of the colors are terrific. It is the job of the salesperson to color-type your skin and to indicate which foundations and which principal color group you should wear. Prescriptives' foundations are grouped in the same color categories used for the entire line: Yellow-Orange, Red-Orange, Red, and Blue-Red. A specific foundation shade is chosen for you by a process the company calls "color printing," which has since been picked up by many other cosmetics lines, including Lancome and Borghese. Potential matches from the four foundation color groups are drawn in a line on your cheek with the Makeup #1 foundation and allowed to dry. The one that seems to disappear into your skin indicates the foundation color group that is best for you. Within that color group, there is a range of shades from light to dark.

What are the drawbacks of color printing? Some of the foundation colors that are "accepted" by your skin may look too pink or orange in the sunlight, and there is the question of proper intensity. Regardless of how scientific color printing sounds, be sure to check the foundation in the daylight to assure true compatibility. As one Prescriptives salesperson told me, "Almost everyone is Yellow/Orange [which isn't orange at all; these shades are all neutral]—there really are no Blue/Red or Red/Orange people," and she's right. Another hitch is that once you know what your principal color group is, you are told that you can wear certain colors in all the other groups for a more natural, dramatic, or intensified look. That's not a concept that everyone would agree with, particularly me, but it's great for selling more products. In spite of this sales tenet, I like the line's color selections. There are beautiful colors in this line, particularly for women of color and women with very light, white skin; you just have to be careful about finding them.

Unique to Prescriptives, and overlooked by me for too long, are their Custom Blended foundations. While this was a passing fad for many other lines, Prescriptives still allows the salesperson to create a specially blended foundation color that can be adjusted as many times as necessary until the color is exactly the way you want it. One salesperson worked with me for over half an hour fine-tuning the color, and when it didn't match to my liking when I got home, I brought it back and she adjusted it again, until it was one of the most perfect matches I've ever had. It is expensive, but if finding just the right color has proved impossible, this option is worth a closer look.

Prescriptives Skin Care

☺ **$$$ All Clean Gentle Lotion** *($18.50 for 6.7 ounces)* contains an exceptionally long list of thickening agents, plant oil, some plant extracts, and preservatives. It can be OK for someone with normal to dry skin, but it can't take off makeup without the aid of a washcloth.

☺ **$$$ All Clean Soothing Cream Cleanser** *($18.50 for 6 ounces)* contains mostly water, slip agent, plant oil, thickeners, water-binding agents, more thickeners, and preservatives. It is best removed by being wiped off with a washcloth, and it can leave a greasy film on the face.

☹ **All Clean Sparkling Clean Gel** *($18.50 for 4 ounces)* is a standard detergent-based, water-soluble cleanser that uses a very strong detergent cleansing agent. It also contains small amounts of lemon oil and spearmint oil, which can irritate or burn the eye area.

☺ **$$$ Eye Makeup Remover** *($15 for 4 ounces)* is a standard eye-makeup remover that contains mostly water, slip agents, detergent cleanser, more slip agent, and preservatives. It will take off makeup, but I don't recommend wiping off makeup, especially around the eye area.

☹ **Skin Balancer No Fragrance, Alcohol-Free** *($16.50 for 6 ounces)* might not contain alcohol, but it does contain magnesium and zinc sulfate at the beginning of the ingredient list. Both of these can cause allergic reactions and irritate the skin. I recommend Milk of Magnesia instead, which is magnesium hydroxide. It not only absorbs oil, but it can soothe the skin and reduce irritation.

☺ **$$$ All You Need Action Moisturizer for Normal to Dry Skin** *($32.50 for 1.7 ounces)* contains mostly water, silicone oil, slip agent, several thickeners, water-binding agents, vitamin E, plant extracts, and preservatives. It doesn't have an SPF rating, so it isn't all you need for daytime. It would be fine as a nighttime moisturizer for someone with normal to somewhat dry skin, but it's nothing exceptional. This is Prescriptives' attempt at an AHA product, but it contains fruit extract, which isn't the same thing as a true AHA. Even if it were, there isn't enough in the product work as an exfoliant.

☺ **$$$ All You Need Action Moisturizer for Dry Skin** *($32.50 for 1.2 ounces)* is similar to the moisturizer above, and the same basic review applies.

☺ **$$$ All You Need Action Moisturizer Oil-Free** *($30 for 1.7 ounces)* is similar to the moisturizer above, give or take a few plant extracts and thickeners, and the same review applies.

☺ **$$$ Line Preventor 3** *($45 for 1 ounce)* won't prevent lines, although it is a good moisturizer for dry skin. It contains mostly water, slip agents, thickeners, silicone oil, water-binding agents, plant extracts, antioxidant, vitamin E, more thickeners, plant oil, more water-binding agents, and preservatives. There is a sunscreen in this product, but it provides only minimal protection from sun damage. There are also antioxidants, but they won't prevent lines.

☺ **$$$ Px Eye Specialist Visible Action Gel** *($35.50 for 0.5 ounce)* may make the lines around your eyes look temporarily diminished, but it can also irritate your skin. It contains mostly silicone oils and a film former. The gel looks convincing when you first put it on, but if you have dry skin you will still need a moisturizer because this product is not all that emollient.

☺ **$$$ Px Comfort Cream** *($37.50 for 1.7 ounces)* is a good moisturizer for someone with dry skin. It contains mostly water, silicone oil, standard water-binding agent, plant oil, several thickeners, plant extracts, more thickeners, plant protein, marine extract, and preservatives. Plant extracts always pose potential problems for someone with sensitive skin. Marine extract and plant protein may sound like interesting water-binding agents, but even if they were superior for the skin (which they aren't), there isn't enough of either to make a difference.

☺ **$$$ Px Comfort Lotion** *($30 for 1.7 ounces)* contains mostly water, slip agent, several thickeners, water-binding agents, anti-irritant, more water-binding agents, silicone oils, more thickeners, and preservatives. This would be a very good moisturizer for someone with dry skin.

☺ **$$$ Px Purifying Scrub** *($18.50 for 3.6 ounces)* is really more of a standard clay mask (which is one of the uses the company recommends) than a scrub. It also contains menthol, which can be a skin irritant.

☺ **$$$ Px Insulation Anti-Oxidant Cream with SPF 15** *($40 for 1.7 ounces)* is one expensive sunscreen. It contains mostly water, silicone oil, slip agent, several thickeners, more silicone oil, vitamin B, water-binding agents, vitamin E, anti-irritant, and preservatives. Plenty of other products contain the same vitamins and cost a lot less.

☹ **$$$ Px Flight Cream** *($28 for 1.7 ounces)* is supposed to help skin subjected to the rigors of flying conditions. It is a good standard moisturizer for dry skin, but nothing more. It contains mostly water, silicone oil, thickeners, plant extracts, plant oil, more thickeners, vitamin E, several more thickeners, and preservatives.

☹ **Px Blemish Specialist** *($17 for 1 ounce)* is just another alcohol- and salicylic acid–based blemish product. It contains some glycerin and a soothing agent, but that won't counteract the irritation from the other ingredients. You can find much cheaper versions at the drugstore, although they won't work any better than this one does.

Prescriptives Makeup

☺ **$$$ FOUNDATION:** Prescriptives reformulated and decreased the number of its foundation types, which is a welcome simplification. There are still about 28 shades for each foundation, and a large number of extremely pink, peach, and coppery colors to wade through, but the neutral shades are some of the most beautiful on the market. The texture has really been improved, too. **Exact Color Makeup #1 Lightweight** *($28.50)* is truly lightweight and water-based (although the salesperson carried on about it being oil-free, it isn't; it contains silicone oil). **These colors are excellent:** Pale Ecru, Antelope, Sepia, Ginger, Sable, Redwood, Pecan, Nutria, Espresso, Mahogany, Extra Light Cool, Extra Light Warm, and Macassar (may turn slightly red). **These colors should be avoided:** Pale, Petal, Camellia, Vellum, Peach, Cameo, Rose, Burnished Gold, Fawn, Blush, Rosewood, Caramel, and Mocha.

☺ **$$$ Exact Color Makeup #2 +** *($28.50)* is more emollient and contains a small amount of vegetable oil, which makes it better for someone with dry skin. **These colors are excellent:** Extra Light Cool, Extra Light Warm, Soft Ecru, Soft Cream, Soft Vellum, Soft Ivory, Soft Bisque, Soft Sepia, Soft Redwood, Soft Rosewood, Soft Pecan, Macassar, Nutria, Espresso, and Soft Gold. **These colors can be good but may turn peach, pink, orange, or ash:** Soft Pale, Soft Peach, Soft Fawn, Soft Taupe, Soft Blush, Soft Rose, Soft Mahogany, Soft Mocha, Soft Antelope, Soft Beige, Soft Ginger, Soft Amber, Caramel, and Sable. **These colors should be avoided:** Soft Petal, Soft Cameo, Soft Camellia, Soft Alabaster, Soft Rose, and Soft Porcelain.

☺ **$$$ Exact Color Makeup 100% Oil-Free with SPF 15** *($28.50)* is a wonderful matte foundation with a dry, nonshiny finish, and SPF 15 is good. **These colors are excellent:** Fresh Extra Light Warm, Fresh Extra Light Cool, Fresh Ecru, Fresh Cream, Fresh Vellum, Fresh Ivory, Fresh Bisque, Fresh Antelope, Fresh Nutria, Fresh Peach, Fresh Taupe, Fresh Fawn, Fresh Sable, Fresh Sepia, Fresh Redwood, Fresh Porcelain, and Fresh Pecan. **These colors can be good but may turn peach, pink, orange, or ash:** Fresh Gold, Fresh Beige, Fresh Ginger, Fresh Pale, Fresh Amber, Fresh Caramel, Fresh Espresso, Fresh Petal, Fresh Mahogany, Fresh Alabaster, Fresh Rose, Fresh Rosewood, Fresh Mocha, and Fresh Macassar. **These colors should be avoided:** Fresh Cameo, Fresh Blush, and Fresh Rose.

☺ **$$$ Instant Face** *($25)* is a talc-based powder that Prescriptives says you can use wet or dry. You can do that with almost any of the new two-in-one face powders. Remember, powder foundations are good only for normal or slightly oily skin types. **All six colors are beautiful and work well.**

☺ **$$$ Custom Blended Foundation Oil Free** *($50)* isn't oil-free (it contains silicone oil), but it has a beautifully natural, smooth matte finish. **Custom Blended Foundation Moisturizing Formula** *($50)*, which is mineral oil-based, has a dewy, moist finish, clearly best for dry skin. Both are both great alternatives to matching existing foundation colors to your skin. Be patient and don't rush the process, and be sure you find a salesperson who has been doing this technique for a while. This may just be the best match in a foundation you've ever found.

☹ **CONCEALER: Camouflage Cream** *($13.50)* comes in 11 shades. Most of the colors are for medium skin tones—only one or two are for fair to medium skin tones—with particularly good choices for women of color. The consistency is somewhat creamy when it goes on and slightly dry when blended, and it can crease into the lines around the eyes. **These colors are very good:** Yellow-Orange Light, Yellow-Orange Medium, Yellow-Orange Dark, Red-Orange Light, Red-Orange Medium, Red-Orange Dark, Blue-Red Light, and Red-Orange Extra Dark. **These colors are too pink or peach:** Red Light, Blue-Red Medium, and Blue-Red Dark.

☺ **$$$ POWDER: All Skins Pressed Powder** *($22.50)* has an impressive array of six colors for a wide range of skin tones. The texture is light and slightly on the dry side, which is great for most skin types.

☹ **All Skins Loose Powder** *($22.50)* is shiny, which defeats the purpose of a setting powder. **Suncolors** *($18.50)* are meant as an all-over dusting of tan color, but they are shiny too.

☺ **$$$ <u>BLUSH:</u> Powder Cheekcolor** *($18.50)* comes in beautiful shades and most have no visible shine, although some of the colors tend to go on quite sheer. The browner tones—Sandalwood, Cherrywood, Tulipwood, and Rosewood—are superb contour colors. **All Skins Face Colors Refillable** *(blush tins $12.50 each; compact $5)* is a two-in-one blush container. What a great concept. You can pick a contour and a blush color, or two different blush colors, or a blush and a pressed powder of your choice. One caution: Most of the colors have a slight amount of shine, although not enough to be a problem. **These colors are intensely shiny and should be avoided:** Peach, Mocha, Bronze, Rose, Rosewood, Cocoa, and Orchid.

☺ **<u>EYESHADOW:</u>** There are some great matte colors in this line. **The Quad Eyeshadow** *($30)* compact colors include three matte shades and one that's shiny, but the strips of color are very thin so that it's hard to get a brush through the color evenly. **Pick 2** *(color tins $10 each; compact $2.50)* is an eyeshadow compact that allows you to insert your own choice of two colors. Great idea, and many of the colors (and there are a lot of colors) are matte and excellent. **These colors are beautiful and matte:** Cameo, Biscuit, Mocha, Pink Sand, Swiss Chocolate, Cocoa, Navy, Stone Mist, Rose Powder, Mushroom, Heather, Rose Smoke, Suede Storm, Midnight Brown, Twilight, Eggplant, Honey, Grey Smoke, Pongee, Toast, Pumpkin, Adobe, Walnut, Tea Leaves, Coal, Peach Dust, Chamois, Clay, Red Earth, Clove, Moss, Seal, Pale Taupe, and Dove. **These colors are too shiny, blue, or green:** Sandalwood, Garnet, Hot Pink, Jade, Mulberry, Violetta, Iris, Bambi, Blue Angel, Henna, Gold, Ink, Canary, Opal, and Hazel.

☹ **<u>EYE AND BROW SHAPER:</u>** The huge selection of **Eye** and **Brow Shaping Pencils** *($12)* come in good colors but are rather crayon-like and go on too greasy.

☺ **$$$ <u>LIPSTICK AND LIP PENCIL:</u> Classic Lipsticks** *($12.50)* have a creamy, slightly glossy finish. **Extraordinary Lipstick** *($15)* comes pretty close to living up to its name. It has a huge color selection, and one of the best series of red shades I've ever seen. The texture is creamy smooth, with a rich feel that is neither greasy or dry. **Stains** *($15)* are misnamed; they don't have much stain and are little more than a gloss in the form of a lipstick. The SPF 18 rating makes them a good sunwear option. **Lipgloss** *($12.50)* is a standard gloss in a tube. **Lip Coloring Pencil** *($12)* comes in a large array of colors and has a great texture, but is not unusual as far as pencils go.

☺ **Matima Sheer Matte** *($15)* isn't in the least bit matte; these lipsticks are all extremely glossy, and they all have shine. **Matte Lipsticks** *($15)* have a nice range of muted colors, but the texture can be a bit dry and they tend to bleed.

☹ MASCARA: Gentle Mascara *($12.50)* may be gentle, but it doesn't build much length or thickness, and it tends to smear.

☺ **$$$** BRUSHES: New to the Prescriptives line is their handsome collection of brushes. The bristles are satiny soft and some of the shapes quite workable, while others are not for everyone. The **Powder Brush** *($30)* is too big for most faces, making it hard to control placement of the powder. The **Eye Lining Brush** *($15)* is a stiff, thin square brush. It would be awfully scratchy and hard to control. The **Cheek Brush** *($28)*, **Eye Shaper Brush** *($18)*, **Eye Shadow Brush** *($18)*, and **Retractable Lip Brush** *($18)* are pricey but good.

Prestige Cosmetics (Makeup Only)

Prestige, a new cosmetics line showcasing only color, has been getting more shelf space at drugstores and small beauty-supply boutiques lately. Not only are the prices absurdly low, but many of the products are surprisingly good, and some are excellent. Unfortunately, the variety of products stocked isn't the same from store to store, so you may not find all the products reviewed below.

☺ POWDER: **Pressed Powders** *($4.51)* are talc-based, have a great dry silky texture, and come in six good neutral shades.

☺ BLUSH: **Blushes** *($2.95)* come in an extremely pretty assortment of colors that are similar to M.A.C.'s shades, and are impressively matte.

☺ EYESHADOW: **Eyeshadows** *($1.90)* are a bit tricky, because the mattes and pearls are hard to differentiate. Choose carefully, because the matte shades are silky and, for the most part, beautiful.

☹ **Eyeshadow Pencils** *($3.95)* are too greasy and hard to sharpen.

☺ EYE AND BROW SHAPER: **Eye Pencils** *($2.75)* are standard pencils that have a good, soft but dry texture and come in every color imaginable.

☹ LIPSTICK AND LIP PENCIL: The standard tube **Lip Glosses** *($3.75)* are fine if you are interested in glosses. The **Lipsticks** *($2.95)* have mediocre staying power and the shades are hidden under color caps that inaccurately represent what you're getting.

☺ **Lip Pencils** *($3.95)*, like the Eye Pencils, come in a huge assortment of colors and are standard but good.

☹ MASCARA: **Mascara** *($2.95)* builds poorly and doesn't make the lashes very thick.

☺ BRUSHES: Prestige has a small but good assortment of **Makeup Brushes** *($2 to $8)*. They are soft and relatively firm, with good flexibility.

Principal Secret (Skin Care Only)

Yes, Victoria, there is still money to be made from being beautiful, even when you no longer have your own TV series. Convincing women that they can look like you by using your skin care routine for three easy payments is a very lucrative business. In fact, Victoria Principal's infomercial is one of the most successful ever.

Actually, Victoria Principal's skin care products are not really hers; they were created by Madame Aida Thibiant, a Beverly Hills aesthetician who has run a successful skin care boutique there for years. (Because Ms. Thibiant was a relative unknown to the American public, Ms. Principal and her partners severed ties with her in 1995.)

Why are we so interested in a product line named after Victoria Principal? I've said it before, but it bears repeating: *Celebrities are not skin care or makeup experts; they are actresses who have signed a good contract to represent a product line.* If you believe they have discovered the perfect products and are sharing them with you, you are not living in the real world. These products aren't why Victoria Principal is beautiful.

Joining her "club" is no bargain either. Every 90 days a club member receives the original "Value Order" she purchased (either the three-piece group for $49.95 or the six-piece group for $79.95), and every fifth shipment is free. That means that for the first year, your bill for skin care alone will be somewhere between $220 and $375, including shipping and handling. If you buy extra products, which are discounted between 20 percent and 50 percent when you belong to the club, the total could soar to more than $500.

I should mention that several of these products aren't bad, and a few are actually quite nice, specifically for someone with normal to dry skin. (Someone with oily, sensitive, or blemished skin could have problems with this skin care routine.) A nice feature is that none of these products are tested on animals. But my opinion about the price remains. And no one needs six to ten different products to take care of her face and body. Did I forget to mention that the claims are exaggerated?

In the following reviews, all prices listed are retail. If you decide to use these products, joining the club is a good idea, because you will need to reorder frequently: most of the products come only in 0.25- to 4-ounce sizes. Four ounces of any cleanser won't last more than a month.

☺ **$$$ Gentle Deep Cleanser** *($16 for 4 ounces)* is a standard detergent-based, water-soluble cleanser. It cleans well but contains two ingredients that can be a problem for the eyes, and it can be drying for some skin types.

☹ **Gentle Exfoliating Scrub** *($20 for 4 ounces)* contains too many irritating ingredients to be called gentle. The third ingredient is polyacrylamide, a potential skin irritant. It also contains salicylic acid, which can peel the skin.

☺ **$$$ Extra Nurturing Cream** *($40 for 2 ounces)* is a good moisturizer for dry skin; it contains mostly water, thickeners, plant oil, silicone oil, more thickeners, water-binding agents, more thickeners, and preservatives.

☺ **$$$ Time Release Moisture with SPF 8** *($35 for 2 ounces)* contains an ingredient that sounds like liposomes. I can't say how truly "time-release" it is, but it should work to keep moisture in the skin. The ingredients are fairly standard: water, thickener, plant oil, several more thickeners, silicone oil, water-binding agents, more thickeners, and, down at the very bottom of the list, vitamin E, glycerin, more water-binding agent, and preservatives. This product is OK for normal to slightly dry skin, but it isn't very emollient and most of the good stuff is at the end of the ingredient list. It is supposed to be applied twice a day, but why apply a product with active sunscreen agents at night?

☺ **$$$ Eye Relief** *($30 for 0.5 ounce)* is a light gel with a light feel. It isn't very emollient, but it does include good water-binding ingredients. It contains mostly water, film former, slip agent, water-binding agent, plant extract, more water-binding agents, and preservatives. It would be good for someone with normal to combination skin. The label claims that it can prevent the formation of wrinkles, which is completely untrue.

☺ **$$$ Alpha Hydroxy Booster Complex** *($49 for 2 ounces)* contains mostly water, thickeners, slip agent, glycolic acid, several more thickeners, silicone oil, more thickeners, plant extracts, anti-irritant, and preservatives. The handful of exotic-sounding ingredients at the very end of the ingredient list are almost nonexistent. However, it is a good, though absurdly overpriced, 3% to 4% AHA product. It would be good for someone with sensitive skin, but it is almost indistinguishable from Pond's Age Defying Cream for Sensitive Skin, which costs one-fourth as much.

☹ **$$$ Intensive Serum with AHAs** *($45 for 0.5 ounce)* contains mostly water, plant extracts, anti-irritant, aloe, slip agents, water-binding agents, thickeners, and preservatives. There is nothing intense about this product except the price. The plant extracts are not AHA ingredients that can exfoliate the skin the way glycolic or lactic acid can.

☺ **$$$ Intensive Serum** *($40 for 0.25 ounce)* is a minuscule vial of some good water-binding ingredients along with quaternium-15, a fairly irritating preservative. It is absurdly overpriced. Forty dollars for 0.25 ounce comes to $2,560 a pound!

☹ **$$$ Time Release Tinted Moisture** *($35 for 2 ounces)* is more like a foundation than a tint providing light to medium coverage. With an SPF of 8, it can't protect from the sun the way an SPF of 15 does, and is best for limited sun exposure only. **The color selection is limited:** Sheer Peach, which is actually quite neutral, but would be good only for a medium skin tone; Sheer Rose, which turns very orange on most skin tones; Sheer Gold, which is a good tan color for medium to dark skin tones, but may appear sallow on some skin tones; and Sheer Bronze, which is too peach for some skin tones.

☹ **Blemish Buster Solution** *($20 for 0.5 ounce)* is just alcohol, sulfur, and zinc. It can irritate the skin and, like many other, much less expensive acne products with the same ingredients, it won't get rid of acne.

☹ **Blemish Buster Mask** *($25 for 2 ounces)* contains cornstarch, which can cause breakouts, as the third ingredient, as well as other ingredients that can clog pores.

☺ **$$$ Invisible Toning Masque** *($23 for 2 ounces)* is unusual for a mask because it doesn't contain clay. Rather, it is a moisturizing mask. Containing mostly water, egg yolk, thickener, glycerin, more thickeners, film former, water-binding ingredients, and preservatives, it closely resembles the Extra Nurturing Cream. It seems unnecessary since so many of the other products contain the exact same ingredients.

Purpose (Skin Care Only)
(Johnson & Johnson)

Prior to 1987 Johnson & Johnson was better known for baby care than for skin care. That has changed. Johnson & Johnson has become better known for their controversial foray into the world of serious wrinkle treatment with Retin-A and Renova. These two products represent over $100 million a year in revenue. Leaving no stone unturned, Johnson & Johnson has made great strides convincing physicians that a prescription for Retin-A and Renova should be accompanied by the Purpose line of products. Your face could easily live without most of the Purpose products, although the Dual Purpose Sunscreen is a consideration.

☹ **Gentle Cleansing Bar** *($3.08 for 6 ounces)* is just a standard bar cleanser that contains tallow and a strong detergent cleansing agent with a little glycerin added, but that won't counteract the drying effect of the soap. Also, the tallow can cause breakouts.

☺ **Gentle Cleansing Wash** *($5.75 for 6 ounces)* is a standard detergent-based, water-soluble cleanser that can be drying for most skin types. However, it may be good for someone with oily skin.

☺ **Dry Skin Cream** *($5.45 for 3 ounces)* is a very standard but good moisturizer for someone with dry skin. It contains mostly water, petrolatum, slip agents, thickeners, plant oil, more thickeners, mineral oil, and preservatives.

☺ **Dual Treatment Moisturizer with SPF 15 Protection** *($7.28 for 4 ounces)* is a good sunscreen for someone with normal to slightly dry skin. It is partly nonchemical and also contains water, glycerin, several thickeners, silicone oil, more thickeners, and preservatives.

Rachel Perry (Skin Care Only)

Health-food stores have been selling Rachel Perry products for years. One of the original "natural" cosmetics lines, it is now also available at some large drugstore chains. Rachel Perry products contain many, if not more, of the same natural-sounding ingredients included in more highbrow natural-product lines such as Aveda, Clarins, and Origins. For the consumer on a budget who is interested in the ballyhoo surrounding botanical skin care products, this line could satisfy that curiosity without hurting the pocketbook or the skin.

☹ **Citrus-Aloe Cleanser and Face Wash** *($10.49 for 4 ounces)* contains plant water, thickeners, plant oil, more thickeners, silicone oil, more oils, and preservatives. The oils make this more of a wipe-off product than a face wash. It can leave a greasy residue on the skin.

☹ **Tangerine Dream Foaming Facial Cleanser with Alpha-Hydroxy Acids** *($10.49 for 6 ounces)* is a standard detergent-based, water-soluble cleanser that contains about 3% AHAs. AHAs are wasted in a cleanser, and it is a problem if you get this kind of concentration in the eyes.

☹ **Peach & Papaya Gentle Facial Scrub** *($10.49 for 2 ounces)* contains mostly plant water, slip agent, thickener, detergent cleanser, more thickener, fruit seeds, sea salt, vitamins A and E, plant oil, soothing agent, menthol, salicylic acid, and preservatives. The menthol and salicylic acid can be irritants, especially if the skin is abraded, which is what a scrub does.

☹ **Sea Kelp-Herbal Facial Scrub** *($10.49 for 2.5 ounces)* contains mostly water, cornmeal, glycerin, slip agent, rye flour, thickener, almond meal, sea salt, plant extracts, and preservatives. This is a pretty thick mess to use as a scrub. It would be cheaper and better for the skin to use plain cornmeal or sea salt all by itself.

☹ **Lemon Mint Astringent for Normal to Oily Skin** *($9.49 for 8 ounces)* contains mostly plant water, AHAs, water-binding agents, peppermint, soothing agent, slip agents, and preservatives. This toner has more than its share of irritating ingredients, including mint, lemongrass, peppermint, and witch hazel. It will irritate the skin, which can make oily skin more oily.

☹ **Perfectly Clear Herbal Antiseptic for Oily or Acne Prone Skin** *($10.49 for 8 ounces)* is mostly alcohol with a host of even more irritating ingredients, including camphor, eucalyptus oil, menthol, peppermint oil, and clove oil. This product is an irritation waiting to happen.

☺ **Violet Rose Skin Toner** *($9.49 for 8 ounces)* contains mostly plant water, water-binding agents, soothing agent, and preservatives. It would be a good irritant-free toner for most skin types.

☺ **Bee Pollen-Jojoba Maximum Moisture Cream** *($12.49 for 2 ounces)* contains mostly bee pollen water; plant water; plant oil; thickeners; silicone oil; more plant oil; vitamins A, D, and E; water-binding agent; more thickeners; and preservatives. If you want to believe that bee pollen can do something for your skin, fine, but there is no research that supports its use for skin care, and there aren't enough vitamins in this cream to work as antioxidants. Still, this would be a good emollient moisturizer for dry skin.

☺ **Elastin and Collagen Firming Treatment** *($10.88 for 2 ounces)* contains mostly plant water, witch hazel extract, water-binding agents (collagen and elastin), more thickeners, more water-binding agent, and preservatives. The collagen and elastin won't firm anything, but the witch hazel can irritate and temporarily swell the skin, which can make it look fuller but can also dry the skin.

☺ **Ginseng and Collagen Wrinkle Treatment** *($14.49 for 2 ounces)* contains plant water; safflower oil; several thickeners; collagen; vitamins A, B, C, D, and E; more oils; and preservatives. The vitamins are way down on the list, but they can provide some antioxidant benefit. This would be a good moisturizer for dry skin, but it won't change wrinkles.

☺ **Calendula-Cucumber Oil Free Moisturizer with SPF 3** *($13.49 for 4 ounces)* contains mostly plant water, slip agent, thickeners, silicone oil, water-binding agents, more thickeners, and preservatives. This isn't oil-free, and the amount of sunscreen is not enough to protect from sun damage.

☺ **Lecithin-Aloe Moisture Retention Cream for Normal-Combination Skin** *($12.49 for 2 ounces)* contains mostly plant water, thickener, several plant oils, more thickeners, vitamins A and D, water-binding agent, more thickeners, silicone oil, and preservatives. The amount of oil in this product isn't good for combination skin. However, it could be a good moisturizer for someone with dry skin.

☺ **Hi Potency "E" Special Treatment Line Control** *($14.49 for 2 ounces)* contains mostly water, vitamin E (16,000 I.U.), thickeners, plant oil, more thickeners, vitamins A and D, more plant oils, aloe, royal bee jelly, and preservatives. Vitamins A, D, and E are good antioxidants, particularly in this concentration, and can prevent dehydration, but they do not nourish the skin. This stuff also won't control lines, but it is a very good moisturizer for dry skin. The royal bee jelly is barely present in this product, which is fine because it serves no purpose for the skin anyway.

☺ **$$$ Immediately Visible Eye Renewal Gel-Cream with Liposomes** *($22.49 for 0.5 ounce)* contains mostly plant water, glycerin, bee pollen extract, plant oil, vitamin A, antioxidant, water-binding agents, more antioxidant, silicone oil, thickeners, and preservatives. Forget the bee pollen; what's interesting about this product are the antioxidants.

☺ **$$$ Visible Transition 5% Alpha-Hydroxy Serum: Patented Prolonged Release Liposomes** *($27.49 for 1.1 ounces)* contains mostly water; AHAs; slip agent; silicone oils; thickeners; plant water; vitamins A, E, and C; water-binding agent; more thickeners; and preservatives. This is a good AHA product for someone with sensitive, dry skin, but the price is absurd. The liposomes are a nice way to keep the moisturizing ingredients in the skin longer.

☺ **$$$ Visible Transition 10% Alpha-Hydroxy Serum: Patented Prolonged Release Liposomes** *($27.49 for 1.1 ounces)* is almost identical to the product above, and the same review applies, except that this one would be better for someone with normal to dry skin.

☹ **Clay and Ginseng Texturizing Mask** *($10.49 for 2 ounces)* contains mostly plant water, clay (supposedly French clay, but clay is clay no matter what country it's from), talc, more clay, thickeners, vitamin E, RNA, plant oil, and preservatives. This is a standard clay mask, and several of the plant extracts may be too irritating, particularly combined with the drying effect of the clay. The RNA won't affect your skin cells, but it sounds impressive.

Revlon

Revlon has been very busy improving its bottom line by becoming a public stock. Revlon models Naomi Campbell, Cindy Crawford, and Elle Macpherson made a personal appearance the day of the initial public offering on the floor of the New York Stock Exchange. You can imagine the commotion that ensued!

Revlon has also added to its bottom line by creating two remarkably successful product lines: first the Age Defying products, and then ColorStay. The ColorStay and Age Defying lines serve two distinct age groups, the former being the 35-and-under crowd and the latter those over 35, and they serve them well with some excellent options. The first ColorStay product was ColorStay Lipstick (which was really a clone of LipSexxxy by Ultima II, a company owned by Revlon). It was advertised as the first lipstick that wouldn't kiss off. Well, it does kiss off if it's a really good kiss, but if it's your average little friendly peck on the cheek, then it pretty much stays on your lips with no telltale imprint. This single product spawned a new generation of lipsticks with a consistency that is ultra-matte and dry.

Revlon Results didn't fare as well as ColorStay and the Age Defying line. These products contain an ingredient complex called Alpha ReCap that is supposed to exfoliate the skin like AHAs but more gently, because it is not an acid. The ingredient— its technical name is methoxypropylgluconamide, and it shows up in many Revlon-owned cosmetics lines such as Ultima II, Monteil (since sold by Revlon), and Charles of the Ritz—is not an AHA. It is a good water-binding agent, which is nice, but it won't function in any way, like a 5% or greater concentration of AHAs.

Revlon's standard lines—Eterna '27', Natural Collagen Complex, and Moon Drops are also still around. They all add up to an interesting group of products for just about every taste, age, and lifestyle.

Revlon Skin Care

☺ **Moon Drops Extra Gentle Cleansing Cream Sensitive/Delicate** (*$6.93 for 4 ounces*) is a standard mineral oil–based wipe-off cleanser that can leave a greasy film on the skin. The vitamins, water-binding agents, and plant extracts in here serve no purpose in a cleanser but help Revlon compete with the fancier lines.

☺ **Moon Drops Replenishing Cleansing Lotion Normal to Dry** (*$6.93 for 8 ounces*) is a standard mineral oil–based cleanser that leaves a greasy residue and requires the aid of a washcloth or tissue to remove all the makeup. Like the product above, this lotion contains several water-binding agents, plant extracts, and vitamins, which actually make it a better moisturizer than a cleanser, but they are wasted in this product.

☺ **Moon Drops Foaming Cleansing Gel Soap-Free Normal to Oily** *($6.93 for 8 ounces)* is a standard detergent-based, water-soluble cleanser that can take off all the makeup without leaving a greasy film on the skin. It can be drying for some skin types, and the menthol and witch hazel can irritate some skin types.

☺ **30 Second Eye Makeup Remover** *($5.50 for 2 ounces)* is a standard detergent-based wipe-off cleanser. It will take off eye makeup, but why wipe and pull at the eyes if you don't have to?

☹ **Waterproof Eye Makeup Remover** *($5.50 for 0.8 ounce)* is a greasy mess. It contains mostly petrolatum, mineral oil, thickeners, and preservatives. It will take off eye makeup, but this step should rarely be necessary.

☺ **Moon Drops One Minute Scrub Skin Polishing Normal to Dry** *($7.14 for 4 ounces)* is an OK scrub, but it can leave a greasy residue on the skin. It contains petrolatum, lanolin oil, and plant oils. It might work for someone with very dry skin, but it could easily clog pores, and you will need another cleanser to get the residue off. I would not even think of recommending this for someone with normal skin.

☺ **Moon Drops Comforting Toner Alcohol-Free Sensitive/Delicate** *($6.59 for 8 ounces)* is a very gentle toner that can be quite soothing and lightly emollient for most skin types.

☺ **Moon Drops Softening Toner Normal to Dry** *($6.93 for 8 ounces)* is similar to the toner above and also contains some good water-binding agents and vitamins A and E. The same review applies.

☹ **Moon Drops Clarifying Astringent Oil Control Normal to Oily** *($6.93 for 8 ounces)* is an alcohol-based toner that also contains some chamomile extract and a soothing agent, but that won't compensate for the irritation caused by the alcohol.

☺ **Moon Drops Nourishing Moisture Lotion SPF 6 Normal to Dry** *($7.59 for 4 ounces)* won't nourish anyone's skin, but it is a good emollient moisturizer for dry skin. It contains mostly water, standard water-binding agents, thickeners, petrolatum, vitamins A and E, shark oil, more water-binding agents, more thickeners, and preservatives. SPF 15 is best for everyday use.

☺ **Moon Drops Lightweight Moisturizer SPF 6 Oil-Free Normal to Oily** *($7.93 for 4 ounces)* is not oil-free (it contains silicone oil), but it is a lightweight moisturizer that would be good for someone with normal to slightly dry skin if it contained a more effective sunscreen. It contains mostly water, standard water-binding agents, thickeners, plant extracts, more water-binding agents, and preservative.

☺ **Moon Drops Soothing Moisture Cream SPF 6 Sensitive/Delicate** *($7.93 for 4 ounces)* would be a good emollient moisturizer except that it doesn't contain enough sunscreen to adequately protect from the sun.

☺ **Moon Drops Soothing Moisture Cream SPF 6 Extra Moist Sensitive/Delicate** *($7.59 for 4 ounces)* is a good moisturizer for dry skin, but it isn't all that soothing; the ingredients are similar to those in many of the other moisturizers in this collection. It would be great if it had an SPF of 15.

☺ **Moon Drops Five Minute Clay Mask Deep-Cleansing Normal to Oily** *($7.49 for 4.8 ounces)* is a standard clay mask that can't deep-clean, but it can help exfoliate the skin. If you're looking for a clay mask, this one is just fine.

☺ **Moon Drops Three Minute Moisture Pack Skin Calming Sensitive/Delicate** *($7.14 for 4.12 ounces)* is similar to many of the other moisturizers in this line. It contains mostly water, thickeners, mineral oil, slip agents, more thickeners, plant extract, soothing agent, water-binding agents, more thickeners, and preservatives. This product is unnecessary if you use any of the other moisturizers in this line, but it would be fine to leave on the face as a mask.

☺ **Eterna '27' All Day Moisture Lotion** *($13.25 for 2 ounces)* is a very emollient, good moisturizer for dry skin. It contains mostly water, slip agent, thickener, plant oil, more thickeners, silicone oil, water-binding agents, more thickeners, more water-binding agents, and preservatives. Several amino acids appear at the end of the ingredient list, but there isn't enough to have much effect, and they are nothing more than good water-binding agents anyway.

☺ **Eterna '27' All Day Moisture Cream** *($13.25 for 1 ounce)* is very similar to the lotion above, but with more thickeners. It would be good for dry skin.

☺ **Eterna '27' with Exclusive Progenitin** *($15 for 2 ounces)* is going to sound strange, but remember, I'm only describing this product; I didn't formulate it. The active ingredient is called pregnenolone acetate. It is derived from the urine of pregnant women and is considered an anti-inflammatory agent. Therefore, this moisturizer is actually a very mild topical cortisone-type cream. In my opinion, unless your dry skin is a result of slight dermatitis, this cream is unnecessary. This very emollient cream is for dry skin only; it contains mostly water, mineral oil, thickener, petrolatum, more thickener, plant oils, water-binding agents, vitamin E, more thickeners, and preservatives.

☺ **Natural Collagen Complex with SPF 15** *($10.49 for 3.85 ounces)* is a lightweight moisturizer with a good SPF; it contains mostly thickeners and water-binding agents. It also contains collagen, which is a good water-binding agent (and nothing more), and some algae extract, which has little to no benefit.

☺ **Natural Collagen Complex Protective Moisture Cream with SPF 6** *($10.49 for 3 ounces)* is similar to the SPF 15 moisturizer above, only more emollient due to the inclusion of mineral oil and petrolatum. It would be good for someone with dry skin, but SPF 15 is the number most dermatologists and skin cancer specialists recommend for daily use, and I do too.

☺ **Natural Collagen Complex Protective Moisture Lotion SPF 6** *($10.49 for 3 ounces)* is similar to the product above, and the same review applies.

☹ **Natural Collagen Complex Protective Eye Cream with SPF 4** *($9.49 for 0.5 ounce)* is a nonchemical sunscreen that would be good for someone with normal to dry skin, but SPF 4?

☺ **Results Day-Light Replenisher SPF 8** *($11.39 for 2 ounces)* contains mostly water, water-binding agent, slip agent, several thickeners, petrolatum, more thickeners, more water-binding agents, vitamin E, and preservatives. This is a good moisturizer with a sunscreen that is adequate only for minimal sun exposure.

☺ **Results Daily Requirement Moisture Cream with SPF 8** *($11.39 for 2 ounces)* is almost identical to the product above, and the same review applies.

☺ **Results Day-Light Moisturizer Oil-Free Fluid with SPF 8** *($11.39 for 2 ounces)* is similar to the Results products above and is oil-free, but some of its other ingredients can be a problem for someone with oily or combination skin. This is a good moisturizer for dry skin, but the SPF isn't high enough for more than minimal sun protection.

☺ **Results Sensitive Regenerating Formula with SPF 8** *($11.39 for 2 ounces)* is similar to the Results products above, and the same reviews apply.

☺ **Results Rest & Renewal Night Cream Concentrate** *($14.29 for 2 ounces)* contains mostly water, water-binding agent, thickeners, slip agents, mineral oil, silicone oil, more thickeners, more water-binding agents, more thickeners, and preservatives. This is a very good moisturizer for someone with dry skin. It is essentially the same as the moisturizers above, just without the sunscreen.

☺ **Results Brighten-Up Eye Cream** *($13.79 for 0.75 ounce)* is almost identical to the product above, and the same review applies.

☺ **Results Line Diminishing Serum** *($13.79 for 0.75 ounce)* won't diminish anything, but it is a very good moisturizer for someone with dry skin. It contains mostly water, water-binding agents, slip agent, silicone oil, mineral oil, vitamin E, more water-binding agents, anti-irritant, thickeners, and preservatives.

Revlon Makeup

FOUNDATION: Revlon provides testers for some of its new foundations, which makes it more likely that you'll be able to find the right color.

☹ **New Complexion Makeup for Normal to Dry with SPF 4** *($8.25)* and **New Complexion Makeup for Normal to Oily with SPF 4** *($8.25)* have been improved. In the past, all the shades for these two foundations were too pink, orange, peach, or rose. However, Revlon has recently added new colors that are much more neutral and impressive. Still, there are never any testers, and SPF 4 is too low to provide much protection. **Touch & Glow Moist Makeup** *($6.30)* is not a product I recommend; all the colors are glaringly pink or peach.

☺ **Springwater Matte Makeup Oil-Free** *($8.25)* is a lightweight foundation that definitely has a matte finish, and all of the colors are wonderfully neutral shades of beige or tan. Unfortunately, there are no testers.

☺ **DoublePlay** *($9.49)* is a lightweight cream-to-powder foundation in stick form. It is an impressive foundation with a handful of good colors, and testers are available in most stores. If you have normal to combination skin, this one is definitely worth a try. **These colors are good:** Bare Buff, Creamy Natural, and Rich Beige. **These colors are OK but may turn peach:** Porcelain Rose, Sandrift, Fresh Beige, Warm Honey, and Bronzing Stick. Ivory may be too pink for most skin tones.

☺ **Age Defying Makeup with SPF 8** *($7.14)* is best for someone with normal to somewhat dry skin (it contains oil), providing light to almost medium coverage. SPF 8 isn't great, but the color selection and texture are both quite good.

☺ **Age Defying Extra Cover Creme Makeup with SPF 12** *($8.99)* comes in colors that are all surprisingly excellent, the texture is very smooth and emollient, and SPF 12 is a nice touch. For someone with normal to dry skin, this is a definite option if testers are available, and they often are.

☺ **ColorStay Makeup** *($8.22)* is beyond matte, beyond no shine, and far beyond the claim of "It won't come off on him." It won't come off even when you want it to. This is one of the most stubborn makeups I've ever seen. Get it on right the first time, because once it dries, it won't budge. I didn't notice in the daylight that I had a bit too much foundation above my mouth and a little streaking on my nose. All the blending in the world, even with my oily skin, wouldn't smooth it out. It was there to stay. Removing it at night takes some effort, including several attempts with your cleanser and a washcloth. ColorStay Foundation is appropriate only for someone with truly oily skin and a deft hand at blending. The colors are superior, except for the lightest shade, Ivory, which can be too pink; the rest are stunning neutral shades, in a range of 12 colors. There are no shades for very light or very deep to dark skin tones, which is a serious limitation, but the medium skin tones have a wide selection.

☺ <u>CONCEALER:</u> **New Complexion Concealer** *($6.75)* comes in three shades: Light, Medium, and Deep. This lightweight concealer leaves a sheer residue that covers beautifully. It is one of the better concealers I have tested.

☹ **Springwater Oil-Free Concealer** *($5.50)* goes on very light, yet covers well. Unfortunately, it has a slight tendency to crease. **Age Defying Concealer with Nonchemical SPF 12** *($6.59)* comes in a nice range of colors, but it creases into the lines around the eyes as the day goes by, and that helps accentuate wrinkles, not diminish them.

☹ <u>POWDER:</u> **Love Pat Pressed Powder** *($6.75)* colors are too pink or peach for most skin tones. **Touch & Glow Pressed Powder** *($7.50)* is almost identical to Love Pat Pressed Powder, and the color selection is also poor. **Springwater Pressed Powder Oil-Free** *($7.53)* has three good colors—Light, Medium, and Dark—but the first ingredient is a skin irritant and can cause breakouts.

☺ **New Complexion Powder Oil-Control Normal to Oily Skin** *($6.59)* is a standard talc-based powder with a decent color selection. It does blend on smooth and soft, but nothing about this product will control oil in the least.

☺ **Age Defying Pressed Loose Powder** *($6.59)* is a puzzle. Pressed loose powder is a contradiction in terms, isn't it? This product is a lightweight pressed powder that goes on rather sheer but slightly chalky. It has a silky texture, and the colors are OK.

☺ <u>BLUSH:</u> **Age Defying Cheek Color** *($8.99)* is a cream blush with a slight powdery finish, no matter what Revlon calls it. Cream blushes are hard to blend and don't hold up all that well during the day. Powder blushes rest on top of the skin, while cream blushes merge into it; that's the nature of creams. Unless you have flawless skin, they tend to accentuate every dent and imperfection. If you have perfect, even skin, you may like this blush—it does have a great texture—but if not, you're likely to have the same problems I did.

☺ **Naturally Glamorous Blush-On** *($6.99)* has a great color selection and a smooth application. **Most of the colors are excellent. These colors are too shiny:** Ginger Gold and Pure Radiance.

☺ **In the Pink Cheek Color** *($3.97)* is similar to the product above. All of the shades are soft and beautiful; it's a great but small assortment of blue-toned blushes.

☹ **EYESHADOW:** The **Single Matte Eyeshadows** *($2.86)* will work for anyone who wants a soft, natural-looking eye design. Be careful—not all of the colors are matte, and many have quite a bit of shine. The only ones I recommend are the matte shades, and they are nicely, and accurately, labeled as matte. **Eye Shaper Duos** *($3.84)* and **Overtime Eyeshadows** *($4.48)* come in sets of two or four colors, respectively, that are either too shiny or strange combinations.

😐 **Age Defying Eye Color** *($6.59)* is a cream eyeshadow that dries to a powder finish, but before it can do that, it seeps into the lines around the eyes and emphasizes every wrinkle. In any case, cream eyeshadows are just hard to work with; they're awkward to blend with the applicator they come with, and even harder to blend with your fingers. They're supposed to blend out softer than powders, but I don't find that to be true. Also, cream eyeshadows crease faster than powders.

😐 **ColorStay Eyecolor** *($4.89)* comes in a tube, which is not my favorite way of applying shadow. Blendability is essential, and that isn't easy with such a dry, immovable eye color. These colors are all about as stubborn as they come: they can make it through the day where others may long since have smeared and disappeared. But again, once on, they are not easy to remove.

☺ **EYE AND BROW SHAPER:** **Time Liner Eye Pencils** *($4.89)* are a good product. Revlon offers an assortment of other pencils, but these are the best. **Jetliner Intense** *($4.84)* is a liquid eyeliner with a soft, pen-shaped tip. It applies a very dramatic, intense line. **Natural Brows Color & Style System** *($4.95)* is a powder that comes in four excellent shades: True Blonde, Rich Brown, Soft Black, and Light Brown. The brush it comes with is terrible, but it is one of those rare cosmetics that come packaged with a good applicator. A professional angled brush would work just fine for applying this powder. **Fine Line Natural Brow Pencil** *($5.99)* is ultra-thin and works like a high-tech pencil with a twist-up applicator. It also takes refills. It can easily stroke on thinner lines than other pens for a more natural-looking brow.

☺ **LIPSTICK AND LIP PENCIL:** Most of the **Moon Drops Moisture Creme** *($5.75)*, **Super Lustrous Creme** *($5.75)*, and **Velvet Touch** *($6.25)* lipsticks have great colors and smooth, moist textures. Velvet Touch is supposed to have a matte finish, but in comparison to ColorStay it isn't the least bit matte. Still, it is a good creamy, opaque lipstick that gives full coverage and has good staying power. It could easily slip into the lines around the mouth, though. The other two are just good creamy lipsticks with the same potential for movement. **Outrageous Creme Lipcolor** *($5.99)* has an unusually creamy, moist texture with surprising staying potential, and feels great. **Moon Drops Color Lock Anti-Feathering Lip Base** *($5.75)* really does keep lipstick from bleeding—what a find! And, of course, **ColorStay Lipstick** *($5.75)*, the most popular of the ultra-matte lip products. It has good staying power and goes on extremely matte and opaque. It can dry out the lips and may feel uncomfortable if you are used to creamy lipsticks. It also tends to peel off instead of just wearing away. Nevertheless, this ultra-matte lip color is certainly worth trying. **Time Liner Lip Pencil** *($4.93)* comes in a nice variety of colors and has a good soft texture. **ColorStay Lipliner** *($4.89)* is undeniably tenacious and less greasy than most.

☹ **Moon Drops Moisture Frost** *($5.75)*, **Super Lustrous Frost** *($5.75)*, and **Outrageous Lipcolor Luminesque** *($5.99)* are all too shiny.

☺ **MASCARA: Impulse Long Distance Mascara** *($3.95)* and **Impulse Quick Thick Mascara** *($3.95)* are both excellent: no smudging, easy and quick application, and they make lashes thick and long. **Lengthwise Mascara** *($3.99)* is excellent, and I strongly recommend it. **Lashfull Mascara** *($5.35)* is another very good mascara that goes on well and really makes it through the entire day.

☺ **Fabulash Big Brush Mascara** *($5.15)* is a good mascara, but it can't compete with Lengthwise Mascara.

☹ **ColorStay Lashcolor** *($5.50)* goes on quickly and definitely lengthens, but it tends to clump.

☹ **BRUSHES:** Revlon has several brushes in good shapes and sizes, but the **Blush Brush** *($6.50)* and **Eyeshadow Brush** *($4.25)* have oversized handles that are cumbersome and hard to carry in a makeup bag for touch-ups during the day. Also, the bristles are too soft to apply the color evenly.

St. Ives (Skin Care Only)

☺ **Swiss Formula Alpine Mint Foaming Facial Cleansing Gel** *($3.25 for 12 ounces)* is a standard detergent-based, water-soluble cleanser that also contains some plant extracts. It can be a good cleanser for some skin types, but it can also be quite drying. Some of the plant extracts can irritate the eyes.

☺ **Swiss Formula Peaches and Cream Extra Moisturizing Facial Beauty Wash** *($2.29 for 12 ounces)* is similar to the product above, except this one also contains a small amount of plant oils, which can help decrease the dryness caused by the detergent cleansing agents. Some of the plant extracts can be irritating for the eyes.

☺ **Swiss Formula Facial Cleanser and Makeup Remover** *($2.29 for 5 ounces)* is a fairly standard mineral oil–based, cold cream–type cleanser that must be wiped off. It can leave a greasy residue on the skin.

☹ **Swiss Formula Pure Glycerin Extra Mild Facial Cleansing Liquid** *($3.04 for 12 ounces)* is a standard detergent-based, water-soluble cleanser that also contains some plant extracts. The detergent cleansing agents are pretty strong, and it can be quite drying for most skin types.

☹ **Swiss Formula Apricot Scrub with Soothing Elder Flower** *($2.30 for 5 ounces)* is a cornmeal scrub that uses sodium lauryl sulfate, which is a strong skin irritant and can also be drying, as its main detergent cleansing agent.

☹ **Swiss Formula Alcohol Free Soothing Mint and Aloe Purifying Facial Toner** *($3.29 for 12 ounces)* contains mostly water, slip agent, plant extracts, and preservatives. The mint and witch hazel can irritate the skin.

☺ **Swiss Formula Alpha-Hydroxy Moisturizing Facial Renewal Lotion** *($3.29 for 12 ounces)* contains mostly water, slip agent, AHAs, glycerin, plant oil, more AHAs, salicylic acid, soothing agent, water-binding agents, more plant oils, aloe, thickeners, silicone oil, more thickeners, mineral oil, and preservatives. This is a good 7% AHA product that also contains about 1% salicylic acid. Depending on your skin type, it can be a fairly potent skin exfoliant, but it does come in a very good emollient base. If you have dry, sun-damaged skin, you may want to consider this product, although I don't recommend salicylic acid as an exfoliant for the face.

☺ **Swiss Formula Collagen-Elastin Essential Moisturizer** *($3.29 for 14 ounces)* is a very good moisturizer for someone with dry skin. It contains mostly water, mineral oil, slip agents, thickeners, water-binding agents, plant oil, plant extracts, thickeners, silicone oil, and preservatives.

☺ **Swiss Formula Peaches and Cream Moisturizing Beauty Lotion** *($2.30 for 5 ounces)* is similar to the moisturizer above, but even more emollient.

☺ **Swiss Formula Raspberry Pearl Night Recovery Cream** *($2.30 for 5 ounces)* is similar to the product above, and the same review applies.

☺ **Swiss Formula Collagen-Elastin Hydrating Facial Firming Gel** *($2.99 for 12 ounces)* contains mostly water, slip agent, several water-binding agents, plant extracts, and preservatives. It won't firm anything, but it is a very good lightweight moisturizer for someone with slightly dry or combination skin.

☹ **Swiss Formula Cucumber and Elastin Stress Gel for Eyes and Face** *($2.30 for 5 ounces)* is similar to the product above, except it also contains alcohol, which is not the best for the face or eyes.

☺ **Swiss Formula Firming Masque with Pure Mineral Clay** *($2.29 for 6.7 ounces)* is a standard clay mask and little else.

Shiseido

Shiseido is the only Japanese name-brand cosmetics line sold in U.S. department stores. This and the reputation the Japanese have for creating excellent, reliable products are probably part of its appeal, but expertise in electronics does not necessarily translate to cosmetics. I was surprised to find that very few of Shiseido's skin care and makeup products had changed since I last reviewed the line two years ago. The makeup line is rather limited, although some products are excellent, especially the foundations, lipsticks, and blushes. The counter displays are attractive but inaccessible.

In contrast, the skin care line is huge. There are several skin care divisions, yet despite these categories, the various cleansers, moisturizers, and toners aren't really all that different. The Pureness group is supposed to be for oily skin, but many products are more suitable for dry skin; Vital Perfection is for normal/combination skin, but many of the products would be a problem for someone with combination skin; and Benefiance, for dry/mature skin, doesn't seem all that different from the others. There is also a group of specialty products for those who think their skin care needs aren't being met by all the other items.

By the way, as this book went to press, Shiseido counters at most Nordstrom stores were sporting a new high-tech device to enhance sales. Called a Multi Micro Sensor Machine, it is nothing more than a video camera with a magnifying lens that takes a mega-closeup picture of your skin's surface, magnified beyond what you really want to see. Unfortunately, some of the salespeople get a bit carried away when they describe this intriguing instrument. Several told me that it can see underneath my skin. It can't. This is surface stuff only. I was also told that you can't trust what you feel on your skin, and the sensor is the only way to get an accurate reading. That isn't true either. On different days at different stores, I was told different things about my skin. That's because my skin is more normal in the morning and gets oilier as the day goes by. Like any snapshot, this closeup captures only a moment in time. It does not give you a complete picture of your skin's needs. It can't tell you anything about irritation, allergies, skin sensitivities, or sun needs, and it may be affected by how you washed your face that morning or by the other skin care products you may be using.

Shiseido Skin Care

☹ **$$$ Benefiance Creamy Cleansing Emulsion** *($27 for 6.7 ounces)* is a standard mineral oil–based wipe-off cleanser that can leave a greasy residue on the skin.

☹ **$$$ Benefiance Creamy Cleansing Foam** *($27 for 4.4 ounces)* is a standard detergent-based, water-soluble cleanser that can be drying for most skin types. This one could be OK for someone with oily skin, but the price makes no sense.

☹ **$$$ Pureness Cleansing Foam Oil-Control** *($15 for 3.7 ounces)* is almost identical to the product above; the reason for the price difference is anyone's guess.

☹ **Pureness Cleansing Gel** *($15 for 5.3 ounces)* is a standard detergent-based, water-soluble cleanser that uses sodium lauryl sulfate, which is extremely drying and irritating for most skin types, as the cleansing agent.

☹ **$$$ Pureness Cleansing Water** *($15 for 5 ounces)* is basically a wipe-off cleanser. It does take off makeup, but wiping at the face is never a good idea.

☹ **$$$ Vital Perfection Advanced Makeup Cleansing Gel** *($23 for 4.2 ounces)* is a mineral oil–based cleanser that can leave a greasy residue and requires a washcloth to get it all off the face.

☹ **$$$ Vital Perfection Cleansing Cream** *($22 for 3.9 ounces)* is a standard mineral oil–based cold cream that must be wiped off the face.

☹ **$$$ Vital Perfection Cleansing Foam** *($22 for 4.5 ounces)* is almost identical to the Benefiance Creamy Cleansing Foam above, and the same review applies.

☹ **Vital Perfection Conditioning Cleansing Soap** *($20 for 5.2 ounces)* is just very expensive soap and can be drying and irritating for most skin types. There is nothing conditioning about it.

☺ **$$$ Benefiance Balancing Softener** *($34 for 5 ounces)* is a good irritant-free toner that contains mostly water, glycerin, several slip agents, and preservatives. There are some water-binding agents at the very end of the ingredient list, which makes them completely irrelevant.

☹ **Benefiance Enriched Balancing Softener** *($34 for 5 ounces)* is similar to the product above except that it contains alcohol, which can irritate and dry the skin.

☹ **Pureness Balancing Lotion** *($18 for 6.7 ounces)* is an alcohol-based toner that won't balance anything, but it will irritate the skin. It also contains a small amount of sodium phenolsulfonate, which can be a skin irritant and cause breakouts.

☹ **Pureness Balancing Lotion Oil-Control** *($18 for 6.7 ounces)* is an alcohol-based toner that also contains clays, sulfur, and salicylic acid. It won't control oil, but it can be drying and irritating for most skin types.

☺ **$$$ Vital Perfection Balancing Softener** *($30 for 5 ounces)* is a good, but ordinary, irritant-free toner that contains mostly water, slip agents, glycerin, water-binding agents, and preservatives.

☹ **Vital Perfection T-Zone Balancing Toner** *($25 for 2.5 ounces)* is similar to the Pureness Balancing Lotion above, and the same review applies.

☺ **$$$ Benefiance Daytime Protective Cream SPF 8** *($35 for 1.4 ounces)* contains mostly water, thickener, glycerin, slip agent, more thickeners, silicone oil, plant oil, petrolatum, more thickeners, fragrance, and preservatives. This is a good but ordinary moisturizer for someone with dry skin, although SPF 8 is good only for minimal sun exposure.

☺ **$$$ Benefiance Daytime Protective Emulsion SPF 8** *($35 for 2.5 ounces)* contains mostly water, silicone oils, slip agents, glycerin, thickeners, fragrance, and preservatives. It is OK for someone with normal to slightly dry skin, but SPF 8 is good only for minimal sun exposure.

☺ **$$$ Benefiance Revitalizing Cream** *($40 for 1.3 ounces)* contains mostly water, plant oil, glycerin, petrolatum, thickeners, silicone oil, water-binding agent, more thickeners, and preservatives. There is trivial amount of vitamin E at the end of the ingredient list. This is a good but standard moisturizer for someone with normal to dry skin.

☺ **$$$ Benefiance Revitalizing Emulsion** *($40 for 2.5 ounces)* is similar to the cream above, and the same review applies.

☺ **$$$ Pureness Moisturizing Cream** *($20 for 1.3 ounces)* contains mostly water, glycerin, plant oil, thickeners, slip agent, more plant oil, more thickeners, and preservatives. This is a good moisturizer for someone with normal to dry skin, but someone with combination or oily skin should stay far away from it.

☺ **$$$ Pureness Moisturizing Emulsion** *($20 for 1.6 ounces)* contains mostly water, glycerin, slip agent, petrolatum, silicone oil, several thickeners, plant oil, more thickeners, and preservatives. This is a good emollient moisturizer for someone with dry skin. It contains a minuscule amount of fruit extract, too little to have any effect.

☹ **Pureness Moisturizing Gel Oil-Free** *($20 for 1.6 ounces)* contains too many irritating and drying ingredients, including alcohol, sodium phenolsulfonate, and a small amount of salicylic acid, to make it worthwhile for any skin type.

☺ **$$$ Vital Perfection Daytime Protection Moisturizer SPF 8** *($30 for 1.4 ounces)* contains mostly water, slip agent, silicone oil, plant oil, petrolatum, thickeners, more plant oil, glycerin, more thickeners, and preservatives. This is a very good emollient moisturizer for someone with dry skin, but the SPF is disappointing.

☺ **$$$ Vital Perfection Moisture Active Cream** *($32 for 1.3 ounces)* is similar to the moisturizer above, minus the sunscreen, and the same review applies.

☺ **$$$ Vital Perfection Moisture Active Emulsion** *($32 for 2.3 ounces)* is similar to the cream above, and the same review applies.

☺ **$$$ Vital Perfection Moisture Active Lotion** *($32 for 2.3 ounces)* is a more lightweight version of the emulsion above. The alcohol it uses to lessen the emolliency can be a slight problem for some skin types.

☺ **$$$ Vital Perfection Daily Eye Primer** *($30 for 0.5 ounce)* contains mostly water, slip agents, glycerin, mineral oil, thickeners, plant oil, more thickeners, and preservatives. This is a good emollient moisturizer for dry skin, but it's incredibly ordinary.

☺ **$$$ B.H-24-Day/Night Essence** *($65 for two 0.5-ounce containers)* consists of two very small bottles, each containing a liquid that is supposed to be worn under your regular moisturizer. The Day Essence contains mostly water, slip agents, alcohol, thickeners, water-binding agents, PABA (a sunscreen that is considered a strong irritant and is rarely used anymore), vitamin E, and preservatives. The Night Essence has essentially the same formulation minus the PABA. The alcohol in both liquids is an irritant. Basically, this is an overpriced toner, and if the moisturizer you are using is good, you shouldn't need a second undercoat. If you have dry skin, you shouldn't be using a moisturizer with alcohol.

☺ **$$$ Benefiance Energizing Essence** *($47 for 1 ounce)* contains mostly water, glycerin, alcohol, slip agents, thickeners, more slip agents, plant extract, fragrance, and water-binding agents. It's an OK lightweight moisturizer for someone with normal to slightly dry skin, but the alcohol can be a problem for some skin types.

☺ **$$$ Benefiance Firming Massage Mask** *($37 for 1.9 ounces)* contains mostly water, glycerin, slip agents, thickener, silicone oil, water-binding agent, plant oil, fragrance, and preservatives. This is a good, but very ordinary, moisturizer; calling it firming is an exaggeration.

☺ **$$$ Benefiance Revitalizing Eye Cream** *($40 for 0.51 ounce)* contains mostly water, plant oil, mineral oil, petrolatum, slip agent, water-binding agent, more thickeners, and preservatives. This is a good but ordinary emollient moisturizer for dry skin.

☺ **$$$ Bio-Performance Advanced Super Revitalizer** *($60 for 1.7 ounces)* contains mostly water, glycerin, silicone oils, thickener, slip agent, more thickeners, more silicone oil, petrolatum, and preservatives. This is a very standard, but good moisturizer for someone with dry skin. But silicone oil and petrolatum for $60 is a burn!

☺ **$$$ Bio-Performance Synchro Serum** *($75 for 0.03 ounce of Powder and 0.5 ounce of Essence)* is incredibly overpriced. You're supposed to combine the contents of the two vials in this package. The Powder contains a thickener, several water-binding agents, and preservatives. The Essence contains water, slip agents, alcohol, more slip agents, and preservatives. Mixed together, these two compounds do make an OK moisturizer, but nothing more, and the alcohol can be drying.

☺ **$$$ Revitalizing Cream** *($125 for 1.4 ounces)* is hopelessly ordinary, and the price is unspeakable. It contains mostly water, plant oil, petrolatum, slip agent, mineral oil, thickener, water-binding agent, more thickeners, more water-binding agent, preservative, fragrance, and more preservative. There are minute amounts of placenta extract and vitamin E, but they come well after the preservatives and are meaningless in both amount and what they can do for the skin.

☹ **Pureness Blemish Control Cream** *($15 for 0.53 ounce)* contains mostly sulfur, water, clay, talc, and alcohol. There are dozens of similar concoctions and none of them work either.

☺ **$$$ Pureness Exfoliating Treatment Gel** *($18 for 3.6 ounces)* uses a piece of synthetic material as the exfoliant in a fairly gentle water-soluble base. It can be a good scrub for most skin types.

☺ **$$$ Pureness Hydra Purifying Masque, Peel-Off** *($18 for 2.7 ounces)* is basically plastic and alcohol. It dries on the face like a film and then peels off. That can make the face feel smooth, but it won't purify anything; also, the alcohol and plastic can be drying and irritating for some skin types.

☺ **$$$ Pureness Oil-Blotting Paper** *($10 for 100 sheets)* is just what the name implies. You press these small sheets over your face to help absorb oil during the day. The sheets are coated with a light layer of clay that can absorb oil. It's an option, but plain old powder and permanent-wave endpapers do essentially the same thing.

☺ **$$$ Vital Perfection Hydro-Intensive Mask** *($28 for 1.4 ounces)* contains mostly water, glycerin, slip agents, alcohol, thickeners, plant oil, more thickeners, and preservatives. This very ordinary mask can be drying for some skin types.

☹ **Vital Perfection Rinse-Off Clarifying Mask** *($25 for 3 ounces)* is basically just clay and alcohol. It can be drying and irritating for most skin types.

☺ **$$$ Vital Perfection Protective Lip Conditioner, SPF 4** *($20 for 0.14 ounce)* doesn't have much of a sunscreen, so there isn't much else to say about this otherwise very emollient lip balm.

☺ **$$$ Sun Block Lip Treatment, SPF 15** *($15 for 1 ounce)* is almost identical to the one above only this one has the proper SPF. It's still overpriced for what you get.

Shiseido Makeup

☺ **$$$ FOUNDATION: Stick Foundation** *($27)* is for dry skin only and goes on fairly greasy; after blending, though, it can be surprisingly sheer, and it does feel great on dry skin. **These colors are excellent:** I2, I4, B2, B4, B6, and G1. **These colors are too orange or pink for most skin tones:** P2, P4, P6, and C1 (this one is a green primer color for the skin, something I never recommend).

☺ **$$$ Fluid Foundation** *($28)* has a great consistency and blends easily on the skin. **These colors are excellent:** Natural Light Ivory, Natural Fair Ivory, Natural Light Beige, Natural Fair Beige, Natural Fair Pink (almost too pink), Natural Warm Beige, Natural Deep Beige, and Warm Bronze. **These colors should be avoided:** Natural Light Pink (no one is this pink) and Natural Deep Pink.

☺ **$$$ Creme Powder Compact Foundation** *($30)* looks like a cream but dries to a silky and light finish; on some skin types, it can look powdery and choppy by the end of the day. It can be used either wet or dry. **These colors are excellent:** Natural Light Beige, Natural Fair Beige, Natural Deep Beige, Natural Light Pink, Natural Fair Pink, Natural Deep Pink, Warm Bronze, Natural Light Ivory, and Natural Fair Ivory.

☺ **$$$ Dual Compact Powdery Foundation** *($27.50)* is basically a talc- and mineral oil-based pressed powder that can be used wet or dry. It comes in an excellent assortment of sheer colors.

☺ **$$$ Oil Control Treatment Compact** *($17.50)* isn't oil-free because it contains plant oil, and although the salesperson told me it's medicated, it isn't. This product won't control oil, but it is a good cream-to-powder foundation with a great light texture and a small but excellent color selection. **These are good neutral colors:** 01, 02, 03, 04, and 05.

☺ **$$$ Natural Matte Foundation Oil-Free with Non-Chemical SPF 8** *($28)* isn't oil-free (it contains silicone oil), but it does go on matte and smooth. It may not be the best for someone with extremely oily skin, but it is a very good foundation. SPF 8 is OK but not great, and the nonchemical protection is less irritating than other sunscreen agents. **These colors are excellent:** Natural Deep Ivory, Natural Fair Ivory, Natural Light Ivory, Very Light Ivory, Warm Bronze, Natural Deep Beige, Natural Fair Beige, Natural Light Beige, Natural Summer Pink, Natural Deep Pink, and

Natural Fair Pink. **These colors should be avoided:** Natural Light Pink and Matte Bronze.

☹ **CONCEALER:** Concealer for Circles *($15)* comes in only two shades; 01 is too peach for most skin tones, and 02 is too gold for most skin tones. I wish the colors were better, because the texture of this product is smooth and it blends well. **Concealer for Lines** *($10)* is a standard pencil that comes in two light shades; one is rather peach and the other pink. They don't hide lines in the least and they can easily crease.

☺ **$$$ POWDER:** **Natural Pressed Powder** *($22)* is a standard talc-based powder that goes on very sheer and soft, and the colors are great.

☺ **$$$ BLUSH:** Singles *($24)* and **Tri-Effect Blush** *($28)* are available in a small number of colors, and they blend on smoothly and evenly. The Tri-Effect is just three blush colors in a row that mix together on the brush to create one color. It looks more clever in the compact than it does on the face. **All of the colors are beautiful.**

☺ **$$$ EYESHADOW:** Single *($18.50)*, **Duos** *($21)*, and **Tri Effect Eye Shadow** *($23)* are available in a limited number of acceptable colors. **These colors are excellent:** Bronze Gold, Soft Brown, Grey Brown, Lemonade, and Melon Matches. **These colors are extremely shiny or too blue or green:** Soft Gold, Blue for Beginners, Roseate, Tortoise Shells, Moss, Teddy Brown, Cinders, Anthracites, Purple Quartz, Raspberry on Fire, Steely Blues, Clove/Violet, Red Madness, Desert Hues, Ultra Violet, Bronze Copper.

☺ **$$$ EYE AND BROW SHAPER:** The **Eye Liner Pencil** *($13)* and **Eye Brow Pencil** *($10)* both have a good soft texture and come in an attractive array of muted colors; however, the brow pencils go on heavier than most and need to be blended carefully. **Eyebrow Shapeliner** *($20)* is a brow gel that goes on just fine, but the only shade is slightly taupe, and how many eyebrows can that match? **Shadow Liner** *($25)* is a trio of eyeshadow colors—black, brown, or navy—that can be used wet or dry.

☺ **Eyebrow Shadow Liner** *($22)* is simply two eyeshadows in a single compact. It's the best way to apply brow color, but the packaging is strange. One set of colors is Light Brown and Chestnut, the other Black and Dark Brown. Since your brow color is one or the other but not both, you are buying an extra color you will probably never use. **Pen Liner** *($18)* is a felt-tip style liquid liner. The color goes on evenly and dries matte, but there is only one shade, sort of a black brown. **Liquid Liner** *($18)* is a traditional liner in a tube that you apply with a tiny eyeliner brush. It too comes in only one shade, black.

☺ **LIPSTICK AND LIP PENCIL:** Advanced Performance Lipstick *($14)* has a wonderful creamy texture with a semi-matte finish that is really beautiful. **Advanced Performance Lip Gloss** *($14)* is a traditional lip gloss that comes in lipstick form; it's nothing special. **Staying Power Lipstick** *($18.50)* is supposed to stay on so well that it even comes with its own **Staying Power Lipstick Remover** *($10 for 1.6 ounces)*. Nice try, Shiseido. It's a decent imitation of ColorStay, but the real thing is better. Also, Staying Power Lipstick comes in only a handful of colors, while ColorStay has a wide range to choose from. The special remover is actually not all that special, and the lipstick comes off all by itself or after wiping with a tissue, just like any other lipstick. The **Lip Liner Pencil** *($12)* has a very good dry texture and comes in a lovely array of colors.

☹ **MASCARA:** Advanced Performance Mascara *($18)* and **Mascara Fiber Blended** *($18)* are just OK but not great, and the fiber mascara can flake and get in the eyes.

Sudden Youth (Skin Care Only)

If you flipped this book open to check out this line first, you need to read the section on skin care; it will remind you that you can't buy youth from the cosmetics industry, despite this product's enticing name. Sure, the before-and-after pictures are enough to make a believer out of many women. But as a professional makeup artist, I know how to create that kind of effect. If you look closely, you'll see that the lighting, facial position, backdrop, and makeup in each "before" photograph are different from those in the "after" photograph. Sudden Youth would like you to believe that its products created the difference in the way these women look, but that is not the whole truth. Also, when you look at the ingredient lists, you'll find that these products are remarkably ordinary. The ingredients are not unique or sufficiently different from those in other face lift–type products or moisturizers to warrant the hoopla.

For your information, the company's telephone number is (800) 542-5537.

☺ **$$$ Deep Pore Cleanser** *($22.50 for 8 ounces)* is a standard wipe-off cleanser that contains nothing more than thickeners, mineral oil, plant oil, more thickeners, and preservatives. It can leave a greasy residue, and wiping off makeup can cause wrinkles.

☹ **$$$ Pearlized Facial Wash** *($22.50 for 8 ounces)* is a standard detergent-based, water-soluble cleanser that can be good for some skin types. It contains several plant oils, which can leave a greasy residue.

☹ **Facial Wash** *($15.75; $40.75 for Pro-Size)* is a standard detergent-based, water-soluble cleanser. The main detergent cleansing agent is TEA-lauryl sulfate, which can be drying and irritating on the skin. Also in this cleanser are plant oils, which can help soften the dryness, but why use such an irritating cleansing agent in the first place?

☹ **Alfalfa-Cleansing Bar** *($8.95)* is a standard bar cleanser that uses fats and lye (sodium hydroxide). This can be very drying and irritating for the skin.

☹ **Oat-Cleansing Bar** *($8.95)* is almost identical to the cleansing bar above, and the same review applies.

☹ **Honey-Cleansing Bar** *($8.95)* is almost identical to the Alfalfa Cleansing Bar above, and the same review applies.

☹ **Celery-Cleansing Bar** *($8.95)* is almost identical to the Alfalfa Cleansing Bar above, and the same review applies.

☺ **Eye Make-up Remover Gel** *($14.75 for 1 ounce)* is a standard wipe-off makeup remover. It can indeed remove eye makeup, but repeatedly pulling at the eye area can cause the skin to sag.

☹ **Skin Freshener** *($16.50 for 8 ounces)* is a very standard detergent-based toner that also contains witch hazel and arnica, both of which can be skin irritants.

☹ **Facial Lift Gel** *($13.95 for 1 ounce)* is nothing more than aloe, water, thickener, and preservatives. It is meant to be mixed with **Facial Lift Powder** *($26.95 for 1 ounce)*, which is nothing more than cornstarch and egg white. There are some plant extracts and water-binding agents listed after the preservatives, which means they are not present in any significant amount. If you're thinking that this expensive little mixture is little more than what you could whip up in your kitchen, you're right. Cornstarch and egg white for $40—how depressing. By the way, cornstarch can be a skin irritant and cause breakouts.

☺ **$$$ Essential Beauty Oils** *($15.95 for 1 ounce)* is, as the name implies, a blend of plant oils. You could easily, and for far less money, mix up something like this from items in your kitchen cabinet and get the same benefits for dry skin.

☺ **$$$ Moisture Lotion** *($15.75 for 8 ounces)* contains mostly aloe, water, mineral oil, thickeners, slip agent, plant oils, more thickeners, water-binding agent, and preservatives. It is a good emollient moisturizer for someone with dry skin.

☺ **$$$ Sleeping Beauty Cream** *($24.95 for 2 ounces)* contains mostly aloe, water, slip agent, thickener, plant oils, more thickeners, and preservatives. This is a good emollient moisturizer for dry skin, but it's incredibly ordinary for the price. There are some vitamins, more plant oils, and collagen at the end of the ingredient list, which in larger quantities could have made this product more interesting, but there aren't enough of them in this cream to have any benefit for your skin.

☺ **$$$ Elastin Elegance** *($42.50 for 2 ounces)* contains mostly water, water-binding agent, slip agent, plant oils, thickeners, more water-binding agent, more thickeners, a tiny amount of AHAs, and preservatives. This is a good but ordinary moisturizer for someone with dry skin. It does contain collagen, but that can't affect the collagen in your skin.

☹ **Mint Julep** *($26 for 4 ounces)* is mostly aloe, alcohol, film former, thickeners, plant oil, soothing agent, plant extracts, and preservatives. This is supposed to be a pick-me-up for the face, but the alcohol can dry out the skin and cause irritation.

☺ **$$$ Eye Cream** *($24.95)* contains mostly aloe, petrolatum, plant oil, thickeners, water-binding agents, and preservatives. This is a very good emollient moisturizer for someone with dry skin.

☺ **$$$ Miracle Moisture Masque** *($32 for 4 ounces)* contains mostly water, aloe, slip agent, water-binding agents, thickeners, plasticizer, and preservatives. This is an OK mask if you're not allergic to the plasticizer.

Trish McEvoy

It isn't easy to put together a new cosmetics line that incorporates both skin care and makeup products. Creating a reliable skin care regime that works for many different skin types is a daunting task in itself, but add to that the requirements of a makeup line— foundations, concealers, blushes, eyeshadows, lipsticks, lip liners, brushes, eyeliners, and powders—and you can literally drown in a sea of products. Very few people develop the whole ball of wax all at once; rather, they often start with skin care and slowly add makeup, or vice versa.

New York makeup artist Trish McEvoy couldn't wait. Instead, she (or whoever worked with her) created an entire line all at once, with a broad variety of products. Unfortunately, due to either the elaborate assembly of products or just plain bad judgment, this has to be one of the most confusing, poorly developed lines I've ever reviewed. Trish, what were you thinking during the selection and design phases for your cosmetics line? There are more strange brush shapes and sizes than I've ever seen before, and most are overpriced and unnecessary. I asked several makeup artists (including the counter salesperson) if they thought the brush choices were an asset, and they all said the same thing: "Are you kidding? Most of them are hard to work with, and it's hard to remember what you're supposed to do with them. Imagine explaining to a consumer why you need three differ-ent brushes just for the crease area."

To add to the confusion, the line has six—yes, *six*—categories of eyeshadows: Glazes, Shapers, Definers, Enhancers, Eye Essentials, and Dual Eyeshadows. It would be great if the Glazes were all softer colors for under the brow, the Shapers were deeper colors for the crease area, the Definers were accent colors or liners, and the Enhancers some other type of accent color, but no such pattern exists. In all the groupings, you'll find colors that are very shiny, slightly shiny, matte, light, *and* dark. Very puzzling.

Surely, given the line's six foundations, all women should be able to find a suitable shade or product, but that is far from the case. Only three of the foundations have as many as nine shades, and even those display wide gaps between light and dark, with almost no colors suitable for someone with fair to medium skin tone. Two of the foundations come in only three colors, all for extremely light skin. When it comes to loose powder, once again you'd better have very light skin, because there are only four colors and they're all light. I could go on, but you've probably got the picture.

I suppose that competing with M.A.C. was a priority for McEvoy. It was for Bobbi Brown, another New York makeup artist with an upscale cosmetics line, but Brown's line is not overwhelming (she started with a small group of makeup products, then slowly branched out to include skin care, more color choices, and additional product options).

Brown, McEvoy, and M.A.C. have much in common, but M.A.C. is way ahead, with McEvoy bringing up the rear (and possibly not even making it across the finish line). It's not that McEvoy's line is all bad: quite the contrary. It is just very badly organized, some products are really disappointing, and they're overpriced, particularly compared to M.A.C. (McEvoy's eyeshadows are $16 each; M.A.C.'s are $10.)

You might expect expensive skin care products to have something distinct or individual you wouldn't necessarily find in similar products. I rarely, if ever, find that the so-called "special" ingredients often found in more expensive cosmetics live up to the claims made about them, but at least their presence shows that the formulator put some energy and research into the products or tried to come up with a unique combination of ingredients.

What do I consider unique? A mixture of interesting water-binding agents such as hyaluronic acid with sodium PCA, perhaps; or an AHA product with a unique anti-irritant ingredient such as green tea; or, although I'm loath to say it, even a bizarre concoction of plants—these would all be more distinctive than the standard stuff in Pond's or Nivea. Not that Pond's or Nivea are bad, but while I expect the standard good stuff in the less expensive products, I hope for more from the expensive stuff—something special that partially justifies the higher cost. Besides, these "special" ingredients and "unique" formulas provide a challenge when I do my research.

Not this line, though. Most of the products go beyond ordinary to downright boring. On one hand, I was thrilled to see a department-store line that didn't include an obnoxious list of plants or sea extracts, but I was disappointed to see such standard formulations with such unreasonable price tags. In any case, overlooking some of these products not only will save you a lot of money, but in many instances will save your face at the same time.

Trish McEvoy Skin Care

☹ **$$$ Gentle Cleansing Lotion** (*$20 for 3 ounces*) may indeed be gentle for some skin types, but it could wreak havoc if you tend to break out, are prone to bumps under the skin, or have blackheads. The second ingredient is isopropyl myristate, notorious for clogging pores. Other than that, this is an OK water-soluble makeup remover.

☺ **$$$ Essential Cleanser** (*$22 for 4 ounces*) is my idea of an essential cleanser, but only because it's a knockoff of Cetaphil Lotion (the sensitive-skin cleanser you can buy for a quarter of the price at the drugstore).

☹ **Astringent Cleansing Bar** (*$20 for 3.7 ounces*) uses sodium tallowate (lard) as the primary ingredient. Tallow can cause eczema and blackheads. I wouldn't recommend this for any skin type, and definitely not for someone with problem skin. It also contains mud, mineral oil, and glycerin. The mud can feel heavy on the skin, and the mineral oil isn't great for someone with oily skin.

☹ **Moisture Retaining Bar** (*$20 for 3.7 ounces*) is almost identical to the bar above, minus the mud. It can be extremely drying, and it has the same potential to cause eczema and blackheads.

☹ **Glycolic Wash** (*$37 for 8 ounces*) can be very drying, and you shouldn't wash your face with a product that contains glycolic acid, because you may inadvertently get it in your eyes. Anyway, one glycolic acid product is enough for any face, and it is best to use one that stays on the skin. In a cleanser, some of the acid may be rinsed off, making for an uneven application.

☹ **Eye Makeup Remover** (*$15 for 2 ounces*) would be a fine eye makeup remover if it didn't contain PVP, a hair fixative, rather high on the ingredient list. It can definitely be a skin irritant and should be avoided around the eyes.

☺ **$$$ Waterproof Mascara Remover** (*$15 for 2 ounces*) is mostly silicone oil with a few additional slip agents. It will work, but this is very expensive silicone oil.

☺ **$$$ Light Moisturizer** *($37 for 2 ounces)* contains mostly water, slip agent, thickeners, silicone oil, more thickeners, water-binding agents, film former, vitamins E and A, and preservative. The vitamins are at the end of the ingredient list, meaning they are practically nonexistent. This is as ordinary a moisturizer as you can find, but that doesn't mean it's bad. It would be a good moisturizer for someone with normal to slightly dry skin; it's just not worth the exorbitant price tag.

☺ **$$$ Extra-Light Moisturizer** *($37 for 2 ounces)* is similar to the moisturizer above, minus the silicone oil. It isn't all that light, but it would be a good moisturizer for someone with normal to slightly dry skin.

☺ **$$$ Enriched Moisturizer** *($37 for 2 ounces)* is almost a joke, at least at this price. All this very expensive product contains is water, mineral oil, thickener, lanolin, vitamins A and D, and preservatives. It is definitely a very rich emollient moisturizer for someone with dry skin, but there are cheaper versions of this product.

☺ **$$$ Protective Shield Moisturizer SPF 15** *($37 for 2 ounces)* is similar to the Light Moisturizer above, but with SPF 15. SPF 15 provides the same protection no matter what price tag is attached to it, and you can find it much more cheaply elsewhere.

☺ **$$$ Dry Skin Normalizer, Extra-Rich Improvement Cream** *($40 for 1 ounce)* contains mostly petrolatum, water, thickener, mineral oil, plant oil, more thickeners, lanolin oil, and preservatives. This is little more than Vaseline with a bunch of oils. For this kind of money, they should at least throw in some interesting water-binding agents. It is indeed a good moisturizer for someone with dry skin, just shockingly expensive for what you get.

☺ **$$$ Line Refiner** *($28 for 0.25 ounce)* contains mostly plant water, slip agent, mineral oil, plant oil, thickener (cornstarch, which can be a skin irritant), petrolatum, slip agent, silicone oil, water-binding agents, thickeners, and preservatives. This won't change a line on your face, but it is a good moisturizer for someone with dry skin.

☺ **$$$ Glycolic Face Cream** *($37 for 1 ounce)* contains mostly water, water-binding agents, thickeners, glycolic acid, several more thickeners, and preservatives. This is about a 4% AHA concentration, which is just fine for someone with sensitive skin. There are much cheaper AHA products on the market; nothing about this one makes it worth the expense.

☺ **$$$ Glycolic Lotion** *($37 for 2 ounces)* has a very simple ingredient list of water, glycolic acid, a buffer, and two thickeners. This would be a very good (but overpriced) 8% AHA product for someone with oily skin.

☹ **$$$ Soothing Exfoliating Mask, Normalizing Mask for All Skin Types** (*$26 for 2 ounces*) contains mostly water, clays, glycerin, thickener, and preservatives. This is a very standard clay mask, and if you want clay with no other irritants, you've found the right mask. I wouldn't call clay soothing, however; it can be drying.

Trish McEvoy Makeup

FOUNDATION: I expected to love Trish McEvoy's foundations. Every makeup artist realizes that nothing is as important as getting the foundation right. Foundation is what you will be putting the rest of the colors on, and it has to be neutral and soft: too heavy and the skin looks caked, too subtle and there really is no base present to use as a canvas. Sadly, there isn't much positive I can say about the makeup bases in this line, and there are seven of them.

☺ **$$$ Enriched Foundation** (*$35*), which isn't all that enriched, is probably the best choice, but the options are limited, even though there are colors for very dark skin tones. **These colors are good:** 1 and 2B (both are great for very light skin tones), 4, and 8. **These colors should be used with care:** 3 (can be slightly pink for some skin tones), 5 (can be too yellow), 6 (can be too gold), 7 (can be slightly ash), and 9 (can be too red).

☹ **Protective Shield Foundation SPF 15** (*$35*) tends to peel and streak. It comes in three colors, all of which are appropriate only for very fair skin.

☹ **Protective Shield Tinted Moisturizer** (*$35*) goes on better than the product above, but the color choices are just as limited. It is an option only if you want very sheer coverage.

☺ **$$$ Natural Tint Foundation Oil-Free** (*$35*) isn't really oil-free—it contains silicone oil. Although this foundation goes on evenly and smoothly, the reliable colors are extremely limited. **These colors are the most neutral:** 1, 3B, and 7. **These colors should be avoided:** 2 is too rose; 2B can be too ash; 3 is too peach; 4, 5, and 6 can be too gold; 8 can be too coppery; and 9 can be too red.

☺ **$$$ Cream Powder Makeup** (*$40*) is just what it says—a creamy-feeling makeup that spreads smoothly, then leaves a dry, soft, powdery finish. It can be OK for some skin types, but could be a problem for someone who tends to break out. It contains plenty of wax (including carnauba), and the second ingredient is isopropyl myristate, which can clog pores. **These colors are quite good:** 1, 2B, 4, 5, 6, and 8. **These colors should be avoided:** 3 can be too rose, 7 can be too ash, and 9 can be too red.

☺ **$$$ Dual Powder** *($25)* is meant to provide all-over face color as an alternative to traditional foundation. In theory, that can be great for someone with normal to slightly oily skin, but this product has a very grainy texture and feels extremely dry and "powdery." The Pressed Powder (reviewed below) works much better and has better colors.

☺ **$$$ CONCEALER: Protective Shield Cover-up** *($20)* gives great coverage, blends out nicely to a subtle finish, and doesn't crease, although the texture seems quite thick and heavy at first. **These colors are great for medium to darker skin tones:** 4 and 5. **These colors should be used with care:** Extra Light (has a slight pink cast), Light (has a slight peach tone), and 1B (can be too yellow for most skin tones).

☺ **$$$ POWDER: Loose Powder** *($18)* is talc-based, with a very silky soft texture, but the four color choices are appropriate only for light to medium skin tones. Did someone forget that this line has foundation colors for dark to very dark skin tones? What are those women supposed to use? **Pressed Powder** *($25)* is also a standard talc-based powder with a silky soft texture (vastly better than the Dual Powder above, which is meant to be used as a foundation). If you want to use a powder as an all-over face color, use the Pressed Powder instead of the Dual Powder. The five colors cover a better range than the Loose Powder.

☺ **$$$ All Over Face Powder** *($25)* is a group of rather ordinary talc-based powders similar in texture to the Pressed Powder. The strange array of colors ranges from neutral beige to a bronzer, along with a rose shade, some shiny shades, and a mulberry color. Why someone would want to brush some of these colors all over her face is anyone's guess. My suggestion is not to.

☺ **$$$ BLUSH: Sheer Blush** *($18)* colors are nice but fairly ordinary, and there are a few strange colors to watch out for. **These colors are all interesting, and quite soft and matte:** 2 through 8. **These colors should be avoided:** 1, a very pale shade of orange, and 6, a very shiny rose.

☺ **$$$ Dual Blush** *($18)* is a strange small round tin split in two colors. Two blushes are nice, but it is very difficult to get a full brush dabbed into one color without getting some of the other color on the brush too.

☺ **$$$** The very fat **Pencils** *($18.50)* are soft enough to be used as lipsticks or blushes. They feel like very creamy lipsticks or cream blushes, and are not unique or special. The pencils are convenient if you can somehow figure out how to keep them sharpened.

☺ **$$$** <u>EYESHADOW:</u> Six types of eyeshadows might sound like overkill, but in this case you can ignore the categories and just look for the colors you like, because they are all pretty much alike. The **Glazes, Shapers, Definers,** and **Enhancers** *($16 each)* are interchangeable, with little to no difference in color arrangement or texture. Go for the matte shadows (there aren't as many as you would expect in a line designed by a makeup artist) and you will do just fine. **These colors are best:** Shapers 102, 107, 108, 109, and 116; Definers 15, 20, 21, 22, 26, and 28; and Enhancers 12, 13, and 16. Most of the eyeshadows, particularly the darker shades, are a bit on the "wet" side and tend to crease.

☻ **$$$** **Dual Eyecolor** *($18)* is a small round tin of eyeshadow split in two. All of the colors are matte, but the combinations are a bit strange. Choices include Navy on one side and Tan on the other; Black and Yellow; Plum and Taupe; and Chocolate Brown with Soft Rust. The last one is the only set that really works together. The others are too contrasting for most skin tones and tastes.

☹ **Essential Kit** *($35)* is a compact quad group with a blush, an eyeliner, and two eyeshadows. The way the colors are organized makes it hard to prevent the blush brush from getting into the eyeshadows, and the colors tend to flake into one another. Additionally, any time you buy sets, you rarely end up using all the colors, which makes this kind of product a waste of money. On the other hand, some of the color groupings are matte, and the color that is meant to be used as the blush can be used around the eyes, so if you find a selection that meets all your needs, this can be an essential kit for you.

☻ **$$$** <u>EYE AND BROW SHAPER:</u> The **Eye Pencils** *($16)* are incredibly standard, in a very typical assortment of colors. With all the brushes in this line, why would someone use a pencil instead of a powder to frame the eye or brow?

☺ **$$$** <u>LIPSTICK AND LIP PENCIL:</u> **Sheers** *($16)* are like a gloss, with the same staying power. These colors lack tints that would make them last longer. **Sheers with SPF 15** *($16)* are identical to the Sheers except they contain sunscreen. **Lip Colors** *($16)* are creamy lipsticks with good staying power, a wonderful texture, smooth application, and a very impressive color selection. **Lip Gloss** *($16)* comes in a tube applicator and offers an interesting array of colors, including red, a shiny lavender, and a shiny gold, as well as soft, pale shades of pink, mauve, and peach. These glosses go on very thick and rich, looking more wet than glossy. **Lip Pencils** *($16)* come in a nice assortment of colors, and one side of the pencil is a lip brush. It's a nice touch, but Max Factor sells almost the exact same pencil for a quarter of the price.

☹ **Matte Over** *($16)* is supposed to be used as a lipstick base to help keep lipstick on longer or as a top coat to make any cream lipstick look matte. Either way, it is a problem. Used as a base it tends to peel, and used over lipstick it is just messy.

☹ **Dual Lip Color** *($18)* is just what the name implies: half of the lipstick is one color, and the other half is a completely different color. What happens when you apply it? It goes on as one color. Why bother? I haven't the vaguest idea.

☹ **MASCARA:** The **Mascara** *($15)* stays on wonderfully and doesn't smear or clump. Unfortunately, it doesn't build much length. To remedy that problem, there is **Lash Builder** *($15)*, a clear mascara that adds length and helps the appearance of the lashes. There are plenty of mascaras on the market that build long, thick lashes without a second product.

BRUSHES: It takes good professional brushes to apply makeup well, but the expense is worth it because they last forever. This line offers 20 or so squirrel or sable brushes (the texture is exquisite). Some are great, but there are so many bizarre ones that I'm concerned you may end up getting the wrong ones, and these are too expensive to make a mistake with.

☺ **$$$ Brush 2B** *($38)* is a blush brush with a great soft texture. **Brush 6** *($23)* is a uniquely shaped brush meant to be used for specific placement of the crease color. This isn't for soft blending, but it is great for controlling dramatic definition. **Brush 12** *($19)* is a small, square eyeshadow brush—very practical and usable. **Brush 13** *($19)* is a standard round eyeshadow brush with a less-than-standard price tag. **Brush 16** *($19)* is supposed to be an ultra-thin liner, but I wouldn't even call it slender. You will not end up with a thin line if you use this brush, but it has some application possibilities. **Brush 17** *($19)* is an interestingly shaped brush meant to be a thicker eyeliner brush. One good thin brush is what's needed, but you won't find it in this collection. **Brush 19** *($19)* is a traditional round eyeshadow brush that is great for almost any eyeshadow application. **Brush 26** *($30)* is a traditional powder brush with an unbelievably silky soft texture. **Brush 32** *($18)* is an angle brush for the brow or for liner. Unless you have huge lids, I wouldn't recommend it for lining, but it would be fine for the brow.

☹ **Brush 7** *($18)* is a lipstick brush, but it isn't retractable, which makes storage in a makeup bag messy. **Brush 9** *($18)* is billed as a special blending brush for eye pencils. It would do the job, but it isn't at all necessary. **Brush 11** *($18)* is a small, thin, square brush that is supposed to be used on its edge to smudge on eyeshadow as a liner. That makes it hard to control and kind of sloppy. It would be an OK eyeshadow brush for someone with a small lid area, but that's about it. **Brush 20** *($58)* is a flat-topped blush/contour brush. For this amount of money, you should be getting a really great brush, but this one tends to make the color application look like a stripe. **Brush 21** *($53)* is a thick, somewhat large eyeshadow brush used to apply a base color all over the eye; it costs an absurd, eyebrow-raising amount of money. **Brush 22** *($25)* is a smaller version of the blush brush, meant to be used with cream blush. It's hard enough to apply cream blush evenly with a sponge; it's even more difficult with a brush. The blush also builds up a waxy layer on the brush. **Brush 23** *($28)* is (are you ready for this?) a thickly angled brush designed for *nose* contouring. It's probably not a bad idea for a makeup artist, but I've gotten along without it for years, and so has every other makeup artist I know. **Brush 27** *($38)*, which is even thicker than 23, is supposed to be for contouring under the cheek-bone. It could make the contour look a bit like a line, so make sure you can use it before you empty your wallet. **Brush 29** *($25)* is a floppy, thick, long-bristled brush meant to be used in the crease. It splatters the powder all over the place and is hard to control.

Ultima II

At some point, Ultima II decided to appeal more to women in their 20s than to the over-50 crowd. The products went from ultra-moisturizing to ultra-fun and clever. New names include The Nakeds and LipSexxxy, the new skin care products are called Interactives, and the shades in the color line are all matte and neutral.

At the forefront of this shift in direction are Interactives, a six-step grouping of products that stack (almost interlocking) on top of each other. Supposedly, the design was influenced by ergonomics, the science of accommodating the human body. As impressive as that sounds, I don't get the feeling that these products relate to the human body in any way. In fact, getting the products unhooked from each other isn't all that easy, and the wide jars encourage bacteria growth. But if storage is an issue, this line is definitely an option; the packaging concept offers an attractive solution to the dilemma of how to store cosmetics in a snug bathroom.

What about the Interactives products themselves? According to the brochure, the six products are supposed to cover three skin care needs: "prevention, protection, and repair." Antioxidants are supposed to provide prevention; protection is tackled by an SPF of 15; and "lipid fluidizers" are supposed to repair "the lipid barrier." Of those three, the only one that really makes sense is the SPF 15. The only way antioxidants could really have an effect on the skin would be if they blocked off all air, and that means suffocation—not a great idea. That's why the theory that antioxidants can prevent free-radical damage is only a theory. Lipid fluidizers, in the form of lecithin and glycerin, are nothing more than lipid water-binding agents added to the product to replace fats (sebum or oil) that may be missing from your skin. Thousands of products contain these ingredients.

Turning to the rest of the product line, the display units are attractive, though it's tough to figure out which are The Nakeds and which are the Sexxxy products. Wherever I went, I found the Ultima II sales staff less aggressive than most, which made shopping at their counters less discouraging. From lipsticks to eyeshadows and blushes, the color range is exceptional and very matte. There are a wide range of lipstick shades that vary from natural to full, bold colors, but the distinctions between the different types of lipstick are unclear.

Ultima II Skin Care

☹ **Interactives Clean Team Cleanser + Toner Normal/Dry** *($16.50 for 5.26 ounces)* is a standard mineral oil–based wipe-off cleanser that lists, among the first four ingredients, two thickening agents that can aggravate acne: isopropyl myristate and isopropyl palmitate.

☺ **$$$ Interactives Clean Team Cleanser + Toner Normal/Oily** *($16.50 for 5.26 ounces)* is an OK cleanser for someone with normal to oily skin, but it can be a bit drying.

☺ **$$$ Interactives Thirst Buster Antioxidant Hydrator with SPF 15** *($20 for 1.73 ounces)* contains mostly water, several water-binding agents, several thickeners, silicone oil, several antioxidants, plant extracts, more water-binding agents, plant oils, and preservatives. Although the antioxidants are far down on the ingredient list, there are plenty of them, and SPF 15 provides good protection. This is an option for someone with normal to dry skin who's interested in trying antioxidants.

☺ **$$$ Interactives Night Cap Antioxidant Skin Smoother** *($25 for 1.72 ounces)* contains mostly water, several thickeners, water-binding agents, silicone oil, more thickeners, a form of acrylate (like hairspray), more water-binding agents, anti-oxidants, plant oil, and preservatives. Acrylates in skin care products can make the skin look smoother, but they can also irritate sensitive skin. This product is similar to the one above, only without the sunscreen, and the same review applies.

☺ **$$$ Interactives Booster Shot Antioxidant Firming System** *($28.50 for 0.7 ounce)* contains mostly water, glycerin, film former, thickener, several antioxidants, water-binding agents, plant extracts, more thickeners, and preservatives. Calling hairspray "firming" is stretching the truth; film formers can make the skin look smoother, but they can also irritate sensitive skin. This is an OK lightweight gel for someone with normal to slightly dry to combination skin, but it isn't a booster shot for any type of skin.

☺ **$$$ Interactives Oil Check Antioxidant Oil-Free Hydrator with SPF 15** *($20 for 1.51 ounces)* contains mostly water, talc, thickener, water-binding agents, more thickeners, silicone oils, vitamin E, salicylic acid, more water-binding agents, plant extracts, more thickeners, vitamins A and D, more thickeners, more water-binding agents, and preservatives. I wish companies would stop calling their products oil-free when they contain silicone oils! Also, salicylic acid doesn't exfoliate as well as AHAs do. One of the thickeners is isopropyl myristate, which can cause breakouts, but there isn't much of it, so it probably won't cause a problem. Some aspects of this product are drying and some moisturizing. It seems confusing, so it's hard for me to recommend it.

☺ **$$$ CHR Extraordinary Cream Cleanser** *($17 for 4 ounces)* is a standard mineral oil–based cleanser that must be wiped off and can leave a greasy film on the skin.

☺ **$$$ CHR Extraordinary Lotion Cleanser** *($17 for 6 ounces)* is similar to the cleanser above, only in lotion form, and the same review applies.

☺ **$$$ CHR Extraordinary Lotion** *($65 for 2 ounces)* contains mostly water, thickeners, collagen, protein, water-binding agents, almond oil, rice oil, mineral oil, more thickeners, and preservatives. This is a good emollient moisturizer for dry skin, but it's very overpriced.

☺ **$$$ CHR Extraordinary Cream** *($65 for 1.125 ounces)* contains mostly water, plant oils, mineral oil, slip agent, thickener, lanolin, more thickeners, water-binding agents, more plant oil, more thickeners, fragrance, and preservatives. This is an overpriced, but extremely emollient, moisturizer for someone with dry skin.

☺ **$$$ CHR Moisture Lotion Concentrate** *($32.50 for 3 ounces)* contains mostly water, slip agent, thickeners, water-binding agents, more thickeners, and preservatives. It would be good for dry skin, but don't expect the collagen and protein to change anything about your skin.

☺ **$$$ CHR Cream Concentrate** *($32.50 for 2 ounces)* contains mostly water, thickener, slip agent, lanolin oil, more thickener, mineral oil, plant oil, more thickeners, water-binding agents, more thickeners, and preservatives. This is a very good moisturizer for someone with exceptionally dry skin.

☺ **$$$ Night Cream** *($42.50 for 2 ounces)* is almost identical to the product above, and the same review applies.

☺ **$$$ Eye Cream** *($22.50 for 0.5 ounce)* is almost identical to the two creams above, and the same review applies.

☹ **The Cleanser for Dry Skin** *($13.50 for 5.8 ounces)* is a standard mineral oil–based cleanser that must be wiped off; it can leave a greasy film on the face.

☹ **The Cleanser for Normal/Combination Skin** *($12.50 for 5.8 ounces)* is a standard detergent-based, water-soluble cleanser that also contains glycerin, which can be soothing, and eucalyptus oil, which can be a skin irritant and can irritate the eyes.

☹ **The Soap for Oily Skin** *($9.50 for 3.8 ounces)* is a standard bar soap that also contains lemon and grapefruit extract, which can irritate and burn the skin and eyes. This product also contains tallow, which can cause breakouts.

☹ **The Remover** *($10.50 for 3.6 ounces)* is a standard detergent-based eye-makeup remover that can be slightly irritating.

☹ **The Toner for Oily Skin** *($12.50 for 7.8 ounces)* contains alcohol and eucalyptus oil; both are very irritating and can make oily skin oilier.

☹ **The Toner for Dry Skin** *($13.50 for 7.8 ounces)* contains witch hazel, eucalyptus oil, and sodium phosphate, which can be very irritating and drying for most skin types, particularly dry skin.

☹ **The Toner for Normal/Combination Skin** *($13.50 for 7.8 ounces)* is similar to the product above, with the addition of menthol, a skin irritant.

☺ **$$$ The Moisturizer for Dry Skin with SPF 8** *($13.50 for 1.8 ounces)* contains mostly water, slip agent, thickeners, glycerin, petrolatum, silicone oil, more thickeners, water-binding agents, vitamin E, shark oil, and preservatives. This would be a good moisturizer for someone with dry skin, but it does contain a small amount of eucalyptus oil, which can be a skin irritant for someone with sensitive skin. The sunscreen is good only for minimal sun exposure.

☺ **$$$ The Moisturizer for Normal/Combination Skin with SPF 8** *($13.50 for 1.8 ounces)* contains mostly water, thickeners, slip agent, more thickeners, silicone oil, more thickeners, vitamin E, soothing agent, water-binding agents, eucalyptus oil, and preservatives. Someone with combination skin will find this too emollient, and the small amount of eucalyptus oil can irritate sensitive skin, but it could be good for normal to dry skin.

☹ **The Oil-Free Moisturizer for Oily Skin SPF 8** *($13.50 for 1.8 ounces)* isn't oil-free; it contains mostly water, silicone oil, slip agent, talc, clay, thickeners, water-binding agents, more thickeners, and preservatives. All of the water-binding agents are useless when you also include water-absorbing agents such as talc and clay.

☺ **$$$ Under Makeup Moisture Cream** *($22 for 2 ounces)* is a very emollient moisturizer for very dry skin, but the second ingredient is isopropyl myristate, which can cause breakouts. The cream contains mostly water, thickener, lanolin oil, slip agent, mineral oil, more thickeners, plant oils, more thickeners, fragrance, and preservatives.

☺ **$$$ Under Makeup Moisture Lotion** *($26 for 4 ounces)* is identical to the cream above except that it is slightly less emollient, and the same review applies.

☺ **$$$ ProCollagen with Sunscreen** *($40 for 2 ounces)* contains mostly water, silicone oil, slip agents, water-binding agent, mineral oil, more water-binding agents, thickeners, and preservatives. Collagen is a good water-binding agent, but that's all. This would be a good moisturizer for someone with dry skin. There isn't enough sunscreen to adequately protect from the sun.

☺ **$$$ ProCollagen Face and Throat with Sunscreen** *($40 for 2 ounces)* is almost identical to the product above, and the same review applies.

☺ **$$$ ProCollagen Eyes with Sunscreen** *($26 for 0.9 ounce)* is almost identical to the product above, and the same review applies.

☺ **$$$ Megadose All Night Moisturizer** *($40 for 1.65 ounces)* contains mostly water, thickener, mineral oil, slip agents, more thickeners, plant oil, more thickeners, water-binding agents, vitamin E, fragrance, and preservatives. This is a good moisturizer for dry skin, nothing more.

☺ **$$$ Brighten Up, Tighten Up Eye Cream** *($19.50 for 0.5 ounce)* contains mostly water, a very long list of thickeners, glycerin, silicone oil, water-binding agents, plant extract, vitamins, anti-irritants, more water-binding agents, plant oil, more water-binding agents, more thickeners, and preservatives. This is a very good moisturizer for dry skin. The ingredient list is immense; if you want to try almost every water-binding agent in the book, this is the product to buy. Of course, it won't do anything a hundred other moisturizers can't do.

☺ **$$$ Smart Move** *($25 for 1.7 ounces)* contains mostly water, water-binding agent, thickener, slip agent, more thickeners, silicone oil, plant oil, more thickener, vitamin E, soothing agent, more thickeners, and preservatives. This is a good moisturizer for someone with dry skin.

☺ **$$$ Going Going Gone Makeup Remover** *($13 for 4 ounces)* is just an expensive cold cream. It contains isopropyl myristate, which can cause breakouts.

☹ **3-Minute Purifying Clay Mask** *($12.50 for 4 ounces)* is a standard clay mask that also contains peppermint oil, menthol, and eucalyptus oil, all of which can cause skin irritation.

☺ **$$$ 5-Minute Rehydrating Moisture Mask** *($12.50 for 4 ounces)* contains mostly water, thickeners, slip agents, more thickeners, water-binding agents, and preservatives. This is an OK mask, but it won't replenish your skin any better than a moisturizer will; also, this one contains a small amount of eucalyptus oil, a skin irritant.

☺ **$$$ 30-Second Refining Scrub Mask** *($12.50 for 4 ounces)* is a lightweight scrub that uses synthetic particles as the scrub agent. It also contains a small amount of eucalyptus oil, which can irritate the skin.

Ultima II Makeup

FOUNDATION: When I reviewed the foundations for Ultima II, it was clear that the line was going through a great deal of change. These products and colors were available at the time this book went to press.

☺ **Ultimate Coverage** *($18.50)* is an accurate self-description; use it only if you really want a heavy makeup to cover a skin discoloration. This is thick stuff, but it does blend easily. It provides medium to heavy coverage with a matte finish. **These colors are very good:** Aurora Beige, Cashew, Ivory Bisque, Manila, Natural Beige, and Tuscan Beige. **These colors are too pink or peach:** Bronze Umber and Dresden Peach.

☺ **The Nakeds Smoothing Line Makeup with SPF 10** *($20)* won't smooth lines, but it is a moist foundation that blends on smoothly with a sheer soft finish. **Almost all of the colors are excellent. This is the only color to avoid:** Cool 103, which is too peach for most skin tones.

☹ **The Nakeds Dual Cover Compact Makeup Wet or Dry** *($20)* has a poor, almost sticky texture and doesn't blend well. It tends to cake and can look uneven.

☺ **The Foundation Moisturizing Formula with SPF 6** *($24)* is a lightweight, soft foundation with great colors. **These colors are excellent:** F1Y, F2P, F3P (may turn pink), F5N, F8Y/N, F9Y, F10N, F11P, F12Y/N (may turn peach), and F13Y/N. F14Y/N and F15Y/N are both excellent colors for darker skin tones. **These colors are too peach for most skin tones:** F4Y, F6P, and F7.

☺ The Foundation Oil-Control Formula SPF 6 *($24)* is lightweight, soft, and matte, and also comes in great colors. Many of these foundations are divided into yellow-, pink-, and neutral-based tones, but you should never wear a pink-toned foundation just because your skin has pink undertones. **These colors are excellent:** F1Y, F2P, F5N, F7Y/N, F9Y (may turn yellow), F10N, F12N, and F13Y/N. F14Y/N and F15Y/N are both excellent colors for darker skin tones. **These colors are too peach, pink, orange, or yellow for most skin tones:** F3P, F4Y, F5, F6P, F8P/N, and F11P.

☹ **Wonder Wear Foundation with SPF 6 Oil-Free Makeup** *($20)* comes in great colors, goes on matte, and it wears and wears and wears. This is Ultima II's version of ColorStay Foundation and they share the same problems: they dry into place quickly and then don't budge, which makes blending difficult; they are hard to get off; and if you get the foundation on your nails it will wreck your manicure. It does last all day for someone with oily skin, but this kind of wear may not be so wonderful. **Most of the colors are quite reliable**; it is easier to list just the colors to watch out for. **These colors are too peach or pink:** 3-Neutral Cool, 6-Neutral Cool, 9-Neutral Cool, 11-Neutral, and 12-Neutral Cool.

☹ **Glowtion with SPF 15** *($20)* is a tinted moisturizer with SPF 15. It would be an OK option for a sunscreen with a hint of color, except that this product has sparkles that make the skin shine, making it good for fun wear only.

☺ <u>CONCEALER:</u> **The Concealer** *($11.50)* has a consistency that is smooth without being too dry or too greasy, and there's only a small chance it will slip into the lines around the eyes. There are only two shades, both good for lighter skin tones only. **Sexxxy Coverup** *($12)* goes on rather thick and dry and provides good coverage, but if you have any lines around your eyes, the matte dry finish will emphasize them. This product is an option only for someone with extremely smooth skin, but at least it doesn't tend to crease into the lines around the eyes. It comes in four very usable colors.

☺ $$$ <u>POWDER:</u> **The Nakeds Pressed Powder** *($16.50)* is a standard talc-based powder that has a great, silky-soft texture. The superior colors are numbered 1 to 6 and range from almost white to bronze.

☹ $$$ **The Nakeds Loose Powder** *($19.50)* has a slight shine, which defeats the purpose of a powder.

☹ <u>BLUSH:</u> **Powder Blush** *($16.50)* is a group of extremely shiny blushes. **Bronzing Duet** and **Cheek Duet** *($18.50)* are two shades in a compact, but one is extremely shiny.

☺ **$$$ Wonder Wear Cheek Color** *($16.50)* goes on smooth and even, and the beautiful colors are all wonderfully matte. **The Nakeds Cheek Color** *($16.50)* comes in a subtle range of colors, all of which are agreeably matte.

☺ **Blushing Cream** *($14)* is a standard cream blush that offers matte shades and some shiny ones. Only the matte ones are a real possibility. Although I generally don't recommend cream blush, this one has a very smooth texture and a slightly powdery finish.

☹ **EYESHADOW:** EyeSexxxy *($12)* eyeshadows come in a lipstick-type applicator and are exceptionally shiny. They come in just a handful of colors, but the shine is more than enough reason to avoid them. **Eye Shimmer Quad** *($20)* is just what the name implies, and I do not recommend it. **Nakeds Eye Color Duet** *($16.50)* comes in colors that are all shiny.

☺ **Wonder Wear Eye Color** *($15.50)* comes in a great selection of neutral matte shades that blend on evenly. These are duo sets, but the color combinations work well together. **These colors are excellent:** Wonder Gold/Wonder Chamois, Wonder Buff/Wonder Bare, Wonder Mocha/Wonder Blush, Wonder Thyme/Wonder Mint, Wonder Lilac/Wonder Lavender, Wonder Slate/Wonder Gray, Wonder Steel/Wonder Silver. **This combination is too green:** Wonder Wear Ivy/Wonder Moss.

☺ **The Nakeds Eye Color Single** *($12.50)* is a beautiful group of matte neutral shades. **All of the colors are worth checking out.**

☺ **EYE AND BROW SHAPER:** EyeSexxxy Liner *($12)* is an extremely standard pencil that comes in a twist-up applicator. The eye pencils have a sponge tip at one end to help soften lines after application. **Kohl Eye Pencil** *($11)* is just another standard eye pencil that goes on smooth. **BrowSexxxy** *($12)* is a standard pencil—talk about capitalizing on a name! **Brow Pencil** *($11)* is the same thing as BrowSexxxy; it just has a different name.

☺ **Brow Control** *($12)* is a brow color you apply like mascara. This is an excellent way to fill in the brow, and it comes in four good shades, one of which is clear.

☺ **LIPSTICK AND LIP PENCIL:** Ultima II has several types of lipstick in a wide range of colors, and there is little difference between some of them. The differences, when they do exist, consist mainly of ranges in texture, from creamy to extremely dry. **The Nakeds Matte & Lipchrome** *($13)* isn't all that matte, but it is a good creamy, opaque lipstick. **The Nakeds Lipchrome** *($13)* is a good creamy lipstick that's slightly on the glossy side. **Double Feature** *($13.50)* has a creamy, rich texture. **Never Wetter** *($13.50)* is fairly glossy but provides opaque coverage. **Super**

Luscious *($12)* is a very shiny lip gloss in the shape of a lipstick. **Couture** *($13)* is a very creamy, almost glossy lipstick. **LipSexxxy** *($12.50)* is the original ultra-matte lipstick; it has a very dry, extremely matte finish. It doesn't feel like a powder, but it definitely doesn't feel like a lipstick, nor is it all that sexy; as it wears off, it tends to peel. The texture isn't for everyone, but it is an ultra-matte look. Be careful with ultra-matte lipsticks during the winter; they make chapped lips worse. **Lip Glossy** *($12)* is a standard lip gloss in a tube applicator. **The LipLiner** *($11)* comes in a nice variety of colors and has a smooth texture, but is strictly standard-issue. **LipSexxxy Lip Liner** *($12)* is a standard lip pencil in a twist-up applicator.

☺ <u>MASCARA:</u> **Flutters Lengthening Mascara** *($13)* is simply sensational. It builds long, thick lashes easily and quickly, without a smudge or smear to be seen all day long. **Big Finish Mascara** *($13)* is excellent; it goes on well, doesn't clump, creates long lashes, and doesn't smear.

☻ **Falsies** *($13)* is an OK mascara that builds some length but very little thickness. It doesn't smudge or smear.

Vaseline Intensive Care and Dermasil (Skin Care Only)

☺ **Aloe Vera Triple Action Formula** *($3.19 for 10 ounces)* contains mostly water, glycerin, thickener, aloe, plant oil, more thickeners, vitamins A and E (antioxidants), several water-binding agents, a tiny amount of AHAs, silicone oil, more thickeners, and preservatives. This is a very good emollient moisturizer for someone with dry skin.

☺ **Aloe & Vitamins** *($3.19 for 10 ounces)* is almost identical to the product above, and the same review applies.

☺ **Dermatology Formula** *($4.99 for 11 ounces)* contains mostly water, petrolatum, mineral oil, glycerin, silicone oil, a long list of thickeners, and preservatives. This is a very emollient, very standard moisturizer for someone with dry skin.

☺ **Extra Strength Formula** *($3.19 for 10 ounces)* is similar to the product above, and the same review applies.

☺ **Extra Strength Triple Action Formula with Petroleum Jelly** *($3.19 for 10 ounces)* is similar to the Dermatology Formula above, and the same review applies.

☺ **Dry Skin Formula** *($3.19 for 10 ounces)* contains mostly water, glycerin, thickeners, mineral oil, more thickeners, silicone oil, more thickeners, and preservatives. This is an OK moisturizer for someone with dry skin.

☺ **Dry Skin Triple Action Formula with Alpha Hydroxy Complex** *($3.19 for 10 ounces)* contains mostly water, glycerin, thickener, plant oil, more thickeners, vitamins A and E, water-binding agents, a tiny amount of AHAs, silicone oil, more thickeners, and preservatives. The amount of AHAs is hardly worth mentioning; nevertheless, this is a good emollient moisturizer for someone with dry skin.

☺ **Sensitive Skin** *($3.19 for 10 ounces)* is basically just thickeners with petrolatum, mineral oil, and silicone oil. It also contains a minute amount of menthol, which doesn't help sensitive skin, but there isn't enough to affect the skin one way or the other. This is a good standard moisturizer for someone with dry skin.

☺ **Sensitive Skin with Vitamin E** *($3.19 for 10 ounces)* is almost identical to the product above, and the same review applies. It contains vitamin E, which can be considered an antioxidant.

☹ **Petroleum Jelly Cream Enriched with Vitamin E** *($2.77 for 4.5 ounces)* has, as its second ingredient, aluminum starch, which can be a skin irritant and cause breakouts.

☺ **Dermasil Dry Skin Concentrated Treatment** *($7.49 for 1 ounces)* contains mostly water, silicone oils, plant oils, and preservatives. This is a very good moisturizer for someone with dry skin.

☺ **Dermasil Dry Skin Treatment Cream** *($7.49 for 4 ounces)* is similar to the product above, and the same review applies.

☺ **Dermasil Dry Skin Treatment Lotion Controls Even Severe Dry Skin** *($7.49 for 8 ounces)* is similar to Dry Skin Concentrated Treatment above, but with petrolatum and mineral oil, which makes it even more emollient for someone with very dry skin.

Victoria Jackson

Victoria Jackson Cosmetics had one of the first cosmetics infomercials to hit the airwaves, and it has been amazingly successful. Almost everything you need to do a complete makeup application and cleansing routine is part of the **Introductory Kit** *($119.85)*. The makeup items include a brush set (no sponge tips), four eyeshadows, two shades of foundation in one compact, a retractable lip pencil, three retractable eye or brow pencils, four shades of lip color that come in a compact, two blushers, pressed translucent powder, mascara and lash conditioner, a packet of instruction cards, an instructional videotape, and reorder forms. Whew! Each item is marked with a price that's higher than what it costs as part of the kit. For example, the foundation is marked $24.95, although you receive it for $12.95 when you get it in the kit. In fact, all the

Victoria Jackson products have two prices. If you order a certain number of products, you can get the cheaper price every time. This is a cosmetics line that likes making deals.

But what about the products? Most of the makeup items are fine, although nothing special; a few don't work well at all. The few skin care products are supposed to be suitable for all skin types. It's an interesting and unusual concept, but skin care products for someone with oily skin cannot be the same as products for someone with extremely dry or even normal skin. This line is best for women with normal to dry skin; women with normal to oily or combination skin are not going to be happy. Still, I liked some of these products very much, and the prices (if you buy more than $20 worth of products at a time) are quite reasonable.

Once you place an order, you also start getting the product catalog. One of the "money-saving" offers includes groups of eyeshadows, eye pencils, blushes, and lipsticks divided into **Morning, Noon, and Night** *($89)*. These are three different intensities of makeup (a total of 15 products) in a color family of Red, Peach, or Pink; Morning is the softest, Noon is a little deeper, and Night is the darkest. This is more makeup than anyone needs, and it also assumes that you need drastically different makeup for morning than you need for afternoon and night. There are easier ways to change morning makeup into night makeup than buying entirely different sets of makeup. And that's not all: the eyeshadows are shiny and the lip colors are greasy. The blushes and pencils are nice enough, but they are fairly pricey when purchased individually.

One other product offered in the catalog is the **Ultimate Space-Saving Makeup Kit** *($49.95)*. It looks great in the picture—all your makeup packaged in a neat little box that unfolds in an organized, orderly fashion. It is indeed small and looks convenient, but the containers are not refillable, so once one runs out, refilling it is an expensive proposition.

The makeup demonstration videotape that came with the introductory kit was good and understandable, although I didn't always agree with Ms. Jackson's application techniques. For example, she recommends applying eyeliner and brow color before the eyeshadows, but that means the eyeshadows would likely undo or mess them up. Those are minor points, though. A more annoying feature is that half of the tape is like sitting through another ad, listening to Ms. Jackson and a guest celebrity talk about how great the products are. If you've got the tape, you've already bought the products; now you want to learn how to use them. I suppose that sometimes it's hard to stop selling.

Beauty Note: The prices listed below are the prices for the individual product, not the lower prices you get if you order a number of products.

Victoria Jackson Skin Care

☺ **Facial Cleanser and Eye Makeup Remover** *($12.50 for 4 ounces)* is a standard detergent-based wipe-off cleanser. You are supposed to wipe off your makeup using this watery cleanser applied to a cotton ball, and then rinse off any residue. Wiping off makeup pulls at the skin and can cause it to sag over time.

☺ **Toning Mist** *($13.50 for 4 ounces)* is a very good nonirritating toner that contains mostly water, aloe, water-binding agents, slip agent, and preservatives.

☺ **$$$ Moisturizer** *($19.50 for 2 ounces)* contains mostly water, thickeners, slip agents, more thickeners, water-binding agents, vitamins E and A, and preservatives. This would be a very good moisturizer for someone with dry skin.

☺ **Skin Renewal System** *($29.95 for 1.4 ounces of Extra-Intensive Eye Cream and 1.25 ounces of Extra-Intensive Night Cream)* is somewhat unusual. The Night Cream is in the bottom half of the jar, and the Eye Cream is in the top half. Very cute. However, the ingredients in each are not all that different, so the division seems unnecessary. The Eye Cream contains mostly water, thickener, tissular extract (it's anyone's guess as to what this is, but it certainly can't change your skin tissue), plant oil, mineral oil, water-binding agents, vitamins, and preservatives. The Night Cream contains mostly water, several thickeners, water-binding agents, anti-irritant, silicone oil, and preservatives. Both creams are very good moisturizers for dry skin.

☺ **$$$ Eye Repair Gel** *($18.50 for 0.5 ounce)* contains mostly water, slip agent, several water-binding agents, and preservatives. This would be a good lightweight moisturizer for the skin around the eyes.

☹ **Firming Gel Masque** *($16.50 for 4 ounces)* won't firm anything, and the second ingredient is a strong skin irritant. If your skin looks tighter after you take this mask off, it's due to the irritation.

Victoria Jackson Makeup

☺ **FOUNDATION:** Victoria Jackson offers only one type of **Foundation** *($24.95);* it comes in a single compact with two shades each for four categories of skin tones: Light, Medium, Tan, and Dark. The colors are good, though the Medium shades are a tad ashy green, the Light shade is a bit pink, and there is only one option for darker skin tones. To create the right color for your skin, you are supposed to mix the two shades together, which is fine if you know how to mix them in the right proportions. If you don't, you're likely to have trouble. The foundation is quite thick, and I would not call the application sheer, as the commercial claims. The foundation is petrolatum-based and therefore somewhat greasy. Oily or combination skins would not do well with this one.

☹ **CONCEALER:** There is no individually packed concealer in the Victoria Jackson line. The line suggests using the lighter shade of foundation in the dual foundation compact for the under-eye area. This would be a great idea if the foundation weren't so greasy. It easily slips into the lines under the eyes, and any liner you use will probably smear.

☺ **$$$ POWDER:** Pressed Powder *($16.95)* comes in four shades—Light, Medium, Tan, and Dark—and is talc-based. The colors are all fine and the texture is sheer and light.

☺ **$$$ BLUSH:** Each color-family kit (Peach, Red, and Pink) comes with a **Blush Compact** *($19.95)* that contains two colors. One is always a pale shade of peachy pink, and the other is more vivid. The textures and colors are very good. The Red kit's blush is a nice shade of coral (which is not red, by the way); the Pink kit's blush is a soft shade of pink; and the Peach kit's blush is a brown-peach shade that is probably too brown for most skin tones.

☹ **EYESHADOW:** The **Eyeshadow Compact** *($19.95)* is a single compact of four different colors. The combinations are excellent; unfortunately, almost all are slightly shiny.

😐 **EYE AND BROW SHAPER:** All of the **Eye Pencils** and **Brow Pencils** *($9.95)* are twist-up and have a great smooth texture, a bit on the dry side. There are three eye or brow pencils in each kit—Black, Chocolate Brown, and Taupe.

☹ **LIPSTICK AND LIP PENCIL:** Each Victoria Jackson color kit includes a **Lip Compact** *($17.95)* that contains three shades of lip cream and a lip-color powder. The colors are fine, but the lip creams are very greasy; if you have any problem with bleeding lipstick, these are not for you. The lip powder is a problem because it tends to cake on the lips and dry them out when used alone or when worn for an extended period of time. Lipsticks that come in tubes are listed on the order sheet, but there are no color swatches to assist you in making a decision. The kit includes a **Lip Pencil** *($9.95)* that matches the color categories of Peach, Pink, and Red.

☺ **MASCARA:** Every introductory kit comes with **Dual Black Mascara** *($13.95):* one end is a clear conditioner, the other a black mascara. The mascara is good, but the conditioner consists mostly of a plastic-like substance and glycerin. It won't do much for the lashes, and I didn't notice any difference when I used it. Victoria Jackson's traditional black **Mascara** *($13.95)* is great just by itself.

☹ **BRUSHES:** Victoria Jackson includes a set of brushes in the introductory kit that are adequate but not great. A **Retractable Brush Set** *($40)* that includes a retractable blush brush and a retractable lip brush is overpriced. The **Professional Brush Set** *($18.95)* includes a lip brush, an eyebrow brush/comb, a two-sided eyeshadow brush, and a blush brush. The brush bristles are sparse and not firm enough to hold the color well. There are better brushes on the market.

Yves Rocher (Skin Care Only)

If you have ever tuned in to the Home Shopping Channel, you've likely encountered a pitch for Yves Rocher products. Like any other cosmetics line, Yves Rocher capitalizes on hyperbole and misleading information. However, unique to Yves Rocher is an elaborate catalog that begins in the most absurd manner. The first page starts off by stating that Yves Rocher's "vision of cosmetics actually changed the world of beauty" and that his product line was the first to use plant essences. But farther down on the same page, Mr. Rocher is quoted as saying, "It's not correct that this idea originated with me." The company also claims that it has conducted research on the use of plant extracts for 35 years, but when I asked to see some of the research, I was told that was impossible. Research is research, and if it is not available publicly it is meaningless.

The catalog claims that Yves Rocher's new product line, Reponse Nature, uses the same mechanisms plants use to defend themselves against the environment. Interesting, but plants do not need to protect themselves from the sun, and they do not worry about wrinkling.

Actually, all of Yves Rocher's products seem to be based on some miraculous skin care breakthrough or miracle. It would seem that no one should have a wrinkle after using even one of these products. Of course that isn't possible, but you would never know it from the product write-ups in the catalog. Perhaps it's an attempt to justify the high prices, which range from $18 to $50 for an average of about 1.5 ounces of product.

Soin Clarifiant is the name of a small group of three products supposedly designed for acne-prone complexions. The company claims that using essential oils can purify your skin. They can't. Besides, there isn't all that much oil in these products, despite the claim, although any amount of oil should make someone with acne-prone skin very nervous. The ingredients are fairly typical of most acne products, and they don't work any better in Soin Clarifiant than they do anywhere else. Alcohol, salicylic acid, and grapefruit extract do nothing more than irritate the skin; they can't get rid of acne.

Yves Rocher's Bionutritive group of skin care products is seemingly designed for individuals with dry skin. The blurb in the catalog states quite clearly that when skin is "robbed of its natural moisture, [it] becomes increasingly vulnerable to the effects of physical aging." That just isn't true. Dry skin and aging are not associated. Although dry skin can look wrinkled, once you apply a moisturizer—almost any moisturizer—the wrinkles go away, and if the skin stays moist, the wrinkles won't come back. Permanent wrinkles that have been caused by sun damage are not affected by moisturizers. Bionutritive is supposed to work by using wheat germ and vitamins. But we know you can't feed the skin from the outside in, and many other Yves Rocher products contain wheat germ and vitamins, so why showcase them here? Probably because it reads so convincingly.

Yves Rocher does have its good points. The products are not tested on animals, all of them have a 100% money-back guarantee, and there are indeed some good products. Still, many of the claims are exaggerated, and the special ingredients make up only a small percentage of the actual products (usually less than 5%). The Yves Rocher customer service number is (800) 321-9837.

☺ **$$$ A.D.N. Vegetal Gentle Cleansing Wash** *($22 for 5 ounces)* is supposed to be a water-soluble cleanser, but with mineral oil and corn oil among the first ingredients, it will leave a film on the skin.

☺ **$$$ Hydra Vegetal Cleansing Wash** *($20 for 6.7 ounces)* is an OK cleanser that tends to leave a greasy film on the skin.

☺ **$$$ Meristem Gentle Cleanser** *($18 for 4.22 ounces)* is a fairly standard mild detergent cleanser that would work well for someone with normal to dry skin. Someone with oily skin might find it is not strong enough to take off makeup.

☹ **Soin Clarifiant Foaming Cleanser** *($15 for 2.7 ounces)* is a standard detergent cleanser that can be fairly drying for most skin types. The goal with oily skin is to clean it, not to dry it out. Creating dry skin doesn't stop oil production; it just creates an extra skin problem. This cleanser also contains salicylic acid, which can burn the eyes, so don't use it over the eye area.

☺ **$$$ Bionutritive Foaming Cleanser** *($21 for 6.7 ounces)* is a standard detergent cleanser that is too drying for most skin types.

☺ **$$$ Bionutritive Cleansing Milk** *($21 for 6.7 ounces)* is a mineral oil–based cleanser that leaves a greasy film on the skin.

☺ **$$$ Meristem Soothing Lotion** *($18 for 4.22 ounces)* contains mostly water, plant extracts, soothing agent, water-binding agents, thickeners, more soothing agent, fragrance (which is not great for sensitive skin types), and preservatives. This could be a good soothing toner for some skin types.

☹ **Soin Clarifiant Purifying Astringent** *($16 for 4.2 ounces)* contains water, alcohol, thickener, sage extract (which can be soothing), fragrance, grapefruit extract, citric extract, and preservatives. The alcohol can dry and irritate the skin.

☺ **$$$ Bionutritive Skin Reviving Fluid** *($21 for 6.7 ounces)* contains mostly water, plant extracts, water-binding agents, castor oil, fragrance, and preservatives. It won't revive the skin, but it is a good nonirritating toner.

☺ **$$$ Hydra Vegetal Moisturizing Toner** *($20 for 6.7 ounces)* contains mostly water, slip agents, water-binding agents, and preservatives. There are some amino acids at the end of the ingredient list; they can be good water-binding agents, but they are practically nonexistent here.

☺ **$$$ Reponse Nature Night Treatment** *($50 for 1.41 ounces)* contains mostly water, standard water-binding agent, plant extracts (including one containing a small amount of vitamin A), urea (an antiseptic and possible irritant), water-binding agent, thickeners, vegetable oils, more thickeners, jojoba oil, more water-binding agents, fragrance, and preservative. There are more ingredients following the fragrance and preservative, but their position this far down on the list makes them practically insignificant. Yves Rocher claims that botanical retinol (vitamin A) can somehow change the skin. There is no evidence that synthetic or natural vitamin A does anything to directly affect the skin. It isn't a bad ingredient, but it doesn't do what this product claims it can. The before-and-after pictures of a woman who used the product are impressive, but the company provides no information regarding the status of the woman's skin before she used the cream. That means her skin could have been parched, burnt, or irritated; in that case, any moisturizer would have made a dramatic difference. Also, without any comparison to a control group, the pictures are meaningless. Despite all that, except for the placement of the urea (which probably causes minor irritation to temporarily plump the skin), this is a very good emollient moisturizer for someone with dry skin.

☺ **$$$ Reponse Nature Daytime Complex Maximal Sun Protection SPF 8** *($35 for 0.99 ounce)* contains mostly water, plant extracts (including one containing a small amount of vitamin A; see the Response Nature Night Treatment review regarding that vitamin), water-binding agents, thickeners, plant oil, more thickeners, fragrance, and preservatives. There are more ingredients following the fragrance and preservative, but their position this far down on the list makes them practically insignificant. This is a good lightweight moisturizer that is good for limited sun exposure.

☺ **$$$ Hydra Vegetal 24 Hour Moisture Concentrate** *($22 for 1.35 ounces)* contains mostly water, standard water-binding agents, several thickeners, more water-binding agents (including several proteins), vegetable oils, preservative, and fragrance. There are more ingredients following the fragrance and preservative, but their position this far down on the list makes them practically insignificant. This is a good emollient moisturizer for dry skin.

☺ **$$$ A.D.N.—A.R.N. Time Defense Intensive Firming Complex for Face and Throat** *($75 for 1.69 ounces)* contains mostly water, plant extracts (supposedly containing DNA and RNA), thickeners, water-binding agents, plant oils, more thickeners, standard water-binding agents, protein, more thickeners, and preservatives. DNA and RNA can't be absorbed into the skin to repair cells or stop aging. This is a good emollient moisturizer, but it won't firm anything; it will just take care of dry skin.

☺ **$$$ Meristem Daytime Defense Lotion SPF 15** *($22 for 1.69 ounces)* contains mostly water, several thickeners, mineral oil, more thickeners, water-binding agents, and preservatives. The SPF 15 is nice, but this is a lot of money for an average moisturizer.

☺ **$$$ Meristem Soothing Night Cream** *($24 for 1.7 ounces)* contains mostly water, mineral oil, coconut oil, plant extracts, thickeners, soothing agent, beeswax, standard water-binding agents, lanolin, vitamin E, fragrance, and preservatives. This would be a good emollient moisturizer for someone with dry to very dry skin.

☹ **Oil-Free Balancing Gel** *($19.95 for 1.7 ounces)* contains mostly water, alcohol, standard water-binding agents, thickeners, grapefruit extract, more thickeners, an antiseptic, more thickeners, vitamins A and E, glycerin, and preservatives. Alcohol and grapefruit can't control oil, but they can irritate the skin.

☺ **$$$ Rich Eye Creme** *($28 for 0.5 ounce)* contains mostly water, standard water-binding agents, corn oil, thickeners (including isopropyl myristate, which may cause blackheads), lanolin oil, plant extracts, more thickeners, fragrance, and preservatives. This is definitely a rich moisturizer, but nothing in here will change or prevent one wrinkle on your face.

☹ **Soin Clarifiant Rebalancing Gel** *($16 for 1.05 ounces)* is an alcohol-based gel that won't rebalance anything, but it can be quite drying and irritating.

☺ **$$$ Bionutritive Activating Concentrate** *($35 for 1 ounce)* contains mostly water, thickener, wheat germ extract, water-binding agent, collagen, corn oil, wheat germ oil, thickener, and preservatives. It would be a very good moisturizer for someone with dry skin.

☺ **$$$ Bionutritive Day Creme** *($24 for 1.4 ounces)* would be a good daytime moisturizer for someone with dry skin if it contained a sunscreen of SPF 15, but it doesn't; this is best used indoors only.

☺ **$$$ Bionutritive Night Creme** *($28 for 1.4 ounces)* contains mostly water, thickener, plant oils, water-binding agents, a lot more thickeners, more water-binding agents, fragrance, and preservatives. This would be a very good moisturizer for someone with dry skin.

☺ **$$$ Hydra Vegetal Moisture Concentrate** *($35 for 1.4 ounces)* contains mostly water, slip agents, water-binding agents, several thickeners, urea, amino acid, several water-binding agents, plant oils, preservatives, and fragrance. It would be a good lightweight moisturizer for someone with normal to dry skin.

Yves St. Laurent

Many of the upper-end (meaning expensive) cosmetics lines have an air of snobbery about them. The salespeople seem to sniff at you in disdain if you look as if you don't have money to spend, ask pointed questions, or seem in any way startled by the prices. Yves St. Laurent fits into this category, which is a shame, because some of its products are quite lovely. I found this snobbish attitude not only at the cosmetics counters but at their customer service department as well. My recommendation to management is to drop the attitude; it will only help you sell more product.

Yves St. Laurent Skin Care

☹ **Foaming Cleansing Gel** *($24 for 6.6 ounces)* is a standard detergent-based, water-soluble cleanser that rinses well and takes off all the makeup. The detergent cleansing agent can be very drying and may cause skin irritation, not to mention burn the eyes.

☺ **$$$ Soothing Creme Cleanser** *($24 for 6.6 ounces)* is a standard mineral oil–based cleanser. It can leave a greasy film on the skin and requires a washcloth to really get off all the makeup, which is not very soothing.

☺ **$$$ Instant Cleansing Milk** *($24 for 6.6 ounces)* is similar to the product above, and the same review applies.

☺ **$$$ Gentle Eye Makeup Remover** *($22.50 for 2.5 ounces)* is a silicone oil–based wipe-off makeup remover. Pulling at the eye area causes the skin to sag and is never a good idea.

☹ **Extra-Gentle Tonic Alcohol-Free** *($24 for 6.6 ounces)* contains mostly slip agents, fragrance, film former, plant extracts, and preservatives. This is mostly fragranced water. It's about as do-nothing a skin care product as I've ever seen.

☺ **$$$ Mild Clarifying Tonic** *($24 for 6.6 ounces)* is a silicone oil–based toner that also contains sodium phosphate, which can be a skin irritant. This isn't all that mild, and it's overpriced for what you get.

☺ **$$$ Oil-Control Tonic** *($24 for 6.6 ounces)* is a standard alcohol-based toner that won't control oil, but will irritate the skin.

☺ **$$$ Day/Night Concentrate, Concentrated Revitaliser** *($90 for two 0.5-ounce bottles)* consists of two products. The Day Concentrate contains mostly water, film former, slip agent, plant extracts, thickener, and preservatives. Several water-binding agents and vitamins are included, but they are present in such minuscule amounts that they don't benefit the skin at all. The Night Concentrate contains mostly plant oils, thickeners, water-binding agents, vitamin E, and preservatives. This is one of the most overpriced combinations of ordinary moisturizers you may encounter. They're not bad for your skin; they're just not very good.

☺ **$$$ Hydro-Light Day Lotion Oil-Free with SPF 15** *($35 for 1.3 ounces)* contains mostly water, slip agent, vitamin E (antioxidant), thickeners, and preservative. There is a long list of other ingredients after the preservative, which means they are barely present. This is an extremely ordinary but good basic daytime sunscreen for someone with normal to oily skin, but it's a waste of money to spend this much for something so dull.

☺ **$$$ Hydro-Light Day Lotion with SPF 15** *($50 for 3 ounces)* contains mostly water, silicone oil, film former, glycerin, thickeners, vitamin E, more silicone oil, plant oil, more thickeners, mineral oil, and preservatives. There are some interesting water-binding agents at the end of the ingredient list, which means they amount to little more than air. This is still a good sunscreen for someone with dry skin, but it's completely standard and hardly worth the price.

☺ **$$$ Absolute Hydration** *($57 for 1 ounce)* contains mostly water, thickener, silicone oils, more thickener, slip agents, more thickeners, plant extract, preservative, and fragrance. There are some interesting water-binding agents at the end of the ingredient list, which means they amount to little more than air. This is a good moisturizer for someone with dry skin, but it's completely standard and hardly worth the price.

☺ **$$$ Prevention + /Time Prevention Day Creme** *($65 for 1.7 ounces)* contains mostly water, thickener, silicone oil, a long list of other thickeners, vitamins E and C, more thickeners, and preservatives. This is a good but standard moisturizer for someone with dry skin. The vitamin C is supposed to be wonderful for the skin; it can be a good antioxidant, but that's it. This cream is one of many vitamin C products making great claims for being a fountain of youth; it isn't.

☺ **$$$ Fruit Jeunesse Firming Renewal Complex Glucohydroxy Acid** *($50 for 1 ounce)* contains mostly water, silicone oil, glycerin, thickener, AHAs, slip agent, more silicone oils, vitamin E, water-binding agent, plant oil, soothing agent, and preservatives. This is a good 4% AHA product that can be good for someone with dry, sensitive skin, but there are plenty of cheaper and equally good, if not better, AHA products on the market.

☺ **$$$ Hydro-Intensive Day Creme** *($50 for 1.6 ounces)* contains mostly water, thickeners, slip agents, water-binding agent, petrolatum, vitamin E, more thickeners, mineral oil, and preservatives. This is a fairly ordinary, but good moisturizer for dry skin, with a small amount of sunscreen. Many of the good moisturizing ingredients come way after the preservatives and don't amount to much.

☺ **$$$ Hydro-Light Day Creme** *($50 for 1.6 ounces)* is identical to the Hydro-Intensive Day Creme above except that it also includes petrolatum and sunscreen. The SPF is too low to protect from the sun, but the petrolatum makes the cream slightly more emollient.

☺ **$$$ Intensive Nighttime Revitalizer** *($55 for 1 ounce)* contains mostly water, thickener, silicone oils, water-binding agents, more thickeners, plant oil, mineral oil, a small amount of sunscreen (which is strange in a night cream), preservatives, and fragrance. Vitamins A and E are in here, but they're too far down on the list to count. This is a good emollient moisturizer for dry skin, but it's nothing special.

☺ **$$$ Nighttime Revitalizer** *($55 for 1 ounce)* is almost identical to the Intensive Nighttime Revitalizer above, with a few minor differences (like no sunscreen) and a tiny amount of AHAs—only enough to be water-binding agents, not exfoliants. This is a good emollient moisturizer for dry skin, but it's nothing special.

☺ **$$$ Smoothing Eye Contour Gel** *($45 for 0.5 ounce)* contains mostly water, slip agent, thickener, plant extract, soothing agent, and preservatives. There are some other interesting water-binding ingredients, but they come well after the preservatives, which makes them useless. Other than that, this is a good lightweight moisturizer for the eye area.

☺ **$$$ Time Interceptor Fortifying Complex** *($65 for 1 ounce)* contains water, slip agent, mineral oil, water-binding agent, preservatives, and fragrance. There are some other interesting water-binding agents, but they come well after the preservatives, which makes them worthless. This is a lot of money for mineral oil and thickeners, but the product can be good for dry skin.

☺ **$$$ Hydro-Active Moisture Masque** *($35 for 1.6 ounces)* contains mostly water, mineral oil, film former, thickeners, plant oil, more thickeners, vitamin E, water-binding agents, and preservatives. This is a good, emollient, though completely ordinary moisturizer/mask for dry skin.

☹ **Instant Clarifying Masque** *($30 for 2.5 ounces)* contains mostly water, glycerin, detergent cleansing agent (one that is known for being very drying and irritating) plant oil, thickeners, film former, and preservatives. The ingredients are rather ordinary and the exotic plants come well after the preservatives, making them totally insignificant.

Yves St. Laurent Makeup

☺ **$$$ FOUNDATION: Teint Sur Mesure Duo De Teint** *($65 for 1 ounce)* is two separate products, foundation and concealer, in the same container. The six shades offered are a limited assortment; clearly, Yves St. Laurent doesn't expect women of color to shop at its counters. The notion is to use the concealer over any area on the face that you want to appear lighter—particularly the lines around the mouth, forehead, and eyes—or all over if you wish, before or after applying the foundation. It's a standard technique that can be accomplished with any good concealer and foundation. The texture is surprisingly light and sheer, with a dry, almost matte finish, even though it blends on rather moist and smooth. This is a very good foundation for someone with normal to slightly oily or combination skin. It doesn't settle into lines or streak. **These colors are excellent:** Golden Blond, Savannah Blond, Sandy Beige, Smoky Beige, and Tender Ivory. **This color is too rose for most skin tones:** Pale Pink.

☺ **$$$ Line Smoothing Foundation** *($44)* doesn't smooth lines, but it does have a lovely silky texture. It goes on easily and blends well with the skin, providing medium to slightly heavy coverage. The sales pitch is that it has light-reflecting properties. One salesperson said that meant it would light up the dark areas in my wrinkles. Please! It simply can't do that. **These colors are excellent:** 3, 5, 7, 8, 9, and 10. **These colors should be avoided:** 1, 2, 4, and 6.

☺ **$$$ Teint Libre Moisturizing Foundation** *($32.50)* comes in only four shades, but the colors are good, and the texture is very light and smooth, with a dewy moist finish.

☹ **$$$ Teint Mat Oil-Free Foundation SPF 12** *($31)* is not oil-free; it contains silicone oil. SPF 12 is a pretty good rating. The fancy marketing language says this product has microparticles that can capture sebum (oil). Well, the ingredients are clay and magnesium—not the least bit fancy or unique. Other than that, it is a good, partially matte foundation, best for someone with normal to slightly oily skin. **These colors are great: 2, 3, 4, and 5. These colors are should be avoided: 1 and 6.**

Teint Perfect Powder *($36.50)* wasn't available for review before this book went to press. I will review it in my newsletter as soon as it is available.

☹ **Premier Teint Matte** *($31)* is supposed to contain self-adapting pigments that even out skin tone. Each of the four colors is shiny and either white, orange, or pink. One color is neutral but still shiny. A matte product that contains shine—what were they thinking?

☹ **Teint Spontane** *($31)* is an ultra-sheer face color/moisturizer that rubs very red or orange color over the face with a slight shine.

☺ **$$$ CONCEALER: Radiant Touch** *($32.50)* is an impressive concealer with only one good color (the only other color available is too peach for most skin tones). It is marketed as a way to touch up makeup at the end of the day, the equivalent of "plastic surgery in less than a minute." The concealer is automatically fed into the brush tip like a pen; it is a very sheer cream, lightweight and moist, and doesn't crease into the lines around the eyes. It really does help to apply this under the eyes or on top of the cheekbones at the end of the day for a lift. If you've ever tried to put under-eye concealer on a second time to touch up your makeup, you know how thick that can feel. This product eliminates that problem. Ignore the plastic surgery comment—it doesn't work *that* well.

☹ **Anti-Cernes** *($32.50)* is a greasy mess and easily creases into the lines around the eyes. The two colors are just OK.

☹ **$$$ POWDER: Silk Finish Pressed Powder** *($33)* has a wonderful silky texture, and some of the colors are quite good. **These are the best colors: 3 and 6. The other colors are too pink or peach. Silk Finish Loose Powder** *($33.50)* has a smooth, satiny feel, and all the colors are very good. **Semi Loose Powder** *($55)* comes in a cake form, but the container shaves off the top layer when you twist it, creating a loose powder. It's less messy than a loose powder, but the reason for a loose powder is to eliminate the waxy ingredients that hold a pressed powder together and tend to create a caked look on the face when you overdo it.

☹ **Sunny Complexion Powder** *($35)* has a great silky texture, but is too shiny.

☹ <u>**BLUSH:**</u> **Variation Blush** *($31)* and **Blushing Powder** *($30)* are way too shiny, even though the textures are quite silky.

☹ <u>**EYESHADOW:**</u> All of the eyeshadows are ultra-shiny or too blue or contrasting. Why would any woman want to wear yellow and blue eyeshadow, or pink and green? What a shame, because the texture is quite nice. **Perfecting Eyeshadow** *($31)* contains at least one shiny eyeshadow in almost every set, which means it's perfect at making the eye area look wrinkly. **These are the only colors worth considering: 3 and 5. Variation Solo** *($31)* is a quad set, but two of the shades are shiny. **Eyeshadow Powder Duo** *($31)* is mostly ultra-shiny colors. **This is the only good combination of matte colors: 3.**

☺ **$$$** <u>**EYE AND BROW SHAPER:**</u> **Eyeliner Moire** *($32)* has six extremely iridescent, vivid colors with matching mascara. I'm sure there's a reason for this fashion statement, but I can't figure out what it might be. The small selection of **Eye Pencils** *($16.50)* and **Eye Brow Pencils** *($15)* are ordinary but fine. The **Automatic Pencil** *($33.50; $10 for a refill)* comes in five shades, is convenient to use, and extremely standard. The Eyebrow Pencil has a dry mascara wand on one end to stroke through the brow after you apply the pencil. Good idea, but a less expensive pencil and an old clean mascara brush can do the same thing for a fraction of the price.

☺ **$$$** <u>**LIPSTICK AND LIP PENCIL:**</u> **Rouge Intense** *($24.50)* is a somewhat matte lipstick with a vivid array of colors; it contains a tint, which means the color stays on somewhat longer. It does tend to feather. **Sheer Conditioning Lipstick** *($22.50)* has a soft, creamy, beautiful texture and feels great. **Pure Lipstick** *($24.50)* is a very greasy cream lipstick that tends to feather easily and doesn't stay well, despite the tint. **Rouge Definition** *($24.50)* is Yves St. Laurent's version of a matte lipstick. It comes in a tube and dries to a flat finish. It's OK, but for the money it can't even begin to compete with Revlon's ColorStay. **Lip Liner Pencil** *($16)* is completely standard and completely overpriced.

☺ **$$$** <u>**MASCARA:**</u> **Conditioning Mascara** *($20.50)* is good, but for this price it should be great.

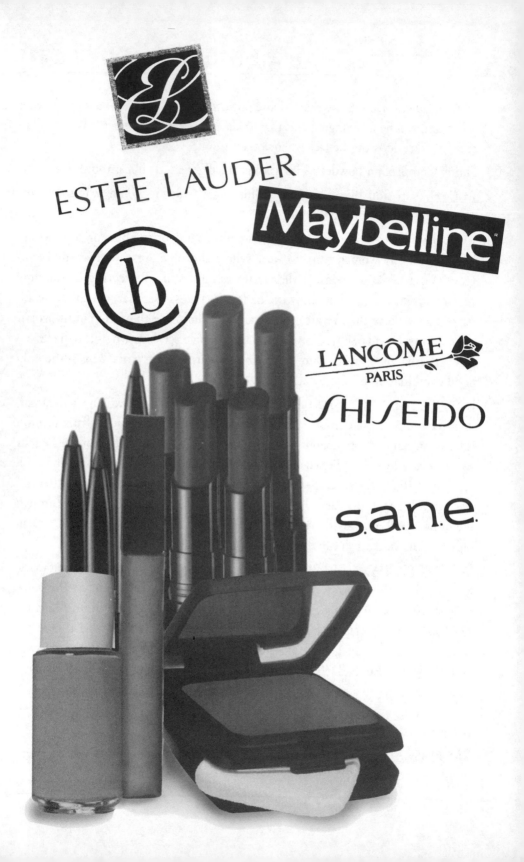

THE BEST PRODUCTS

The following product lists summarize the individual reviews in Chapter 7. Be sure to read these more-detailed product evaluations before making any decisions. I hope all of these recommendations will make you feel informed and confident when shopping for makeup and skin care.

Beauty Note: Most cosmetics companies recommend skin care routines for specific skin types. It is my strong suggestion that you ignore their categories and the corresponding products. A person with dry skin who follows the cosmetics companies' recommendations could end up using too many products that will overgrease the skin and cause buildup, making the skin look dull. Someone with oily skin will most likely be sold products that contain strong irritants that can make oily and acned skin worse. **Please consider each product individually for its quality and value to your skin, instead of its placement in a series of products, its promotional ads or brochures, and the sales pitches you are likely to hear.**

Best Cleansers

Perhaps I was too emphatic years ago when I began nagging about the need for water-soluble cleansers. In those days, the only products available to clean the face were wipe-off cleansers and bar soaps (which were all drying, regardless of the claims on the packaging). Now there are more water-soluble cleansers than I ever thought possible. Not all of them are really water-soluble and many are too drying, but several are very gentle on the skin, remove all the makeup without causing irritation or dryness, do not burn the eyes, and leave no greasy residue. It is also essential that a water-soluble cleanser can be removed easily by splashing and not by being wiped off with a damp washcloth.

Using a washcloth might prevent the water from dripping all around the sink after you're done splashing, but washcloths can cause irritation, and that's not great for the skin.

One thing most water-soluble cleansers have in common, regardless of price, is the basic ingredient list. Cleansers designed for dry skin often contain oils and leave a greasy residue. The problem when someone with dry skin uses a cleanser supposedly designed for her skin type, and then follows that with a rich creamy moisturizer, is that too many emollients can build up, causing the skin to look dull and preventing cell turnover. Cleansers designed for normal to oily skin can contain one or more standard detergent agents that will dry out the skin. Using a drying cleanser on oily skin inevitably means using a moisturizer, and moisturizers used on a regular basis all over the face are almost always a problem for someone with oily or combination skin. Besides, this cycle of drying out oily or combination skin and then following up with a moisturizer is the fastest way I know to cause more skin problems.

Most of the cleansers listed below are for normal to oily/combination skin types. A number of cleansers are made for drier skin types, but they are almost all greasy and require being wiped off. I have found only a handful that are not drying and rinse off completely without leaving any residue.

For normal to oily/combination skin types, the best water-soluble cleansers are: **Adrien Arpel** Aromafleur Petal Daily Cleanser; **Alexandra de Markoff** Complete Foaming Cleanser; **Alpha Hydrox** Foaming Face Wash; **Artistry by Amway** Clarifying Cleansing Gel for Normal to Oily Skin; **Aveda** Purifying Gel Cleanser; **Avon** Anew Perfect Cleanser, Daily Revival Oil-Clearing Cleanser Oily Skin, and Daily Revival Gentle Cleanser for Normal/Combination Skin; **Basis** Facial Cleanser for Normal to Dry Skin; **BeautiControl** Purifying Cleansing Gel; **Beauty Without Cruelty** Alpha Hydroxy Facial Cleanser; **Black Opal** Oil Free Cleansing Gel; **Bobbi Brown** Face Cleanser and Gel Cleanser; **The Body Shop** Tea Tree Oil Facial Wash, Balancing Cleansing Gel for Normal to Oily Skin, and Oil-Free Cleansing Wash for Oily Skin; **Clarins** Oil-Control Cleansing Gel Oily Skin; **Clean & Clear** Sensitive Skin Foaming Facial Cleanser and Sensitive Skin Foaming Facial Cleanser; **Clinique** Wash-Away Gel Cleanser; **Fashion Fair** Gentle Facial Shampoo Mild for Dry, Sensitive Skin; **Flori Roberts** Optima Gel Cleanser Gold Oil-Free; **Guerlain** Evolution Purifying Foaming Gel; **H$_2$O Plus** Cleansing Gel; **Lancome** Clarifiance Oil-Free Gel Cleanser; **M.A.C.** pH Balanced Cleanser; **Marcelle** Gentle Foaming Wash for Sensitive Skin Types Hypo-Allergenic, Liquid Cleanser for Combination Skin, Aquarelle Oil-Free Purifying Cleansing Gel for Oily Skin, and Cleansing Milk for Combination Skin Hypo-Allergenic; **Murad** Refreshing Skin Cleanser; **Nivea Visage** Hydro-Cleansing Gel; **Neutrogena** Fresh

Foaming Cleanser Soap-Free Cleanser for Combination Skin; **Oil of Olay** Sensitive Skin Foaming Face Wash; **Orlane** Detoxinating Purifying Gel Cleanser; **Paula's Choice** One Step Face Cleanser for Normal to Oily/Combination Skin; **Sea Breeze** Foaming Face Wash for Normal to Oily Skin, Foaming Face Wash for Sensitive Skin, and Whipped Facial Cleanser; **Stridex** Clear Antibacterial Face Wash, Maximum Strength.

For normal to dry/sensitive skin, the best cleansers are: BeautiControl Chamomile Balancing Cleansing Lotion; **Beauty Without Cruelty** Herbal Cream Facial Cleanser; **The Body Shop** Foaming Cleansing Cream for Normal to Dry Skin; **Donna Karan** Formula for Clean Skin; **Estee Lauder** Instant Action Rinse-Off Cleanser; **Galderma** Cetaphil Cleanser; **Hydron** Best Defense Gentle Cleansing Creme; **M.D. Formulations** Facial Cleanser Basic; **Monteil** Ice Super Soft Rinse-Off Cleanser; **Paula's Choice** One Step Face Cleanser for Normal to Dry Skin; **Trish McEvoy** Essential Cleanser; **Ultima II** Interactives Clean Team Cleanser + Toner Normal/Oily; **Yves Rocher** Meristem Gentle Cleanser.

Best Exfoliants

This used to be an easy area of discussion. Most beauty experts, as well as dermatologists and plastic surgeons, agree that exfoliating is a wonderful way to take care of both oily and dry skin. A few years back, before Retin-A, there weren't many options when it came to getting dead skin cells off the face. During most of the '70s and '80s the only choices were scrubs with ingredients such as honey and almond pits, cleansers with scrub particles, facial masks, and irritating toners. Most of these options took a toll on the face, and irritation was a typical problem. Then and now my favorite recommendation for a scrub is mixing Cetaphil Lotion with baking soda to create an effective, gentle, and inexpensive scrub. Other scrubs, with their detergent cleansing agents and wax bases, just can't compare, not to mention the extraordinarily reasonable price of baking soda and Cetaphil Lotion. But now the topic has gotten more complicated with the addition of alpha hydroxy acid products, which exfoliate the skin chemically instead of physically.

If you decide to use an AHA product, particularly one from my list of recommendations, the question is, Do you still need to use a physical scrub? The answer isn't all that easy, and you will have to judge for yourself. Most women with normal to dry/sensitive skin should probably use only the AHA product and no other exfoliant. Someone with normal to oily skin should probably still use a scrub on areas with breakouts. Stick with Cetaphil Lotion and baking soda for the most gentle results and listen closely to your skin; irritation is never the goal.

For **normal to oily/combination skin**, the best scrubs are: The Body Shop Foaming Gel Scrub for Normal to Oily & Oily Skin; **Fashion Fair** Gentle Facial Polisher for All Skin Types; **Physicians Formula** Beauty Exfoliating Scrub; **Sea Breeze** Exfoliating Facial Scrub.

For **normal to dry skin, the best scrubs are:** Christian Dior Equite Exfoliating Gel; **Guerlain** Evolution Exfoliating Creme for the Face; **Hydron** Best Defense Micro-Exfoliating Creme; **La Prairie** Essential Exfoliator.

For **normal to oily/combination skin, the best alpha hydroxy acid products are:** **Artistry by Amway** Moisture Essence Serum with Alpha Hydroxy Acids; **Color Me Beautiful** Refining Toner; **Elizabeth Arden** Alpha-Ceramide; **La Prairie** Age Management Line Inhibitor, Age Management Serum, and Age Management Intensified Serum; **M.D. Formulations** Facial Lotion with 12% Glycolic Compound and Forte I Facial Lotion with 15% Glycolic Compound; **Paula's Choice** 8% Alpha Hydroxy Acid Solution; **Trish McEvoy** Glycolic Lotion.

For **normal to dry skin, the best alpha hydroxy acid products are:** Alpha Hydrox Enhanced Creme All Skin Types 10% AHA, Sensitive Skin Creme 5% AHA, Lotion for Normal to Dry Skin 8% AHA, Hand and Body Lotion 8% AHA, and Creme 8% AHA for Normal Skin; **Avon** Anew Perfecting Complex for the Face and Anew Intensive Treatment for the Face; **Black Opal** Skin Retexturizing Complex with Alpha-Hydroxy Acids; **BeautiControl** Regeneration Face and Neck Complex, Regeneration Face and Neck Complex 2, Regeneration for Oily Skin, and Regeneration for Oily Skin 2; **Bobbi Brown** Face Lotion; **Color Me Beautiful** Glycolic Treatment for the Face and Visible Results for All Skin Types; **La Prairie** Age Management Night Cream; **Lubriderm** Moisture Recovery Creme; **M.D. Formulations** Smoothing Complex with 10% Glycolic Compound, Night Cream with 14% Glycolic Compound, and Forte I Facial Cream with 15% Glycolic Compound; **Monteil** Skin Reform Fluid Energizer; **Murad** Advanced Skin Smoothing Lotion and Advanced Skin Smoothing Cream; **Neostrata** Skin Smoothing Cream, Skin Smoothing Lotion, and Sensitive Skin AHA Face Cream; **Neutrogena** Healthy Skin Face Lotion; **Nivea** Inner Beauty Daytime Renewal Treatment Natural AlpHA Complex: **Paula's Choice** 8% Alpha Hydroxy Acid Solution; **Pond's** Age Defying Complex, Age Defying Complex for Delicate Skin Age Defying Lotion, and Age Defying Lotion for Delicate Skin; **Principal Secret** Alpha Hydroxy Booster Complex; **Rachel Perry** Visible Transition 5% Alpha-Hydroxy Serum: Patented Prolonged Release Liposomes and Visible Transition 10% Alpha-Hydroxy Serum: Patented Prolonged Release Liposomes; **Trish McEvoy** Glycolic Face Cream; **Yves St. Laurent** Fruit Jeunesse Firming Renewal Complex Glucohydroxy Acid.

Best Toners

I have been preaching for years about the need to use only nonirritating, alcohol-free toners, and I am pleased to say that the cosmetics industry has finally listened. But keep in mind that alcohol-free does not mean irritant-free. Unfortunately, many cosmetics lines stick other irritating ingredients in their toners.

Toners and all the products that fall into this category (refining lotions, clarifying lotions, soothing tonics, stimulating lotions, fresheners, and astringents) are an extra cleansing step and sometimes they can be soothing and moisturizing. I evaluated these products strictly on how soothing and clean they felt on the face without drying the skin or leaving a greasy residue. It is not best to use toners that exfoliate the skin because they almost always contain extra irritants that can do more damage than the skin handle.

Does it make sense to spend a lot of money on a toner if it doesn't contain irritating ingredients? No. I found excellent toners that had very gentle ingredients and were relatively inexpensive. Many women enjoy using these products, and because of the soothing, fresh feeling many irritant-free toners can provide, I feel they can be beneficial for many skin types.

For normal to oily/combination skin, the best toners are: Aveda Skin Firming/Toning Agent; **Black Opal** Purifying Astringent; **The Body Shop** Honey Water and Tea Tree Oil Freshener; **Clarins** Toning Lotion for Dry to Normal Skin; **EsteeLauder** Clean Finish Purifying Toner N/O; **Hydron** Best Defense Botanical Toner; **Lancome** Tonique Douceur Non-Alcoholic Freshener for Dry/Sensitive Skin; **La Prairie** Age Management Balancer; **L'Oreal** Plenitude Hydrating Floral Toner; **M.A.C.** PA-3 Phyto-Astringent Purifying Toner; **Mary Kay** Gentle Action Freshener; **Neutrogena** Alcohol-Free Toner; **Paula's Choice** Final Touch Toner for Normal to Oily/Combination Skin; **Rachel Perry** Violet Rose Skin Toner.

For normal to dry skin, the best toners are: Artistry by Amway Moisture Rich Toner for Normal to Dry Skin; **BeneFit** Benevitale; **The Body Shop** Hydrating Freshener for Normal to Dry & Dry Skin and Cucumber Water; **Chanel** Firming Freshener; **Circle of Beauty** Skin Refiner Dry Type 4 and Skin Refiner Dehydrated Type 5; **Clarins** Extra-Comfort Toning Lotion for Very Dry or Sensitized Skin; **Erno Laszlo** HydrapHel Skin Supplement Freshener for Extremely Dry and Dry Skin; **Estee Lauder** Clear Finish Purifying Toner N/D and Verite Soothing Spray Toner; **Forever Spring** Ambrosia Skin Refresher; **La Prairie** Cellular Refining Lotion; **Marcelle** Hydractive Alcohol-Free Reviving Toner for Normal to Dry Skin; **Nivea** Alcohol Free Moisturizing Facial Toner; **Origins** Comforting Solution If Your Skin Acts Sensitive and Drenching

Solution; **Orlane** B21 Bio-Energic Vivifying Lotion for All Skins; **Paula's Choice** Final Touch Toner for Normal to Dry Skin; **Physicians Formula** Gentle Refreshing Toner for Dry to Very Dry Skin and Purifying Facial Toner for Normal to Dry Skin; **Revlon** Moon Drops Comforting Toner Alcohol-Free Sensitive/Delicate and Moon Drops Softening Toner Normal to Dry; **Shiseido** Benefiance Balancing Softener and Vital Perfection Balancing Softener; **Victoria Jackson** Toning Mist; **Yves Rocher** Meristem Soothing Lotion, Bionutritive Skin Reviving Fluid, and Hydra Vegetal Moisturizing Toner.

For skin prone to breakouts, the best toners and gels are: **Clean & Clear** Dr. Prescribed Acne Medicine Extra Strength and Dr. Prescribed Acne Medication Maximum Strength; **Fostex** 10% Benzoyl Peroxide Vanishing Gel; **Mary Kay** Acne Treatment Gel; **M.D. Formulations** Benzoyl Peroxide 5% for Extremely Oily and Acne-Prone Skin and Benzoyl Peroxide 10% for Extremely Oily and Acne-Prone Skin; **Oxy 10** Maximum Strength Vanishing Acne Medication and Sensitive Vanishing Acne Medication; **ProActiv** Revitalizing Toner and Repairing Lotion.

Best Moisturizers

Women always ask me which moisturizer is the best or what one product will really do something about wrinkles. Wrinkle creams are a fairy tale (except for sunscreens), but what isn't a fantasy is the fact that there are a lot of great moisturizers to be found. This category includes lotions, creams (even so-called wrinkle creams), specialty creams, day creams, replenishers, liposome creams, and every imaginable cream for the purpose of eliminating dry skin. All these concoctions and combinations do the same thing— moisturize the skin—and they do an excellent job. The repetitive ingredients found in product line after product line just don't warrant the outlandish claims, ridiculous prices, or your attention.

Surprisingly enough, when I ignored the claims and price tags, I liked most of the moisturizers I reviewed. There are some remarkably emollient moisturizers on the market, in all price categories, with great ingredients that can take care of varying degrees of dry skin. Only a handful contain ingredients that I thought were potentially harmful to the skin or would dry it out and cause irritation.

The problem for most women is finding a moisturizer that is right for their skin type. Some moisturizers contain extremely rich ingredients such as lanolin, vegetable oil, mineral oil, petrolatum, shea butter, cocoa butter, or protein that are best only for women with very dry skin. Lighter-weight moisturizers that contain only one or two oils further down on the ingredient list and a selection of water-binding agents are best for skin that is normal to dry. Finding the appropriate type of moisturizer for your skin will be easier if you turn to Chapter Two and review the ingredients listed as appropriate for particular skin types.

When it comes to day creams versus night creams, my recommendation is to ignore those categories and go by what your skin needs. If your skin is extremely dry, products rich in oils, lanolin, and water-binding agents may be necessary for your skin day and night, but the daytime moisturizer must have an SPF of 15 (unless your foundation has a good sunscreen). If your skin is dry but not excessively so, you may want to use a light moisturizing lotion that contains one or two oils and an SPF of 15 for daytime and a more emollient cream at night. If you have slightly dry skin, a lightweight moisturizer or a moisturizing gel should be perfect for both morning and night, but you must absolutely use a product with a good SPF rating during the day.

We won't get into eye or throat creams, because you already know how unnecessary they are. The moisturizer you use on your face will almost always work around your eyes, throat, chest, or wherever. Try to disregard the scare tactics at the cosmetics counters and the brochures that carry on about special formulations designed exclusively for the eye area. These claims are usually not substantiated by the ingredients in the products, which are practically identical to creams supposedly designed just for the face.

Women with oily skin should not get sucked into believing that all skin types, even oily skin types, require a moisturizer to prevent the skin from wrinkling or to combat surface dehydration. Unless we are talking about a sunscreen with an SPF of 15 or dealing with isolated areas of dryness, there is every reason for someone with oily skin to avoid moisturizers. Also, if you avoid using drying and irritating skin care products, that should help reduce your need for a moisturizer. Remember that the words "oil-free" don't mean a product won't feel slick, greasy, or oily. Many ingredients that don't sound like "oil" have a very slick, oily texture. (Oily skin types should wear an oil-free foundation with a high SPF rating to protect their skin from the sun.)

So, does it really make sense to spend a lot of money on moisturizers? Does a woman who spends $50 really get a much better product than one who spends $10? Those of you who have read this whole book already know the answer. Those of you who didn't read the first half of the book and skipped ahead to this section needn't wait in suspense. The best moisturizers for dry skin can be found in almost every skin care line. Yes, that's right, almost every line has its share of good moisturizers, so spending a lot of money does not make sense. As you read the following suggestions, understand that when I say best, I mean best. "Best" moisturizers by Almay or Avon are the equivalent of "best" moisturizers by Chanel or Borghese. Read the reviews in Chapter Seven to evaluate the particular products you are considering, get used to reading skin care ingredients, and ignore words like "lift," "firm," "energizing," or "anti-wrinkle."

For normal to oily/combination skin, the best moisturizers are: Almay Stress Eye Gel; **Beauty Without Cruelty** Green Tea Nourishing Eye Gel; **The Body Shop** Tea Tree Oil Moisturizing Gel; **Borghese** Spa Lift for Eyes; **Circle of Beauty** De Puff Eye Gel; **Color Me Beautiful** Multi-Active Booster Vitasome Energizing Treatment; **Erno Laszlo** Total Skin Revitalizer and pHelitone Firming Eye Gel; **Freeman** Beautiful Skin Chamomile & Allantoin Lite Moisturizer; **H$_2$O Plus** Botanical Nite Gel and Hydrating Eye Cream; **Jafra** Skin Firming Complex; **Lancome** Forte-Vital Serum Raffermissant Skin Firming Serum; **L'Oreal** Plenitude Eye Defense Gel and Plenitude Firming Facial Serum; **M.D. Formulations** Vit-A-Gel with Vitamin A Propionate; **Mon Amie** Intensive Eye Serum; **Nivea Visage** No Oil All Moisture Hydrogel and Eye Contour Gel with Liposomes; **Nu Skin** Enhancer Skin Conditioning Gel and HPX Hydrating Gel; **Oil of Olay** Hydro-Night Renewal Gel and Hydro-Gel; **Paula's Choice** Completely Non-Greasy Moisturizing Lotion; **Principal Secret** Eye Relief; **St. Ives** Swiss Formula Collagen-Elastin Hydrating Facial Firming Gel; **Ultima II** Interactives Booster Shot Antioxidant Firming System; **Victoria Jackson** Eye Repair Gel.

For normal to somewhat dry and dry skin, the best moisturizers are: Adrien Arpel Swiss Formula Day Eye Creme with Vitamin A Palmitate and Collagen, Swiss Formula Day Eye Creme with Vitamin A Palmitate and Collagen, and Skinlastic Lift; **Almay** Moisture Renew Cream for Dry Skin, Moisture Renew Firmasome with Ceramide Liposomes for Dry Skin, Moisture Renew Eye Cream for Dry Skin, Time-Off Age Smoothing Moisture Lotion, Time-Off Wrinkle Defense Capsules with Micro-Fillers, Time-Off Wrinkle Defense Cream with Micro-Fillers, and Replenishing Lotion; **Artistry by Amway** Delicate Care Hydrating Fluid for Sensitive Skin Types, Progressive Emollient, and Revitalizing Night Treatment; **Arbonne** Rejuvenating Cream for All Skin Types; **Aveda** Pure Vital Moisture Eye Creme; **BeautiControl** Microderm Oxygenating Nighttime Line Control and Microderm Oxygenating Firming Gel; **BeneFit** Mrs. Robinson Hyaluronic Creme; **Black Opal** Oil Free Moisturizing Lotion; **Bobbi Brown** Face Cream and Eye Cream; **The Body Shop** Hydrating Moisture Lotion for Normal to Dry Skin and Light Moisture Lotion for Normal to Oily Skin; **Borghese** Dolce Notte ReEnergizing Night Creme and Skin Energy Source; **Chanel** Creme No. 1, Skin Recovery Cream, Emulsion No. 1, Skin Recovery Emulsion, Daily Protective Complex, Hydra-Systeme Maximum Moisture Cream, Hydra-Systeme Maximum Moisture Lotion, Lift Serum Extreme, Advanced Corrective Complex, and Firming Eye Cream;

Chantal Ethocyn Hydrating Complex Moisturizer and Ethocyn Essence Vials; **Charles of the Ritz** Timeless Essence Night Recovery Cream, Age-Zone Controller, Biocharge Replacement Therapy Serum for Changing Skin, Line Refine for Eyes, Timeless Difference Eye Recovery Cream, and Self Protection for Eyes; **Christian Dior** Hydra-Star Dry Skin Moisture Creme, Hydra-Star Dry Skin Moisture Creme Emulsion, Hydra-Star Dry Skin Moisture Emulsion, Hydra-Star Dry Skin Night Treatment Creme, Hydra-Star Normal and Combination Skin Night Treatment Creme, Hydra-Star Normal and Combination Skin Moisture Creme, Hydra-Star Normal and Combination Skin Moisture Fluide, Capture Lift, Firming Night Treatment for the Face, Capture for Face, and Capture for Eyes; **Circle of Beauty** Overnight Eye Treatment; **Clarins** Hydration-Plus Moisture Lotion All Skin Types, Multi-Active Night Lotion for All Skin Types, Multi-Active Night Lotion Very Dry Skin, Multi-Regenerante Treatment Cream for All Skin Types, and Double Serum Total Skin Supplement, Plant Based Concentrate Hydro Serum and Lip Serum; **Clinique** Dramatically Different Moisturizing Lotion, Sub-Skin Cream, Moisture Surge Treatment Formula, Skin Texture Lotion, Skin Texture Lotion Oil-Free Formula, and Daily Eye Saver, Quick Eye-Area Fix; **Color Me Beautiful** Triple Action Eye Cream; **Elizabeth Arden** Visible Difference Eyecare Concentrate, and Micro 2000 Stressed-Skin Concentrate; **Erno Laszlo** Antioxidant Moisture Complex Cream for Extra Dry to Normal Skin, HydrapHel Emulsion, pHelityl Lotion AM Moisturizer for Slightly Dry to Slightly Oily Skin, pHelitone Replenishing Eye Cream for All Skin Types, Total Skin Revitalizer for Eyes, and Total Skin Revitalizer for Night; **Estee Lauder** Verite Moisture Relief Creme, Verite Calming Fluid, Advanced Night Repair, Resilience Eye Creme, and Time Zone Eyes Ultra-Hydrating Complex; **Galderma** Cetaphil Moisturizing Lotion, Nutraderm Original Formula, and Nutraderm; 30; **Guerlain** Evolution Sublicreme No. 1 Light Day and Night Care, Evolution Sublicreme No. 2 Rich Day and Night Care, Evolution Sublifluide Day and Night Care, Issima Anti-Wrinkle Eye Contour Fluid, Issima Intenserum Beauty Treatment, Odelys Perfect Care #1 Day and Night (Light), and Odelys Perfect Care #2 Day and Night (Rich); **Hydron** Best Defense Moisture Balance Restorative Overnight Liposome Complex and Best Defense Fragile Eye Moisturizer; **Jafra** Night Cream Moisturizer for Dry to Normal Skin and Eye Revitalizing Concentrate; **Jergens** Replenaderm Moisturizing Therapy Cream and Replenaderm Moisturizing Therapy Lotion; **Kiehl's** Panthenol Protein Moisturizing Face Cream; **La Prairie** Age Management Eye Repair, Cellular Balancing Complex, Cellular Skin Conditioner, Essence of Skin Caviar Cellular Face Complex with Caviar Extract, and Essence of Skin Caviar Cellular

Eye Complex with Caviar Extract; **Lancome** Nutriforce Double Nutrition Fortifying Nourishing Creme, and Niosome + Perfected Age Treatment; **L'Oreal** Plenitude Advanced Wrinkle Defense Cream; **Lubriderm** Dry Skin Care Lotion Fragrance Free, Dry Skin Care Lotion Original Fragrance, Moisture Recovery GelCreme, Seriously Sensitive Lotion for Extra Sensitive Skin, and Seriously Sensitive Lotion for Extra Sensitive Dry Skin; **M.A.C.** CR-1 Cellular Recovery Night Emulsion, CR-2 Cellular Recovery Night Emulsion, and EZR Eye Zone Repair; **Marcelle** Hydractive Hydra-Repair Night Treatment, Moisture Cream Hypo-Allergenic, Moisture Lotion Hypo-Allergenic, Night Cream, Anti-Aging Cream with Collagen and Elastin Hypo-Allergenic, and Eye Care Cream Ultra-Light Hypo-Allergenic; **Mary Kay** Balancing Moisturizer; **Maybelline** Revitalizing Optimum Eye Treatment Cream; **M.D. Formulations** Forte Advanced Hydrating Complex Cream Formula; **Merle Norman** Luxiva Collagen Support, Luxiva Hydrosome Complex, and Luxiva Protein Cream; **Monteil** Ice Fundamental Emulsion; **Murad** Murasome Skin Perfecting Lotion; **Neutrogena** Intensified Eye Moisture 12-Hour Hydration, Light Night Cream Won't Clog Pores, and Moisture Non-Comedogenic Facial Moisturizer for Sensitive Skin; **Nivea Visage** 12-Hour Deep Moisture Liposome Creme with Vitamin E and Advanced Vitality Creme; **Noevir** 95 Herbal Skin Cream, 105 Herbal Enriched Moisturizer, 105 Herbal Skin Cream, 505 Herbal Skin Cream, and Eye Treatment Gel; **Nu Skin** Celltrex Skin Hydrating Fluid, NaPCA Moisturizer, and Rejuvenating Cream; **Origins** Constant Comforter, Steady Drencher, Time Mender, Starting Over, and Urgent Moisture; **Orlane** B21 Bio-Energic Absolute Skin Recovery Care, B21 Ultra-Light Cream for the Day, B21 Protective Oxytoning Cream For All Skins, Extrait Vital Eye Contour Cream, Extrait Vital Vital Biological Cream, Extrait Vital Vital Biological Emulsion, Soin Hydratant Moisture Skin Care, Hydratant Riche Enriched Moisture Care, Hydralane Moisture Skin Care, Continuous Hydro-active System, and Nutrilane Total Nutrition System for Dry or Delicate Skin; **Paula's Choice** Completely Emollient Moisturizer; **Physicians Formula** Collagen Cream Concentrate for Dry to Very Dry Skin, Oil Free Nourishing Eye Gel for Normal to Oily Skin, Captyane Replenishing Gel-Cream with Microparticles for Normal to Oily Skin, and Captyane Replenishing Night Treatment for Normal to Oily Skin; **Pond's** Nourishing Moisturizer Cream Oil-Free, Nourishing Moisturizer Lotion Oil-Free, Overnight Nourishing Complex Cream Oil-Free, Dramatic Results Skin Smoothing Capsules with Nutrium, and Revitalizing Eye Capsules, Delicate Eye Area; **Prescriptives** Line Preventor 3, Px Comfort Cream, and Px Comfort Lotion; **Principal Secret** Extra Nurturing Cream; **Rachel Perry** Bee Pollen-Jojoba Maximum Moisture Cream, Ginseng and Collagen Wrinkle Treatment, Hi Potency "E" Special Treatment

Line Control, and Immediately Visible Eye Renewal Gel-Cream with Liposomes; **Revlon** Eterna '27' All Day Moisture Lotion, Eterna '27' All Day Moisture Cream, Eterna '27' with Exclusive Progenitin, Results Rest & Renewal Night Cream Concentrate, Results Brighten-Up Eye Cream, and Results Line Diminishing Serum; **Shiseido** Pureness Moisturizing Cream, Pureness Moisturizing Emulsion, Vital Perfection Moisture Active Cream, Vital Perfection Moisture Active Emulsion, Bio-Performance Advanced Super Revitalizer, and Vital Perfection Daily Eye Primer; **St. Ives** Swiss Formula Collagen-Elastin Essential Moisturizer, Swiss Formula Peaches and Cream Moisturizing Beauty Lotion, and Swiss Formula Raspberry Pearl Night Recovery Cream; **Sudden Youth** Elastin Elegance; **Trish McEvoy** Light Moisturizer and Extra-Light Moisturizer; **Ultima II** Interactives Night Cap Antioxidant Skin Smoother, Brighten Up, Tighten Up Eye Cream, and Smart Move; **Vaseline Intensive Care** Aloe Vera Triple Action Formula, Aloe & Vitamins, Extra Strength Triple Action Formula with Petroleum Jelly, Dry Skin Triple Action Formula with Alpha Hydroxy Complex, Sensitive Skin, Sensitive Skin with Vitamin E, Dermasil Dry Skin Concentrated Treatment, and Dermasil Dry Skin Treatment Cream; **Victoria Jackson** Moisturizer and Skin Renewal System; **Yves Rocher** Reponse Nature Night Treatment, Hydra Vegetal 24 Hour Moisture Concentrate, A.D.N.—A.R.N. Time Defense Intensive Firming Complex for Face and Throat, Bionutritive Activating Concentrate, Bionutritive Day Creme, Bionutritive Night Creme, and Hydra Vegetal Moisture Concentrate; **Yves St. Laurent** Absolute Hydration, Prevention + /Time Prevention Day Creme, Hydro-Intensive Day Creme, Hydro-Light Day Creme, Intensive Nighttime Revitalizer, Nighttime Revitalizer, and Time Interceptor Fortifying Complex.

For dry to very dry skin, the best moisturizers are: **Adrien Arpel** Swiss Formula Day Cream #12 with Collagen and Vital Velvet Moisturizer, Moisturizing Blotting Lotion, Freeze-Dried Collagen Protein Night Creme and Freeze-Dried Collagen Protein Eye Creme; **Alexandra de Markoff** Compensation Skin Serum and Skin Tight Firming Eye Cream; **Almay** Moisture Renew Moisture Lotion for Dry Skin, Moisture Renew Night Cream for Dry Skin, Moisture Balance Eye Cream for Normal Skin, Perfect Moisture, Sensitive Care Cream for Super Sensitive Skin, Time-Off Age Smoothing Night Cream, Time-Off Age Smoothing Moisture Cream, Time-Off Age Smoothing Eye Cream, Stress Cream, and Anti-Irritant; **Arbonne** Moisture Cream for Normal to Dry Skin, Night Cream for Normal to Dry Skin, Skin Conditioning Oil, Bio Hydria Night Energizing Cream, and Bio Hydria Eye Cream; **Aveda** Miraculous Beauty Replenisher, Calming Nutrients, and Energizing Nutrients; **Avon** Hydrofirming Cream Night Treatment, Dramatic Firming Cream for Face and Throat, and Hydrafirming

Cream Night Treatment; **BeautiControl** Essential Moisture Lotion AM/PM; **Beauty Without Cruelty** All Day Moisturizer, Nutrient Rich Maximum Moisture Cream; **BeneFit** Vita Hydrating Creme; **The Body Shop** Rich Moisture Cream for Dry Skin, Aloe Vera Moisture Cream, Jojoba Moisture Cream, Moisture Cream with Vitamin E, Rich Night Cream with Vitamin E, and Under Eye Cream; **Chanel** Creme No. 1, Skin Recovery Eye Cream; **Charles of the Ritz** Moisture Balancing Day Care Skin Soother, Revenescence Cream, and Special Formula Emollient; **Christian Dior** Resultante Moisturizing Day Cream for Wrinkles, Resultante Revitalizing Wrinkle Cream, and Icone Principe Regulateur for All Types of Dryness; **Clarins** Face Treatment Cream for Dry or Reddened Skin, Face Treatment Plant Cream for Dehydrated Skin, Face Treatment Plant Cream for Dry or Extra Dry Skin, Gentle Night Cream for Sensitive Skin, Multi-Regenerante Treatment Cream "Special" for Very Dry, Very Devitalized Skin, Revitalizing Moisture Cream with Plant Marine "Cell Extract," Revitalizing Moisture Base with Plant Marine "Cell Extract" for All Skin Types, and Eye Contour Balm "Special" for Very Dry Skin; **Clinique** Advanced Cream, Self Repair System, Very Emollient Cream, Moisture Stick, and Daily Eye Benefits; **Coty** Vitamin A-D Complex Cream and Vitamin Moisture Balancer Emollient Daytime Lotion; **Elizabeth Arden** Millenium Day Renewal Emulsion, Millenium Night Renewal Creme, Millenium Eye Renewal Cream, Skin Basics Beauty Sleep, Skin Basics Velva Moisture Film, Special Benefit Orange Skin Cream, and Eight Hour Cream; **Erno Laszlo** Active pHelityl Cream PM Moisturizer for Sensitive/Slightly Dry Skin, and HydrapHel Complex PM Moisturizer for Extremely Dry and Dry Skin, pHelityl Cream; **Estee Lauder** Estoderme Creme, Estoderme Emulsion, Swiss Performing Extract Moisturizer, European Performing Cream, Age Controlling Creme, Enriched Under-Makeup Creme, Skin Perfecting Creme Firming Nourisher, Re-nutriv Creme, Re-nutriv Firming Eye Creme, Maximum Care Eye Creme, Extra Forte, Re-nutriv Liquid, and Re-nutriv Replenishing Creme; **Eucerin** Original Moisturizing Creme; **Fashion Fair** Enriched Night Creme, Moisturizing Creme with Aloe Vera for Dry Skin, Dry Skin Emollient for Excessively Dry Skin, and Special Beauty Creme with Collagen; **Flori Roberts** My Everything Creme; **Forever Spring** Ginseng Facial Feed, Super Rich Emollience, and Petal Soft Eye Cream; **Freeman** Beautiful Skin Honey and Vitamin E Night Creme and Beautiful Skin Honey & Vitamin E Revitalizing Antioxidant Creme; **Guerlain** Evolution Specific Eye Contour Care; **H₂O Plus** Day Lotion; **Iman** PM Renewal Cream; **Jafra** Extra Care Cream Unscented; **Jergens** Advanced Therapy Lotion, Aloe Enriched, Advanced Therapy Lotion Daily Care Moisturizer with Original Scent, Advanced Therapy Lotion, Dry Skin Care with Vitamin E & Lanolin, Advanced Therapy Lotion, Light Care, Advanced Therapy

Lotion, Ultra Healing Extra Dry Skin Treatment, Advanced Therapy Dual Healing Cream; **Kiehl's** Creme d'Elegance Repairateur Superb Tissue Repairateur Creme and Imperiale Repairateur Moisturizing Eye Balm with Pure Vitamins A & E; **La Prairie** Cellular Day Creme, Cellular Night Cream, Cellular Wrinkle Cream, and Cellular Eye Contour Creme; **Lancome** Hydrative Continuous Hydrating Resource, Noctosome Renewal Night Treatment, Nutribel Nourishing Hydrating Emulsion, Trans-Hydrix, Nutrix Soothing Treatment Creme, Progres Eye Creme, Renergie Double Performance Treatment, and Hydrix Hydrating Creme; **L'Oreal** Plenitude Action Liposomes, Plenitude Advanced Overnight Replenisher, Plenitude Hydra Renewal, and Plenitude Revitalift Anti-Wrinkle Firming Care for Face and Neck; **Marcelle** Eye Cream Ultra Rich Hypo-Allergenic; **Mary Kay** Extra Emollient Moisturizer, Extra Emollient Night Cream, Advanced Moisture Renewal Treatment Cream, and Eye Cream Concentrate; **Merle Norman** Intensive Moisturizer, Luxiva Eye Cream, and Aqua Lube; **Monteil** Firming Action Night Treatment, Super Moist Night Creme, Super Moist Line-Stop Creme Concentrate, Acti-Vita Enriched Eye Creme, Acti-Vita Enriched Moisture Creme, Acti-Vita Multi-Nutritive Creme, and Ice Ultimate Cream Concentrate; **Noevir** Special Night Cream, Eye Treatment Stick; **Nu Skin** Intensive Eye Complex; **Orlane** Anagenese Eye Contour Cream, Anagenese Total Time Fighting Care, and B21 Absolute Skin Recovery Care Eye Contour; **Physicians Formula** Elastin Collagen Moisture Lotion, Deep Moisture Cream, Emollient Oil, Enriched Dry Skin Concentrate for Dry to Very Dry Skin, Extra Rich Rehydrating Moisturizer, Gentle Moisture Lotion, Intensive Therapy Moisture Cream for Dry, Rough Skin, Intensive Therapy Moisture Lotion, Nourishing Night Cream for Dry to Very Dry Skin, Luxury Eye Cream, Captyane Replenishing Eye Complex for All Skin Types, Captyane Replenishing Gel-Cream with Microparticles for Normal to Dry Skin, and Captyane Replenishing Night Treatment for Normal to Dry Skin; **Pond's** Dry Skin Extra Rich Skin Cream; **Purpose** Dry Skin Cream; **Shiseido** Benefiance Revitalizing Cream, Benefiance Revitalizing Emulsion, and Benefiance Revitalizing Eye Cream; **Sudden Youth** Essential Beauty Oils, Moisture Lotion, Sleeping Beauty Cream, and Eye Cream; **Trish McEvoy** Enriched Moisturizer, Dry Skin Normalizer, Extra-Rich Improvement Cream, and Line Refiner; **Ultima II** CHR Extraordinary Lotion, CHR Extraordinary Cream, CHR Moisture Lotion Concentrate, CHR Cream Concentrate, Night Cream, Eye Cream, Under Makeup Moisture Cream, Under Makeup Moisture Lotion, and Megadose All Night Moisturizer; **Vaseline** Dermatology Formula, Extra Strength Formula, Extra Strength Triple Action Formula with Petroleum Jelly, and Dermasil Dry Skin Treatment Lotion Controls Even Severe Dry Skin; **Yves Rocher** Meristem Soothing Night Cream and Rich Eye Creme.

Best Sunscreens

I've discussed at length why sunscreens are essential for skin care and why I prefer SPF 15 to other numbers, but the bottom line is that sun protection is crucial for everyone. If you want to select a sunscreen with a lower rating that's up to you, but please do not venture out with anything less than SPF 8. (For my "best sunscreen" listing I've included only products rated SPF 10 or greater. In Chaper 7 I review products with SPF 8, but I chose to leave them out of this best compilation.) The only thing left to explain is why the lists below are so disproportionate, with vastly more sunscreens for normal to dry skin than for normal to oily. The answer is not reassuring, at least not to those with oily skin or skin prone to breakouts. Sunscreen agents work better in an emollient emulsion than in a matte base or liquid. A few sunscreens work quite well in a liquid or gel, but they are almost all alcohol-based, which doesn't help the face. The sunscreens I prefer for normal to oily skin use a silicone oil-based liquid that dries to a matte finish, or, as is the case for Almay Oil-Control Lotion, an extremely matte base. This is one area of skin care that is difficult for someone with oily skin, and it takes experimentation to find what works well for you.

For normal to oily/combination skin, the best sunscreens are: Almay Oil Control Lotion for Oily Skin SPF 15; **Clinique** Zero-Alcohol Sun Block SPF 25; **Cover Girl** Protective Skin Nourishing Moisturizer SPF 15; **Lancome** Body Protective Spray SPF 15; **Origins** Silent Treatment SPF 15; **Paula's Choice** Essential Non-Greasy Sunscreen SPF 15.

For normal to slightly dry and dry skin, the best sunscreens are: Adrien Arpel Morning After Moisturizer SPF 20; **Almay** Moisture Balance Moisture Lotion SPF 15 for Normal/Combination Skin, Moisture Renew Moisture Lotion for Dry Skin SPF 15, and Time-Off Age Smoothing Moisture Lotion SPF 15; **Alpha Hydrox** SPF 15 Moisturizing Daily Lotion; **Avon** Anew Perfect Eye Care Cream with SPF 15, Anew Perfect Eye Care Cream with SPF 15, and Sun Seekers Sunblock Lotion SPF 15; **Beauty Without Cruelty** SPF 12 Daily Facial Lotion; **BeneFit** Dayscreen 15; **The Body Shop** Watermelon Sun Block SPF 20; **Chanel** Protection Totale Total Defense Moisture Lotion SPF 15 and Protection Totale Total Defense Oil Control Moisture Lotion SPF 15; **Charles of the Ritz** Any Age Self Protection for Face SPF 15; **Clarins** Hydration-Plus Moisture Lotion SPF 15 for All Skin Types and Sun Care Cream SPF 15; **Clinique** City Block SPF 15, Full-Service Sun Block SPF 20, and Special Defense Sun Block SPF 25; **Coppertone** Skin Selects Sun Protecting Lotion for Sensitive Skin SPF 15 Nonirritating and Skin Selects Sun Protecting Lotion for Dry Skin SPF 15 Rehydrating; **Dermablend** Maximum Moisturizer SPF 15, PABA-Free; **Dermalogica** Intensive

Moisture Balance SPF 10, Solar Shield SPF 15, and Solar Block SPF 15; **Donna Karan** Formula for Facial Moisture; **Elizabeth Arden** Immunage UV Defense Cream SPF 15, Immunage UV Defense Lotion SPF 15, Daily Moisture Drink Lotion SPF 15, and Sunwear Daily Face Protector SPF 15; **Erno Laszlo** Daily Moisture Protection Lotion SPF 15 AM Moisturizer for All Skin Types and Antioxidant Moisture Complex SPF 15 Oil-Free Moisturizer for All Skin Types; **Estee Lauder** Day Wear Super Anti-Oxidant Complex SPF 15, Advanced Suncare No Chemical Sunscreen SPF 15, and Advanced Suncare SunBlock Lotion Spray No Chemical Sunscreen SPF 15; **Eucerin** Daily Facial Lotion SPF 20; **Hydron** Best Defense Facial Moisturizer Oil-Free with SPF 15; **Jafra** Sunblock Cream SPF 15; **Kiehl's** Ultra Moisturizing Eye Stick with SPF 18 and Vitamin E; **La Prairie** Time Management Moisturizer with SPF 15; **Lancome** Protective Eye Creme Anti-Wrinkle with Non-Chemical SPF 15 and Protective Face Creme SPF 15; **Marcelle** Multi-Defense Cream Daily Moisturizer SPF 15 Perfume-Free, Oil-Free Multi-Defense Lotion Daily Moisturizer SPF 15 Perfume-Free, and Sun Block Cream SPF 15 PABA-Free, Perfume-Free; **M.D. Formulations** SPF 20 Sunblock; **Merle Norman** Daytime Moisturizer Replenishment Complex SPF 15; **Murad** Murasun Spectrum 15 Daily Defense; **Neutrogena** Intensified Day Moisture SPF 15 and Moisture Non-Comedogenic Facial Moisturizer SPF 15 Untinted; **Nivea** UV Care Daily Facial Moisture Lotion SPF 15; **Noevir** Sun Defense SPF 15; **Nu Skin** Sunright 15 Maximum Protection Sunscreen; **Origins** Let the Sunshine SPF 14 No Chemical Sunscreen and Let the Sunshine SPF 21; **Paula's Choice** Essential Moisturizing Sunscreen SPF 15; **Physicians Formula** Self Defense Protective Moisturizing Lotion with SPF 15 for Normal to Dry Skin, Vital Defense Moisture Concentrate with SPF 15 for Dry to Very Dry Skin, Vital Defense Moisture Lotion with SPF 15 for Normal to Dry Skin, and Vital Defense Oil Free Lotion with SPF 15 for Normal to Oily Skin; **Pond's** Nourishing Moisture Lotion with SPF 15 and Nourishing Moisturizer Lotion Oil-Free with SPF 15; **Prescriptives** Px Insulation Anti-Oxidant Cream with SPF 15; **Purpose** Dual Treatment Moisturizer with SPF 15 Protection; **Revlon** Natural Collagen Complex with SPF 15; **Trish McEvoy** Protective Shield Moisturizer SPF 15; **Ultima II** Interactives Thirst Buster Antioxidant Hydrator with SPF 15; **Yves Rocher** Meristem Daytime Defense Lotion SPF 15; **Yves St. Laurent** Hydro-Light Day Lotion Oil-Free with SPF 15 and Hydro-Light Day Lotion with SPF 15.

Best Facial Masks

Although I am rarely a woman of few words, I feel quite comfortable stating that there are no facial masks on the market that I think are particularly exceptional for the skin or worth the extraordinary or even reasonable price tags. Most facial masks use clay as their main ingredient. The added thickeners, standard water-binding agents, and new and improved water-binding agents are found in all masks, and several also include a nice array of irritating ingredients. Obviously, I don't recommend facial masks, but some women feel that applying a mask is a great way to pamper themselves.

For normal to oily skin, the best masks are: Arbonne Mild Masque; **Beauty Without Cruelty** Purifying Facial Mask; **Circle of Beauty** Pore Purge Clay Mask; **Clarins** Absorbent Mask; **Erno Laszlo** Sea Mud Mask; **Estee Lauder** Quick Lift 4-Minute Mask N/D, Quick Lift 4-Minute Mask N/O, and Stress Relief Eye Mask; **Forever Spring** Baby Soft Facial Clay.

For normal to dry skin, the best masks are: Artistry by Amway Hydrating Masque; **BeneFit** Soothing Gel Mask and Seaweed Mud Mask; **The Body Shop** Peanut & Rosehip Face Mask; **Chanel** Maximum Moisture Mask and Natural Exfoliating Mask; **Charles of the Ritz** Moisture Intensive Facial; **Clarins** Purifying Plant Facial Mask and Revitalizing Moisture Mask with Plant Marine "Cell Extract" for All Skin Types; **Dermalogica** Skin Hydrating Masque and Intensive Moisture Masque; **Erno Laszlo** pHelitone Firming Eye Gel Mask for All Skin Types; **Estee Lauder** Triple Creme Hydrating Mask and Soothing Creme Facial; **Freeman** Beautiful Skin Avocado & Oatmeal Facial Masque; **Guerlain** Evolution Fresh Complexion Mask, Issima Aquamasque, and Odelys Moisturizing Creme Mask; **Jafra** Refreshing Moisture Mask for Dry and Dry to Normal Skin; **Kiehl's** Soothing and Cleansing Algae Masque for Balancing Skin Types and Imperiale Repairateur Moisturizing Masque; **Mary Kay** Moisture Rich Mask; **Shiseido** Benefiance Firming Massage Mask; **Yves St. Laurent** Hydro-Active Moisture Masque.

Best Specialty Products

The only small group of products that fit this category were skin-lightening products. There aren't many available, probably because they don't work all that well, but the ones that do exist almost all use the same lightening agent: hydroquinone.

The best skin-lightening products are: Black Opal Advanced Dual Complex Fade Gel; **Flori Roberts** Chromatone Fade Creme Plus Gold; **M.D. Formulations** Forte Skin Bleaching Gel with 2% Hydroquinone in a Base Containing 10% Glycolic Compound; **Murad** Advanced Age Spot and Pigment Lightening Gel; **Neostrata** Gel for Age Spots and Skin Lightening.

Best Foundations

Perhaps no area of makeup is more treacherous and just plain hard to get exactly right than finding the perfect foundation. The problems are many, but the most difficult to overcome are hopes, color choice, and texture. Women want a foundation that fits like a second, secret skin; it should look invisible, but still provide coverage, camouflage, and a radiant look. That is no short order. Foundations have their limitations, and some women find that hard to accept. For instance, some women make a personal quest of finding an oil-free foundation that will last through the evening. If you have oily skin, that just isn't possible without serious touch-ups several times during the day. Some expectations can be fulfilled, but not all.

Choosing the right foundation color is not only time consuming, it is exceedingly frustrating. How many foundations can you test on one face before it becomes raw from wiping off the one you don't like and then trying another, and another, and another? Yet that is what it takes to zero in on the right color.

The last hurdle is finding a pleasing texture that feels soft and silky but doesn't streak, cake, or look thick. Now tell me that isn't a challenge!

Be patient when it comes to finding the right foundation. Try it on before you buy it. Take the time to check the color and texture in daylight. There is no way around this if you want to get the best foundation possible for your skin's needs. Testing a foundation is crucial to get the right color and texture.

If you can splurge on only one product, foundation is it. This is the one area where spending a little bit more is the best option. Of course, you can find some great inexpensive foundations. However, shopping for a foundation at the drugstore is only an option if there are testers.

Please note that the category for normal skin includes only those foundations that are best for that skin type alone. In reality, women with normal skin can wear almost any foundation they want to, determined more by the finish they prefer than anything else.

For very oily skin, the best foundations are: Clarins Le Teint Mat Multi Eclat Matte Finish Foundation; **Fashion Fair** Fragrance-Free Oil-Free Liquid; **Iman** Second to None Oil-Free Makeup with SPF 8; **Lancome** MaquiControle; **Prescriptives** Exact Color Makeup 100% Oil-Free with SPF 15; **Revlon** ColorStay Makeup; **Ultima II** Wonder Wear Foundation with SPF 6 Oil-Free Makeup.

For normal to oily/combination skin, the best foundations are: Artistry by Amway Oil-Free Foundation; **Aveda** Equilibrium Fluide Foundation; **Avon** Oil-Free Foundation and Self Adjusting Foundation; **BeautiControl** Oil-Free Liquid Sheer Foundation;

BeneFit matte makeup and matte tint; **Bobbi Brown** Oil-Free Foundation; **The Body Shop** Every Day Foundation; **Chanel** Teint Pur Matte SPF 8; **Charles of the Ritz** Superior Foundation for Normal to Oily Skin; **Circle of Beauty** Skin Image Soft Matte Makeup SPF 8; **Clinique** Stay True Oil-Free; **Color Me Beautiful** Soft Focus Skin Perfecting Oil-Free Foundation SPF 8; **Cover Girl** Balanced Complexion for Combination Skin Makeup; **Elizabeth Arden** Flawless Finish Complete Control Matte Makeup SPF 10; **Erno Laszlo** Oil-Free Normalizing Base; **Estee Lauder** Demi-Matte; **Flori Roberts** Maximum Matte Souffle Oil-Free Makeup; **Jafra** Supertone Makeup Oil Controlling SPF 6; **Lancome** MaquiMat and MaquiLibre SPF 15; **La Prairie** Cellular Oil-Free Matte Foundation with SPF 8; **Mary Kay** Day Radiance Formula III Oil-Free for Oily and Combination Skin; **Max Factor** Rain All Day Hydrating Makeup and Balancing Act Skin Balancing Makeup; **Monteil** Habitat Natural Foundation with Chemical-Free SPF 4; **Prescriptives** Custom Blended Foundation Oil Free; **Shiseido** Natural Matte Foundation Oil-Free with Non-Chemical SPF 8; **Ultima II** The Foundation Oil-Control Formula SPF 6.

For normal skin, the best foundations are: **Aveda** Dual Performance Creme Powder; **The Body Shop** All-in-One-Face Treat SPF 15; **Borghese** Molta Bella Liquid Powder Makeup SPF 8; **Chanel** Teint Facettes Lumiere Perfecting Compact Makeup; **Clinique** Sensitive Skin Makeup SPF 15; **Jane** True to You Sheer Finish Foundation; **Lancome** MaquiLumine; **L'Oreal** Luminair Cream-Powder Makeup; **Revlon** DoublePlay; **Shiseido** Creme Powder Compact Foundation and Oil Control Treatment Compact.

For normal to dry skin, the best foundations are: **Adrien Arpel** Powdery Creme Foundation; **Alexandra de Markoff** Countess Isserlyn Soft Velvet Makeup Oil-Free and Countess Isserlyn Powder Creme Finish Makeup; **Artistry by Amway** Liquid Foundation; **Avon** Face Lifting Foundation, Hydrating Foundation, and Anew Perfect Foundation; **Borghese** Effetto Bellezza Targeted Treatment Makeup SPF 8; **Chanel** Teint Naturel SPF 8 and Teint Extreme Lumiere with Non-Chemical SPF 8; **Charles of the Ritz** Superior Moisture Foundation for Normal to Dry Skin; **Christian Dior** Teint Dior Eclat Satin; **Circle of Beauty** Skin Image Dewy Moist Makeup SPF 8; **Clarins** Satin Finish Foundation; **Clinique** Balanced Makeup Base and Soft Finish Makeup; **Color Me Beautiful** Liquid Foundation; **Elizabeth Arden** Flawless Finish Every Day Makeup SPF 10; **Erno Laszlo** pHelitone Fluid; **Estee Lauder** Lucidity Light Diffusing Makeup, Just Perfect Light Diffusing Makeup, and Enlighten Skin-Enhancing Makeup with SPF 10; **Guerlain** Issima Foundation; **Jafra** Supertone Moisturizing Makeup SPF 6; **La Prairie** Cellular Perfection Flawless with SPF 8; **Lancome** MaquiVelour Hydrating Foundation; **L'Oreal** Hydra Perfecte Protective Hydrating Makeup SPF 10 and Lightnesse Light

Natural Makeup; **M.A.C.** Satin Finish; **Make Up For Ever—Paris** Soft Modeling Film; **Mary Kay** Day Radiance Formula II for Normal to Dry Skin; **Maybelline** Natural Defense Makeup with SPF 15; **Mon Amie** Foundation; **Monteil** Soft Cover Liquid Makeup SPF 8; **Origins** Some Coverage, More Coverage, and Most Coverage; **Orlane** Satilane; **Prescriptives** Exact Color Makeup #1 Lightweight, Exact Color Makeup #2 +, and Custom Blended Foundation Moisturizing Formula; **Revlon** Age Defying Makeup with SPF 8 and Age Defying Extra Cover Creme Makeup with SPF 12; **Shiseido** Stick Foundation and Fluid Foundation; **Ultima II** The Nakeds Smoothing Line Makeup with SPF 10 and The Foundation Moisturizing Formula with SPF 6; **Yves St. Laurent** Teint Sur Mesure Duo De Teint and Line Smoothing Foundation.

For dry to seriously dry skin, the best foundations are: **Alexandra de Markoff** Countess Isserlyn Creme Makeup; **Chanel** Teint Lumiere Creme with Non-Chemical SPF 8; **Christian Dior** Teint Actuel; **Clinique** Extra Help; **Elizabeth Arden** Flawless Finish Hydro Light Foundation; **Estee Lauder** Country Mist and Re-nutriv Souffle Makeup; **Fashion Fair** Liquid Sheer Foundation; **Lancome** MaquiDouceur; **Monteil** Soft Cover Creme Makeup SPF 8; **Merle Norman** Luxiva Liquid Makeup SPF 16 and Luxiva Ultra Foundation with HC-12; **Yves St. Laurent** Teint Libre Moisturizing Foundation.

The best alternatives to liquid foundations are: **Artistry by Amway** Powder Foundation; **Avon** Perfect Match Wet/Dry Powder; **BeautiControl** Perfecting Wet/Dry Finish Foundation; **The Body Shop** All-in-One Face Base; **Charles of the Ritz** Perfect Finish Solid Powder Foundation; **Christian Dior** Teint Poudre; **Clarins** Compact Powder Foundation; **Clinique** Super Double Face Powder Foundation; **Color Me Beautiful** Perfection Microfine Powder Foundation; **Coty** Line Minimizing Makeup; **Elizabeth Arden** Flawless Finish Dual Perfection Makeup and Flawless Finish Control Matte Powder Makeup; **Estee Lauder** More Than Powder and Compact Finish Double Performance Makeup; **Flori Roberts** Compact Face Powder with Oil-Control; **Lancome** Dual Finish Powder; **L'Oreal** Dualite Powder; **M.A.C.** Studio Fix Foundation; **Merle Norman** Luxiva Ultra Powder Foundation; **Prescriptives** Instant Face; **Shiseido** Dual Compact Powdery Foundation; **Ultima II** The Nakeds Dual Cover Compact Makeup Wet or Dry.

For maximum coverage regardless of skin type, the best foundations are: **Clinique** Continuous Coverage Makeup SPF 11; **DermaBlend**; **Estee Lauder** Maximum Coverage with Non-Chemical SPF 10; **Merle Norman** Aqua Base; **Ultima II** Ultimate Coverage.

Best Concealers

Trying to find a good under-eye concealer is still not an easy task, but it has improved a great deal since the last edition of this book. A concealer shouldn't be too dry or too creamy, shouldn't crease into the lines under the eye (this requirement cannot be ignored, particularly by those of us with an increasing number of under-eye lines), and should provide good coverage. I found some good concealers in all price categories, and this time I even have rave reviews for some inexpensive options. I also found a lot of concealers that are still too thick, too greasy, too peach, too pink, too dark, or too expensive.

High ratings for concealers go to: Almay Cover-Up Stick, Extra Moisturizing Undereye Cover Cream, and Time-Off Age Smoothing Concealer; **Avon** Face Lifting Moisture Firm Concealer with SPF 8; **Circle of Beauty** No Flaw Maximum Cover Concealer; **Clinique** Quick Corrector and Soft Concealer Corrector; **Jafra** White Souffle; **Jane** Clueless Two Way Concealer; **Lancome** MaquiComplet; **L'Oreal** Mattique Conceal Oil-Free Cover-Up and Hydra Perfecte Concealer SPF 12; **M.A.C.** TV Touch; **Mary Kay** Perfecting Concealer; **Max Factor** Erase Colour Precise; **Maybelline** Undetectable Creme Concealer; **Origins** Original Skin Concealer; **Revlon** New Complexion Concealer; **Ultima II** The Concealer and Sexxxy Coverup; **Yves St. Laurent** Radiant Touch.

Best Powders

It doesn't make sense to spend a lot of money on a finishing powder because there is so little difference between products. More than 95 percent of them are talc-based; the rest of the ingredients vary only slightly, although the companies make absurd claims about light-reflecting properties and micro-encapsulated color, all of which is nonsense. When I think of the number of pressed powders priced between $16 and $30, I just shake my head at the audacity of the cosmetics companies. Unfortunately, after recommending that you go inexpensive for this product group, I can't muster much enthusiasm for the finishing powders available at the drugstore. Some of these are superior products, but there is no way to test the color. In regard to drugstore finishing powders, I make my suggestions based on what I think are the safest choices for the products with the best texture, but if you are inexperienced or haven't had luck finding the best color, trying on a powder is generally the best way to make a decision, and that means resorting to the cosmetics counters or in-home sales. If you go one of those routes, I definitely recommend the less expensive lines.

The best finishing powders, both loose and pressed, are: **Adrien Arpel** Real Silk Powder; **Artistry by Amway** Loose Powder; **Aveda** Pure Finish Pressed Powder and Pure Finish Loose Powder; **Avon** Translucent Pressed Powder and Oil-Control Pressed Powder; **BeautiControl** Loose Perfecting Powder and Oil-Free Translucent Pressed Powder; **Black Opal** Oil Absorbing Pressed Powder; **The Body Shop** Soft Pressed Face Powder and Color Balance Loose Powder; **Borghese** Powder Milano; **Charles of the Ritz** Translucent Pressed Powder and Blemish Control Powder; **Christian Dior** Pressed Powders and Loose Powders; **Clarins** Pressed Powder; **Clinique** Soft Finish Pressed Powder, Stay Matte Sheer Pressed Powder, and Blended Face Powder with Brush; **Color Me Beautiful** Translucent Pressed Powder and Translucent Loose Powder; **Erno Laszlo** pHelitone Concentrating Pressed Powder; **Guerlain** Treatment Powder Foundation; **Iman** Luxury Pressed Powder Oil-Controlling; **Jane** Oil-Free Finishing Powder; **Lancome** Poudre Majeur Pressed Powder and Poudre Majeur; **La Prairie** Protective Pressed Powder and Foundation Finish Loose Powder; **L'Oreal** Visuelle Pressed Powder; **M.A.C.** Pressed Powder and Loose Powder; **Make Up For Ever—Paris** Poudre Libre and Compact Powder; **Marcelle** Pressed Powder; **Mary Kay** Powder Perfect Loose Powder and Powder Perfect Pressed Powder; **Maybelline** Revitalizing Translucent Powder, Shine-Free Oil-Control Translucent Pressed Powder Finish Matte Pressed Powder, and Shades of You 100% Oil-Free Pressed Powder; **Merle Norman** Remarkable Finish Loose Powder and Remarkable Finish Pressed Powder; **Mon Amie** Pressed/Translucent Powder; **Monteil** Supreme Pressed Powder; **Origins** Original Skin Pressed Powder and Original Skin Loose Powder; **Prescriptives** All Skins Pressed Powder; **Prestige** Pressed Powders; **Trish McEvoy** Pressed and Loose Powder; **Revlon** New Complexion Powder Oil-Control Normal to Oily Skin; **Shiseido** Natural Pressed Powder; **Ultima II** The Nakeds Pressed Powder; **Victoria Jackson** Pressed Powder.

The best bronzing powders (matte shades only) are: **The Body Shop** Tinted Bronzing Powder; **Christian Dior** Sun Powders; **Clarins** Duo Soleil; **Clinique** Bronze Doubles.

Best Blushes

Blush is probably one of the easiest cosmetics to get right. It is hard to buy a bad blush. Not that there aren't some real losers out there, but there are far more winners. The problem with blush is usually application, and that is where good brushes come into play. Using the proper brushes is essential for getting blushes (and eyeshadows) to go on correctly.

Blushes received high marks if they were matte, had a soft nongrainy texture, blended on smoothly, did not fade or dissipate with time, and had a good selection of colors. There are plenty that qualify, so don't spend a lot of money on blush unless you need to test the color first. Many drugstore blushes are of a superior quality and provide the same results as those at the department store.

The best blushes are: **Adrien Arpel** Mix & Match Cheek Color and Powdery Creme Blush; **Alexandra de Markoff** Cheek Chic; **Almay** Cheek Color and Brush-On Blush; **Artistry by Amway** Powder Blush; **Aveda** Silk Powder Blush; **Avon** True Color Powder Blush; **BeautiControl** Unbelievable Blushes; **Black Opal** Natural Color Blush; **The Body Shop** Cream Blush, Powder Blush, Brush-On Rose, Brush-On Bronze, Twist & Bronze, and Twist & Blush; **Borghese** Blush Milano; **Charles of the Ritz** Moistureful Cheeks; **Christian Dior** Blush Final; **Circle of Beauty** Blush Creamy Cream to Powder; **Clarins** Cream-to-Powder Blush; **Clinique** Beyond Blusher and Soft Touch Creamy Blush; **Estee Lauder** Just Blush! Eye and Cheek Powder; **Fashion Fair** Blush; Il Makiage Color Rouge; **Guerlain Powder** Blush and Meterorites; **Iman** Blush; **Jafra** Powder Blush and Water Colour Blushing Gel; **Jane** Blushing Cheeks; **L'Oreal** Visuelle Softly Luminous Powder Blush and Blushesse; **M.A.C.** Blush; **Make Up For Ever—Paris** Colors; **Marcelle** Moisturizing Blush; **Mary Kay** Powder Perfect Cheek Color; **Max Factor** High Definition Blush; **Maybelline** Shades of You 100% Oil-Free Powder Blush; **Mon Amie** Blushes; **Monteil** Silk Powder Blush; **Origins** Brush on Color; **Physicians Formula** Matte Blush; **Prescriptives** Powder Cheekcolor; **Prestige** Blushes; **Revlon** Naturally Glamorous Blush-On and In the Pink Cheek Color; **Shiseido** Singles, Duos, and Tri Effect Blush; **Trish McEvoy** Sheer Blush; **Ultima II** Wonder Wear Cheek Color and The Nakeds Cheek Color; **Victoria Jackson** Blush Compact.

Best Eyeshadows

By now I am well known for my opinions about shiny eyeshadows as well as blue and green eyeshadows (or any brightly colored eyeshadows, for that matter). It still is my goal to find the best matte shades available, and I am thrilled to say that the cosmetics industry has caught on. There are more than enough matte shades available in all price ranges. You can shop both the drugstore and cosmetics counters and find wonderful textures and colors. There is no reason to wear shiny eyeshadows, so why not give them up forever; your skin will look less wrinkly, not to mention more fashionable.

Be aware that almost all of the lines listed below have some shiny eyeshadows mixed in with their matte colors. Avoid the shiny ones at all costs.

The best matte eyeshadows can be found in the following lines: **Alexandra de Markoff** Professional Palette Eyeshadow Singles; **Almay** Long Lasting Eyecolor Singles, Duos, Quads, and Amazing Lasting Eyecolor; **Artistry by Amway** Eye Colour; **Aveda Velvet Powder** Eye Shadow; **Black Opal** Color Rich Eyeshadows; **Borghese** Singles, Duales, and Trios; **Charles of the Ritz** Moistureful Eye Color; **Clinique** Soft Pressed Eyeshadow; **Estee Lauder** Just Blush! Eye and Cheek Powder, Compact Disc Eyeshadows, and Singles and Duos; **Iman** Eyeshadow; **M.A.C.** Eyeshadow; **Make Up For Ever— Paris** Colors; **Marcelle** Eyeshadows; **Mary Kay** Powder Perfect Eye Color; **Merle Norman** Creamy Powder Rich Eyeshadows Singles, Duos, and Trios; **Mon Amie** Eyeshadows; **Monteil** Rich Powder Eyeshadow Singles and Duos; **Origins** Eye Accent Eyeshadows; **Physicians Formula** Matte Collection Singles and Duos; **Prescriptives** The Quad Eyeshadow and Pick 2; **Prestige** Eyeshadows; **Shiseido** Single, Duos, and Tri Effect Eye Shadow; **Trish McEvoy** Glazes, Shapers, Definers, and Enhancers; **Ultima II** Wonder Wear Eye Color and The Nakeds Eye Color Single.

Best Eye and Brow Shapers

Some cosmetics companies sell two different eye pencils, one for the brow and the other for lining the eye. Other cosmetics companies are more straightforward and sell only one that does both jobs. That is the practical and honest approach. There is usually little to no difference between eye and brow pencils. The contrasts mainly involve color choice.

An eye pencil with a dry texture makes it difficult to line the eyelid after you've applied your eyeshadows; if the pencil is on the greasy side, it will line the lid more easily, but it is also more likely to smear under the lower lashes in a very short time. (Actually, both kinds have problems with smearing.) I have always preferred lining the eyes with regular eyeshadow powder and a small, thin eyeliner brush. I usually line my lower lashes with a soft brown eyeshadow and my eyelid with a black or dark brown eyeshadow. You can also wet the brush and apply the eyeshadow as you would a liquid liner in a more vivid line. In fact, even when I line my eyes with a pencil, I go over it with an eyeshadow to make sure it has a better chance of staying all day. The difference in the look and in how long it lasts compared with using a pencil alone, is amazing— particularly if you have oily or combination skin. If, however, the technique of lining your eyes with an eyeshadow and a tiny brush has eluded you and you prefer pencils, there are still many good ones. You can shop the more expensive lines, but it is a waste of money, because regardless of the price almost all the pencils I tested in all price ranges had more similarities than differences.

Eyebrow pencil has long been the standard method for making eyebrows appear thicker or more defined and it still is, but greasy pencils look overly made-up and dry ones are not that easy to apply and can still look thick and heavy. It is my strong recommendation that you fill in the brow with a powder, either an eyeshadow or a specific eyebrow powder.

Several companies sell colored eyebrow gels as a way to fill, lift, and define the brow. There are also a few companies that make a clear brow gel that isn't much different than using hairspray on a toothbrush and brushing it through the brow. For the most part the natural-colored brow gels are great. I strongly recommend them as another way to make eyebrows look fuller but not artificial. If you can learn how to use the eyebrow gels, they can be a great alternative to pencils.

The best pencils that can be used for both lining the eyes and filling in the brows are: Black Opal Precision Eye Definer; **Charles of the Ritz** Classic Liners for Eyes; **Elizabeth Arden** Slender Liners Eye Pencils, Dual Perfection Brow Shaper and Eye Liner, and Smoky Eyes Powder Pencil; **Fashion Fair** Slim Line Eye Liner Pencils and Brow Pencil; **Flori Roberts** Eye Contour Pencils; **Il Makiage** Slim Pencils; **Iman** Perfect Eye Pencils, Perfect Brow Pencils, and Shaping Sticks; **Jafra** Eye and Brow Pencils; **Jane** Eye and Brow Pencils; **Lancome** Le Crayon Poudre for the Brows; **L'Oreal** Le Grand Kohl Perfectly Soft Liners and Brow Elegance; **M.A.C.** Eye Pencils; **Make Up For Ever—Paris** Demographic Pencils; **Marcelle** Eye Pencil; **Maybelline** Expert Eyes Brow and Eye Liner Pencil; **Merle Norman** Trim Line Eye Pencils; **Mon Amie** Brow Pencil and Eye Liner Pencil; **Prescriptives** Eye Pencils; **Prestige** Eye Pencils; **Revlon** Time Liner Eye Pencils and Fine Line Natural Brow Pencil; **Ultima II** EyeSexxxy Liner, Kohl Eye Pencil, BrowSexxxy, and Brow Pencil.

The best liquid liners are: Almay Eye Defining Liquid Liner and I-Liner; **Cover Girl** Liquid Pencil Soft Precision Liner; **Estee Lauder** Liquid Liner; **Jafra** Liquid Eyeliner; **Lancome** Maquiglace Liquid Liner and Automatic Eye Lining Felt Pen; **L'Oreal** Lineur Intense; **M.A.C.** Creme Liner; **Maybelline** Lineworks Felt-Tip Eye Liner Lineworks and Liquid Liner Washable; **Revlon** Jetliner Intense.

The best eyebrow powders are: Elizabeth Arden Great Color Brow Makeup; **The Body Shop** Eye Brow Powder Makeup; **Flori Roberts** Matte Brows; **Max Factor** Brush & Brow Eyebrow Color; **Maybelline** Ultra-Brow Brush-On Brow Color; **Revlon** Natural Brows Color & Style System.

The best brow gels are: Borghese Brow Milano; **Chanel** Brow Shaper; **Max Factor** Brow Tamer; **Origins** Just Browsing; **Ultima II** Brow Control.

Best Lipsticks

By now we are all over the search for lipsticks that will last all day, right? We also know that the greasier or glossier the lipstick, the less likely it is to last, and the more matte the lipstick, the longer it is likely to stick around, although it may be too drying. If you don't have a problem with dry lips and you want to try a matte look, mattes and ultra-mattes are certainly an option.

The best creamy lipsticks are: Almay Lip Opaque Lip Color; **Aveda** Fresh Essence Lip Matte and Fresh Essence Lip Colour; **Black Opal** Matte Plus Moisture Lipstick and True Tone Vitamin Rich Lipstick; **Borghese** Superiore State-of-the-Art and La Moda Concentrate; **Christian Dior** Rouge a Levres and Rouge Accent; **Clinique** Re-Moisturizing Lipstick; **Color Me Beautiful** Classic Lipstick; **Cover Girl** Remarkable Lip Color SPF 15; **Estee Lauder** Perfect Lipstick, All Day Lipstick, True Lipstick, Double Matte Lipstick, and Polish Performance; **Flori Roberts** Matte Lipstick and Gold Hydrophillic Lipstick; **Guerlain** Kiss Kiss with SPF 8; **Iman** Luxury Moisturizing Lip Colors; **Jafra** Lasting Lip Color; **Lancome** Hydra-Riche Hydrating Lip Colour, Rouge Absolu Hydrating Long Lasting Lip Colour, and Rouge Superb Matte Lip Colour; **La Prairie** Matte Lipstick; **L'Oreal** Colour Supreme Long Wearing Lip Colour and Colour Riche Hydrating Creme Lip Colour; **M.A.C.** Satin Lipstick and Cream Lipstick; **Max Factor** Moisture Rich Lipstick, New Definition, and Lasting Color Lipstick; **Maybelline** Shades of You Lipstick and Shades of You Long Wearing Lipstick; **Mon Amie** Lipstick; **Prescriptives** Extraordinary Lipstick; **Revlon** Moon Drops Moisture Creme, Super Lustrous Creme, Outrageous Creme Lipcolor, and Velvet Touch; **Shiseido** Advanced Performance Lipstick; **Trish McEvoy** Lip Colors; **Ultima II** The Nakeds Matte & Lipchrome and Double Feature; **Yves St. Laurent** Sheer Conditioning Lipstick.

The best lipsticks that are more glossy than creamy are: Almay Color Basic Lipstick; **Aveda** Uruku Lip Colour; **BeautiControl** Lasting Lip Color; **The Body Shop** Lipsticks and Lip Treats; **Borghese** Lip Treatment Moisturizer SPF 15; **Circle of Beauty** Rich Lasting Cream Lipstick; **Clinique** Different Lipstick; **Cover Girl** Continuous Color Self Renewing Lipstick SPF 15, Continuous Color Self Renewing Lipstick (No SPF), and Soft Radiants; **Elizabeth Arden** Luxury Moisturizing Lipstick and Lip Spa; **Estee Lauder** Double Color Lipstick; **Flori Roberts** Lipstick; **Jafra** Moisturizing Lipstick SPF 6; **Lancome** Rouge Sensation Superb Sheer Lip Colour and Stylo Sport Lipstick with SPF 15; **La Prairie** Sheer Lipstick and Moisturizing Tint; **L'Oreal** Sheer Colour Riche SPF 15; **M.A.C.** Sheer Lipstick; **Make Up For Ever—Paris** Transparents and Nacre; **Marcelle** Lipsticks; **Maybelline** Moisture Whip Lipstick and Long Wearing Lipstick;

Prescriptives Classic Lipsticks; **Ultima II** The Nakeds Lipchrome, Couture and Never Wetter; **Yves St. Laurent** Pure Lipstick.

   The best lip glosses and lip treatments are: Adrien Arpel Freeze-Dried Protein Lip Peel and Salve; **Almay** Glossy Lip Shine and Demi Sheer SPF 15 Lip Color; **BeautiControl** Lip Apeel; **Black Opal** Simply Sheer Lipstick with SPF 15; **Chanel** Maximum Moisture Lip Treatment; **Circle of Beauty** Sheer Treat Lipstick, Crystal Cream, and Lip Comfort; **Clarins** Lip Beauty Multi-Treatment; **Clinique** Gloss Wear SPF 8, Almost Lipstick, Semi-Lipstick, Sun Buffer Lipstick, and Lip Block, SPF 15; **Color Me Beautiful** Lip Conditioner SPF 15; **Coty** Lip Doctor Color Therapy Stick with AHA and Sheer to Stay 6 Hour Lip Color; **Cover Girl** LipSlicks LipGloss SPF 15; **Elizabeth Arden** Special Benefit, Eight Hour Cream Lip Protectant Stick, SPF 15; **Guerlain** Multicolor Lip Gloss; **Jafra** Lip Gloss; **Kiehl's** Lip Balm #1; **Lancome** Lip Balm; **Max Factor** Restorative Lip Care SPF 15; **Maybelline** Shades of You See Through Gloss and Moisture Whip Gloss; **Merle Norman** LipSoother Plus and Lip Moisture; **Neutrogena** Lip Moisturizer, SPF 15, With PABA-free Sunblock Protection; **Prescriptives** Stains and Lipgloss; **Shiseido** Advanced Performance Lip Gloss and Sun Block Lip Treatment, SPF 15; **Trish McEvoy** Sheers, Sheers with SPF 15, and Lip Gloss; **Ultima II** Super Luscious and Lip Glossy.

   The best matte lipsticks are: Circle of Beauty Satin Matte Lipstick; **Color Me Beautiful** More Than Matte Lipstick; **Clinique** Long Last Lipstick; **Coty** '24' Hour Creme Lipstick; **Make Up For Ever—Paris** Matte; **Yves St. Laurent** Rouge Intense.

   The best ultra-matte lipsticks are: Avon Perfect Wear Lip Color; **The Body Shop** Lipstain and Continual Lip Color; **Charles of the Ritz** LipSTICK; **Coty** Self-Sealing Lip Makeup and Lip Writer Stayput Lipstick; **L'Oreal** Endure Stay-On Lip Colour; **M.A.C.** Matte Lipstick and Liptone; **Maybelline** Great Lip Lip Color; **Revlon** Color Stay Lipstick; **Shiseido** Staying Power Lipstick; **Ultima II** LipSexxxy; **Yves St. Laurent** Rouge Definition.

   Preventing lipstick from feathering into the lines around the mouth is of interest to many women, including myself.

   These products can stop almost any lipstick from wandering into lines: **BeautiControl** Lip Control Creme; **The Body Shop** No Wander; **Coty** Stop It Anti-Feathering Stick for Lips and Hold It Wear Extending Base for Lips; **Revlon** Moon Drops Color Lock Anti-Feathering Lip Base.

Best Lip Pencils

   There is no reason to spend more than a few dollars on lip pencils. I can say without any hesitation that lip pencils priced over $6 are a waste of money. There is little to no difference between a higher-priced pencil and a less expensive one. You can spend $22 on Estee Lauder's very attractive retractable lip pencil in the metallic blue case or you can spend $4 or $5 on Almay's or Revlon's lip pencils and get the same look. The decision is up to you. The only real difference is that a few are greasier than others. I recommend staying away from them because they can smear and may not last as long as pencils that are a bit drier. Rather than listing every cosmetics line I've reviewed, I will just say that all of them have great lip liners; some have more color choices than others.

Beauty Note: Lip liner shapes the mouth before you apply lipstick. Lip pencils do not stop lipstick from bleeding. They can slow it down a little, but that's about it. I would also like to put in a vote for ignoring the fashion of outlining the lips in a darker color and then filling in with a lighter shade. Besides being strangely obvious, it also tends to look ghoulish when the lip liner is brown. I rarely have time for lip liner and I like the shape of my mouth, so I skip to the chase and use one of the anti-feathering products mentioned above with my lipstick. It looks just as good, and I'm the only one who knows I haven't lined my lips.

Best Mascaras

I am still surprised by how many good mascaras there are at both drugstores and department stores. In fact, I think they've improved all around. All price ranges include excellent mascaras. Obviously, it is foolish to buy the most expensive mascara when reasonably priced ones are equally good. Given that this is one product you can't readily test at the counters, try a few of the inexpensive ones I suggest and see what works for you. It really is the most sensible and beautiful decision.

The best mascaras are: Almay Triple Thick Mascara, One Coat Mascara, and Mascara Plus; **Avon** Voluptuous Full-Figured Mascara, Incredible Lengths, and Pure Care Mascara; **Borghese** Maximum Mascara for Sensitive Eyes and Superiore State of the Art Mascara; **Chanel** Instant Lash Mascara and Fragile Lash Mascara; **Charles of the Ritz** Perfect Finish Lash; **Christian Dior** Lengthening Mascara with Cashmere and Mascara Parfait; **Clarins** Mascara; **Color Me Beautiful** Lush Lash; **Cover Girl** Extension Waterproof Mascara, Remarkable Washable Waterproof Mascara, Long 'n Lush, and Thick Lash; **Elizabeth Arden** Twice as Thick Two Brush Mascara, Two Brush Mascara Regular, Really Great Mascara, and Defining Mascara; **Estee Lauder** More Than Mascara and Luscious Creme Mascara; **Jane** Flashes Ultra Rich Mascara; **La Prairie** Lash Out Extending Mascara; **Lancome** Defincils, Intencils, and Keracils; **Make Up For Ever—Paris** Mascara; **Marcelle** Ultimate Lash Mascara; **Max Factor** 2000 Calorie

Mascara; **Maybelline** Great Lash Pro Vitamin, Illegal Lengths Mascara, and No Problem Mascara; **Origins** Fringe Benefits Mascara; **Revlon** Impulse Long Distance Mascara, Impulse Quick Thick Mascara, Lengthwise Mascara, and Lashfull Mascara; **Ultima II** Flutters Lengthening Mascara and Big Finish Mascara; **Victoria Jackson** Mascara; **Yves St. Laurent** Conditioning Mascara.

Best Brushes

More than ever before, professional-sized brushes are available in all price ranges. Keep in mind that the texture of the brush is more important than the source of the bristles. While many cosmetics companies love bragging about the type of animal hair used, you are not buying a mink coat. What counts is softness and firmness, no matter where it came from.

These companies make the best brushes: Aveda; BeneFit; The Body Shop; Estee Lauder; Expressions Brushes; Joan Simmons Brushes; M.A.C.; Maybelline; Prescriptives; Prestige; Trish McEvoy.

BEAUTY THAT RESPECTS NATURE

Cruelty-Free Makeup

It is a remarkable tribute to earnest consumers that fewer and fewer cosmetics companies still test their products on animals. However, despite this significant victory, most cosmetics companies continue to get the raw ingredients for their products from companies that persist in conducting animal testing. Consumers erroneously blame the manufacturers for continuing these tests and sometimes even criticize the cosmetics companies themselves for purchasing from these manufacturers instead of from those that don't do animal testing. What consumers don't realize is that the manufacturers have no choice. The FDA and the National Health and Welfare Canada (the Canadian equivalent of the FDA) require cosmetics companies and manufacturers of cosmetic ingredients to use animal testing to establish safety standards. According to Dr. John Bailey, head of the FDA's Office of Cosmetics and Colors, "Though animal testing isn't perfect, it is the best we have right now." That makes it legally difficult for companies that may need to resort to animal research to prove safety and reliability to the FDA when a product is called into question. Even if the FDA refuses to change its mind on this one, that won't stop the cruelty-free trend. Consumers all over the world care about the issue of animal testing, and consumer demand drives the marketplace. More often than not, especially in this case, it is a good thing it does.

As long as these governmental regulating bodies require animal testing as a prerequisite for judging safety, little change will take place. Who wants to take the risk of using data from nonanimal testing at such a basic level (the ingredients that go into a formula) when the FDA and NHWC say that is inadequate proof?

According to an article in the August 1995 issue of *Drug and Cosmetics Industry* magazine, Dr. Albert Kligman, the well-known dermatologist who invented Retin-A, presented a paper titled "Human Skin, An Alternative to Animals for Assessing Irritation" at a symposium where guests from the FDA and the NHWC and other researchers were present. According to Dr. Kligman, no animal has skin that closely resembles human skin. Human skin seems to have a much more diverse and complicated response to irritating substances than animal skin. In other words, why use animals when they can't give us accurate information about human skin? Animal-rights groups have been saying this for years, and now that a well-respected traditional dermatologist like Kligman has come up with similar findings, it is possible that the FDA and NWHC may eventually change their requirements for product safety, which presently include extensive animal testing. With this kind of support, completely cruelty-free cosmetics may become a reality.

Echoing that sentiment was an article in *The Wall Street Journal*'s "Marketplace" on October 23, 1995, about a Dr. Marque Todd's work to find alternatives to animal testing, which is being funded by Mary Kay Cosmetics Inc. Dr. Todd is one of many researchers working in this field in the United States and abroad as a result of pressure from animal-rights groups. Even more consequential is an upcoming ban in Europe, starting in 1998, on the sale of any cosmetic tested on animals. Another incentive that encourages cosmetics companies to find other methods of safety testing is the cost and time involved in animal testing. In vitro tests are much less expensive to perform, and the results are often more accurate and quicker to ascertain.

The eighth edition of *Personal Care For People Who Care* is now on my reference shelf, and it's a must-read source for any consumer interested in purchasing products that have not been tested on animals. Published by the National Anti-Vivisection Society (NAVS), this comprehensive guide lists which companies do and do not test their products on animals. According to the book, "frequently cosmetic companies purchase ingredients for their products from outside sources. With or without the company's knowledge, these ingredients may be subject to animal testing. As a result, it [is] only fair to distinguish "cruelty-free" companies from those unsure of ingredient and supplier testing status." Companies that do not test their final products on animals, do not use ingredients from suppliers who test on animals, and do not contract for such testing are indicated by a red heart. You can obtain the book by calling NAVS at (800) 888-NAVS; communicating via e-mail at navs@navs.org; or by writing them at P.O. Box 94020, Palatine, IL 60094-9834. The book is $4.95 (and an extra donation is good karma and helps NAVS to continue its work). NAVS even has a World Wide Web site at *http://www.navs.org*.

The following cosmetics companies do not use animal testing:

Adrien Arpel

Alexandra de Markoff (Revlon)

Almay (Revlon)

Arbonne

Artistry by Amway

Aveda

Avon

Basis

BeautiControl Cosmetics

Beauty Without Cruelty

Beiersdorf

The Body Shop

Bonne Bell

Borghese

Chanel

Charles of the Ritz (Revlon)

Christian Dior

Clarins

Clinique (Estee Lauder)

Color Me Beautiful

Estee Lauder

Freeman Cosmetics

Guerlain
(ingredients may be tested on animals)

H₂O Plus

Il Makiage
(ingredients may be tested on animals)

Jafra

Jergens

Kiehl's
(ingredients may be tested on animals)

Lancome

L'Oreal

Lubriderm

M.A.C. Cosmetics

Mary Kay Cosmetics

Maybelline (L'Oreal)

Merle Norman Cosmetics

Monteil of Paris

Murad

Neutrogena Skincare

Nivea

Nu Skin International

Origins

Orlane

Paula's Choice

Prescriptives (Estee Lauder)

Prestige Cosmetics

Rachel Perry

Revlon

St. Ives Labs

Shiseido

Ultima II (Revlon)

Victoria Jackson

Yves Rocher

Yves St. Laurent
(ingredients may be tested on animals)

The following cosmetics companies continue to use animal testing:

Chesebrough-Pond's

Clearasil

Clean & Clear

Coty

Cover Girl

Dermasil

Dove

Elizabeth Arden

Erno Laszlo

Fostex

Galderma

Johnson & Johnson

Max Factor (Procter & Gamble)

Noxzema

Oil of Olay

Oxy Products

Pond's

Procter & Gamble

Sea Breeze

Vaseline Intensive Care

Appendix

Customer Service Phone Numbers:

Adrien Arpel
(212) 333-7700

Almay
(800) 4-Revlon
In Canada (905) 276-4500

Alpha Hydrox/Neoteric
(800) 55-ALPHA

Alexandra de Markoff
(800) 4-Revlon

Arbonne
(800) 272-6663

Aveda
(800) 283-3224
(800) 328-0849

Avon
(800) 367-2866
In Canada (800) 265-2866

Basis (Beiserdorf)
(800) 926-4832

BeautiControl
(800) 624-4573

Beauty Without Cruelty
(707) 769-5120

BeneFit
(800) 781-2336

Black Opal
(718) 937-4039

Bobbi Brown
(212) 980-7040

The Body Shop
(800) 541-2535

Borghese
(212) 572-3100

Chanel
(212) 688-5055

Chantal Ethocyn
(800) 920-5577

Charles of the Ritz
(800) 4-Revlon
In Canada (919) 603-2000

Christian Dior
(212) 759-1840

Circle of Beauty
(212) 838-8384

Clarins
(212) 980-1800

Clean & Clear
(800) 526-3967

Clinique
(212) 572-3800

Color Me Beautiful
(800) 533-5503

Coty
(212) 850-2300

Cover Girl
(800) 426-8374

DermaBlend
(905) 660-0622

Dermalogics
(310) 352-4784

Donna Karan
(800) 647-7474

Dove
(800) 451-6679
In Canada (416) 461-9432

eB5
(503) 230-8008

Elizabeth Arden
(212) 261-1000

Erno Laszlo
(415) 341-0925

Estee Lauder
(212) 756-4801

Eucerin
(800) 227-4703
In Canada (203) 853-8008

Fashion Fair
(312) 322-9444

Flori Roberts
(800) 631-2158

Forever Spring
(800) 523-4334

Freeman
(310) 286-0101

Galderma
(800) 582-8225

Guerlain
(212) 751-1870

H2O Plus
(800) 242-2284

Hydron
(800) 449-3766

Iman
(212) 750-6776

Il Makiage
(800) 722-1011

Jafra
(800) 551-2345

Jane
(800) 820-JANE
(619) 634-4250

Jergens
(800) 222-3553

Johnson & Johnson
(800) 526-3967
In Canada (800) 265-8383

Kiehl's
(800) KIEHLS-1

La Prairie
(800) 821-5718

Lancome
(800) 526-2663
(212) 984-4444

L'Oreal
(800) 322-2036

Lubriderm
(800) 223-0182
In Canada (416) 288-2200

M.A.C.
(800) 387-6707

Marcelle
(514) 631-7710

Mary Kay
(800) 627-9529
In Canada (800) 268-2342

Max Factor
(800) 862-4222

Maybelline
(901) 320-4778

Merle Norman
(800) 348-8889

M.D. Formulations
(800) 55-FORTE

Herald Pharmacal
In Canada (408) 723-3350

Mon Amie
(800) 983-3000

Monteil of Paris
(212) 593-7400

Murad
(800) 242-1103
In Canada (310) 568-1940

NeoStrata
(800) 628-9904
In Canada (215) 624-4224

Neutrogena
(800) 421-6857

Nivea
(800) 233-2340
In Canada (203) 853-8008

Noevir
(800) USA-8888
In Canada (800) 465-4655

Nu Skin
(801) 345-1000

Oil of Olay
(800) 285-5170
In Canada (800) 668-0151

Origins
(800) ORIGINS

Orlane
(800) 775-2541

Physicians Formula
(818) 334-3395

Pond's
(800) 243-5804
In Canada (203) 661-2000

Prescriptives
(212) 756-4801

Principal Secret
(800) 545-5595

Purpose
(800) 526-3967
In Canada (800) 265-8383

QVC
(800) 345-1515

Rachel Perry
(800) 966-8888

Revlon
(800) 4-REVLON
In Canada (919) 603-2000

Shiseido
(212) 805-2300

St. Ives
(800) 421-9231

Sudden Youth
(800) 628-6471

Trish McEvoy
(212) 758-7790

Ultima II
(800) 4-REVLON
In Canada (919) 603-2000

Vaseline Intensive Care
(800) 743-8640

Victoria Jackson
(800) V-MAKEUP

Yves Rocher
(800) 321-9837

Yves St Laurent
(212) 621-7300

Bibliography

A Consumer's Dictionary of Cosmetics Ingredients by Ruth Winter, Crown Trade Paperbacks

International Cosmetic Ingredient Handbook, published by The Cosmetic Toilietry and Fragrance Association

International Cosmetic Ingredient Dictionary, published by The Cosmetic Toilietry and Fragrance Association

Drug and Cosmetics Industry magazine

Cosmetics & Toiletries magazine

Cosmetics & Toilietries Applied Research Series, published by Allured Publishing

Personal Care For People Who Care, 8th Edition, published by the National Anti-Vivisection Society

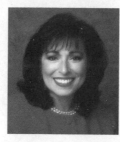

Meet
Paula Begoun

Best-selling author Paula Begoun has sold close to a million books, educating women about the facts and secrets the beauty industry doesn't want consumers to know. Her other books include *Blue Eyeshadow Should Be Illegal* and *Don't Go Shopping For Hair Care Products Without Me*.

Paula spent ten years as a successful professional makeup artist, four years as the owner of a small chain of cosmetics stores, and two years as a cosmetic salesperson at various department stores (where she frequently was fired for telling the truth). Currently, she writes a bimonthly newsletter called *Cosmetics Counter Update* and is a syndicated journalist for **Knight Ridder News Tribune Service.** Her weekly "Dear Paula" column has been gaining popularity across the country in such newspapers as the *New York Daily News* and the *Houston Chronicle*.

Paula has been a guest on hundreds of talk shows including more than 12 appearances on the **Oprah Winfrey Show.** She has also appeared on the **Today Show, Dateline NBC, 20/20, CBS This Morning**, and **Leeza.** Paula is applauded by women across the country as a reliable source for straightforward answers to all of their cosmetics questions.